APHASIA

APHASIA

Edited by

F. Clifford Rose

Director
Academic Unit of Neuroscience
Charing Cross and Westminster Medical School
London

Renata Whurr

Chief Speech Therapist
National Hospital for Nervous Diseases
London

Maria A. Wyke

Senior Lecturer in Neuropsychology
Institute of Psychiatry
University of London
London

W

Whurr Publishers

London Jersey City

19b Compton Terrace
London N1 2UN
England

First published 1988

British Library Cataloguing in Publication Data
Aphasia
1. Aphasia
I. Rose, F. Clifford II. Whurr, Renata
III. Wyke, Maria A.
616.85′52 RC425

ISBN 1-870332-00-8

Library of Congress Cataloging-in-Publication Data
Aphasia
Includes bibliographies and indexes.
1. Aphasia. I. Rose, F. Clifford (Frank Clifford)
II. Whurr, Renata. III. Wyke, Maria A.
[DNLM: 1. Aphasia. WL 340.5 A6438]
RC425-A6 1987 616.85′52 87-25342
ISBN 1-870332-00-8

Typeset by Maggie Spooner Typesetting, London
Printed in Great Britain by LR Printing Services Limited, Crawley, West Sussex

Foreword

During the past century interest in aphasia has waxed and waned; it originally blossomed as a major focus for the study of the interrelationship of brain and behavior during the golden era of clinical-pathological correlation that characterized late 19th century medicine. Interest in language pathology then waned, almost disappearing in the first half of the 20th century, an era that stressed an holistic overview of all brain functions including language. The past three decades have witnessed a strong resurgence of interest in aphasia and a considerably broader approach has been developed, encompassing a number of divergent disciplines. Aphasia has again achieved importance in the study of language and human brain function.

Starting with a recycling of knowledge available from the 19th century clinical-pathological approach, modern neurologic techniques were applied to aphasia. The clinical approach was strongly enhanced by incorporation of the newly devised brain imaging techniques such as isotope brain scans, computed tomography and magnetic resonance imaging. For the clinician, the ability to correlate the clinical phenomenology of aphasia with other phenomenological and laboratory evidence has rekindled a strong interest in language disorder as a medical sign. In addition, a great deal of the information garnered from the clinical studies has proved useful for more academic studies of language and brain function.

Advances in aphasia research have been greatly augmented by the steady progress that has been made in psychology, particularly the relatively new field of neuropsychology that has developed in step with the increased clinical knowledge of aphasia. Language has been, and remains, the single most investigated faculty (module) of neuropsychology, and disordered language — aphasia — represents a major aspect of this effort. While the utilization of aphasia has been greatest in neuropsychology, other branches of psychology (e.g., experimental psychology, physiological psychology, cognitive psychology) investigate language function and have found disordered language a useful approach.

Aphasia has also attained an increasingly important status in the study of linguistics during the past few decades. Two relatively new subspecialties, neurolinguistics and psycholinguistics, have utilized findings derived from the investigation of acquired language disorder to devise and support major theories of language function. In recent years even theoretical linguists have used aphasic individuals as a tool for dissecting the complexities of human verbal discourse. Aphasia has become a significant interest of linguists.

During this same period language therapy has developed from virtual nonexistence to the position of a large, vigorous and successful field of endeavor. Therapists specially trained in aphasia now routinely evaluate and treat individuals who have become aphasic. Many new techniques have been devised for improving language function in the aphasic; some have proved successful and even the failures have added to the understanding of language. Because language therapy approaches aphasia from yet another totally different viewpoint, it has added to the richness of current knowledge and theory concerning language and language disorders. The discipline has firmly established itself in both pragmatic and intellectual domains.

Finally, in the past decade or so a number of individual investigators have been able to approach language disorders from crossed specialty viewpoints. A purely clinical, psychological, linguistic or language therapy approach is no longer an adequate base from which to understand current concepts, base coherent research or plot future directions for aphasia investigation. Information from multiple fields must be utilized. While advances are still being made in each of the individual approaches to aphasia, more and more often the truly significant new advances are accomplished by the amalgamation of ideas garnered from two or more of the disciplines.

In the present volume, the editors have clearly recognized both the problem and the potential; they have accomplished the task of presenting multiple approaches to aphasia. The three editors, themselves experts in three different approaches to the study of aphasia, have collected chapters by world-recognized authorities whose fields of expertise cover quite divergent approaches to language disorders. With these chapters, plus the input of the editors themselves, a single volume has been produced in which many of the most important approaches to language disorder are authoritatively presented. This volume represents a state-of-the-art discussion of the multiple facets of language disorder. For anyone interested in the study of aphasia, from almost any vantage point, this volume provides an excellent compendium of background information, the more valuable because it is deliberately cross-disciplinary. In addition, much of the information provided will prove useful for those undertaking investigation of language function. The volume will be of equal value to clinicians, psychologists, language therapists, linguists, educators, and others truly interested in language and its disorders.

D. Frank Benson, M.D.
The Augustus S. Rose Professor of Neurology
UCLA School of Medicine
Los Angeles

Contributors

John Boeglin, *Faculté de Médecine, Université de Montreal, Quebec, Canada*

Jason W. Brown, *Department of Neurology, New York University Medical Center, New York, New York, U.S.A.*

F. Clifford Rose, *Academic Unit of Neuroscience, Charing Cross and Westminster Medical School, London, U.K.*

David Crystal, *Department of Linguistics, University College of North Wales, Bangor, U.K.*

Patricia Emery, *Speech-Language Pathology, Boston University School of Medicine and Boston Veterans Administration Medical Center, Boston, Massachusetts, U.S.A.*

M.L.E. Espir, *Department of Neurology, Charing Cross Hospital, London, U.K.*

Pierre Feyereisen, *National Fund of Scientific Research, University of Louvain, Belgium.*

Uri Hadar, *Academic Unit of Neuroscience, Charing Cross and Westminster Medical School, London, U.K.*

Nancy Helm-Estabrooks, *Audiology-Speech Pathology Service, Boston Veterans Administration Medical Center and Department of Neurology, Boston University School of Medicine, Boston, Massachussetts, U.S.A.*

Ruth Lesser, *Department of Speech, University of Newcastle upon Tyne, Newcastle upon Tyne, U.K.*

A. Damien Martin, *Department of Communication, Arts and Sciences, New York University, New York, New York, U.S.A.*

I.C. McManus, *Department of Psychology, University College, London, and St. Mary's Hospital Medical School, London, U.K.*

M.J. Morgan, *Department of Psychology, University College, London, U.K.*

David J. Mulhall, *Plymouth Health Authority, Devon, U.K.*

Costanza Papagno, *Department of Neurology, University of Freiburg, Federal Republic of Germany.*

Klaus Poeck, *Department of Neurology, RWTH Aachen, Federal Republic of Germany.*

Andre Roch Lecours, *Faculté de Médecine, Université de Montreal, Quebec, Canada*

Elliott D. Ross, *Department of Neurology, University of Texas Health Science Center at Dallas, Dallas, Texas, U.S.A.*

John F. Stein, *University Laboratory of Physiology, University of Oxford, Oxford, U.K.*

Marie-Josèphe Tainturier, *Faculté de Médecine, Université de Montreal, Quebec, Canada.*

Luigi A. Vignolo, *Clinica Neurologica dell' Universita, Brescia, Italy.*

Claus-W. Wallesch, *Department of Neurology, University of Freiburg, Federal Republic of Germany.*

Renata Whurr, *Speech Therapy Department, National Hospital for Nervous Diseases, London, U.K.*

Maria A. Wyke, *Department of Psychology, Institute of Psychiatry, University of London, London, U.K.*

Dahlia W. Zaidel, *Department of Psychology, UCLA, Los Angeles, California, U.S.A.*

Contents

Preface

Russell Brain claimed that his small book *Speech Disorders* was on a large subject, growing still larger as it expanded into linguistics, phonetics and communication theory. The key to understanding speech and language (and the pathology of both) was physiology, which was the link between the anatomy of the brain, in terms of the description of the lesion, and psychology, in terms of the understanding of the communication disorder.

This book is based on Brain's model: the theoretical aspects of aphasia are followed by the examination of the patient and the treatment of aphasia. It provides, in a single volume, coverage of the most recent developments in all three spheres.

Brain observed that aphasia was a confusing subject, partly because it was inherently complex, partly because conflicting interpretations were often made of the available facts, and partly because it was multidisciplinary; this confusion encouraged the presentation of discrete facts from which it was difficult to discern guiding principles. We have attempted to avoid these problems in this volume. Theory, assessment and treatment are given equal emphasis, and contributors are multidisciplinary in their backgrounds — neurologists, psychologists, linguists, psycholinguists and speech pathologists, all with a special interest in and experience of aphasia. This provides insight into the nature of aphasia for readers who have a similar broad variety of backgrounds, both professional and geographical, from which the contributors themselves come.

F. Clifford Rose
Renata Whurr
Maria A. Wyke

London
Autumn 1987

I

The Background

1

Classification of Aphasia

Andre Roch Lecours, Marie-Josèphe Tainturier and John Boeglin

> 'Round and round like a stage army moves the procession: the clinical appearances are identical, but each fresh group of observers views them with new eyes and with different preconceptions.'
>
> (Henry Head, 1926)

On occasion, clinicians of aphasiology will readily claim that there are as many clinical forms of aphasia as there are aphasic patients (or else as many aphasiological taxonomies as there are aphasiologists). The taxonomical undertaking may then be perceived as futile and illusory, but there are other occasions when the language behaviours of a given patient strongly bring to mind those of another, in view either of striking similarities or of apparently meaningful oppositions. Albeit with variation in levels of skepticism or dogmatism, anyone with experience in clinical aphasiology will acknowledge, on the one hand, that aphasic semeiology varies widely from one patient to another but, on the other, that certain symptom complexes seem to be shared by subgroups of patients. Obviously, the latter can be taken to indicate that brain–language relationships are to some extent constant within the species.

Broca's two initial case studies — those of Leborgne (Broca, 1861a) and Lelong (Broca, 1861b), whose names were as similar and dissimilar as were their brain lesions — have proven productive enough to found a surviving doctrine. They were not the first ones (see below) and the bibliography of Moutier's (1908) dissertation, which is comprised of no less than 1488 entries (Lecours and Joanette, 1984), refers to an astoundingly high number of single-case reports. After several decades of relative discredit, such reports have recently regained popularity: it is once again generally agreed upon — silently if one is a genuine cognitivist — that, when clearly supported by data, claims about the nature of brain dysfunction in a given individual with given biological and social characteristics imply claims about a human subgroup with comparable characteristics. None the less, in order to teach with appropriate conviction that the human brain 'honours' this or that psycholinguistic distinction, an exercise to which many scholars willfully lend themselves these days (open-class versus closed-class lexicon, reversible versus non-reversible sentences, animates versus inanimates, and so forth), it feels more comfortable when reference is made to more than one case. Unless adhering to Pierre Marie's (1906a) view that there is only one form of aphasia, this means resorting to an aphasiological taxonomy (whether or not on a temporary basis).

The editors of this book, apparently not unconditional adherents of Marie's teachings on aphasia, thought it appropriate to include a chapter on classification of the aphasias, and we have taken up their challenge.

The term 'aphasia', used by Plato to designate the state of speechlessness and inability to respond to a definitive argument or to verbally react to an emotionally overwhelming situation, was resurrected by Armand Trousseau (1864) who — after consulting both his colleague Emile Littré, the author of the famous dictionary, and a Greek friend, Monsieur Chrysaphis, the keeper of a Parisian restaurant — gave the term its contemporary meaning. Paul Broca's 'aphemia' was then pushed out of the limelight, so that our story begins with Trousseau's terminological victory (Hécaen and Dubois, 1969; Ryalls, 1984).

On Aphasiological Taxonomies

According to Webster's dictionary, taxonomy is 'the science of classification', the 'laws and principles covering the classifying of objects' (Guralnik and Friend, 1964). An overview of aphasiological taxonomies since the 1860s warrants some preliminary comments:

1. Concerning 'objects' taken as the primary matter to be classified,
   - (a) these have almost always been semeiological in nature. This is where 'laws and principles' have appeared from the beginning and still appear to be immediately applicable. This semeiological basis has been explicitly acknowledged in some cases (*see* Alajouanine below), or has been presented as subsequent to preoccupations concerning either dysfunctions of the mind or structures of the brain; or, more recently, concerning either structures of the mind or dysfunctions of the brain.
   - (b) In a few instances, taxonomizing has been attempted by direct reference to mechanisms of the mind rather than to observation of aphasic behaviour (*see* Freud below).
   - (c) There have also been instances when the objects have become

tenuous to the point that the only legitimacy of the taxonomy has been that of the paper on which a boxes-and-arrows geometry was created (*see* Grasset below).

2. The taxonomical undertaking, which will no doubt remain healthy as long as we know so little about the mutual relationships of brain and language, has been and is being constantly revamped: the pretext is usually a 'new' point of view, or better yet, a hypothesis (formulated or reformulated), almost always of a psychological nature (with or without the consent of its author).
3. In Boston or elsewhere, the best taxonomies are able to account unequivocally for about a third of all cases of aphasia (Albert *et al.*, 1981; Prins *et al.*, 1978), the other two thirds remaining, for the time being, 'mixed aphasias'.

Before Trousseau — Part I (Broca)

Pierre Paul Broca — Broca's (1861b) basic idea concerning localization was that a phrenology of the convolutions of the brain stood a better chance of survival than Gall's phrenology of the bumps of the skull. The third frontal convolution of the left hemisphere — as opposed to Bouillaud's (1825) 'anterior lobules' of the brain — and the 'faculty of articulated language' —as opposed to the 'general faculty of language' (Broca, 1865) — were but a mere example of Broca's conception. He knew, at least when he carefully edited the 1868 version of his yearly updated vitae (Broca, 1968), that deviant language behaviour could take on various forms (*alogia, amnesia, aphemia*, and *alalia*: acquired disorders of thought, verbal memory, language production, and speech) and probably stem from various sources, but he did not feel any need for a unifying label. As for Trousseau, his main intention was apparently to replace Broca's term with one of his own coining. None the less, his remarkable 1877 *Clinique Médicale de l'Hôtel-Dieu de Paris* suggests that he anticipated that his 'aphasia' was bound to encompass eventually more than his young rival's 'aphemia': whether or not 'the illustrious Professor of Montpellier' had been 'under an illusion' (Trousseau, 1877) when he reported his personal experience of 'alalia' (see Lordat below), it seems that his report had a most attentive reading by Trousseau.

Pioneering Taxonomies of the Aphasias

Jules Gabriel François Baillarger — Given the time when Trousseau coined the word 'aphasia' or, rather, given the time when, as the uncontested medical leader of l'Hôtel-Dieu de Paris, he imprinted the minds of his colleagues with its contemporary significance, the earliest explicit classification of the 'aphasias' is, as far as we know, that of Baillarger (1865). Ignoring the anatomical issue, Baillarger established his classification on the basis of clinical observations and rightly qualified it as 'psychological'. His taxonomy is presented under two main headings: on the one hand, *aphasie simple*, which includes two subtypes, depending on whether or not written expression is spared; on the other hand, *aphasie avec perversion de la faculté du langage* (literally: 'aphasia with perversion of the faculty of language').[1] Baillarger's 1865 work on aphasia shows that he deserves the credit for establishing the basic taxonomical dichotomy between fluency and non-fluency, a dichotomy that has never been challenged since, although not everybody will agree that defining an official cut-off point in relation to fluency always makes it easy to decide whether a given patient belongs to the fluent or to the non-fluent category.

John Hughlings Jackson — A few years after Baillarger, Jackson also recognized the clinical existence of three symptom complexes which largely overlapped with those of his French colleague, although he suggested a significantly different taxonomical division in arguing a clear distinction between *articulatory difficulties due to paresis* and *true affections of speech* (Head, 1926). He isolated 'paralytic' articulation disorders under a first main heading which conceivably encompassed several other forms of arthric disorders besides Baillarger's simple aphasia with preservation of written expression. His second main heading, 'true affections of speech', regrouped two sympton complexes, one with and one without reduction of verbal fluency. The two main headings are opposed by the existence of automatic–voluntary dissociation in the second condition although not in the first (in which Jackson's conceptions differ from Baillarger's); whereas the fluency/non-fluency dichotomy allows to oppose, on the one hand, paralytic disorders and true aphasia where 'the patient is speechless or nearly so' and, on the other, true aphasia where the patient utters 'plenty of words but mistakes in words' (Head, 1926).

Associationist Taxonomies

Associationist taxonomies are all derived from more or less elaborate psychological models which, until recently, their authors insisted on correlating with cerebral anatomy. The basic contention behind these taxonomies is that the various aspects of linguistic behaviour are specifically linked to the activities of highly specialized cortical areas and of their mutual axonal connexions. The diverse clinical forms that aphasia can assume thus

1. In contemporary terminology: *pure anarthria* and *Broca's aphasia*, on the one hand, *Wernicke's jargonaphasia*, on the other.

appear to be the result of selective lesions at given levels of one complex neuronal network or another.

Beginning with Baginski (1871), associationist taxonomies proliferated, for instance: Bastian's (1898) in England, Wernicke's (1874, 1886) and Lichtheim's (1885) in Germany, Charcot's (1884) and Dejerine's (1914) in France. The best known and no doubt the most influential of these taxonomies, even to this day, are those of Wernicke.[2]

Carl Wernicke and Ludwig Lichtheim — In 1874, Wernicke acknowledged the existence of two major types of aphasia:

1. *Motor aphasia*, the result of a lesion of the third frontal convolution of the left hemisphere (a tip of the hat to the French surgeon). This region of the cortex is a 'verbo-motor centre' and contains stored memories of movement sensations — 'Bewegungsvorstellungen' — corresponding to the encoding of articulate speech, hence the characteristic production disorder.
2. *Sensory aphasia*, the result of a lesion of the first temporal convolution of the same hemisphere. This region of the cortex is an 'auditivo-verbal centre' and contains stored memories of auditory sensations corresponding to the decoding of articulate speech, hence the characteristic auditory comprehension disorder.

Moreover, Wernicke, then only 28 years old and very clever indeed, postulated the existence of a third symptom complex:

3. *Conduction aphasia* ('Leitungsaphasie') — the result of a lesion of an axonal pathway associating the auditivo-verbal centre with the verbo-motor one. In this type of aphasia, predicted Wernicke, the memories of both motor and auditory sensations should be intact and the patient should present neither articulatory nor auditory comprehension disorders; fluent paraphasic speech should bear witness to the lesion of the associative pathway.

Finally, Wernicke recognized that other posterior lesions could impair reading and writing abilities but these disorders were 'asymbolias' rather than aphasias.

In spite of the term Wernicke created to designate the frontal component of his 1874 speech area, he explicitly conceived of both his centres as being mnemonic-sensory: the rostral one was labelled as 'motor' by reference to symptoms, not to mechanisms.[3] With early associationist taxonomies such as Wernicke's (1874), still another basic classificatory dichotomy was established, that between symptom complexes with impairment of auditory

2. The legend goes that Bastian, apparently on the basis of the results of an autopsy which cruelly contradicted his associationist predictions (Head, 1926), lost a great deal of his enthusiasm for diagram-making.
3. One wonders how this point escaped Luria many years later (cf. below).

comprehension versus those without (*sensory* versus *motor* and *conduction aphasias*).

In 1885, Lichtheim elaborated a model which allowed for the functional description of seven types of aphasia, either already described or yet to be observed. Two symptom complexes corresponded to lesions of specific brain centres. The five others, dubbed *commissural aphasias*, were attributed to lesions of the associative links between these two centres, of links between these centres and the (non-localized) biological basis of ideation and, finally, of links between these centres and the input and output systems.

Wernicke's 1886 taxonomy is comprised of the same seven entities. Anatomical labels are now prominent: while conduction aphasia remains unchanged, the original motor and sensory headings are broken down into *subcortical*, *cortical*, and *transcortical* subtypes.[4] Wernicke thus clearly indicates his belief that associationism should be understood both in psychological and in anatomical terms: he sees no reason to doubt (perhaps with lesser conviction in the case of the transcortical aphasias) the existence of a one-to-one correspondance between the components of his psychological model and various anatomical components of the brain.

Lichtheim's and Wernicke's seven forms of aphasia[5] are to be found in all but a few contemporary classifications, albeit often under different headings. As a rule the two cortical types have become, respectively, *Broca's aphasia* and *Wernicke's aphasia*, and the two subcortical ones *pure anarthria* and *pure verbal deafness*. As for the two transcortical types, they have usually kept both their cryptic names and their poor clinical definitions.

Joseph Jules Dejerine — The influence of Wernicke's classification on Dejerine's (1914) is quite obvious (and Dejerine did indeed acknowledge this influence). In a way, Dejerine's taxonomy, like those of Bastian (1898) and a few others, was clinically more appropriate than Wernicke's since it incorporated disorders of written language: the presence versus the absence of reading and/or writing disorders were thus introduced as pertinent oppositions in aphasiological taxonomy.

Another opposition, albeit an incongruous one from the semantic point of view, was also introduced by Dejerine between the notion of *true* versus that of *pure* aphasia, the first impairing 'internal language' and the second leaving it intact. This opposition served as the basis for defining two of the three major headings of Dejerine's typology. His *true aphasias* included *Broca's aphasia*, *Wernicke's aphasia*, and *global aphasia*, as well as several other clinical entities[6] such as *Wernicke's word deafness* and *Wernicke's word*

4. Apparently satisfied with its clarity, Wernicke also applied his anatomical trichotomy to the alexias.

5. As well as several forms of Wernicke's alexias.

6. Conduction aphasia was not included in this classification, which is surprising given Dejerine's remarkable knowledge of the associative connections of the cerebral hemispheres (Dejerine, 1901).

blindness which, on account of an association of the predominant modality-related comprehension disorder with other manifest, although relatively minor, language disturbances, Dejerine distinguished from *pure word deafness* and *pure word blindness*.[7] The latter two types, together with *pure motor aphasia* (which Dejerine also called *aphemia*) constituted the *pure aphasias*. Exner's pure agraphia (1881) was excluded on anatomical grounds: Dejerine argued oddly that the very existence of a 'writing centre' and therefore of pure agraphia could be only a myth since one can write on ice while skating just as well as with a pencil on paper.

Although Broca, Wernicke and others were obviously interested in brain convolutions, Dejerine and his wife, Augusta Klumpke (Lecours and Caplan, 1984) were no doubt the first to undertake detailed anatomo-clinical studies of aphasia, using the method of whole-brain serial sections[8], and although they were, to a certain extent, cautious enough to avoid compromising labels, to introduce documented neuroanatomy as a fundamental parameter of aphasiological taxonomy. This remains true even if Dejerine's third category, comprised of *amnestic aphasia* and of several forms of *transcortical aphasia*, is rightly headed *other varieties of aphasia without discrete neuroanatomical substrata* ('sans valeur de localisation').

Jean Martin Charcot — Superficially similar in many respects to the classifications of Bastian and Wernicke, Charcot's (1884) taxonomy was original in that the Master of the Salpêtrière insisted that lesions of the same anatomical structures could result in different clinical pictures depending on the patient's cultural background and/or mental structure. The potential importance of this conception on aphasiological taxonomy will be emphasized toward the end of this chapter.[9]

Bernard Grasset — Some of the associationist taxonomies turned out to be mere paper-and-pencil confabulations, sometimes esthetic, but generally devoid of any cognitive or biological foundation as well as of any clinical reality. Grasset's (1880) classification, with its *motor* and *sensory subpolygonal, polygonal, suprapolygonal* and *transpolygonal aphasias*, is a good example.

A Taxonomy of Holisms

As eloquently argued by Henry Head (1926), efficacious reaction to associationism was bound to occur. Given the origin of the doctrine, and given the fact that Fulgence Raymond was to leave Charcot's chair (to Dejerine or to Pierre Marie?) soon after the turn of the century, it was only

7. Or *alexia without*, as opposed to *alexia with, agraphia* (Dejerine, 1892).
8. As far as we know, nobody has done better since.
9. In any case, it is certain that no occipital-splenial lesion can cause alexia in an illiterate, although an illiterate with such a lesion might not be the ideal candidate to include in an alphabetization program.

natural that such reaction should come from France and, specifically, from La Salpêtrière (the School if not the Hospital). Aphasia was a topic of great interest at the Faculty. Dejerine and his wife were identified with associationism and Marie felt as though he should react (Marie, 1906a, b), i.e. formulate a 'new conception of aphasia' (Piéron, 1909), and it should be added that he had a good resident, François Moutier, to assist him in carrying out this mission (Lecours and Joanette, 1984).

Pierre Marie and Charles Foix — A strict holist does not classify, and Pierre Marie came very close to doing just that. His conception of aphasia, as expressed in 1906 and which came to be known as 'Pierre Marie's law', was as follows:

Aphasie de Broca = Aphasie de Wernicke + anarthrie

In other words: (1) there is only one Aphasia, that being *Wernicke's aphasia*; (2) there is a paralytic disorder of speech, *anarthria*, which is fundamentally different from aphasia; and (3) the so-called *Broca's aphasia*[10] is the co-occurrence of anarthria and aphasia.

It remains a small mystery how Charles Foix, Alajouanine's 'Maître incomparable' (Lhermitte *et al.*, 1981), could manage, on the one hand, to leave everybody under the impression that he was unconditionally faithful to the teachings of Pierre Marie and, on the other hand, to propose a four-part anatomically (very well) documented subdivision of Wernicke's aphasia (Marie and Foix, 1917). This included a conduction-aphasia-like nosological entity, *supramarginal gyrus aphasia*, explicitly attributed to damage of a specific part of the cortical region which Marie qualified as 'Wernicke's area'[11] and considered to be functionally homogeneous.

Goldstein — Although regularly quoted as one of the most vigorous supporters of the holist theory of Aphasia, Kurt Goldstein did not consider such a theoretical position to be incompatible with the division of aphasic behaviour into numerous semeiological constellations. Indeed, Goldstein's (1948) 'classification', at least in the way we have attempted to reconstitute it (Lecours and Lhermitte, 1979), includes no fewer than 30 headings, which seems a surprising number when the modest three headings of the original classification of the father of aphasiological associationism (Wernicke, 1874) are considered. Geschwind's (1964) paper on the 'paradoxical position of Kurt Goldstein' is very informative in this respect.

Eberhard Bay — Whether groping for sound, or logorrheic, or behaving somewhere in between, aphasics experience 'word-finding difficulties' (WFD), that is, difficulties in accessing their mental lexicon. According to Bay (1964), WFD is 'die genuin Aphasie' and Pierre Marie was right about the nosological individuality of *anarthria*, at least if it is relabelled as *cortical*

10. Global aphasia in this context.
11. That is, the first two temporal, the angular, and the supramarginal gyri (Marie, 1906a).

dysarthria (which it is in certain cases: Alajouanine, Pichot and Durand, 1949; Ladame, 1902; Lecours and Lhermitte, 1976). Thus, several laws are possible:

WFD + Nothing = Pitres' Aphasia (amnestic aphasia, anomia)
WFD + Cortical dysarthria = Broca's aphasia
WFD + Cortical acoustic disorder + General mental disorder = Wernicke's aphasias
WFD + Lack of ideas ('Einfallsleere') = Transcortical sensory aphasia

and so forth. This way of parsing reality is appealing, especially as it is clinically based.

A Psychophysiological Taxonomy

Sigmund Freud — Freud's (1891) avant-garde monograph on aphasia was a flop at publication and remained so for at least half a century, more than 70% of the original printing being pulped by the editor in 1900 (Anzieu, 1975). The section on taxonomy was not as penetrating as those in which Freud presented his views on the biology of language, or in which he formulated his 'Kritische Studie' of most of his contemporaries' teachings (Charcot included, but with the notable exception of Jackson). Freud deduced the principle of his aphasia classification from a conceptual scheme in which he opposed the notion of 'word concept' to that of 'object concept', each corresponding to a complex network of 'associations' — *psychological* ones — between bits of information of multimodal nature, and each associated to the other through other (psychological) associations. Founded on psycho-physiological rather than on clinical considerations, Freud's classification includes three headings: (1) *verbal aphasia*, which impairs the associations constitutive of the word concepts; (2) *asymbolic aphasia*, which impairs the associations between the word concept and the object concept and (3) *agnostic aphasia*, which impairs the associations constitutive of the object concept. A sensible man, Freud also provided ample room for 'mixed' forms of aphasia, but it remains a hazardous venture to attempt drawing parallels between Freud's taxonomy and any other that we know of.

A Pseudolinguistic Taxonomy

Henry Head — Henry Head (1926), officially a holist (globalist), did not avoid the pitfalls so well characterized in the sentence quoted in the epigraph to this chapter. His taxonomy includes four labels, each of which firmly evokes some aspect of language behaviour:

1. *Verbal aphasia* (Broca's aphasia).
2. *Syntactic aphasia* — Wernicke's aphasia, surprisingly enough, given the syntactic competence of Wernicke's aphasics.
3. *Anomia* — according to Tissot (1966), and we agree, a mild form of Wernicke's aphasia rather than anomia.
4. *Semantic aphasia* — for which we did not succeed in finding an equivalent in any other taxonomy, including Luria's (see below).

At first sight, Head's labels, with their limpid linguistic connotations, appeal since, after all, aphasia does impair language, but the short definition he provides of each of his labels leaves the reader in a state of perplexity. For instance, *verbal aphasia* is characterized as 'a defective power of forming words, whether for external or internal use'. As we decode it, this definition could apply not only to Broca's aphasia, but also to Wernicke's aphasia, conduction aphasia, and so on. Of course, it is entirely possible that we did not correctly interpret Head.

Atheoretical Taxonomies

Théophile Alajouanine — With the mentality of one born in 1890, the son of the ironmaster of Montluçon, a village in the French province of Bourbonnais (Lhermitte *et al.*, 1981), as well as with that of a legitimate son of the Salpêtrière (through Pierre Marie and Charles Foix), Alajouanine fully exerted his inborn creativity when his patients were Ravel, Gernez, or Valéry Larbaud (Alajouanine, 1948) but, when it came to serious matters such as aphasiological taxonomies, Alajouanine was cautious and did not take kindly to the use of alien neologisms such as 'associationisme' and 'aphasie de conduction'. Not only are his taxonomical teachings in considerable accord with those of Charcot, Dejerine, and, of course, Charles Foix, but they also manage to remain compatible with Pierre Marie's views. As a result, Alajouanine's 1968 classification of 'aphasia' consists of 11 items under three major headings:

1. Aphasia without impairment of verbal articulation:
   (a) Complete temporal aphasia (complete Wernicke's aphasia and transcortical sensory aphasia, elsewhere).
   (b) Temporal aphasia with sensory predominance (Wernicke's aphasia with predominance of verbal deafness).
   (c) Angular gyrus syndrome (Wernicke's aphasia with predominance of written language disorders, alexia with agraphia).
   (d) Jargonaphasia (conduction aphasia, oddly enough).
   (e) Pitres' aphasia (anomia).

2. Aphasia with impairment of verbal articulation:
   (a) Full Broca's aphasia or Dejerine's total aphasia (global aphasia).
   (b) Broca's aphasia.
3. Pure aphasia:
   (a) Pure anarthria.
   (b) Pure agraphia.
   (c) Pure word deafness.
   (d) Pure alexia.

Alajouanine's contribution to the study of arthric disorders of left brain-damaged subjects, whether among Broca's aphasics (Alajouanine, Ombredane and Durand, 1939) or in its 'pure' form (Alajouanine *et al.*, 1949; Lecours and Lhermitte, 1976), have become classics, and his 1939 monograph can be considered as marking the birth of 'neurolinguistics' (Lhermitte *et al.*, 1981). The number of contemporary occidental aphasiological taxonomies which are not in quasi-total agreement with Alajouanine's 11-item scheme is indeed very limited.

Harold Goodglass — No doubt the most influential of contemporary aphasiological taxonomies, and by far, is that of the Bostonians of the Geschwind school (Goodglass and Kaplan, 1972). This classification is based on an exceptionally rigorous method of clinical observation and is reminiscent, to some extent, of Alajouanine's. It also comprises 11 items: besides Broca's, Wernicke's, conduction, alexic-agraphic and anomic aphasias, the Boston classification includes four 'pure' entities and two 'transcortical' ones. As Dejerine did before them (see above) and no doubt with similar intention of paying tribute to the memory of Broca, Harold Goodglass and Edith Kaplan talk of 'aphemia' when it comes to labelling the behaviour of left-hemisphere lesioned dextrals with isolated arthric disorders and normal written expression.

Andrew Kertesz — Andy Kertesz' (1979) taxonomy is derived from the application of what he qualifies as 'the numerical approach' to the problem of classifying aphasias. This consists in submitting a large group of aphasic patients to a standardized aphasia examination battery (the oral language subtests of the Western Aphasia Battery (Kertesz and Poole, 1974)) and letting statistical wizardry (i.e., cluster analysis) regroup the patients according to their various scores. According to Kertesz (1979), the numerical approach can provide 'objective clusters of aphasics on the basis of test scores, free from the constraints of previous classifications'. Obviously, the main result of this approach is that most patients will find a place in the scheme (since all contribute to its definition); of course, another consequence is that patients whom clinicians perceive as quite dissimilar will be given the same nosological label (Basso *et al.*, 1985). As to the labels themselves, they remain on the whole conservative although Kertesz distinguishes between an 'afferent' and an 'efferent' variety of 'conduction aphasia' (Kertesz, 1979), without any obvious kinship to Luria's use of these attributes (see below).

A Partially Neurolinguistic Taxonomy

Henry Hécaen — As it is for a large part based both on anatomoclinical correlations and on various structural aspects of language, Hécaen's taxonomy may rightly be qualified as 'neurolinguistic' (Hécaen, 1972). As a rule, Hécaen's headings are meant to underline a particular linguistic dysfunction and, contrary to Henry Head's, his labels are, on the whole, potentially meaningful. For example:

1. *Broca's aphasia* is identified as *aphasia of phonematic realization* when arthric disorders dominate the clinical picture, and *agrammatic* or *syntactic realization aphasia* in cases where agrammatism becomes apparent after a period of favourable evolution.
2. *Conduction aphasia* is appropriately classified among the *expressive aphasias*[12] and is labelled as *sentence programming aphasia.*[13]
3. The group of the *amnestic aphasias* are renamed *morpheme selection disorders.*

In spite of an unprecedented resurgence of synonymy, Hécaen's taxonomy is very much related to classic taxonomies such as those of Dejerine, Foix, and others, as well as to the Bostonian one (see above). This no doubt reflects the fact that, rather from a preconceived hypothetical scheme, this classification stems from systematic clinical observation and bears witness to a laudable effort to unify aphasiological terminology.

Aphasiological Taxonomy Rediscovered

Aleksandr Romanovich Luria — Bewegungsvorstellungen are not Bewegungsvorstellungen but rather 'articulemes' and, moreover, they are not located in the third frontal convolution but rather in the postcentral one, 2.5 cm caudally, to your left as you enter (Jarry, 1962): both Broca and Wernicke were therefore wrong (Luria, 1964). Although Luria's contribution to neuropsychology has been among the most significant of this century, his aphasiological taxonomy (Luria, 1964) has not proved particularly useful outside the Soviet Union. It comprises six headings (see Jakobson below),

12. Implicitly, Hécaen thus rejects the anterior/posterior dichotomy, and we agree.

13. The authors of this chapter do not understand why Hécaen thus chose to underline the abundant production of aborted sentences in the spontaneous discourse of conduction aphasics rather than their characteristic production of phonemic deviations.

each of which designates the dysfunction of a specific psychological mechanism. Luria claims, for instance, and this represents in our opinion his most original contribution to aphasiology, that a lesion of the opercular third of the postcentral gyrus causes a particular type of aphasia which he identifies as *afferent motor aphasia*, the result of a 'disturbance of the articuleme', that is, of a disruption of the 'continual afferent correction' which is normally ensured through proprioceptive feedback generated by the activity of the phonoarticulatory musculature. This obviously makes sense, as it has since Wernicke (see above); none the less, the correspondence between Luria's afferent motor aphasia and previously discussed clinical pictures is a subject that remains highly controversial (Valdois, Ryalls, and Lecours, 1987).

A Linguistic Taxonomy

Roman Jakobson — For those interested in aphasia primarily or solely from the linguistic standpoint, Roman Jakobson's (1956, 1964) taxonomies are certainly of the greatest interest. In 1956, when his aim was to characterize the Broca/Wernicke anterior/posterior dichotomy in structuralist terms, Jakobson opposed *contiguity* to *similarity disorders*. In 1964, he further specified his characterization of the aphasias by reference to his friend Luria's taxonomy, and this was brilliantly achieved, following the 'distinctive-features methodology' (so to speak), on the basis of three oppositions. The 1956 dichotomy is replaced by one opposing *encoding* to *decoding disorders* (Luria's *motor afferent, motor efferent*, and *dynamic aphasias* versus his *semantic, sensory*, and *acoustic–amnestic aphasias*). Disorders of *sequence* are then opposed to disorders of *concurrence* (Luria's *dynamic, efferent motor*, and *acoustic–amnestic aphasias* versus his *afferent motor*,[14] *semantic*, and *sensory aphasias*). Finally, aphasias by *disintegration* are opposed to aphasias by *limitation* (Luria's *efferent motor* and *sensory aphasias* versus his *dynamic* and *semantic aphasias*).

One wishes that Jakobson had found the time to concoct a linguistic characterization of more encompassing classification of, say Goodglass and Kaplan (1972).

Interlude: On Terminological Confusion

Since the Broca–Trousseau etymological debate on 'aphemia' (Broca, 1864;

14. Luria's *afferent motor aphasia* is thus characterized as a disorder of the encoding of simultaneously produced units, that is, a disorder in combining features into phonemes. In our opinion, this strikingly fits Alajouanine's *phonetic disintegration syndrome* (Alajouanine *et al.*, 1939).

Trousseau, 1864), aphasiologists have consistently acted as addicts of terminological ambiguity. More than any other discipline, with the possible exception of psychiatry, aphasiology has generated and tolerated terminological confusions in its vocabulary and, particularly, in its classifications. Although the reported facts have long remained essentially the same, the issue of classification has been and remains flawed by three lexical phenomena, namely: synonymy, homonymy, and malapropism.

Synonymy

Reviewing the aphasic literature, the creativity demonstrated in coining terms designating clinical entities previously named by others is astounding. For example, the nosological entity that Broca renamed *aphemia*, a label which he himself was ready to change to *aphrasia* had Trousseau been willing to make a compromise, has also been designated under the following terms (among others); verbal amnesia, motor aphasia, central motor aphasia, nuclear motor aphasia, cortical motor aphasia, efferent motor aphasia, polygonal motor aphasia, true motor aphasia, atactic aphasia, apraxia of speech, cortical dyslalia, glossopsychic aphasia, kinesthetic aphasia, laloplegia, verbal aphasia, aphasia of phonematic realization... and Broca's aphasia.

Homonymy

In contrast to synonymy, and perhaps even more confusing, is that the same labels have occasionally been employed to refer to different clinical phenomena. For example, depending on whether one accepts or rejects the concept of 'centre', the term *central aphasia* can designate a syndrome that attests to the lesion or dysfunction of a particular 'centre' (e.g., Lichtheim, 1885), or else a syndrome due to the lesion of the middle part — the centre — of the speech area (e.g., Brain, 1961). Still another interpretation of the term is found in Goldstein (1948) who uses 'central' — as opposed to 'peripheral' — to designate aphasias characterized by an impairment of the 'abstract attitude'.

Malapropism

All too often, the terms chosen do not mean what they say. An 'aphasic' patient should not talk at all, and most of us are therefore guilty of using a malapropism but Henry Head (see above), with his *nominal, verbal, syntactic*, and *semantic aphasias* probably remains an all-time champion in spite of strong and persistent competition.

Parameters of Aphasiological Taxonomy

It has been questioned to what extent the currently popular version of the 'speech area' integrally applies to the 75% of the human population (according to UNESCO statistics, 1977) which does not conform to the following prototype: a right-handed unilingual adult who speaks a language without tonal oppositions, nor agglutinations, and who has learned to write it following an alphabetic or syllabic convention (Lecours, 1980).[15] One might *a fortiori* formulate a similar argument concerning the Occidentals taxonomies of the aphasias. Consequently, a valuable goal of future taxonomic research would be to try to incorporate certain parameters that have been neglected, or at least not explicitly nor systematically acknowledged in the past. The nature of such parameters might be:

1. *Biological* — Age ('logorrhoeic neologistic jargon' does not really qualify as a regular taxonomic heading for childhood aphasia); sex, although we find it hard to conceive why and how the neural devices subtending human language should be as strongly sex-linked as certain data apparently indicate (Kimura, 1981; McGlone, 1980)[16]; degree of hand dominance (a classic preoccupation of aphasiology but never included as a classification parameter).
2. *Biopathological* — Including aetiology as a parameter of classification, as Luria (1964) hinted and as Kertesz (1979) began doing systematically, is obviously pertinent (typical agrammatism is seldom observed in a patient with an astrocytoma or a degenerative disease).
3. *Socio-environmental* — Typology of spoken languages (is paragrammatism the same in English as in Turkish or Cree?); typology of written languages; why is *Gogi aphasia* (Kimura, 1934) so seldomly diagnosed at Queen Square? And why should one from Mysore recover written English before written Kanadda (Karanth, 1981)?); unilingualism versus multilingualism; literacy.

Moreover, many aphasic patients will often resist being permanently labelled: from Wernicke's aphasia to conduction aphasia to amnestic aphasia, for instance, if things go well after a posterior temporal infarct, or else from amonia to transcortical sensory aphasia if the causative disease is progressive.

15. This argument was formulated without evoking the vorgestalt of the slightest doubt as to the fact that left hemisphere dominance for language is genetically determined and shared by the species as a whole.
16. As suggested by Kinsbourne (1980), this could be in part a political rather than a biological issue.

The New Cognitivist Approach

If it is agreed that the test of brain and language relationships must rely upon theories of biology and of behaviour that have independent empirical warrants and, if this premise is applied to aphasiological research on taxonomy, this is the 'new' approach to the taxonomic question which is inherent in the scientific trend known as cognitive neuropsychology (or 'boxology').

Thereby differing from those whom Head (1926) qualified as 'diagram makers', modern boxologists do not wish to legitimize their psychological diagrams by mapping them onto the brain: so much the better if they turn out to have meaning from the biological point of view, but this is not a prerequisite. The new way stems from a fundamentally explicit tenet: classifying aphasic behaviours can and should be done through characterization of symptoms and symptom complexes by reference to models of normal language processing. Another significant fact concerning the new cognitive approach to aphasiological taxonomy is that, at least for the time being, classifications concern specific aspects of language behaviour (e.g., reading isolated words) rather than whole syndromes. This leads to taxonomical atomization. Theories are specific to encapsulated aspects of language behaviour and, if tested, say, for reading, repetition and writing, the same patient may well be given three different taxonomical labels (dyslexia of type X + dysechophemia of type Y + dysgraphia of type Z), and none of these, nor *a fortiori* their combination, need correspond to a classic label.

Clinicians may find this annoying but, until new and more powerful tools for biological research in the domain of neuropsychology are developed, it might be the best way for aphasiologists to progress further in the domain of taxonomy. Given that clinicians already know, for instance, that *Broca's aphasia* can, at least diachronically, be observed with or without *phonetic disintegration*, with or without *agrammatism* and with or without *deep dyslexia*, it would not take such a big step to find great interest in observing that *deep dyslexia* can also occur in the context of *logorrheic Wernicke's jargon* (Sheperd *et al.*, 1986). Whether a new label will be created to designate this association is of relatively lesser importance.

Before Trousseau — Part II (Lordat or the old cognitivist approach)

Before Trousseau's terminological triumph over Broca (see above), people had been interested in classifying the 'alalias'. Thus, between 20 and 40 years before Broca first met Leborgne, during the 1840s and probably earlier,

Jacques Lordat, who did not care much about Gall's teachings, explicitly taught his students at the Faculté de Médecine de Montpellier that the study of alalia could only be pursued by reference to a clear conception of the various steps of normal language processing, i.e. that the characterization of alalic syndromes could only be derived from a model of normal function (Lordat, 1843). In this respect, he proposed that, from its decision to communicate a thought to the embodiment of this thought into conventional sounds, the human mind accomplishes a succession of ten modular acts: 'each of which should be studied separately' (Lordat, 1843; Lecours *et al.*, 1987). Various types of pathological linguistic behaviour can result from an impairment of these acts. 'Incoherence' results when the impaired acts are 'exclusively mental' and pre-linguistic, as in typhus, alcoholic intoxication, and somniloquia. Impairment of the 'admirable mental operations'[17] behind human speech and language behaviour can lead, depending on the level of impairment, to several types of alalia and paralalia, such as 'asynergetic alalia' (*anarthria*), 'alalia by verbal amnesia' (*Broca's aphasia*), and 'incorrigible and unconscious paralalia' (*Wernicke's jargonaphasia*). In the latter, Lordat tells his students, two types of faulty utterances are typically produced: in the first, the idea is mapped onto an existing word but not the target one; in the second, the target is retrieved but, in production, 'the letters and syllables are inverted'. And then Lordat (1843) wonders why he has not as yet observed patients with a specific impairment of grammar: following a method that was to gain popularity a century and a half later, and just as Wernicke was to predict the existence of conduction aphasia some 30 years later, Lordat thus predicted the existence of agrammatism.[18]

Acknowledgement

The activities of the Centre de Recherche du Centre Hospitalier Côte-des-Neiges are funded by the Medical Research Counsil of Canada and by the Fonds de la Recherche en Santé du Québec.

References

ALAJOUANINE, TH. Aphasia and artistic realization. *Brain* (1948), **71**, 228–242.

ALAJOUANINE, TH. *L'aphasie et le langage pathologique* (1968). Paris: Baillière.

ALAJOUANINE, TH., OMBREDANE, A. and DURAND, M. *Le syndrome de désintégration phonétique dans l'aphasie* (1939) Paris: Masson.

17. Apparently including a whole set of buffer-like specialized memories.

18. And improvised for his students a rather convincing simulation: 'Moi aimer vous, désirer beaucoup vous être utile'.

ALAJOUANINE, TH., PICHOT, P., and DURAND, M. Dissociations des altérations phonétiques avec conservation relative de la langue la plus ancienne dans un cas d'anarthrie pure chez un sujet français bilingue. *Encéphale* (1949), **28**, 245-265.

ALBERT, M., GOODGLASS, H., HELM, N.A., RUBENS, A.B., and ALEXANDER, M.M. *Clinical aspects of dysphasia* (1981) New York: Springer-Verlag.

ANZIEU, D. *L'autoanalyse de Freud et la découverte de la psychanalyse* (1975) Paris: PUF.

BAGINSKI 'Aphasie in Folge schwerer Nierenerkrankungen.' *Berliner Klin. Wft.* (1811; quoted in Moutier, 1908).

BAILLARGER, J.G.F. *Recherches sur les maladies mentales* (1865) Paris: Masson.

BASSO, A., LECOURS, A.R., MORASCHINI, S., and VANIER, M. Anatomo-clinical correlations of the aphasias as defined through computerized tomography: On exceptions. *Brain and Language* (1985), **26**, 201-229.

BASTIAN, H.C. *A Treatise on Aphasia and Other Speech Defects* (1898) London: Lewis.

BAY, E. Principles of classification and their influence on our concepts of aphasia. In A.V.S. De Reuck and M. O'Connor (eds), *Disorders of Language* (1964) pp. 122-142. London: Churchill.

BAYLE, J.M.J. *Les fondateurs de la doctrine française de l'aphasie* (1939) Bordeaux: Bière.

BOUILLAUD, J.B. Recherches cliniques propres à démontrer que la perte de la parole correspond à la lésion des lobules antérieurs du cerveau, et à confirmer l'opinion de M. Gall sur le siège de l'organe du langage articulé. *Archives Générales de Médecine* (1825), **8**, 25-45.

BRAIN, W.R. *Speech Disorders* (1961) London: Butterworths.

BROCA, P. Remarques sur le siège de la faculté du langage articulé, suivies d'une observation d'aphemie (perte de la parole). *Bulletin de la Société Anatomique de Paris* (1861a), **6**, 330-357.

BROCA, P. Nouvelle observation d'aphémie produite par une lésion de la moitié postérieure des deuxième et troisième circonvolutions frontales. *Bulletin de la Société Anatomique de Paris* (1861b), **6**, 398-407.

BROCA, P. Sur les mots aphémie, aphasie, aphrasie. Lettre à Monsieur le Pr. Trousseau. *Gazette des hôpitaux* (1864), January 23.

BROCA, P. Du siège de la faculté du langage articulé. *Bulletin de la Société d'Anthropologie* (1865), **6**, 377-393.

BROCA, P. Recherches sur la localisation de la faculté du langage articulé. *Exposé des titres et travaux scientifiques de Paul Broca* (1868; quoted in Bayle, 1939).

CHARCOT, J.M. *Differente formi d'afazia; lezioni fatte nella Salpêtrière nel semestre d'estate dell'anno 1883* (1884) Milan: Vallardi.

DEJERINE, J.J. Contribution à l'étude anatomo-pathologique et clinique des différentes variétés de cécité verbale. *Mémoires de la Société de Biologie* (1892), **9**, 61-90.

DEJERINE, J. avec la collaboration de Dejerine-Klumpke, A. *Anatomie des Centres Nerveux*, (1901) Paris: Rueff.

DEJERINE, J. *Séméiologie des affections du système nerveux* (1914). Paris: Masson.

EXNER, S. *Untersuchungen uber die Lokalisation der Funktionen in der Grosshirnrinde des Menschen* (1881). Vienna: Wilhelm Braumuller.

FREUD, S. *Zur Auffasung der Aphasien* (1891), Vienna: Deuticke. (English translation: Freud, S. (1953). *On Aphasia*, New York: International Universities Press.)

GESCHWIND, N. The paradoxical position of Kurt Goldstein in the history of aphasia. *Cortex*, (1964), **1**, 214-224.

GOLDSTEIN, K. *Language and Language Disturbances* (1948). New-York: Grune & Stratton.

GOODGLASS, H. and KAPLAN, E. *The Assessment of Aphasia and Related Disorders* (1972). Philadelphia: Lea & Febiger.

GRASSET, B. *Des localisations dans les maladies cérébrales* (1880). Paris: Delahaye.

GURALNIK, D.B. and FRIEND, J.H. *Webster's New World Dictionary of the American Language* (1964). Cleveland: College edition.

HEAD, J. *Aphasia and Kindred Disorders of Speech* (1926). London: Cambridge University Press.

HÉCAEN, H. *Introduction à la Neuropsychologie* (1972). Paris: Larousse.

HÉCAEN, H. and DUBOIS, J. *La naissance de la neuropsychologie du langage* (1969). Paris: Flammarion.

JAKOBSON, R. Two aspects of language and two types of aphasic disturbances. In R. Jakobson and M. Halle (eds), *Fundamentals of Language* (1956) pp. 55-82. The Hague: Mouton.

JAKOBSON, R. Towards a linguistic typology of aphasic impairments. In A.V.S. de Reuk and M. O'Connor (eds), *Disorders of Language* (1964) pp. 21-42. London: Churchill.

JARRY, A. *Tout Ubu* (1962). Paris: La Librairie Générale Française.

KARANTH, P. Pure alexia in a Kannada English bilingual. *Cortex* (1981), **77**, 187-198.

KERTESZ, A. *Aphasia and Associated Disorders* (1979). New York: Grune & Stratton.

KERTESZ, A. and POOLE, E. The aphasia quotient: The taxonomic approach to measurement of aphasic disability. *The Canadian Journal of Neurological Sciences* (1974), **1**, 7-16.

KIMURA, D. Sex differences in speech organization within the left hemisphere. *Research Bulletin 548* (1981), Psychology, University of Western Ontario.

KIMURA, K. Aphasia: Characteristic symptoms in Japanese. *Journal of Psychiatry and Neurology* (1934), **37**, 437-459.

KINSBOURNE, M. If sex differences in brain lateralization exist, they have yet to be discovered. *The Behavioural and Brain Sciences* (1980), **3**, 241-242.

LADAME, P.L. La question de l'aphasie motrice sous-corticale. *Revue Neurologique* (1902), **10**, 13-18.

LECOURS, A.R. Corrélations anatomo-cliniques de l'aphasie. La zone du langage. *Revue Neurologique* (1980), **136**, 591-608.

LECOURS, A.R. and CAPLAN, D. Augusta Dejerine-Klumpke or 'The lesson in anatomy'. *Brain and Cognition* (1984), **3**, 166-197.

LECOURS, A.R. and JOANETTE, Y. François Moutier or from folds to folds. *Brain and Cognition* (1984), **3**, 198-203.

LECOURS, A.R. and LHERMITTE, F. The 'pure form' of the phonetic disintegration syndrome (pure anarthria). Anatomo-clinical report of a historical case. *Brain and Language* (1976), **3**, 88-113.

LECOURS, A.R. and LHERMITTE, F. *L'aphasie* (1979). Paris: Flammarion (English translation: Lecours, A.R., Lhermitte, F., and Bryans, B. *Aphasiology* (1983). London: Baillière Tindall).

LECOURS, A.R., NESPOULOUS, J.L. and PIOGER, D. Jacques Lordat or the birth of cognitive neuropsychology. In E. Keller and M. Gopnik (eds), *Motor and Sensory Processes of Language* (1987), Hillsdale: Lawrence Erlbaum.

LHERMITTE, F., LECOURS, A.R. and SIGNORET, J.L. Théophile Alajouanine (1890-1980). *Brain and Language* (1981), **13**, 191-196.

LICHTHEIM, L. On aphasia. *Brain* (1885), **7**, 433-484.

LORDAT, J. Leçons tirées du cours de physiologie de l'année scolaire 1842-1843: Analyse de la parole pour servir à la théorie de divers cas d'alalie et de paralalie que les nosologistes ont mal connus. *Journal de la Société de Médecine Pratique de Montpellier* (1843), **7**, 333-353, 417-433, and **8**, 1-17 (reprinted in Hécaen and Dubois (1969), pp. 129-167).

LURIA, A.R. Factors and forms of aphasia. In A.V.S. de Reuck and M. O'Connor (eds) *Disorders of Language* (1964) pp. 143-167. London: Churchill.

MARIE, P. Revision de la question de l'aphasie: la troisième circonvolution frontale gauche ne joue aucun rôle spécial dans la fonction du langage. *Semaine Médicale* (1906a), **26**, 241-247.

MARIE, P. L'aphasie de 1861 à 1866. Essai de critique historique sur la genèse de la doctrine de Broca (1906b). (Reprinted in: Marie, O. *Travaux et Mémoires: Vol. I* (1926). Paris: Masson.)

MARIE, P. and FOIX, C. Les aphasies de guerre. *Revue Neurologique* (1917), **1**, 53-87.

MCGLONE, J. Sex differences in human brain asymmetry: A critical survey. *The Behavioural and Brain Sciences* (1980), **3**, 215-227.

MOUTIER, F. *L'aphasie de Broca* (1908). Paris: Steinheil.

PIÉRON, H. La conception nouvelle de l'aphasie. *Rivista di Scienza* (1909), **6**, 3-10.

PRINS, R.S., SNOW, C. and WAGENAAR, E. Recovery from aphasia: spontaneous speech versus language comprehension. *Brain and Language* (1978), **6**, 192-211.

RYALLS, J. Where does the term 'aphasia' come from? *Brain and Language* (1984), **21**, 358-363.

SHEPERD FLEET, W., ROTHI, L., RAADE, A. and HEILMAN, K. Deep dyslexia in a Wernicke's aphasic. Communication presented at the 24th annual meeting of the *Academy of Aphasia* (1986), Nashville, Tennessee, October 19-21.

TISSOT, R. *Neuropsychopathologie de l'aphasie* (1966). Paris: Masson.

TROUSSEAU, A. De l'aphasie, maladie décrite récemment sous le nom impropre d'aphémie. *Gazette des Hôpitaux* (1864; quoted in Moutier, 1908), January 12.

TROUSSEAU, A. *Clinique Médicale de l'Hôtel-Dieu de Paris: Vol. 2* (1877). Paris: Baillière.

UNESCO *Statistical Yearbook* (1977). New York: UNESCO.

VALDOIS, S., RYALLS, J. and LECOURS, A.R. (1987). Luria's aphasiology: A critical review. *Journal of Neurolinguistics* (in press).

WERNICKE, C. *Der aphasische Symptomenkomplex* (1874). Breslau: Kohn and Weigert.

WERNICKE, C. Einige neuere Arbeiten über Aphasie. *Fortschritte der Medicin* (1886; quoted in Freud, 1891).

2

Linguistic Levels in Aphasia

David Crystal

The Need for Description

'Empirical work must come first'. It is discomfiting, but salutary, to begin with such a quotation — discomfiting, because it was a remark of Hughlings Jackson, made in the 1880s at a British Medical Association meeting, as apposite today as it was a century ago. Much has happened meanwhile. Yet there still remains a pressing need for a comprehensive and systematic description of the linguistic behaviour of aphasic patients, made at a level of detail that would be considered routine in, say, human anatomy or physiology. Compared with medical case studies, where are the published accounts of the *whole* of aphasic patients' linguistic behaviour, as manifest in a sample of their conversation? There are many partial studies and illustrations, of course, which give sample utterances, snippets of dialogue, test results, and linguistic observations. These help to build up a clinical character of the condition, and they provide input for formulating aphasia theories and therapies, but the goal of a comprehensive and precise description of a patient's linguistic strengths and weaknesses is still far from routine, and is usually missing from accounts of research investigations or of therapeutic practice.

Nevertheless, the demand for adequate descriptions continues. Some years ago, it was voiced primarily with reference to questions of diagnosis and assessment; more recently, with reference to procedures of treatment and rehabilitation; and more recently still, with reference to the problem of how to evaluate aphasia therapy. Indeed, these days the role of an initial linguistic description seems to take on the status of an axiom, in the accounts of many scholars. For example, in the introductory chapter of a recent volume on aphasia therapy (Code and Muller, 1983), the editors remark that 'a description of the patient's communicative abilities along linguistic parameters would appear to be essential before treatment can be planned', and in the concluding chapter to the same volume, Coltheart (1983) remarks that 'any study intending to obtain information about the efficacy of any form of treatment should begin with the assembling of a good description of the patient'. In another recent review, the author states: 'A detailed analysis of a patient's spontaneous speech is the first step in planning a treatment programme' (Ludlow, 1981). Such comments are widespread in the aphasia literature, making the almost complete absence of comprehensive descriptions all the more regrettable.

The need for detailed descriptions is not motivated solely by the demands of therapy, but also by the requirements of differential diagnosis. It is now something of a truism to point to the terminological uncertainty and the competing typologies that characterize the field of aphasiology. 'There is still no universally agreed definition of aphasia' complains Lesser (1978) on her opening page, and, after reviewing various syndromes, she concludes that 'it would be a mistake to give the impression that these syndromes are easily recognized in a clinical population'. Whurr (1982) begins similarly, with reference to typology: 'There is still no universally agreed classification. Terminological confusion exists, due, in part, to the multidisciplinary interest in the subject (clinical, physiological and behavioural), but also due to the diversity of philosophical and psychological theories on which much of the work has been based'. She concludes: 'In the absence of such descriptive statements, the traditional aphasiological foci of attention on matters of definition, diagnosis and classification seem positively misguided'. The role of accurate linguistic description of patient behaviour as a means of resolving these problems has long been appreciated: Jakobson, for instance, has argued the importance of the point for 30 years (*see*, for example, Jakobson, 1954). As recently as 1980, Jakobson still found it necessary to say: 'The further development of linguistic inquiry into aphasia demands a greater concentration on the description and classification of the purely verbal syndromes.' His own pioneering application of linguistic concepts to aphasia is rightly regarded as monumental, but his classifications remain extremely general, and have not, it seems, been followed by detailed subclassifications carried out at appropriate linguistic levels, or by applications relating his intentions to the specific demands of routine clinical practice.

The reasons for the lack of descriptive progress are not hard to find. The talk presupposes an adequate descriptive framework, and knowledge of how to use and apply it. In so far as linguistics is concerned with the provision of descriptive frameworks for language, it should be pointed out that reasonably comprehensive frameworks have only recently been devised, and there are still many gaps to be filled by pure research. Similarly, the training of those people most involved in the study of aphasia has until recently lacked components in which such descriptive frameworks are routinely taught and practised. It is only as recently as 1974, after all, that a course on linguistic theory and description became an obligatory feature of speech therapy training in Britain; and many training courses in other parts of the world still lack this feature. Even in centres where the frameworks are available, and where the willingness to learn and use them is present, there are problems — primarily that of finding time and opportunity to carry out the descriptions of patient behaviour required before systematic advances in diagnosis and treatment can be made (*see further* Crystal, 1982b). Consequently there is a marked lack of publicly accessible data, and no guarantee that the data that are available have used the same descriptive framework, enabling comparative statements to be made clearly and consistently.

The theoretical framework required to solve the descriptive problem has been appreciated for a long time — a model of language which recognizes and interrelates a set of linguistic *levels*, or dimensions of linguistic analysis capable of independent study. The importance of this model is once again summarized by Jakobson (1980):

> 'The question of levels is relevant indeed. Too often, attempts to treat the linguistic aspect of aphasia suffer from inadequate delimitation of the linguistic levels. One could even say that today the most important task in linguistics is to learn how to delimit the levels . . . But in all linguistic questions and especially in the case of aphasia, it is important to approach language, and its disruption in the framework of a given level, while remembering at the same time that . . . the totality and the interrelation between the different parts of the totality have to be taken into account.'

Reference to at least the main levels of linguistic inquiry is now commonplace in aphasia studies. It is conventional to recognize the levels of phonology, grammar and semantics (Lesser, 1978; Albert *et al.*, 1981; Whurr, 1982). But this recognition of the theoretical importance of the model has not been accompanied by a corresponding readiness to provide descriptions in terms of the model. The idea of levels has proved its worth by providing a framework in which clinical observations can be placed somewhat more neatly than previously, and it has acted as a reminder to clinicians of the potential complexity of language; but in fact hardly any publications illustrate its systematic, detailed descriptive use, and there is a real danger of misleading conclusions being drawn about aphasia, when the limitations of the model fail to be understood, and the notion of level comes to be applied in an oversimplified way.

Some cautionary remarks are in order before proceeding to a descriptive approach. In particular, it must not be forgotten that the concept of 'level' is a linguistic fiction, with both the number of levels and the nature of their boundaries being the outcome of specific linguistic theories. It is fashionable to search for neurological or psychological correlates of linguistic levels, but one does not need to commit oneself to a 'God's truth' view of these constructs in order to use them, and indeed there are interesting arguments against adopting such a view (*see further* Crystal, 1982a). The three-level approach, for example, is only one such possibility. There are two-level models (e.g. form v. meaning, structure v. use), four-level models (e.g. recognizing a separate level of phonetics alongside phonology, or morphology alongside syntax), five-level models (e.g. phonetics/phonology/morphology/syntax/semantics), etc. In some approaches, different kinds of levels are recognized, as in Halliday's notion of 'inter-levels' (of phonology and semantics) relating the primary levels of substance, form and context (Halliday, 1961). The linguistics literature has devoted much space to considering the question of how levels of analysis are motivated and applied, and it is generally recognized that levels ought not to be presented as if they had some kind of life of their own, but rather ought to be seen within a particular theoretical frame of reference. For instance, there is no single answer to the question: 'Is there a level of prosody?' Some approaches see prosody as a sub-level within phonology ('non-segmental' as opposed to 'segmental' phonology); some see it as separate from phonology (they would talk about a 'phonological and prosodic analysis', for example); others see it as best subsumed under the level of grammar; and there are other possible positions. To make a decision, one must first know something about the range of forms and functions that are designated by the term 'prosody' — the variations in pitch, loudness, speed and rhythm of speech — and reflect on the extent to which these variations operate in language as do the phonemes or distinctive features of phonology, or the syntactic rules of grammar. Only after one has made a judgement about their linguistic role and significance will one decide whether to 'promote' them to the status of a linguistic level, and give them some kind of autonomy in one's description (*see further* Crystal, 1969).

It must be remembered, too, that linguistics is concerned with the properties of language in general (not just English, or modern European languages), and that its models have to be tested against the variety of languages encountered in the world. It is not enough to devise a levels model that works quite well for English, and to assume its psycholinguistic or neurolinguistic reality, forgetting that the model may not work so well for structurally unrelated languages (whose speakers none the less have to be credited with isomorphic brains). Aphasia studies must also be generalizable in this way, and they usually are not. To take just one example, Lesser (1978) decides that in her book, 'as is more usual in aphasiology, the term *syntax* will be used to include morphology as well as sentence structure'. Now it is certainly possible to devise a theory in which a level of morphology has no separate representation (generative grammar, for instance), and such a theory does not do too much harm to the facts of English, where inflectional endings are few, but it is most unlikely that such a theory would do justice to aphasic behaviour in, say, Turkish or Japanese (which are agglutinating languages, with complex word-structure), or Arabic or Greek (which are languages with a complex inflectional system). In such cases, the morphological component of the description would be so important that it would have to be recognized in one's general approach as a major level, and not be swallowed up as a junior aspect of the syntax. Similar issues arise in relation to any of the other linguistic levels.

A further cautionary observation relates to the notion of 'autonomy' of levels, referred to above. As Jakobson and many other theoreticians have emphasized: 'The various levels of language are autonomous. [But] Autonomy doesn't mean isolationism; all levels are interrelated' (Jakobson, 1980). Indeed, the convenience of a framework in which one is permitted to study a single aspect of linguistic form or function to the exclusion of others must not be allowed to obscure the artefactual nature of this manoeuvre, nor to minimize the importance of expounding the nature of the relationships which obtain between levels, and which define the language system as a whole. Points of contact between levels are frequently noticed in clinical investigation, e.g., the functional load of the phoneme /s/ at the grammatical level (where it realizes plurality, possession, 3rd person present, etc.), or the use of rising intonation as an alternative to syntactic forms of question, or the way in which lexical problems interfere with the construction of sentences (as in so-called 'word-finding' difficulties). What has to be appreciated is that these are not isolated topics: in principle, *all* descriptive statements made at a given level must be related to the corresponding statements made at other levels, the interactions noted, and some kind of integrated account arrived at. One should never take language apart without the intention of putting it back together again (*see further* Crystal, 1987).

The Importance of Transcription

An integrated description in terms of levels is an important goal of aphasia studies, but it cannot even begin to be achieved without a firm transcriptional foundation — and this is usually lacking. Whenever one obtains a sample of language from a patient (spontaneous speech, test results, reading aloud, or whatever), the first step should be to transcribe it; and the whole of one's analytic edifice depends on the accuracy of the transcription. If a transcription is unclear, partial or inconsistent, it becomes impossible to verify the analyst's descriptive claims. A good transcription, in essence, is an account of the sample which makes it unnecessary to refer back to the tape from which it derived. It 'replaces' the tape, in the sense that any analyst trained in the conventions of the transcription can read it and 'hear' what was said as clearly as if he were listening to the tape itself. Few transcriptions ever reach this degree of autonomy, but all should strive to attain a reasonable level of accuracy and consistency. Unfortunately, transcriptions of aphasic speech are rarely complete and usually ambiguous.

The kind of transcription generally encountered in published work on aphasia can be illustrated by the following (taken from Goodglass, 1968):

> Yes . . . . ah . . . . Monday . . . ah . . . Dad and Peter Hogan, and Dad . . . ah . . . . Hospital . . . and ah . . . Wednesday . . . Wednesday, nine o'clock and ah Thursday . . . ten o'clock ah doctors . . . two . . . two . . . an doctors and . . . ah . . . teeth . . . yah. And a doctor . . . an girl . . . and gums, and I.

It is impossible to derive from such a transcription a clear auditory impression of how the patient must have spoken this utterance. The punctuation is partly conventional (periods and commas), partly unconventional (the use of triple dots, but in two cases the use of quadruple dots). Are the dots intended to represent a *system* of pauses, in the sense that all triple dots are the same length? What exact value has the comma in relation to the other punctuation? What was it in the data that led the analyst to use a period after *yah* and not a comma or a triple dot? Or (to move to lexico-grammatical issues), what is the evidence to support the transcription of *an* in two places, instead of *and*? Does the fact that *Hospital* is written with a capital letter mean that the analyst is seeing this word as a proper noun, or as the beginning of a new sentence, or both? A transcription of this kind raises many such questions; none are trivial, for analytic decisions will later be made to depend on them. If one wishes to measure the length of this patient's sentences, for example, the decisions that led the transcriber to assign periods will be crucial.

There seems to have been no change in this kind of loose transcriptional practice since the 1960s. Ludlow (1981), for example, illustrates the following Broca's utterance:

> Me . . . my wife . . . went . . . school, no, speech, speech, speech therapy. Oh, I don't know, I went . . . and work, work.

The same problems recur. Why is there a comma after school, and not a period? What motivated the period after *therapy*? Why no period after *know*?

The use of punctuation supplemented by an arbitrary and idiosyncratic list of graphic devices seems to be standard practice in aphasia studies still, and it will not do. Such an approach leaves out far too much relevant information — information that is prerequisite for anyone wishing to sharpen their instruments for diagnosis and assessment, or to improve their techniques of therapy. Most obviously, these transcriptions omit to tell us anything about the intonation, stress, rhythm and other prosodic and paralinguistic features of spoken language — features that are central to our understanding of the organization and progress of aphasic speech. Indeed, it is the particular combination of one of these features (stress) with certain word clusters which, in the view of Goodglass (1968), 'forms the essential feature of the agrammatism of Broca's aphasia' (see also the balanced comments in Lesser, 1978). If this is the case, one would at least expect aphasic transcriptions to contain stress marks to enable researchers to check the hypothesis — and this is not routinely done.

It is not simply a matter of stress. The multiple functions of intonation in the organization and processing of speech are also strongly implicated in the search for an explanation of aphasic disturbance. Is each word in a given sequence spoken with a separate intonation unit (a 'word-at-a-time' intonation) or do the words group themselves intonationally (and rhythmically) in certain ways? If the latter, the particular groupings can tell us a great deal about the way the patient is processing language, and where his difficulties lie. An example is the abnormal chunking introduced by prosody into one of Mr J's sentences (Crystal *et al.*, 1976). Mr J would say, at a certain stage in his treatment.

the bòy is/ . èating a/ . àpple/

Later, he was able to say:

the bòy/ is . èating/ a . àpple/

still somewhat hesitant, but at least now the main prosodic units correspond to the main grammatical elements of the sentence. To show this improvement, one requires a transcription in which at least tone unit boundaries, tonicity, and nuclear tone type are marked, along with stress and pause conventions, where needed.

The kind of transcription illustrated here is of course still only a crude level of phonological representation. A much more detailed level of transcription is required to capture the whole range of non-segmental phonological features available in a language, in which such variables as increases and decreases of tempo and loudness, alterations in the pitch range of stretches of utterance, rhythmical variations, and the many kinds of vocal paralinguistic effect (e.g. breathy, creaky, nasal, tense tones of voice) are taken into account. The level of detail of such a transcription has been illustrated elsewhere, for normal varieties of English, where it is possible to identify the salient phonological characteristics of, say, a sermon, or a sports commentary, or

1. / marks tone-unit boundaries; ò represents a falling tone; . represents a brief pause; all other syllables are unstressed. These conventions are taken from the transcriptional system presented in Crystal (1969), used in full in Crystal and Davy (1969), and in simplified form in Crystal, Fletcher and Garman (1976) and elsewhere.

everyday conversation, using such a combination of variables. It is my view that the nonsegmental variability of aphasic language is no less complex than that encountered in other varieties of English, and deserves a comparably serious treatment. This is most obviously the case for the more 'fluent' forms of aphasia, where variations in pitch range, loudness and speed are often important cues to our awareness of the patients' comprehension and control of what they say. Thus one patient (Mrs W) used to produce fairly well-formed sentences, consisting of main clause and subordinate clause as follows:

well I used to go down there whenever I could you see

which, lacking any prosodic transcription, tells us nothing about her problems of expression, and her listener's problems of comprehension. In fact, what Mrs W said was:

'well I/'used to/'go down thére/' 'when/ever I còuld you sée/'
'low, piano, allegro' *'ascending, crescendo, lento'*

where the inverted commas indicate that the first, main clause was spoken in a low-pitched, quiet and rapid tone of voice, and the second, subordinate clause was spoken with the voice level increasing and slowing. In short, the overall auditory effect was something like:

.... whenever I could you see.

This consistent obscuring of the main clauses in Mrs W's speech was an important feature of her assessment, and an early target for treatment. Similar forms of prosodic complexity can be demonstrated for other tyes of aphasia, e.g. the variations in the tempo of utterance of syllables and segments in 'non-fluent' speech.

It should be noted, at this point, that my requirement of a reasonably full prosodic and paralinguistic transcription of aphasic speech is not an abnormally strong one. It is no more than I would expect as a foundation for the description of any sample of spoken language, but in the case of aphasia the requirement has an added significance in that it is a prerequisite for an adequate symptomatology. I take it as axiomatic that an aim of aphasiology is a comprehensive statement of clinical symptoms. It is often said, impressionistically, that aphasic prosody is disturbed. But little effort has been made to build an appropriate bridge between these last two sentences. Thus, for example, in a recent synthesis representing the influential Boston approach, we have an account of Melodic Intonation Therapy (MIT), and an interesting case report, on the one hand (Albert *et al.* 1981); but on the other hand, the authors do not give any intonational transcription of their patient's speech, and in their introduction the section on 'linguistic aspects of dysphasia testing' makes no mention of intonation or prosody at all. There are several valuable hypotheses about prosody in aphasia, and several experimental studies (cf. Lesser, 1978), but there is a remarkable lack of naturalistic empirical data on the point. We urgently need descriptions of patients' prosodic and paralinguistic features, both in a range of linguistic settings, and longitudinally; equally, we need similar transcriptions of the prosody and paralanguage of the patients' interlocutors, the prosodic character of whose stimuli exercises so much influence on the patients' response. Until a level of prosodic transcription becomes routine, the claims made about other levels of the patients' linguistic organization are inevitably to some extent arbitrary and uncertain.

Segmental phonological transcriptions of spontaneous or elicited speech samples (that is, of the vowel/consonant sequences that constitute the 'verbal' aspect of utterance), although somewhat more familiar than prosodic ones, are not made routinely. Here, too, we need an objective transcription, not simply to describe the patient's articulation problems (if any), but also to provide a data-base to verify grammatical and semantic hypotheses. Even the most experienced analysts have to be on their guard against reading grammatical or semantic information into what they hear on a tape. A phonetic sequence such as [an] could be a realization of *and, an, in, on*, or other words; and if contextual clues are ambiguous or absent, as is often the case in patients' conversations about themselves or their backgrounds, what justification has the analyst for assigning one rather than another of these interpretations to the sounds in question? In the transcript illustrated on page 28, for example, what grounds were there for a transcription of *an doctors* and *an girl*, as opposed to, say, *and doctors . . . and girl*? Was there something in the phonetics which motivated Goodglass' decision? If the phonetic evidence was [an], it would have been better to transcribe it thus, to enable other analysts to judge the matter for themselves, and perhaps argue for alternative grammatico-lexical interpretations. One of my own commonest problems, in this respect, is what to do with a final [s] following a noun, in non-fluent speech. A patient talks about a car and then says *brother*[*s*]: does he mean *brothers* (plural), *brother's* (possessive), *brothers'*, *brother's* (i.e. 'brother is' or 'brother has'), and so on? It is easy to underestimate the amount of analytical indeterminacy in the description of disordered speech. Indeed, it is only in recent years that the concept of phonetic indeterminacy has received investigation at all, in the attempts by various groups to set up new conventions for phonetic transcription, in which uncertainty is formally recognized (*see* Grunwell *et al.*, 1980).

The Primary Levels

On the basis of an adequate transcription, and bearing in mind the

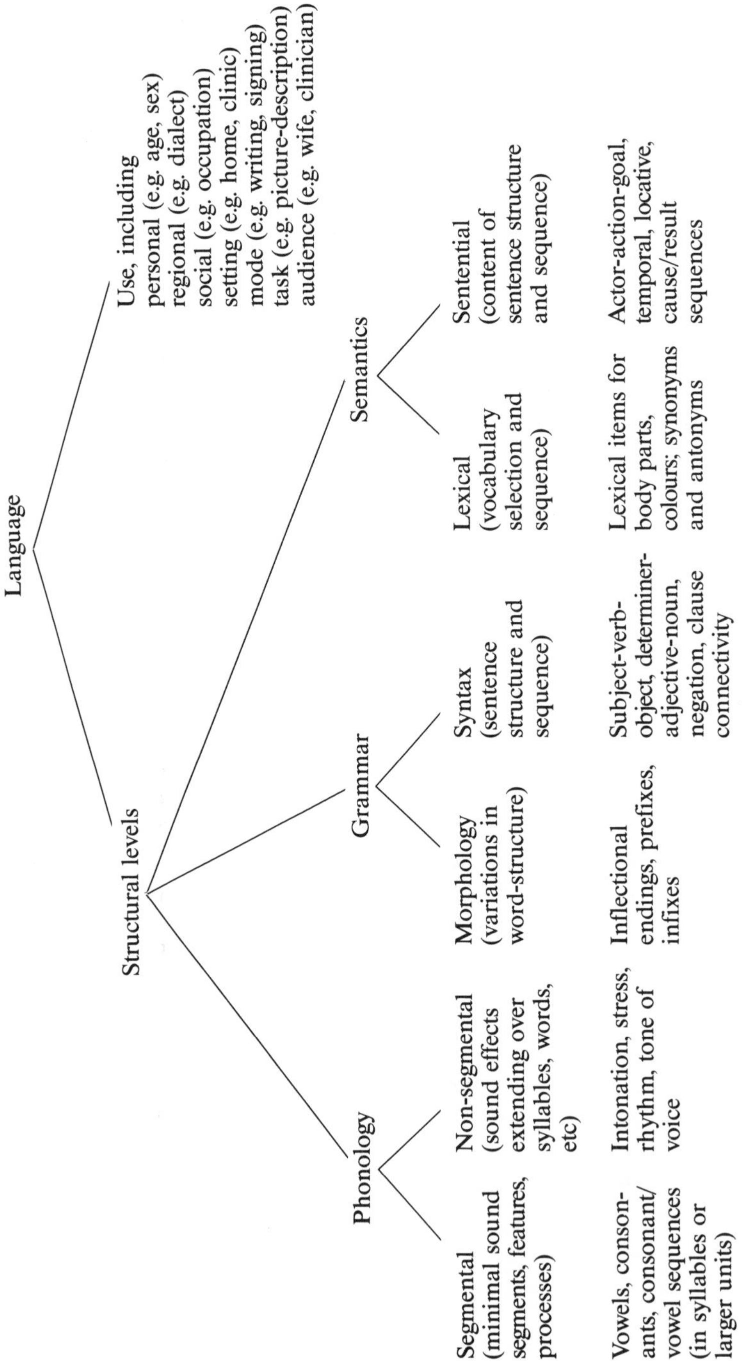

Figure 1. Levels of Language Analysis, with examples of each category

artefactual nature of the exercise, it is usual to approach the description of aphasic disturbance using the three primary levels of *phonology*, *grammar* and *semantics*. These are three dimensions of the structural analysis of language — the 'structure' of language here being contrasted with the 'use' of language in social situations (which is sometimes loosely referred to as a *pragmatic* 'level'). These levels, with their main subdivisions (as most widely recognized) and some examples of the data which would be subsumed under each heading, are illustrated in *Figure 1*. A detailed discussion and clinical application of the theoretical issues relating to each level is presented in Crystal (1981). A complementary set of profiling procedures is given in Crystal (1982c). For present purposes, it will perhaps be most useful to focus on those issues that would seem to have particular relevance for aphasia studies, especially in so far as they relate to concepts that have been inadequately investigated.

The central question is to determine the depth of detail at which useful descriptive statements should be made. At one extreme, there are the maximally general characterizations of the disorder which ignore levels altogether (such as 'fluent' v. 'non-fluent'). At the other extreme, there are the maximally detailed specifications of all the linguistic variables encountered in a sample, as presented in a set of profiles (*see* Crystal 1982c). Between these two extremes, there are innumerable possibilities. Some scholars are satisfied with a classification of aphasic errors which recognizes only the three primary levels, with little or no further subclassification: 'phonological' or 'phonemic' errors are seen alongside 'grammatical' or 'syntactic' errors, and 'semantic' or 'lexical' errors. One often has to 'see through' traditional clinical terminology to establish that a levels approach is in use — for example, the notion of *paraphasia* at first glance seems to be defined in a way that cuts across the various levels e.g. 'the production of unintended syllables, words or phrases during the effort to speak' (Goodglass and Kaplan, 1972), but the real use of this notion recognizes them through its classification of *phonemic paraphasia* (phonological level), *verbal* and *neologistic paraphasias* (semantic level).

Some classifications collapse into a single category notions that belong to different levels; for example, Ludlow (1981, *Table 1*) has as two of his categories 'impaired articulation and melody' (which seems to bring together an aspect of phonetics and one of phonology) and 'impaired fluency and syntax' (an aspect of grammar plus an aspect of phonetics/phonology). Others operate neatly with binary classifications within levels, probably the most well-known one being the distinction between *agrammatic* and *paragrammatic* speech within the level of grammar (though the involvement of semantic factors in this distinction must not be ignored). A classification in terms of levels of use is routinely made in aphasia tests, recognizing such distinctions as mode of communication (speaking, listening comprehension, reading, writing) and task (repetition, confrontation naming). Coltheart (1983), addressing the question of what counts as a useful descriptive level at which to work, considered the following specifications (among others) to be helpful; 'using function words in spontaneous speech', 'non-verbal behaviour assisting conversational speech', 'speech comprehension at the single-sentence level' and 'reading comprehension at the paragraph level'.

However, when one considers the properties of an 'ideal' aphasia theory, it is plain that the depth of descriptive detail presented by these approaches is still a long way from what is required. A theory of aphasia ought to be predictive, in the sense that from a precise specification of neurological damage it should be possible to derive predictions concerning the patient's linguistic behaviour at any point in time during the recovery process. Such a theory would also have to take into account the facilitating or hindering effects of formal interventions, in the course of therapy or rehabilitation. Now, despite the limited progress that has been made in this direction, everyday clinical work has no alternative but to proceed as if the theory existed. Clinicians will make assumptions to guide their therapy, on the basis of the medical case history and accompanying general observation, and their intention will be to change the patient's behaviour in a controlled manner, through the use of treatment hypotheses deriving from an ongoing analysis of their own stimuli and their patient's response. I see no point in an aphasia theory that is unable to make predictions about therapy, and it is in relation to therapy that the descriptive detail of the classification referred to above proves to be inadequate.

For, how would a clinician be able to interpret such notions as 'paraphasia' or 'word-finding problem' in order to carry out treatment? Even the more detailed specifications suggested by Coltheart are too general in this respect: a much more precise statement about such notions as 'function words', 'non-verbal behaviour' or 'single sentence' is required before a clinician could devise a treatment programme based on this rationale. Which function words are strong, which weak, and in which contexts? Which features of non-verbal behaviour are strong, which weak, and related to which aspects of conversation? Which kinds of single sentence? Which kinds of paragraph? Clinicians have to begin a session of treatment with a specific interaction, using specific sentences of a particular type, and they must monitor the patient's response, which also uses specific sentences (whether normal or abnormal) of a particular type. The treatment session does not deal with 'function words'. It deals with a particular function word, or set of words, in conditions that ought to be carefully specified. The goal is to establish the use of one or other of these words in the patient's behaviour, and it is by no means uncommon for whole sections of a session to be devoted to the eliciting and training of a single item. An assessment made at the beginning and end of such a training period has therefore to be sufficiently detailed to capture the progress that may have been made, and to guide decisions as to how the next stage in therapy might proceed. At this level of concern, the task of description is inevitably an extremely detailed one, and the gap between it and the level of generality illustrated above is enormous.

It is not solely aphasia therapy that is undermined by the lack of appropriately detailed descriptions. Theoretical research into aphasia is being hindered by a reluctance to look beneath the general labels and to provide a more precise specification of the disorder. The point can be illustrated from one of the most frequently cited diagnostic criteria — *agrammatism* — which is often used as if it were a well-defined notion, but which is not the case. The imprecision hinges on the 'amount' of grammar that can be subsumed under the term. At one extreme, the term seems to refer to the whole of the grammatical level, as in the definition of Critchley (1970): 'An aphasic disorder which impairs syntax rather than vocabulary'. Most of grammar is implicated in Jakobson's account of agrammatism as a contiguity disorder: 'The syntactical rules organizing words into higher units are lost', and this 'causes the degeneration of the sentence into a mere "words heap"' ... 'Word order becomes chaotic; the ties of grammatical co-ordination and subordination ... are dissolved', 'words endowed with purely grammatical functions, like conjunctions, prepositions, pronouns, and articles, disappear first ...' and a 'typical feature ... is the abolition of inflection' (Jakobson, 1954).

At the other extreme, agrammatism is used to refer to just one aspect of grammatical analysis, the factor of so-called 'grammatical' or 'function' words (another example of the bias introduced by the English language, incidentally, for there are many languages to which this concept does not readily apply). For example, Eisenson (1973) says: 'Typically, agrammatism is characterized by the patient's errors or omissions in the use of functional words ... which serve to establish contextual relationships (grammatical context) of spoken and written content'. Albert *et al.* (1981) describe it as 'a near total absence of the "small grammatical words" of the language'. Some definitions stress the morphological aspect of the problem, by drawing attention to the loss of inflections (e.g. Albert *et al.* (1981)), others ignore morphology and give a definition solely in terms of syntax (e.g. Nicolosi, Harryman and Kreshek's 1978 definition as 'impairment of the ability to produce words in their correct sequence' — a definition they have based on Wood (1957)). Albert *et al.* (1981), begin with morphology, but end up with an account that implicates the whole of the system of grammatical relationships: 'Closer inspection of agrammatic speech suggests that this style has a more complex explanation than a mere dropping out of grammatical elements. In fact there appears to be a basic loss of the concept of words as having a functional role in a sentence. The severe agrammatic uses words as disconnected, nominalized ideas, which can be placed contiguously without any expressed grammatical connection between them'.

Several problems present themselves, as one tries to make sense of such a range of definitions. To take the statement of Albert *et al.* — to what extent is this last characterization a matter of 'agrammatic speech' in general, or, as they say, 'severe' agrammatic speech in particular? And would they wish to maintain that, from the observation that there is no 'expressed' grammatical connection, there is no underlying grammatical connection made at all? Or, to take Eisenson's (1973) statement: 'In severe form, agrammatism may be expressed as *telegrammatism*. All functional words and grammatical markers may be omitted'. The *all* seems to be the point at issue, for he gives as a 'more typical' example of agrammatic production the sentence *I eggs and eat and drink coffee*. If this is typical, how does it square with the various accounts that mention the omission of pronouns and conjunctions in agrammatism? In fact, there is considerable uncertainty about the function words which are omitted in agrammatic speech. Albert *et al.* (1981) list them as 'the customary articles, pronouns, noun and verb inflections [sic], auxiliaries'; Goodglass (1976) says 'articles, connective words, auxiliaries, and inflections'; Eisenson (1973) says 'articles, prepositions and conjunctions'; Robbins (1951) says 'auxiliaries and relational words' in one definition, 'conjunctions and other subordinate [sic] words' in another, and adds that 'words are uttered in incorrect sequence, infinitives are misused'.

Rough characterizations of this kind may be generally satisfactory for impressionistic clinical purposes, but as soon as a more rigorous approach is required, a clearer and more comprehensive description becomes essential. Research studies in neurolinguistics and neuropsychology, for example, cannot afford to be loose in their handling of the notion of agrammatism, especially when statistical studies are involved, or in case studies where the meticulous analysis of lists of examples and counter-examples is routine. Yet, the looseness is universal. In a valuable review of deep dyslexia, for example, Coltheart (1980) asks whether such patients are agrammatic; points out that several of those studied in his paper were not; and concludes that 'agrammatism of speech is *not* one of the symptoms of deep dyslexia'. A little later in the same volume Morton begins his paper with the words, 'In spite of their trouble with reading, their agrammatism and non-fluency . . .', referring to his group of patients (1980), and Saffran *et al.* (1980) state that 'almost all of the patients would be classified as agrammatic'. What are the descriptive criteria used in this debate? Coltheart (1980) defines agrammatism as 'function words and inflections . . . selectively absent from speech which is still relatively meaningful and communicative'; Saffran *et al.* (1980) say that it 'consists mostly of concrete nouns . . . contains relatively few verb forms . . . and is notably lacking in functors'. Whatever the reality of the situation, it is plain that with overlapping definitions of this kind, points of similarity and difference may be obscured. Unless everyone uses precisely the same set of descriptive criteria, comparisons can be weakened to the point of vacuity.

What must be appreciated is that there is no 'correct' definition of a notion such as 'function word', and it is certainly not possible to take it as self-evident. The distinction between 'content words' and 'function words' (or whatever terminology is used) is not clear-cut, as has long been recognized in the linguistics literature (*see*, for example, the special volume of *Lingua* (1966) devoted to the topic of word-classes). Function words are said to be empty of meaning, to have solely grammatical function. In fact, hardly any of the words considered functional have no referential meaning (the clearest cases are the infinitive particle *to*, and the 'empty' uses of *there* and *it* in *there's a horse in the street* and *it was yesterday I saw him* respectively). Most function words have some kind of referential meaning (consider all the prepositional or pronominal items, for example), and some lists of such words contain many items whose supposed grammatical status is open to question. In *Deep Dyslexia* (Coltheart, Patterson and Marshall, 1980), referred to above, there is an Appendix listing function word paralexias used by certain patients. They include items such as *had, was, to, the, not, or, am, are*; but they also include *on, down, most, while, where, just, neither, both, almost*, which seem to be semantically at a remove from the first set; And also *perhaps, sometimes, something, ever, generally, instead, never, seldom, therefore, usually* and *several*, which are really somewhat unexpected. After all, if such are included, where does one draw the line between function and content word? If *sometimes* and *seldom* are included, why not *often, frequently, regularly*, and thousands more of the adverbials available in English (*see* Quirk *et al.*, 1985)? A line may have to be drawn to enable research to proceed, but in our present state of knowledge of the areas of grammar involved it is going to be an arbitrary one. It certainly cannot be left to take care of itself.

Agrammatism is not an isolated example. A concept such as 'word-finding' is likewise implicated, in view of how this notion may be made to depend on a word classification principle similar to the above. Albert *et al.* (1981), for example, see word-finding as 'an estimate of the balance between contentive words and grammatical filler words', contentive words being 'nouns, principal verbs, adjectives and adverbs'. They would presumably class *sometimes, usually*, etc. as content words, compared with the approach cited in the previous paragraph. Most discussions of word-finding problems are not even so specific, most authors apparently seeing the concept of 'word-finding' as so self-evident that it does not require definition. Yet one has only to ask 'What is it that is to be found?' to see that the term hides a nest of methodological and theoretical problems. At one extreme, *all* the words in a language can be said to present difficulties of retrieval, including all classes of 'content' words and all the 'grammatical' words containing some degree of specifiable meaning. At the other extreme, only one subclass of 'content' words is considered relevant, as when word-finding difficulties are cited only as part of the discussion of anomia (as in the Index to Eisenson (1973), for example). In some contexts, it would seem to be the word in a specific grammatical and phonological form which has to be found (*take, takes, took, taken, taking*). In other contexts, a more abstract sense of 'word' is clearly intended — the 'underlying form' of the various grammatical and phonological possibilities (the *lexical item*, or *lexeme* TAKE). A lexeme is the minimal unit of meaning in the semantic system of a language (*see* Lyons, 1977), and the notion has proved valuable in enabling the semantic analysis of vocabulary to proceed independently of the complications introduced by the constraints of grammatical form, although its potential as a means of refining and making precise the concept of 'word-finding problem' has yet to be appreciated.

We can see this if we look at just some of the possibilities that the notion of 'word-finding' can subsume. A particular form of lexeme may be 'lost', such as the noun *switch* as opposed to the verb *switch*, or the 3rd person form of the verb (*switches*), or the first part of a (multi-word) lexeme (saying *on* for *switch on*, for instance); or the whole of a lexeme may be 'lost', as when all forms of the lexeme, regardless of context, are unusable (*switch, switches, switching, switch on*, etc.); or again, a particular use of a lexeme may be lost (*switch* in the sense of 'electric switch', but not in the sense of 'change direction'), or a particular relationship between one lexeme and another (oppositeness, for example, *switch on* v. *switch off, big* v. *small*). The study of the way in which the lexemes of a language are organized into *semantic fields*, and are linked by specific *semantic* (or *sense*) *relations*, such as synonymy, oppositeness and hyponymy (the relationship of inclusion), constitutes one of the major themes of contemporary semantics, but it is an approach which has not been systematically applied to the analysis of aphasia. Aphasia tests often inquire after particular synonyms or antonyms, of course, but the tasks are always somewhat artificial, and do not take account of the range of contextual factors which constitute the real difficulty in handling a language's vocabulary. As an example of the 'decontextualized' approach, one might consider the kind of question put to patients in which they are asked (in so many words) for the opposite of, say, *run*. An inadequate response may well be due to the fact that there is no single 'correct' opposite for this lexeme: *run* has several opposites, depending on the context in which it is used, as the following examples illustrate:

> It's not enough to run round the track; you have to *jump* the hurdles as well.
>
> I *walked* towards the bus-stop; but when I saw the bus coming I started to run.

The engine was running nicely, but then there was a sharp noise and it *stopped*.
My horse isn't running; it's been *scratched*.
The buses aren't running; they're *on strike*.
The play's not running any more; it's been *taken off*.

Most lexemes in the language have many such 'opposites', and the commonest words have most of all. Without adequate contextual awareness, then, it is not possible to make sense of a patient's responses. Therapists may present a task in which they assume that the opposite of *run* is *walk*; the patient however may respond by saying *scratch*, which might easily be interpreted either as a comprehension difficulty with *run*, or a word-finding problem with *walk*, or both, unless one thought to check the horse-racing context. Similar problems arise when one considers the way in which patients might be using synonyms, or any other sense relation. The only solution, of course, is to ensure that the clinicians' approach to lexical assessment and remediation is given an adequate descriptive foundation: they must be aware, in principle, of the range and complexity of the semantic factors involved, and have available, as a matter of routine, a systematic description of the lexical possibilities being drawn upon by the patient. Primitive lexical descriptions, more than adequate for basic clinical needs, already exist: they are called dictionaries and thesauri, but are such books ever seen as being essential pieces of clinic equipment? Are they ever routinely consulted as a preliminary to condemning a patient's lexical response as 'random', or to constructing a lexical teaching programme?

The Tip of the Iceberg

The cases of agrammatism and word-finding are only two of the notions which have received inadequate description in terms of the main linguistic levels and their subdivisions. Agrammatism is primarily a grammatical notion, but it has been only partially explicated in its reliance on function words and morphological structure. It now needs to be investigated using a more abstract set of syntactic relations within the frame of reference of a reasonably comprehensive descriptive model, e.g. such relations as subject, object, complement, verb, used in association with the clause, phrase, and other aspects of grammatical hierarchy (*see further* Crystal, 1981). Word-finding is primarily a semantic notion, but it too has been only partially explicated, in terms of simple quantitative notions such as word frequency, word length, and word association forms (Lesser, 1978); it now needs to be investigated using a set of qualitative semantic relations, both syntagmatic and paradigmatic, so that lexical assessment and treatment can be seen within the frame of reference of an emerging system of structured semantic fields (*see further* Crystal, 1981). The descriptive refinement of already available aphasiological notions is only the tip of the iceberg of linguistic enquiry into the disorder, using the model of levels. There remain wholly uncharted areas of aphasic linguistic behaviour —areas that are undoubtedly central to our understanding and treatment of the condition, but which have received little or no study because of the limited account that has been taken of theoretical linguistic insights in clinical training and practice. The point can be briefly illustrated from each of the main linguistic levels.

Within phonology, the neglect of non-segmental characteristics of language, especially of intonation, has already been pointed out in relation to the need for transcriptional accuracy. In the absence of non-segmental transcriptions, there will obviously be little precise study of the way in which patients control the forms and functions of intonation, stress, rhythm, pause, etc. in relation to the rest of their language, and to the kinds of task they are called upon to perform. Equally, the way in which clinicians make use of non-segmental variation in order to organize their stimuli, or to highlight a particular feature of language, has received little description. Recommendations about interaction remain controversial (e.g. whether one should increase or decrease the tempo of speech stimuli to facilitate the patient's response), and diagnostic characterizations remain vague (e.g. using general impressions about 'melody' or 'colour' of speech, and relying on a notion of 'dysprosody' whose phonetic or phonological status it is never possible to determine (*see* Crystal, 1981)).

The segmental (vowel, consonant, syllable) aspect of phonology is a more familiar area, but even here there are glaring gaps. To begin with, there is a marked bias towards the study of consonant errors, often to the exclusion of vowels. This is presumably a consequence of the tradition in articulation testing, where only consonants are investigated; but it cannot be justified in relation to aphasia, where errors of vowel length and quality are common. While consonant errors are of course the majority, it must not be forgotten that vowel values can play an essential part in the distinguishing of pairs of consonants — final [p] and [b], for instance, are primarily distinguished in terms of the length of the preceding vowel, as in *cap/cab*, etc. Secondly, there has been little sign of the importance of taking into account a sound's *distribution* in relation to larger linguistic units, such as syllable, word, tone unit, phrase. There is still a marked tendency to talk about sounds globally — a patient's 'difficulty with [l]', for example, instead of a 'difficulty with [l] in word-initial position'. Indeed, despite all the use made of the term *phoneme*, there is still a predominance in the aphasia literature to think of phonemes as sounds, as physical entities, instead of what they are — abstract classes of sounds, contrasting units within a sound system.

The almost universal focus on the phoneme as the key to the understanding of aphasic phonology is clear from a review such as that of

Lesser (1978), but this is by no means a satisfactory state of affairs. There are many other ways of studying phonological systems, and while some attention has been paid to the use of one of these (the distinctive feature frame of reference used in generative phonology), there are further approaches of considerable relevance to the analysis of aphasic errors, whose application has hardly begun. For example, one might examine those phonological processes that extend beyond the individual phoneme, and which apply to whole syllables, words or larger units — what have been variously referred to as 'prosodies' (Firth, 1948), or 'phonological processes' (Ingram, 1976). The idea that a single process can explain the selection of certain sounds made by a speaker at different points in an utterance has proved to be helpful in studies of normal language acquisition and of child language disability (Grunwell, 1981), and it seems likely that it would also be illuminating in the study of adult disorders. Several aphasiological notions seem tailor-made for analysis in terms of processes (e.g. 'perseveration'), and the approach might help to resolve some of the puzzles left by previous characterizations of disorders. Conventional accounts of apraxia, for example, refer to inconsistency of phonological errors (*see* Lesser, 1978). Yet is there really inconsistency, or is this the result of using only a phonemic model to investigate the disorder? Faced with a set of data where an item such as *pig* is recorded as [pig], [kig] and [sig], there seems to be inconsistency; but widening the scope of the enquiry may lead to explanations for the alternative forms. The /p/ may be realized as [k] under the influence of a following /k/, for example, as in *the pig is coming* (what is often referred to as an instance of 'consonant harmony'); the [s] may be the consequence of a preceding phoneme, as in *I see a pig*. We are not at the stage when it is possible to predict classes of error, or define the constraints on such processes as harmony; but there is a great deal to be gained by making use of the notion of process in analysing aphasic speech samples.

From the point of view of grammar and semantics, apart from the issues already noted, there is a considerable neglect of the hierarchical properties of sentence construction, especially the relationships between sentence and clause, and between clause and phrase (phrase and word, and word and morpheme, as we have seen, are routinely investigated). To illustrate the problem, first at the grammatical level, we may take the following sentence sequence:

You.
You asked.
You asked John.
You asked my brother.

Each sentence increases by one word, but there is a qualitatively different jump between the third and the fourth sentence. The fourth sentence is not simply a linear string of four separate words: the relationship between *my* and *brother* is closer than that between *my* and *asked*, or *my* and *you*. This is conventionally illustrated in the form of a constituency diagram, such as:

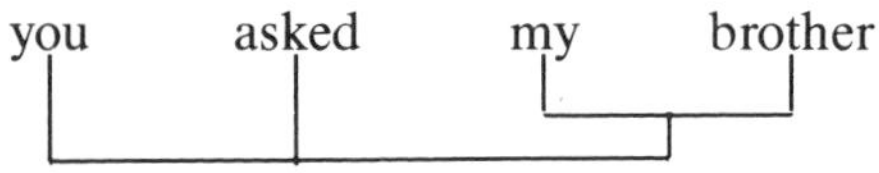

(though this is only one way of representing the structural relationships involved). However we calculate the 'processing load' involved in these sentences, it should be evident that the jump from the third to the fourth sentence involves two extra factors — the extra word, and the extra level of sentence structure. It would not therefore follow that, because patients could handle some four-word sentences (such as *I saw John today*, where there is no hierarchical structure), they would be able to handle this one. They may be able to say (or comprehend) *you asked John* and *my brother* as separate utterances, but the conflating of the two might be beyond them. Moreover, it does not follow that because patients can handle hierarchy after the verb (as in *you asked my brother*), they can handle it before the verb (as in *my brother asked me*); indeed, differential ability in this respect is the norm for both adults and children (cf. Quirk *et. al.*, 1985). Also, the possibility of interference from other grammatical and semantic factors must be considered (in statement v. question, positive v. negative construction, using animate v. inanimate nouns, following static v. dynamic verbs (e.g. *see* v. *hit*), etc., as well as phonological factors, such as placement of nuclear tone). Whether one is studying comprehension or production, the relationship between clause and phrase elements always needs to be systematically taken into account. A similar set of factors needs to be borne in mind when one looks at more complex clauses, and the sequencing of clauses within sentences (*see* Crystal, 1981).

In recent years, some progress has been made in the analysis of aphasic speech using the concept of grammatical hierarchy, but the potentially more fruitful corresponding analysis in semantic terms has not been much invoked. The distinction between grammar and semantics here is best illustrated with a sentence, analysed from both points of view:

	John	kicked	the ball.
Grammar	Subject	Verb	Object
Semantics	Actor	Action	Goal

That the two levels are not the same notions masquerading under different labels can be shown by using other sentences:

	The ball	was kicked	by John.
Grammar	Subject	Verb	Adverbial
Semantics	Goal	Action	Actor

In the first sentence, the Subject is the semantic Actor; in the second, it is the semantic Goal of the Action. The clauses and clause elements of grammar play a number of semantic 'roles', which have been variously labelled by different scholars, and this constitutes an illuminating avenue of enquiry into the nature of aphasic disability. This is especially the case in relation to the more 'fluent' speech characteristic of Wernicke's aphasia, where a grammatical analysis is often unilluminating, as a wide range of sentence patterns is in use. Such speech is often said to be semantically 'empty', 'low in information', containing 'unnecessary words', 'circumlocutions' and various kinds of 'jargon'. On the other hand, there seems to have been little attempt to provide a qualitative analysis of these notions — to describe the kinds of circumlocution, to see whether certain semantic elements are more prone to circumlocution, and so on. Nor does anyone seem to have investigated these issues in relation to the semantic load carried by the therapists' verbal stimulus to the patient (though, for some programmatic suggestions, *see* Crystal, 1981). Yet this kind of information is surely central to any real understanding of the condition. Faced with a question such as *What is a key?*, patients may respond by keeping their meaning mainly constant, and varying their grammar (*A key opens a door, A door is opened by a key, It's a key to open a door*, etc.); or by keeping the grammar mainly constant, and varying the semantic content (*I open a door, You open cupboards, You lock a door*, etc.); or of course by some combination. Similarly, clinicians may vary the grammatical ways in which they ask the same question (*What can you do with a key?, What's a key for?*, etc.); or vary the meaning while maintaining the same grammatical form (*Do you eat things with it? Do you open things with it?*, etc.); or of course vary both factors at once.

Patients may be unable to process certain semantic elements, and have a facility in coping with others, e.g. they might be unable to handle lexemes when they have an Actor role to play in a sentence, but able to handle them when they function as Goal (*cat bite* vs. *bite cat*). They may have a preference for certain semantic roles, tending to focus on these first, to the neglect of other elements in the sentence; this may happen as part of comprehension or production. For example, one patient focused on any element that had a temporal role to play: in answer to a question such as *Where did you go yesterday?* he would focus on *yesterday* and talk about when it was, which day it was, etc.; in his own spontaneous speech, he would tend to begin a sentence with a temporal expression and use such expressions repeatedly in his speech (*well sometimes/ I like to quite often really/ — on Sundays/ I go you see/ often/...*). Rather than discount this kind of monologue as 'empty', 'stereotyped' or 'automatic', it makes more sense to investigate it systematically, and arrive at a description of the semantic roles and patterns that are being used and those being avoided. Only in this way can a norm be established for patients, which can act as a baseline for suosequent evaluation of their linguistic progress.

There are, then, several major areas within each of the linguistic levels which have yet to be applied in an appropriately detailed and systematic way to the description of aphasic language. The iceberg metaphor is currently an apt one. Far more remains to be described than has been described already. The next step is to generate sufficient motivation and resources to get the descriptive job done, so that linguistically more sophisticated experiments and therapeutic programmes may be carried out, and the foundations of a genuine theory of aphasia laid. It would be nice if the iceberg metaphor turned out to be archaic by the end of the century.

References

ALBERT, M.L., GOODGLASS, H., HELM, N.A., RUBENS, A.B. and ALEXANDER, M.P. *Clinical Aspects of Dysphasia* (1981). Vienna and New York: Springer.

CODE, C. and MILLER, D. (eds) *Aphasia Therapy* (1983). London: Edward Arnold.

COLTHEART, M. Deep dyslexia: a review of the syndrome. In M. Colheart., K. Patterson and D. Muller (eds) *Deep Dyslexia* (1980), pp. 22-47. London: Routledge and Kegan Paul.

COLTHEART, M. In C. Code and D. Muller (eds) *Aphasia Therapy* (1983), pp. 193-202. London: Edward Arnold.

COLTHEART, M., PATTERSON, K. and MARSHALL, J.C. (eds) *Deep Dyslexia* (1980). London: Routledge and Kegan Paul.

CRITCHLEY, M. *Aphasiology* (1970). London: Edward Arnold.

CRYSTAL, D. *Prosodic Systems and Intonation in English* (1969). Cambridge: Cambridge University Press.

CRYSTAL, D. *Clinical Linguistics* (1981). Vienna and New York: Springer; (1987), London: Edward Arnold.

CRYSTAL, D. Pseudo-controversy in linguistic theory. In D. Crystal (ed.) *Linguistic Controversies* (1982a), pp. 16-24. London: Edward Arnold.

CRYSTAL, D. Towards a bucket theory of language disability: taking account of interaction between linguistic levels, *Clinical Linguistics & Phonetics* (1987), [pages not yet known].

CRYSTAL, D. Terms, time and teeth. *British Journal of Disorders of Communication* (1982b), **17.1**, 3-19.

CRYSTAL, D. *Profiling Linguistic Disability* (1982c). London: Edward Arnold.

CRYSTAL, D. and DAVY, D. *Investigating English Style* (1969). London: Longman.

CRYSTAL, D., FLETCHER, P. and GARMAN, M. *The Grammatical Analysis of Language Disability* (1976). London: Edward Arnold.

EISENSON, J. *Adult Aphasia: Assessment and Treatment* (1973). Englewood Cliffs: Prentice-Hall.

FIRTH, J.R. Sounds and prosodies. *Transactions of Philosophical Society* (1948), 127-52.

GOODGLASS, H. (1968) Studies on the grammar of aphasics. In S. Rosenberg and J.H. Koplin (eds) *Developments in Applied Psycholinguistics Research*, pp. 177-208. New York: MacMillan.

GOODGLASS, H. (1976) Aggrammatism. In H. Whitaker and H.A. Whitaker (eds) *Studies in Neurolinguistics* Vol. 1, pp. 237-260. London: Academic Press.

GOODGLASS, H. and KAPLAN, E. *The Assessment of Aphasia and Related Disorders* (1972). Philadelphia: Lea & Febiger.

GRUNWELL, P. *The Nature of Phonological Disability in Children* (1981). London: Academic Press.

GRUNWELL, P. *et. al.* Progress report: the phonetic representation of disordered speech. *British Journal of Disorders of Comm.* (1980), **15**, **3**, 215-220.

HALLIDAY, M.A.K. Categories of the theory of grammar. *Word* (1961), **17**, 241-292.

INGRAM, D. *Phonological Disability in Children* (1976). London: Edward Arnold.

JAKOBSON, R. Two aspects of language and two types of aphasic disturbances. Reprinted in *Selected Writings*, Vol. 2 (1954), pp. 239-259. The Hague: Mouton, 1971.

JAKOBSON, R. On aphasic disorders from a linguistic angle. In R. Jakobson (ed.) *The Framework of Language*, (1980) pp. 93-111. Ann Arbor: Michigan Studies in the Humanities.

LESSER, R. *Linguistic Investigations of Aphasia* (1978). London: Edward Arnold.

LINGUA *Word-classes* (1966). Amsterdam: North-Holland Publishing Company.

LUDLOW, C.L. Recovery and rehabilitation of adult aphasic patients: relevant research advances. In R.W. Reiber (ed.) *Communication Disorders* (1981), pp. 149-177. New York: Plenum Press.

LYONS, J. *Semantics* (1977). Cambridge: Cambridge University Press.

MORTON, J. Two auditory parallels to deep dyslexia. In M. Coltheart, K. Patterson and J.C. Marshall (eds) *Deep Dyslexia* (1980), pp. 189-196. London: Routledge and Kegan Paul.

NICOLOSI, L., HARRYMAN, E. and KRESHEK, J. *Terminology of Speech Disorders* (1978). Baltimore: Williams & Wilkins.

QUIRK, R., GREENBAUM, S., LEECH, G. and SVARTVIK, J. *A Comprehensive Grammar of the English Language* (1985). London: Longman.

ROBBINS, S. *A Dictionary of Speech Pathology and Therapy* (1951). Cambridge, Mass.: Sci-Art Publishers.

SAFFRAN, E.M., BOGYO, L.C., SCHWARTZ, M.F. and MARIN, O.S.M. Does deep dyslexia reflect right-hemisphere reading? In M. Coltheart, K. Patterson and J.C. Marshall (eds) *Deep Dyslexia* (1980), pp. 381-406. London: Routledge and Kegan Paul.

WHURR, R. Towards a typology of aphasic impairment. In D. Crystal (ed.) *Linguistic controversies* (1982), pp. 239-257. London: Edward Arnold.

WOOD, K.S. Terminology and nomenclature. In L.E. Travis (ed.) *Handbook of Speech Pathology* (1957), pp. 44-71. Englewood Cliffs: Prentice-Hall.

3

Non-verbal Communication

Pierre Feyereisen

Introduction

The term 'non-verbal communication' usually refers to deliberate or non-deliberate use of bodily movements during social interactions. It is assumed that some non-verbal behaviour — hand gestures, facial and vocal expresssions of emotions, gaze orientations — can communicate like speech, transmitting information, either by influencing the audience or by activating mental representations (Feyereisen and de Lannoy, 1985). Thus to some extent the term is an oxymoron, expressing contradictory meanings: non-verbal communication is not a language but it may function as a language. A more precise picture of the relationship between verbal and non-verbal communication can be obtained by examining the consequences of cerebral lesions resulting in aphasia: is there simultaneous impairment or selective sparing of non-verbal behaviour?

The question is of therapeutic as well as of theoretic interest. It could be supposed that aphasics could bypass their difficulties in language processing by non-verbal communication, and indeed clinical experience does suggest that at least some aphasics can compensate for their verbal impairment by using non-verbal substitutes either spontaneously, for example by gesturing the use of an object they are unable to name, or as a result of rehabilitation training. Similarly, disorders of verbal comprehension might be circumvented by residual abilities, processing of affective information, direct access to the meaning of non-symbolic signs, or general knowledge of social rules. In this sense, it is said that aphasics communicate better than they speak (Holland, 1982).

For this reason, several therapeutic plans aim at improving the communicative effectiveness of aphasic patients by training them to use non-verbal signals (e.g. Davis and Wilcox, 1981) or by systematic teaching of sign languages (Christopoulou and Bonvillian, 1985; Moody, 1982; Peterson and Kirshner, 1981) the assumption being that language can be restored more easily in the visuo-gestural, than in the oral, modality. To understand how these achievements are possible, and to appreciate their limits, it is necessary to put non-verbal behaviour in a theoretical framework that stresses commonalities with, and differences from, language. If a non-verbal system can be mastered, why could not language be learned again? What are the respective properties of verbal and non-verbal communication that explain the impairment of one and the sparing of the other? On what processes does compensatory use of non-verbal signals rely when language is defective? Moreover, clinical intuition seems to be contradicted by the systematic analysis of the processing of non-verbal signals by aphasic subjects. Aphasia is often associated with perceptual or motor deficits outside the language domain, so that the basis for therapeutic training of non-verbal communication remains unclear, even if the apparent contradiction between clinical and experimental data probably reflects conceptual ambiguity in defining non-verbal communication, differences in assessment methods and subject sampling, or reduced severity of non-verbal impairments relative to language disorders.

These questions in clinical practice are echoed by theoretical discussions concerning the nature of aphasic impairments, of hemispheric specialization, and of mental representations underlying speech production. Data on the non-verbal behaviour of aphasic subjects in these different fields of research have indeed been used to raise the issue of the specificity of language processes.

Is Aphasia a Language Disorder?

Since the end of the nineteenth century, there has been controversy concerning the relationship between language and thought disorders in aphasia (Ombredane, 1951). As to whether aphasia should be considered a pathology of language use or the consequence of a more general intellectual deficit, critical observations have been provided by the analysis of spared or impaired non-verbal abilities. The hypothesis of asymbolia, a supramodal deficit in symbolic functioning, has inspired a great deal of research on non-verbal communication in aphasia.

Is the Left Hemisphere Specialized in the Processing of Verbal Materials?

While data on the lateralization of cognitive functions in normal and brain-damaged subjects accumulated, different ways of characterizing the respective competence of the cerebral hemispheres were proposed (for reviews *see* Bertelson, 1982; Bradshaw and Nettleton, 1981; Cohen, 1982). The early dichotomy between verbal and visuospatial functions was substituted by dichotomies stressing modes of processing information (serial versus parallel, analytic versus holistic). It was thus suggested that the left hemisphere control of language could occur as a consequence of more fundamental specialization. In such a perspective, the observation of non-verbal behaviour of aphasic subjects is relevant from two points of view. On the one hand, Kimura (1976) suggested that 'brain regions considered to be important for symbolic-language processes might better be conceived as important for the production of motor sequences'. In left-hemisphere damage, apraxia is regularly associated with aphasia. Gesture and speech production might both suffer from defective temporal organization of position changes in oral or manual musculature. The interference of verbal behaviour with concurrent right-hand motor performance in dual-task paradigms by normal subjects would also suggest linkage between language and motor control rather than functional separation (Kinsbourne and Hiscock, 1983). On the other hand, Sergent (1983, 1984) argues for the co-operation of both the right and left cerebral hemispheres in the processing of visual input and an advantage of the left hemisphere in extracting fine-grained information. Consequently, left-hemisphere damaged subjects would show impairments in visual perception not only when reading or when a verbal mediation is required but also when task difficulty is increased, i.e. when the task requires in-depth information processing. From such a perspective, aphasia is expected to be associated with perceptual deficits affecting the comprehension of non-verbal signals.

Are Gestures and Speech Parallel Manifestations of a Common Conceptual Representation?

It has recently been argued from data on aphasic behaviour that parallel disruptions of gestural and verbal processes would reveal the existence of a common mechanism underlying speech and gesture production (Bates *et al.*, 1983; Kendon, 1983; McNeill, 1985). Different aspects of the process of putting thoughts into words or hand movements are underlined. Kendon (1983) stressed the potential communicative value of gestures. Gestures and speech constitute two separate modes of representation that are co-ordinated in the communication process 'because both are being guided by the same overall aim' (p. 20). Brain lesions may disrupt the single central organizer and lead to parallel impairments of gesture and speech. Bates *et al.* (1983) analysed the emergence of symbols in infancy in the gestural and the vocal modality. Some gestural conventions are conceived as a kind of naming and called 'manual names'. For these authors, non-verbal impairments in aphasics also suggest a modality-free breakdown of the symbolization process by which signs 'stand for' their referents. McNeill (1985) argued for a common computational stage in the production of gestures and speech. The differences between sub-types of aphasia would be similar in oral and gestural output: the use of referential gestures would parallel sparing of content-word vocabulary. From these different points of view, the processes of communicating, naming, or sentence formulating would only be partially modality-specific.

The object of this chapter is to examine the disputed issue of specificity by stressing the heterogeneity of the clinical and experimental data on non-verbal behaviour of aphasic patients and by identifying the empirical evidence for supramodal deficits in the different domains. The notion of non-verbal communication encompasses a great variety of behaviour that might differ in relationship to language, for example, gestures that may convey meaning like language, and speech-related hand movements accompanying speech might be more related to linguistic behaviour than emotional expression. These different kinds of non-verbal behaviour will be distinguished, and the question of association to language disorders will be treated separately. In these different domains, specificity does not simply mean dissociation of impairments. Cases of dissociation may be interpreted in two ways: as selective impairment of distinct modality-specific processes or as differences in task requirements that render, for example, comprehension easier than production, gesture easier than language processing, or automatic processes less disrupted than voluntary ones. In the latter case, aphasia without non-verbal impairments could be observed but not the reverse. Conversely, non-specificity will be supported by regular association of verbal and non-verbal deficits and correlation in their severity as well as by evidence of similar influence of some independent variables on verbal and non-verbal behaviour.

There are problems in the analysis of non-verbal impairments. First, a statistically significant association with language disorders is not sufficient to demonstrate that both verbal and non-verbal impairments depend on the defective functioning of a single mechanism. Rare cases of double dissociations would be enough to indicate separation of the underlying mechanisms. Second, associations might be due to impairments on different levels of processing, for example, non-verbal disorders of aphasic subjects might depend on amodal disruptions in conceptual representations, on linguistic mediations in the assumed non-verbal processing, or on sensorimotor impairments on a lower level. Thus, defective operations must be specified in a model of the cognitive system.

Gestural Representations

Deictic movements like pointing, descriptive gestures like pantomime or illustrative hand movements, and symbolic gestures whose meaning is fixed by social conventions may theoretically substitute for words, and deaf signing people have admirably succeeded in exploiting this mode of communication. Such compensation is not commonly observed in aphasic people and it has been suggested that, unlike speech- and hearing-impaired subjects, brain-damaged subjects might be as defective in the gestural as in the oral modality. The problem is to identify the basis for the association of gestural and verbal deficits: either in the disruption of some supramodal mechanism or in the casual simultaneous impairment of separate modality-specific processes. Empirical data and theoretical interpretations bear on the production and comprehension of gestures by aphasic subjects.

(A) Gestural Expression

Sometimes brain-damaged people are unable to produce symbolic gestures on request (verbal command or instruction to imitate), although the same gestures are executed spontaneously in natural contexts. Similarly, pantomime of object use may be impaired in spite of correct object manipulation. These gestural disorders are part of a deficit called 'ideomotor apraxia', which also includes impaired imitation of meaningless movements. Ideomotor apraxia is more frequent after left than after right hemisphere lesions and usually occurs in association with aphasia (de Ajuriaguerra, Hécaen and Angelergues, 1960; De Renzi, Motti and Nichelli, 1980). The relationship between aphasia and apraxia is examined by Poeck in this volume, and the relevant data will be reviewed here as far as gestural representations are concerned. Indeed, ideomotor apraxia has received different explanations that, to some extent, also apply to the communicative behaviour of aphasic subjects.

Theoretical interpretations

Four concepts of gestural deficit may be identified (Roy, 1982).

(1) The conceptual deficit hypothesis

From the observation of impairments of aphasic subjects in gesture imitation, Marie (1906; cited by Signoret and North, 1979) suggested the existence of a general cognitive deficit underlying both verbal and gestural performance. Two versions of that hypothesis are currently espoused: apraxia as a result of intellectual deterioration or as a consequence of general communication disorders. The first is supported by significant correlations of scores in apraxia examination with age and psychometric intelligence (WAIS performance score, for example). Support for the second hypothesis was offered by Duffy and Duffy (1981) on the basis of multiple correlations between Raven's matrices intelligence test, the Porch Index of Communicative Ability, and pantomime performance. The authors admit that these data do not rule out an alternative explanation, namely, a verbal mediation in motor control (Luria, 1961).

(2) The motor deficit hypothesis

Left-hemisphere-damaged subjects show impaired performances in a variety of motor tasks that do not imply symbolic processing: tapping (e.g.

Carmon, 1971), rapid pointing (e.g. Wyke, 1968), tracking (e.g. Heilman, Schwartz and Geschwind, 1975), manipulating apparatus created for experimental purpose (e.g. Kimura, 1977), and copying meaningless hand positions or movements (e.g. Kimura and Archibald, 1974; Jason, 1983, 1985). Ideomotor apraxia might simply result from this motor impairment.

(3) The perceptual deficit hypothesis

Earlier interpretations of apraxia suggest that the impairment in mental representation of the body can be the possible source of disorders in gesture production (*see* J. Lhermitte, 1939; Morlaas, 1928; Schilder, 1935, cited by Signoret and North, 1979). From such a perspective, an association of ideomotor apraxia is expected with impairments in perceptual tasks involving the body schema. Similarly, defective pantomime or object manipulation might result from impaired conceptualization of objects whose use has to be shown, so this impairment would appear in perceptual and motor tasks.

In fact, the motor deficit hypothesis and the perceptual deficit hypothesis constitute refinements of the conceptual deficit hypothesis by specifying the nature of the mental representations underlying gesture planification.

(4) The disconnection hypothesis

Some cases of apraxia show unilateral impairments, usually an inability to execute left-hand gestures on request while right-hand behaviour is normal. This pattern has been interpreted as resulting from a disconnection between the speech area and the motor cortex due to a callosal lesion (Liepmann, 1900, cited by Geschwind, 1975), an interpretation that has been extended to cases of bilateral apraxia under the assumption that the intra-hemispheric asociations between speech and motor regions were interrupted. From such a perspective, apraxia and aphasia may dissociate, but the fact that gestures are also impaired in imitation tasks cannot be explained by this kind of dissociation. The model also assumes a specialized mechanism for motor control that may be disconnected from mechanisms of visual analysis or itself disrupted, so that the motor deficit hypothesis is also partially accepted.

The first two hypotheses strongly assume that aphasia is not a modality-specific disorder, but depends on a general impairment of either the conceptual or the motor system. The disconnection hypothesis assumes specific language or gestural disorders. Examination of supportive empirical evidence will thus provide an initial answer to the question of specificity of mechanisms underlying speech and gesture production, but few attempts have been made to specify the domain validity of these different hypotheses, each of which may be true for individual cases. CT scan correlates also suggest that the label of ideomotor apraxia may well cover disturbances appearing in diverse forms for different reasons. There is no precise localization of the lesions producing ideomotor apraxia, which results not only from large lesions involving the parietal cortex and subcortical structures but also from small lesions in different parts of the brain (Agostini *et al.*, 1983; Basso, Luzzatti and Spinnler, 1980; DeRenzi *et al.*, 1983; Heilman, Rothi and Kertesz, 1983; Kertesz and Ferro, 1984). Varieties of gestural impairments may be defined on the basis of performance differences in eliciting conditions and movement parameters, by error analysis, or by correlations with associated deficits.

The data

(1) The influence of eliciting conditions

Production of gestures in response to verbal instruction is often more impaired than gesture imitation (Pickett, 1974; Hécaen, 1978; Lehmkuhl, Poeck and Willmes, 1983). That aphasics simply do not understand the verbal request, a trivial explanation, is ruled out by the observation of a parallel advantage of the imitation condition in subjects whose auditory comprehension is not impaired. Two explanations remain plausible. The first suggests that these brain lesions hinder the transfer of information from the speech decoding system to the motor planning system (the disconnection hypothesis). An inverse dissociation has been described in a woman who could produce gestures on verbal request but was unable to gesture the use of an object shown to her (Assal and Regli, 1980).

The alternative explanation for the advantage of the imitation condition assumes that more information on the parameters of the movement to be planned is available when a model is provided than in the verbal condition. Similarly, poorer performances in pantomime of object use are observed in the visual than in the tactile presentation of the object (DeRenzi, Faglioni and Sorgatto, 1982). These modality effects suggest deficits in motor planning rather than in conceptualizing object functions.

(2) The parameters of the elicited gestures

Apraxia examination usually involves elicitation of gestures belonging to different categories (Poeck, 1986). Performances vary according to the body parts used (face, hands, legs), and a possible dissociation of mechanisms for the motor control of oral and manual movements is suggested on the basis of differential impairments in imitation of meaningless positions or sequences (Kolb and Milner, 1981a; Kimura, 1982). Movements of the axial musculature (eyes, head, torso) are no less impaired than those of the distal musculature (Poeck, Lehmkuhl and Willmes, 1982). Bimanual movements are more disturbed than unimanual movements, but it is not known whether the difference is the simple consequence of hemiplegia or the result of higher task demands in bimanual co-ordination.

Imitation of meaningful movements does not differ from that of meaningless movements, and thus the expected results from the conceptual deficit hypothesis are not found (DeRenzi *et al.*, 1980; Lehmkuhl *et al.*, 1983). Among the meaningful gestures, descriptive, expressive and symbolic gestures sometimes have to be distinguished. Goodglass and Kaplan (1963) found natural and conventional gestures less impaired than pantomimed use of objects. Performance of subjects impaired in the verbal condition only or in the verbal condition and in imitation did not correlate across categories of gestures (Hécaen, 1978). Accordingly, two kinds of ideomotor apraxia might be distinguished, the one impairing pretended or actual use of objects, the other impairing communication by expressive and/or conventional movements.

(3) Nature of errors

Gestural performance is usually rated on scales assessing the severity of praxic disorders but not the nature of the errors. Imitation tasks or the elicitation of gestures by pictures of movements allow finer measures because the performance may be compared on particular dimensions to the specified target. For example, Roy (1981) distinguished position, order, perseveration, and omission errors whose distribution differed among aphasic subjects, left-hemisphere damaged subjects without aphasia, and right-hemisphere damaged subjects. Similarly, during the imitation of pantomime, more errors in arm orientation and the use of body parts as objects were observed in left- than in right-hemisphere damaged subjects but no differences in the partial execution of movements (Haaland and Flaherty, 1984).

Lehmkuhl *et al.* (1983) also had different categories of errors, but their results did not lead to the identification of characteristic patterns. These attempts to distinguish varieties of gesture disorders on the basis of error analysis probably fail because the error types are not defined on specified theoretical grounds. The study of apraxia in relation to theoretical models of motor control, as suggested by Paillard (1982) and by Kelso and Tuller (1981), permits the identification of stages in gesture production or factors influencing motor preparation. From such perspectives, it remains to be determined whether apraxia stems from execution problems, resulting in clumsiness, or from problems in action planning, leading to omission errors or execution of inappropriate movements. Similarly, deficits in the representation of actions, specification of the parameters of movement (direction, amplitude, timing, etc.), co-ordination of body segments, or any other operation required in gesture production would result in distinctive error patterns.

(4) Associated deficits

Another way to distinguish varieties of apraxia is to examine association with other perceptual and motor impairments. For example, Haaland (1984) found no differences between three groups of apraxic subjects, defined according to the severity of their impairment in gesture imitation, in motor tasks like tapping or maze co-ordination. This suggests that the extent of motor disorders does not account for apraxia.

Heilman, Rothi and Valenstein (1982) proposed defining two kinds of ideomotor apraxia in which the mental representation of movement as assessed in perceptual tasks is impaired in one case and spared in the other. Their subjects had to select the gesture corresponding to a specified target from three successive presentations. The distractors were either the incorrect execution of the intended gesture or the correct performance of inappropriate gestures. Apraxic subjects with posterior lesions made more errors than those with anterior lesions, mostly in the incorrect execution condition. In these subjects, gestural impairment could result from a disturbance of visuokinesthetic representations of the movement. The observed difficulty of apraxic–aphasic subjects in acquiring new gestures in a gesture memory task (the Buschke paradigm of selective reminding) was also interpreted as evidence of defective visuokinesthetic representation of movement in memory, but this can still be explained by a performance deficit hypothesis (Rothi and Heilman, 1984).

In fact, several studies have compared gesture comprehension and production in the context of the asymbolia hypothesis and found disorders on the receptive and expressive levels to be moderately associated (Gainotti and Lemmo, 1976; Kadish, 1978; Ferro *et al.*, 1980; Duffy and Duffy, 1981; Rothi, Heilman and Watson, 1985) but as suggested by Heilman *et al.* (1982), the performances may dissociate. First, task requirements differ and comprehension is less impaired than production (Netsu and Marquardt, 1984). Second, cases have been reported of normal gestural performance in spite of impaired comprehension of gesture (16 subjects out of the 53 in the series of Gainotti and Lemmo, 1976). Therefore, some subjects can imitate gesture they do not understand (Rothi, Mack and Heilman, 1986).

The relationship between aphasia and gesture production deficits

Since both result from left-hemisphere lesions, ideomotor apraxia is often observed in association with aphasia. Correlations between the severity of praxic and linguistic disorders provide the main empirical support for the hypotheses of a motor or a central symbolic deficit, although some findings conflict with these correlations because different measures of severity yield different patterns of correlation. Nor are specific associations with sub-types of aphasia observed, other than a generally more severe gestural deficit in global aphasia than in milder forms (Kertesz and Hooper, 1982; Lehmkuhl *et al.*, 1983). Dissociations between verbal and gestural deficits have also been described. Aphasics are less impaired in gestural than in verbal expression (Davis, Artes and Hoops, 1979). Aphasia without apraxia is common, and Kertesz, Ferro and Shewan (1984) have described the anatomical basis for such dissociation. This phenomenon has also been reported among deaf-signing patients, who produce language in the gestural modality (Poizner, Bellugi and Iragui, 1984). To some extent, the task demand to produce movements on request seems to be lower for non-linguistic than for linguistic signs, be they oral or manual. A related observation is the advantage of sign languages over oral languages in the acquisition of communicative skills by mentally handicapped children (Abrahamsen, Cavallo and McCluer, 1985); different variables like sign transparency or the concreteness of the referent may explain this effect (Luftig, 1983).

The inverse dissociation of apraxia without aphasia is much less common when verbal behaviour is carefully assessed, but it is sometimes observed: five cases have been reported in the series of de Ajuriaguerra *et al.* (1960), one case by Heilman, Gonyea and Geschwind (1974), and two cases in the series of De Renzi *et al.* (1980). Separation of the underlying mechanisms is also observed in left-handed people recovering from aphasia but not from apraxia (Selnes *et al.*, 1982). Other arguments against the hypothesis of a unitary disturbance of language and gesture are provided by evidence that rehabilitation in one modality does not influence performance in the other, for example, training the production of pantomimes does not improve verbal performance (Helm-Estabrooks, Fitzpatrick and Barresi, 1982), and teaching Amerind signs does not facilitate retrieval of words that have equivalent meanings (Drummond and Rentschler, 1981).

Moreover, the different interpretations of apraxia suggest several explanations for the observed association with aphasia (Feyereisen and Seron, 1982, 1984). The limited knowledge we have of the disturbed operations in ideomotor apraxia does not allow us to identify a supramodal deficit that would also be responsible for verbal impairments. Thus the significance of the co-occurrence of verbal and gestural deficits in left-hemisphere-damaged patients is open to discussion: is it a spurious correlation due to the simultaneous impairment of distinct control centres, or does the association indicate the existence of common, underlying mechanisms? If the latter, then the question arises of the nature of the impaired mechanism: are gesture and speech disturbed because of incomplete specification of the input at the conceptual level or because of disrupted control of the motor programs? Examination of performance on the receptive side might partially answer this question, since a conceptual deficit is assumed to impair both comprehension and production of symbolic gestures.

(B) Comprehension

Pantomime comprehension is usually studied with a gesture-to-picture matching task (*see* e.g. Duffy, Duffy and Pearson, 1975; Ferro *et al.*, 1980b; Gainotti and Lemmo, 1976; Pickett, 1974). This task requires the interpretation of gestures, i.e. transcoding them into a format that is compatible with the result of picture interpretation. It is not, as has sometimes been argued, a recognition task involving delayed judgement of identity. Compared with other brain-damaged subjects, aphasics show impaired performances, and the extent of the deficit correlates with the severity of naming and auditory comprehension deficits. Disorders of gesture comprehension have been interpreted in the context of the asymbolia hypothesis first formulated by Finkelnburg in 1870 (Duffy and Liles, 1979), but this interpretation is not unanimously accepted and alternative explanations have been proposed.

One problem concerns the identification of defective operations in asymbolia. Different disorders may be distinguished, as follows.

(1) Disorders of the semiotic function

According to a strong version of the asymbolia hypothesis, a severe comprehension deficit would involve the loss of the general knowledge that conventional signs can substitute for things. Yet, the gesture comprehension difficulty of aphasic subjects is only moderately correlated with ratings of gesture arbitrariness (Duffy and McEwen, 1978). Moreover, aphasics are impaired to a similar extent in processing facial expression of emotions and symbolic gestures (Goldblum, 1980). Thus conventional gestures are not more poorly understood than natural signals or iconic representations. Nor is the strong hypothesis supported by error analysis studies showing a partial processing of gestural signs (Daniloff *et al.*, 1982; Seron *et al.*, 1979; Varney and Benton, 1982). Indeed, the most frequent error in matching tasks involves the choice of a picture that relates to the picture of the pantomimed object. Studies in which no semantic distractors are presented find a higher proportion of aphasic subjects with normal performance than studies with semantic foils in the response array, an effect confirmed in a controlled experiment by Duffy and Watkins (1984). Thus aphasics may understand a part of the meaning of the gesture but not enough to discriminate related concepts. Similarly, impaired subjects can understand some gestures, while failing to understand others (Daniloff *et al.*, 1982; Feyereisen, Seron and de Macar, 1981).

(2) Impairment of analytic competence?

A weaker version of the asymbolia hypothesis can be formulated according to which semantic confusions result from loosened links between signs and referents and from blurred boundaries of concepts. Related phenomena would be the typicality effect in the categorization of words and pictures, resulting from a spared ability to categorize the central items of a natural class but an impairment in processing atypical instances or related non-members (for examples, in decisions concerning the bird category, penguin and bat; *see* Grober *et al.*, 1980). A similar view stresses the generality of non-verbal impairments of aphasic subjects in matching tasks involving pictures, colours, or sounds as well as gestures. The deficit would be in identifying the feature that is relevant for the conceptual matching (*see* e.g., Cohen, Kelter and Woll, 1980), and so errors in gesture comprehension would result from inappropriate weighting of features that distinguish related items.

The error analysis in gesture-to-picture matching is consistent with these interpretations. There is, however, no systematic control for the hypothesis that holistic processing of configurational or structural properties is spared while analytic processing is impaired. Without such a control, there is a risk of formulating circular explanations and ad hoc interpretations (Morais, 1982).

(3) Defective inferential processes

A peculiarity of the experiment devised by Feyereisen *et al.* (1981) also suggests a third interpretation of conceptual disorders in asymbolia. In order to compare comprehension of pantomime, symbolic, and expressive gestures, the pointing-to-object task was modified, and the subjects were requested to identify the picture of a context in which the gesture might occur. In these conditions, a greater difficulty in processing expressive gestures was interpreted as resulting from a defective inferential process, i.e. an impaired evaluation of the probability of the gesture ocurring in a given context. Preliminary observations suggest that aphasic subjects are more impaired in matching gestures to context than in matching a video recorded gesture to a photograph of the gesture taken from a slightly different perspective (Feyereisen, data on file). Thus some perceptual processes concerning gestures seem to be spared.

Effects of experimental conditions on gesture comprehension can be interpreted from such a perspective. Gestures describing actions are better understood than gestures referring to objects (Daniloff *et al.*, 1982) and pointing to pictures of actions with objects is easier than pointing to pictures of isolated objects (Netsu and Marquardt, 1984). It might be that some gestures lead more readily to correct inferences than others.

Gestures would present intrinsic ambiguity and aphasic subjects would be more sensitive than normal subjects to that polysemy by understanding pantomimes less well than names of objects (Duffy and Watkins, 1984). The results of Seron *et al.* (1979), indicating that aphasic subjects' errors are considered by normal judges 'plausible but improbable', also support such an interpretation, which, however, remains to be tested with gestures whose characteristics have been appropriately selected.

More experimentation is needed to identify the defective operations in gesture comprehension, but two problems must be faced whatever hypothesis is chosen. The first concerns modality effects in comprehension disorders. Since Varney (1978), several authors have reported higher correlations of pantomime comprehension scores with reading comprehension than with auditory comprehension, although both are significantly positive (Seron *et al.*, 1979; Feyereisen *et al.*, 1981). Accordingly, it is suggested that 'defects in pantomime recognition are the result of specific information processing disturbance' (Varney, 1982, p. 38). The second problem concerns dissociations between verbal and non-verbal comprehension. In all studies where individual data are reported, cases exist of aphasic subjects whose gesture comprehension is spared in spite of language comprehension deficits. Moreover, the recovery rate differs in the two modalities (Ferro *et al.*, 1980). Much less frequent are the cases of inverse dissociation (gesture comprehension impairment without reading comprehension deficit). Ferro *et al.*(1983) describe the anatomical basis of the dissociation that results from differences in localization of lesions. Moreover, differences in CT scan correlates of gesture comprehension deficits in acute and chronic stages suggest multiple representation of gestures. Large lesions, disrupting several mechanisms involved in gesture comprehension, would be necessary to produce long-term impairments. CT scan correlates, however, do not allow a clear distinction between two explanations for the frequent cases in which verbal and non-verbal disorders associate: the overlapping of distinct specific processing units or the presence, in addition to modality-specific processes, of some 'symbolic/conceptual', modality-free mechanism.

In conclusion, the very general approach adopted so far to describe gestural impairments in aphasia does not allow firm conclusions on the specificity of the conceptual structure underlying the use of verbal and non-verbal symbols. Most of the evidence favours the hypothesis of a supramodal deficit. Cases of dissociation do occur, but they show more often aphasia with intact gestural behaviour than the reverse. It is thus suggested that task requirements are lower in producing or understanding gestures. Nevertheless, we have no clear idea of the nature of a modality-free impairment showing these task effects. Gestural representations might be spared because of the influence of variables like iconicity, reliance on visual guidance, or reference to procedural knowledge. Thus if the role of variables affecting the use of gestures and words differently is not made precise, the hypothesis of a general conceptual deficit cannot be considered verified. Nor should one reject an alternative model specifying different operations leading to the production or comprehension of words and gestures.

A distinction between a 'surface form' and more abstract representations underlying the processing of verbal and non-verbal information has been suggested in different domains: sentence production (Garrett, 1982), picture categorization (Snodgrass, 1984), and object recognition (Ratcliff and Newcombe, 1982). This distinction might be extended to the case of gesture processing. If different stages are identified, dissociations can be explained by selective impairments or modality-specific low-level operations. The analysis of other gestural behaviours more closely connected to speech production but not necessarily expressing symbolic meanings raises similar problems.

Non-verbal Activity During Speaking

(A) Theoretical Frame

Speaking people show a great deal of head, eye, and hand movements, so it has been suggested that the analysis of the relationship between the verbal utterances and these movements might shed new light on the processes underlying speech production. From the observation of lateral differences in the manual activity of normal subjects during conversation, Kimura (1973) suggested the existence of common cerebral control of speech and hand movements and, thus, the non-specificity of some mechanisms underlying speech production. In order to identify the nature of this interaction, two questions should be answered.

First, is right-hand preference related to left hemisphere activation during speech planning or to the use of the higher competence of the left hemisphere in motor control (Feyereisen, 1986a)? The activation hypothesis assumes that the more one hemisphere is involved in a task, the more the contralateral movements are elicited. This hypothesis accounts for observations of mouth asymmetry (Graves, Goodglass and Landis, 1982; Graves, Landis and Simpson, 1985; Hager and Van Gelder, 1985) and for changes of hand preference in several movement categories during verbal and visuospatial tasks (Hampson and Kimura, 1984), but it is only partially supported by the analysis of lateral differences in conjugate lateral eye movements during various cognitive activities (for a review, see Ehrlichman and Weinberger, 1978). The motor control hypothesis is supported by qualitative analysis, which shows a greater number of direction changes in the movements of the right hand during speaking (Kimura and Humphreys, 1981). Second, the problem arises concerning the locus at which gesture and speech production interact. Co-activation of gestures and speech might result either from properties of the thinking process by which the conceptual structure of the message is computed (*see* e.g., McNeill, 1985) or from lower level interactions during the programming of movements (cf. Kelso *et al.*, 1983). Observations on the non-verbal behaviour of aphasic subjects during speaking may be reviewed from these perspectives.

(B) Empirical Evidence

(1) Quantitative studies

Systematic analysis of aphasic behaviour in spontaneous non-verbal activity are few in number. Several group studies have been conducted comparing normal and language-impaired subjects with different measures: global judgements on non-verbal activity or amount of face, eye, and head movements. For instance, Golper and Gordon (1984) made silent films of subjects during conversations and reported that more right-hemisphere damaged subjects were recognized by naïve judges as neurological patients than were aphasics. The percentage of subjects suffering from facial weakness was equal in the two brain-damaged groups, but aphasic subjects maintained a normal appearance more often. Kolb and Milner (1981b) systematically observed spontaneous facial expressions — like eyebrow raising, lip tightening, and sticking out the tongue — produced during neuropsychological testing. The subjects with left- or right-frontal lesions produced fewer movements than patients with temporal or parietal lesions, but no differences emerged in function of the hemispheric side of the lesion. Similarly, administration of sodium amytal reduced facial expression regardless of the side of the injection. During conversation on selected topics, no statistical differences between aphasic and normal subjects appeared when rate, duration, and mean duration of six co-verbal behaviours were compared: head nod, head tilt, head shake, eye contact, eyebrow raising, and smiling (Katz, Lapointe and Markel, 1982). Correlations with linguistic performance as assessed by the Porch Index of Communicative Ability indicated an inverse relationship between verbal scores on the one hand and smile rates and duration of eye contact on the other. These non-verbal signals could serve as compensatory devices to maintain the social bond in conversation when speech is impaired. Conversely, Feyereisen and Lignian (1981) reported a reduced duration of eye contact in non-fluent aphasics during the central part of speaking turns whose duration exceeded 15 seconds. This behaviour has also been observed in normal subjects during speech planning and might serve to regulate turns in conversation. This 'communicative competence' of aphasic patients is in accordance with the pragmatic adjustment shown by these patients in experimental tasks (*see* review in Foldi, Cicone and Gardner, 1983) and with the assumption of right-hemisphere dominance in emotional expression (*see* below).

A different picture is expected for manual activity. Under the assumption of a common control mechanism for speech and gesture production, two predictions are formulated: first, similarity in ranking aphasic subjects on the fluency dimension for verbal and gestural measures; second, similarity in use of content words and referential gestures as opposed to function words and non-propositional accompanying movements. Contradictory findings have been reported, and differences in subject sampling and in verbal and gestural measures do not at present allow definitive conclusions.

Parallels between speech fluency and rate of gesture production are described in two studies. Cicone *et al.* (1979) analyzed small portions of a conversation for four subjects, two being described as 'anterior' or Broca's aphasics, the other two as 'posterior' or Wernicke's aphasics. The posterior aphasics produced more movements per time unit than the anterior aphasics and their gestural units showed greater complexity, i.e. greater chaining of several components. Duffy, Duffy and Mercaitis (1984) devised a different situation, but obtained similar results. One non-fluent Broca's aphasic and one fluent Wernicke's aphasic participated in a referential task where information on a picture of an object was pantomimed while no vocalization was allowed. The two subjects showed similar accuracy (about 55%), but differed in the number of movements per pantomime or per second. Analyses of larger samples of aphasic subjects, however, do not confirm the results of these preliminary investigations. Feyereisen (1983) found no significant differences in movement duration or frequency between four non-fluent and eight fluent aphasics. These measures were not correlated with speech rate, but when the movements were analyzed into elementary components, a correlation with fluency was observed. Replication with another sample of twelve aphasic subjects and time sampling of gestural behaviour (instantaneous record of presence or absence of gestures every five seconds) did not show correlation with speech rate (Spearman's Rho = $0 \cdot 08$; Feyereisen and Bouchat, unpublished observations). The total number of gestures per minute did not correlate with mean length of utterances in a mixed sample of five control and ten aphasic subjects (Glosser, Wiener and Kaplan, 1986).

Consistent results are provided by studies using gesture-to-word ratios, but such a measure leads to interpretation problems because it is affected by gesture and speech production; indeed, a high ratio may indicate either an increased gestural rate or a decreased verbal fluency. Nevertheless, the hypothesis of a common mechanism for gesture and speech control predicts an absence of between-group differences if a reduction in fluency is associated with a decline in gesture production. In fact, higher gesture-to-word ratios than in control groups were found by Goldblum (1978) in four anterior aphasics and by Herrmann *et al.* (1985) in five non-fluent aphasics. A similar but non-significant trend was noted by Glosser *et al.* (1986). Inconsistent relations between speech fluency and rate of gesture production probably reflect the heterogeneity of symptomatologies characterized by a slow speech tempo, for example, fluency does not correlate with other measures of aphasic speech such as the proportion of content words (Feyereisen, 1984; Feyereisen *et al.*, 1986).

It is also hypothesized that referential value of manual activity correlates with the informative content of speech production. A higher proportion of gesture carrying information was found in anterior than in posterior aphasics (Goldblum, 1978; Cicone *et al.*, 1979; unpublished data of Pedelty cited by McNeill, 1985). The percentage of interpretable gestures correlated positively with auditory comprehension and naming scores, and the percentage of uninterpretable gestures negatively (Glosser *et al.*, 1986). However, Feyereisen and Bouchat (unpublished observations) did not find correlations between the proportion of illustrative gestures and the proportion of nouns in story telling. Some dissociations did occur in very reduced aphasic subjects who were unable to produce names in high proportion but could use descriptive gestures. Case reports of gestural behaviour in two jargonaphasics yielded similar results (Nespoulous, 1979; Butterworth, Swallow and Grimston, 1981), and it was concluded from the ability to express meanings gesturally in spite of severe word finding difficulties that the conceptual structure underlying speech production had been spared in these subjects. Thus, there is a contradiction between observations of simultaneous impairments of referential activity in the verbal and gestural modalities and observations of dissociated performances. Moreover, a methodological problem arises in assessing the communicative value of gestures. Movements are usually said to be 'illustrative' when they relate by their form to the verbally expressed content. Thus, judgements of representational value are not independent of the characteristics of speech content and it might be that the gestures of Broca's aphasics are considered more illustrative, not because of gesture quality, but because of the greater proportion of content words in their speech.

(2) Functional analysis of co-verbal behaviour

The assumption of a common cerebral basis underlying speech and spontaneous co-verbal activity sometimes relies on the idea that gesture and speech serve similar functions. Thus in the study of human communication, both channels should be considered and their co-ordination analyzed. Several studies describe the communicative value of aphasics' non-verbal behaviour from such a perspective. Gesture may serve different pragmatic functions and be used to refer, to express feelings, requests, and comments, or to regulate social exchanges. It has been suggested that aphasic subjects could rely on the gestural mode of communication to achieve these pragmatic functions (Nespoulous, 1979; Labourel, 1982). It is not clear, however, that the meaning of gestures can be identified outside the context of verbal utterances and of conventional situations. Furthermore, the communicative value of aphasics' behaviour depends largely on characteristics of the residual linguistic ability. Thus, non-fluent aphasics use more gestures that substitute for speech, and fluent aphasics use more accompaniment gestures (Behrmann and Penn, 1984). Similarly, non-fluent aphasics more often rely on partners' verbalizations and assent to, or disagreement with, their guesses in producing yes/no gestures. Hence, communicative functions of gesture relate to content of verbal utterances, and it is not certain from the functional analysis that gesture can offer an alternative way of communicating when language is impaired.

Correlatively, there are methodological problems in assessing non-verbal communicative abilities. Aphasia can be described in brain-damaged people because some standard language uses are assumed in the population: every unimpaired person is believed able to say 'oven' when asked to do so when presented with the corresponding picture, and there is a conventional pronunciation of the word that is understood in the English-speaking community. Small variations may cause loss of meaning and 'oben', fo example, will be called a non-word. The morphology of gestural behaviour is much less constrained by formative rules, and diverse configurations may be observed when the attempt is made to represent objects or actions by gesture. Moreover, considerable individual differences exist in the disposition to gesture spontaneously during speech. Thus there is a problem in defining the normal appearance of non-verbal signals.

From such a perspective, it may be considered that the only true compensatory use of gesture is the creation of sign languages, as is the case among deaf-mute people. There is another problem with the functional value of the non-verbal behaviour in the normal population. Language uses are organized according to pragmatic rules allowing for agreement on topics of reference and for mutual comprehension through co-operation. Numerous linguistic devices allow understanding in spite of the unavoidable ambiguity of natural language in ordinary use. It may be that spontaneous gestural activity during speech is not produced to aid understanding and even that it is noticed by the listener. The primary function of co-verbal activity would then be not to communicate, but rather to assist the speaker in the task of planning verbal utterances (Rimé, 1983). The lack of constraints on the morphology and function of non-verbal signals is a reason for the underdevelopment of models tracing the path of information flow underlying motor and perceptual processes in coverbal activity. There may be diverse kinds of relationships between gestures and speech as there are diverse types of aphasic disturbances and thus no simple way to describe modifications of gestural behaviour in cases of language impairment. Studies showing the effects on gesture use of alterations that restrict to some defined components of the speech production process have yet to be done.

Emotional Behaviour

The hypothesis of right hemisphere superiority in emotional processing has oriented most of the studies on non-verbal expression and comprehension of emotion by aphasic subjects (Heilman and Satz, 1983). Right-and left-hemisphere lesions have different effects on both the expressive and the receptive levels in the processing of facial, vocal, and verbal expressions of emotions, but the question as to whether the differential contributions of the cerebral hemispheres in emotional behaviour relate to other cognitive processes remains open.

On the one hand, the problem arises of the interpretation of the observed lateral differences that could relate either to the emotional nature of the process or to the involved perceptual and motor processes (Feyereisen,

1986b; Gainotti, 1984). In one case, emotion is considered a specific domain. Similar consequences of unilateral brain damage for the emotional processing of vocal and facial cues are expected but not for the non-emotional processing of the stimuli. In the other case, the different emotional behaviours may relate to non-emotional ones, for instance, comprehension of facial expressions of emotion may relate to the recognition of facial identity, or the production of emotional prosody to the production of prosodic features that are linguistically determined.

On the other hand, the dissociation of representational and emotional non-verbal behaviours of aphasic subjects might result either from a reduced task demand in emotional processing or from a specificity of affective evaluation. Intact emotional behaviour of aphasic subjects has traditionally been interpreted as the result of automatic or sub-propositional processing. The assumption of specific mechanisms for affective evaluation seems to offer an alternative explanation for the spared behaviours, but the very nature of emotion would make the distinction between these two interpretations impossible. If emotional experience results from irruption of spontaneous motor scripts into controlled action (*see*, for example Leventhal, 1980), emotion is necessarily an automatic process. From such a perspective, affective motor or perceptual reactions are emotional when automatic, while the posing of facial expressions of emotion or interpreting verbal or non-verbal stimili as emotional cues would not constitute emotional but rather controlled processes. Accordingly, the behaviour of aphasic subjects might show impairment in these tasks while spontaneous emotional behaviour would be spared.

(A) Expression of Emotion

Clinical and experimental observations suggest intact spontaneous expression in left-hemisphere-damaged aphasic subjects and lack of expression in right-hemisphere-damaged patients. For example, Borod *et al.* (1985) presented pleasant and unpleasant scenes to normal and brain-damaged subjects who were instructed to 'describe their feelings and reactions'. The records of the session were shown to judges who rated the utilization of three channels: facial expression, intonation, and speech. The analysis of variance of the rating scores showed a group-by-channel interaction: the left-hemisphere-damaged subjects were judged to use facial and vocal channels most and the speech channel least. In the left-and right-hemisphere-damaged groups, facial expressiveness correlated with the use of emotional intonation, but neither measures correlated with speech expressiveness. Analyses of facial activity accompanying speech during interview or neuropsychological examination may also be noted in this context, even if the emotional nature of the recorded movements was not specified (Golper and Gordon, 1984; Katz *et al.*, 1978; Kolb and Milner, 1981b).

A systematic investigation of facial expressivity in brain-damaged subjects was conducted with the slide-viewing paradigm, where the inadvertent facial behaviour of the subject is filmed during presentations of different categories of slides (Duffy and Buck, 1979; Buck and Duffy, 1980). The film was then presented to judges who were asked to rate expressiveness and to guess the kind of slide viewed. The number of correct responses and the expressiveness measures were the independent variables. Aphasics did not differ from normal subjects and their performance did not correlate with their scores in the Porch Index of Communicative Ability or with their scores in a pantomime expression test. When severe aphasics were excluded, the right-hemisphere-damaged subjects were found significantly less accurate than normal and aphasic subjects. Whereas normal subjects showed decreasing accuracy from familiar, pleasant, unusual, to unpleasant slides, the performance of aphasics was above 40% accuracy in the four categories. Different results were observed in a similar experiment, where facial movements were recorded during the presentation of films arousing emotions (Mammucari *et al.*, 1986). A reduced number of adequate facial reactions to unpleasant films was found in both left- and right-hemisphere-damaged subjects, but reduced gaze avoidance only in the right-hemisphere-damaged group. This suggests that the reason for the difference between aphasics and right-hemisphere-damaged subjects lies more in the ability to experience negative emotions than in the control of facial activity.

Vocal expression of emotion is also assumed to be mainly controlled by the right hemisphere and, therefore, is spared in cases of aphasia. Some cases of right-hemisphere-lesioned patients have been reported in which the ability to express feelings by the tone of the voice was impaired (Ross, 1981, 1984). The objective analysis of vocal parameters confirmed the clinical judgement of speech monotony, but the deficit was not restricted to emotional prosody, and similar impairment in the use of propositional prosody, for example, the interrogative rise, was observed (Shapiro and Danly, 1985). Aphasics also show a modification of the prosodic features that are linguistically determined in relation to deficits observed in speech production (*see*, for example, Cooper and Zurif, 1983; Danly and Cooper, 1983; De Bleser and Poeck, 1985; Ryalls, 1982, 1984; Weniger, 1984). Very few comparable studies measuring parameters of vocal expression of emotion — speech tempo, pitch, loudness — are available, and evidence for the dissociation of affective and non-affective prosody in aphasia is still lacking. It might be that the peculiarities of vocal expression requires integration with speech production and thus bi-hemispheric control (Ross *et al.*, 1981). Nevertheless, the control mechanisms for speech production and vocal expression may dissociate, at least in a repetition task. Two cases of mixed transcortical aphasia could repeat the content, but not the emotional tone of sentences and spontaneous emotional behaviour was normal (Speedie,

Coslett and Heilman, 1984). Thus there is a left-hemisphere contribution in the control of emotional prosody but the extent to which it relates to the control of speech production and propositional prosody remains unknown.

The normal spontaneous facial activity of aphasic subjects contrasts with their impairments as demonstrated by oral apraxia tests, in which subjects are instructed to produce emotional or arbitrary movements like tongue protrusion and blowing (De Renzi *et al.*, 1966; Kolb and Milner, 1981a; Lehmkuhl *et al.*, 1983; Mateer and Kimura, 1977; Tognola and Vignolo, 1980). Similarly, the observation of facial asymmetry in brain-damaged subjects support the hypothesis of an intervention of the left cerebral hemisphere in the voluntary control of facial motility. Bruyer (1981a) analyzed facial asymmetry in brain-damaged subjects with normal judges choosing left or right composites as the most expressive. For sad and neutral poses, composites contralateral to the lesion were judged less expressive, which could be due to mild motor weakness of the hemiface controlled by the damaged hemisphere. No asymmetry appeared in posing for smiles in any of the groups. When the asymmetry of the mouth opening was measured in aphasic subjects, lateral differences appeared to vary with the nature of the elicited behaviour: singing and serial speech were left-sided, whereas greater right opening was observed during word-list generation, repetition, and conversation. This asymmetry was interpreted as an indication of contralateral hemispheric involvement (Graves and Landis, 1985). Thus both hemispheres might intervene in the control of facial movements depending on the different task demands.

Data on facial asymmetry in normal subjects have been discussed in the context of differences for spontaneous and posed emotional expression (*see* reviews in Borod and Koff, 1983; Campbell, 1986; Rinn, 1984). It is suggested that spontaneous movements are more symmetrical than deliberate ones; furthermore, the asymmetry of deliberate movements favours either the right or the left hemi-face (Hager and Ekman, 1985). In brain-damaged subjects, disorders of spontaneous or voluntary motility might result from different lesions. A lesion of the motor cortex would impair voluntary movements (facial hemiparesis) but spares spontaneous smiling (Monrad-Krohn, 1924), whereas damage to the supplementary motor area (medial part of the frontal lobe) would cause the inverse: more facial asymmetry in spontaneous emotional movement than in voluntary movement (Laplane *et al.*, 1976, 1977). However, comparison of posed and spontaneous expressions of positive and negative emotions in the same brain-damaged subjects revealed main effects of group and condition resulting from higher accuracy in left- than in right-hemisphere-damaged subjects and in posed than in spontaneous expression, but no group-by-condition interaction (Borod *et al.*, 1986). Thus, the pattern of lateralization did not change with the posed or spontaneous nature of the movement. Furthermore, accuracy in emotional expression did not correlate with performance on the oral apraxia test in aphasic subjects.

In summary, there are still interpretation problems concerning the respective role of each cerebral hemisphere in the control of emotional expression. On the one hand, emotional inexpressivity of right-hemisphere-damaged subjects could be due either to a disturbance of the control mechanisms of movements or to an inability to experience emotions in experimental or everyday situations. On the other hand, there are conflicting data from aphasic subjects showing intact emotional expressivity and impaired control of the oro-facial musculature involved in vocal or facial expression, but it is not certain that the discrepancy results from dissociation between posed and spontaneous behaviour. The difference seems rather due to methodological reasons: impairments are observed mainly when the quality of movement execution is rated or when expressive behaviour is objectively analyzed, but normality in appearance is suggested by studies assessing the communicative value of facial or vocal expression. Thus aphasic subjects might still remain able to convey feelings non-verbally even though their means are impaired.

(B) Comprehension of Emotion Cues

The hypothesis of right-hemisphere dominance in emotional processing has also inspired several studies on the interpretation of emotional expressions in brain-damaged subjects. The first systematic observations bore on the comprehension of intonation.

(1) Prosody

Better performance of aphasic than of right-hemisphere-damaged subjects in decoding paralinguistic cues of emotion have been reported by several authors (*see*, for example Heilman, Scholes and Watson, 1975; Tucker, Watson and Heilman, 1977). This advantage may be interpreted in two non-exclusive ways. The difference could result from a dissociation between comprehension of prosody and of words: aphasic subjects could still understand prosodic feature that are linguistically determined (interrogation, stress, etc.). There could also be a dissociation between the emotional and the propositional processing of the utterance. Access to affective meaning would be spared in cases of auditory comprehension disorders, but decoding the linguistically determined prosodic features would be impaired.

The hypothesis of independent processing of prosody and verbal content suggests a dissociation between disorders of paralinguistic and linguistic comprehension, although several studies report impairments in understanding prosodic cues of emotion in aphasics (Schlanger, Schlanger and Gerstman, 1976; Seron *et al.*, 1982). Comprehension of non-emotional prosody is also impaired, sometimes even in subjects with good verbal comprehension. Conversely, an aphasic subject with impaired comprehension and repetition was reported to be able to process normally emotional and non-emotional prosody (Heilman *et al.*, 1984). Dichotic presentation of intonation contours (transmitting emotional or non-emotional information) identified in a multiple-choice task resulted in impaired performance of aphasic as compared with normal subjects when the responses to right-ear stimulation were analyzed, whereas the responses to the left ear did not significantly differ in the two groups (Hartje, Willmes and Weniger, 1985). In a parallel task of dichotic presentation of syllable triplets, stimulation to both ears resulted in impaired performances. Thus, in aphasic subjects the intact right hemisphere performed at a normal level only when the prosodic information from the left ear was processed. Similarly, right-hemisphere-lesioned subjects showed less impaired performance in prosodic tasks when stimulations to the right ear than when stimulations to the left ear were analyzed ($p = 0.048$, judged to be non-significant by the authors, versus $p<0.001$). This suggests two sources of impairments in aphasic subjects: first, a degradation of input transiting by the left hemisphere (right ear stimulation), and second a genuine contribution of the left hemisphere to the processing of prosody, as shown by the better performance of right-hemisphere-damaged subjects when the stimulation to the right ear was analyzed. This contribution of the left hemisphere could vary with task demands. Left posterior lesions impaired identification, but not discrimination of emotional prosody (Denes *et al.*, 1984). Similarly, left-hemisphere-damaged subjects processed emotional prosody as efficiently as normal subjects in a discrimination task and in identification between two alternatives but performed more poorly when the response had to be selected from four labels (Tomkins and Flowers, 1985).

Some observations suggest that the emotional content of a sentence facilitates speech understanding by aphasic subjects. If so, attribution of emotional meaning would be easier when the speech content and the prosody of a sentence are congruent then when they are not, even for subjects suffering from verbal comprehension disorders; this expected result was observed by Seron *et al.* (1982). Intermediate performance was noted for neutral sentences when the judgements were based on prosody only. The other control sentences — neutral prosody and emotionally loaded content — were not presented. Also consistent with the hypothesis is the group-by-type of prosody interaction observed by Heilman *et al.* (1984). Although impaired in both conditions when compared with normal subjects, aphasic subjects better understood emotional than non-emotional prosody. In summary, both hemispheres intervene in the comprehension of vocal expression, but the extent to which their contribution relates to other emotional or prosodic processing remains unknown.

(2) Facial expressions

Analysis of the comprehension of facial expressions of emotions in brain-damaged subjects typically shows superior performances of aphasic subjects as compared with right-hemisphere-damaged subjects but impairments of both lesioned groups as compared with normal subjects. The impairment of aphasic subjects was first reported by Cicone, Wapner and Gardner (1980) and by De Kosky *et al.* (1980) and then confirmed by Goldblum (1980) and Blunk (1982). In Katz' (1980) study, the aphasics did not differ as a group from normal subjects, but a deficit was observed in the five most severe cases. This study suggests that discrepant results reported by Borod *et al.* (1986) and Etcoff(1984a), who found no differences in the perception of facial expressions by normal and aphasic subjects, could be due to population sampling and possible exclusion of severe aphasias.

Apart from studies showing more severe disturbances in interpreting facial expressions in right-hemisphere-damaged than in left-hemisphere-damaged subjects, other data do not show statistical differences between these two groups (Kremin, 1980; Kurucz *et al.*, 1980; Prigatano and Pribram, 1982). The results of the two last studies are difficult to interpret because of the verbal nature of the experimental task, which could have disturbed aphasic subjects, and because of the small size of the sample, which could have favoured the type II error in the statistical inference (non-significant results do not necessarily demonstrate the absence of true differences). More interesting is the fact that the most impaired population turned out to be that of the bilateral brain-damaged subjects. Along with the very poor performance of split-brain subjects in interpreting facial expression (Benowitz *et al.*, 1983), these observations suggest that both hemispheres have to co-operate to understand emotion in facial movements. The conditions for such co-operation cannot be identified until the nature of the contribution of each hemisphere is specified.

Different results suggest disturbances of different natures in right-hemisphere-damaged and in left-hemisphere-damaged subjects. For example, Cicone *et al.* (1980) examined the processing of facial expressions in a task where the subjects chose from four photographs the item corresponding to the target face representing positive emotions (joy, surprise) or negative emotions (sadness, disgust, fear, anger). The multiple choice gave the correct response, an expression of the same polarity, an expression of the opposite polarity, and a neutral expression. A significant group-by-emotion interaction was observed, the happy face being often correctly interpreted by the normal and left-hemisphere-damaged subjects but rarely so by the right-hemisphere-damaged subjects. The groups also differed by the nature of their errors: most of the subjects chose the face of the same polarity more often than the face of the opposite polarity, but the right-hemisphere-damaged subjects showed the reverse pattern. It is thus suggested that the conceptual structure of emotion could be spared in aphasia but not by right-hemisphere lesions, but this hypothesis is not supported by several studies on right-hemisphere-damaged subjects showing normal emotional processing in other modalities than facial expression. These subjects could be helped by the verbal nature of the task (Kolb and Taylor, 1981; Etcoff, 1984b) and could be less impaired when they had to process vocal or postural cues than facial expressions (Benowitz *et al.*, 1983). Furthermore, their deficit in processing facial expressions of emotions did not relate to their reduced emotional arousal measured by the electrodermal response (Zoccolotti *et al.*, 1982).

Another difference between aphasic and right-hemisphere-damaged subjects is in the processing of facial identity, which would be spared in the former, but impaired in the latter. In the study by De Kosky *et al.* (1980), three groups of subjects (nine right-hemisphere-damaged subjects with hemi-neglect, nine conduction aphasics, and nine neurological controls) processed facial expressions in same/different judgements of identity or of expression on two photographs, naming the emotion shown on a face and pointing to the face expressing a given emotion. When the groups were equalized by taking into account their scores in the facial identity judgement, the two brain-damaged groups showed similar impairments in the three emotional tasks. It was thus suggested that the impairments evidenced by the right-hemisphere-damaged subjects related to other visual processing of faces, while they did not in aphasics.

An experimental analysis of the relationship between the interpretation of facial expressions and facial recognition partially supported this hypothesis (Etcoff, 1984a). Separation of the processes was shown in normal and aphasic subjects, i.e. subjects with an intact right-hemisphere, since right-hemisphere lesions disrupt both, but some cases of dissociation were observed among right-hemisphere-damaged subjects. Similarly, Bowers *et al.* (1985) did not replicate the results of the co-variance analysis by De Kosky *et al.* (1980) but observed again impairments in left hemisphere-damaged subjects in the two most difficult conditions: discrimination of facial identity when expressions differed and emotion discrimination when identities differed. It may be accepted that interpreting facial expression dissociates from processing facial identity. This specific process could be impaired by a left-hemisphere lesion but less severely than by a right-hemisphere lesion.

Divergent explanations for the aphasic behaviour in processing emotional faces have been proposed. On the basis of significant correlations between the verbal and the non-verbal matching of facial expressions and of gestures, Kremin (1980) argued for a general disturbance of comprehension that would not be material specific. Similarly, an inability to match facial expressions could be related to other well-documented non-verbal impairments in matching tasks involving sounds, colours, pictures, or pantomimes (*see* above). De Kosky *et al.* (1980) observed that the aphasic subjects performed normally in the two judgement tasks but not in the verbal tasks. This result was expected as far as naming is concerned, but the impaired pointing in subjects with spared comprehension of isolated words was more surprising. The authors suggested a disconnection between the language area and the 'emotional areas' of the right hemisphere. But such an explanation would not account for the deficit observed in other studies using non-verbal tasks. Some authors have suggested a covert linguistic mediation in matching facial expressions, but left-hemisphere-damaged patients without aphasia do not score significantly better than aphasic subjects in these tasks (Goldblum, 1980; Kremin, 1980). In these cases, perceptual processes might be disturbed by posterior lesions, but a visual field defect does not seem to be a critical factor in left-hemisphere-damaged subjects (Goldblum, 1980; Bruyer, 1981b). Finally, the most satisfactory interpretation could be that the left hemisphere plays a significant role in processing visual information, as suggested by Sergent (1983, 1984). Variations of aphasic performances with characteristics of input and task demands have yet to be analyzed from such a perspective.

Conclusions

Regarding the problematic issue of specificity of emotional processing, one might consider that emotions constitute a special cognitive domain. Zajonc (1980, 1984) argues for very rapid affective categorization and that 'preferences need no inferences'. To some extent, emotional evaluation has the properties of a module as an input system in Fodor's (1983) sense: they are rapid, mandatory, and give only limited access to consciousness. Inconclusive evidence from the neuropsychological study of emotion probably results from methodological problems in eliciting emotions in experimental situations. It is not certain, therefore, that impairments shown by brain-damaged subjects, more particularly after right-hemisphere lesions, relate to emotional processing. Correlatively, defective performances of aphasic subjects may be due to either a genuine left hemisphere contribution or to ineffective elicitation of emotion in the task.

General Conclusions

There is little doubt at present that aphasia is often associated with non-verbal disorders. The discussion bears on the interpretation of that association. Either the verbal, gestural, and perceptual deficits are different aspects of a single impairment that manifests itself in several modalities (common representations are assumed to underly word finding, gesture production, or comprehension, and a disruption on this level explains the several observed disorders) or the different elements of the syndrome are to be considered statistically, but not necessarily, associated, and the fact that impairments sometimes dissociate would demonstrate the fractionation of the cognitive system into separate processing units for modality-specific representations. An intermediate position would be to consider that some cases of aphasia are explained by general conceptual deficit, and others by modality-specific disorders. For example, difficulties in naming, semantic errors in word comprehension, and an inability to establish semantic relationships between pictures of objects could, when associated, all depend on a disorganization of the conceptual system underlying these operations (Gainotti, 1982). Isolated impairments might also occur (naming difficulty without comprehension deficit, for instance) and these cases would show defective functioning of lower level modality-specific processes. Thus identification of defective operations is partly an empirical question and different patterns of dissolutions in individual case studies should be described (Marshall, 1986) in relation to models of normal functioning and by the experimental analysis of the variables influencing verbal and non-verbal behaviour.

References

ABRAHAMSEN, A., CAVALLO, M.M. and MCCLUER, J.A. Is the sign advantage a robust phenomenon? From gesture to language in two modalities. *Merrill-Palmer Quarterly* (1985), **31**, 177-209.

AGOSTINI, E., COLETTI, A., ORLANDO, G. and TREDICI, G. Apraxia in deep cerebral lesions. *Journal of Neurology, Neurosurgery and Psychiatry* (1983), **46**, 804-808.

ASSAL, G. and REGLI, F. Syndrome de disconnexion visuo-verbale et visuo-gestuelle. Aphasie optique et apraxie optique. *Revue Neurologique* (1980), **136**, 365-376.

BASSO, A., LUZZATTI, C. and SPINNLER, H. Is ideomotor apraxia the outcome of damage to well-defined regions of the left hemisphere? Neuropsychological study of CAT correlations. *Journal of Neurology, Neurosurgery, and Psychiatry* (1980), **43**, 118-126.

BATES, E., BRETHERTON, I., SHORE, C. and MCNEW, S. Names, gestures, and objects: Symbolization in infancy and aphasia. In K.E. Nelson (ed.) *Children's language, Vol. 4* (1983) pp. 59-123. Hillsdale, N.J.: Lawrence Erlbaum Associates.

BEHRMANN, M. and PENN, C. Non-verbal communication of aphasic patients. *British Journal of Disorders of Communication* (1984), **19**, 155-168.

BENOWITZ, L.L., BEAR, D.M., ROSENTHAL, R., MESULAM, M.M., ZAIDEL, E. and SPERRY, R.W. Hemispheric specialization in non-verbal communication. *Cortex* (1983), **19**, 5-11.

BERTELSON, P. Lateral differences in normal man and lateralization of brain function. *International Journal of Psychology* (1982), **17**, 173-210.

BLUNK, R. Recognition of emotion and physiognomy in right- and left-hemisphere damaged patients and normals. Deauville: Presented at the International Neuropsychological Society Meeting (1982).

BOROD, J.C. and KOFF, E. Asymmetries in affective facial expression: behavior and anatomy. In N. Fox and R. Davidson (eds), *The Psychobiology of Affective Development* (1983), pp. 293-323. Hillsdale, N.J.: Lawrence Erlbaum Associates.

BOROD, J.C., KOFF, E., PERLMAN, M. and NICHOLAS, M. Channels of emotional expression in patients with unilateral brain damage. *Archives of Neurology* (1985), **42**, 345-348.

BOROD, J.C., KOFF, E., PERLMAN-LORCH, M. and NICHOLAS, M. The expression and perception of facial emotion in brain-damaged patients. *Neuropsychologia* (1986), **24**, 169-180.

BOWERS, D., BAUER, R.M., COSLETT, H.B. and HEILMAN, K.M. Processing of faces by patients with unilateral hemisphere lesions. I. Dissociation between judgment of facial affect and facial identity. *Brain and Cognition* (1985), **4**, 258-272.

BRADSHAW, J.L. and NETTLETON, N.C. The nature of hemispheric specialization in man. *The Behavioral and Brain Sciences* (1981), **4**, 51-91.

BRUYER, R. Asymmetry of facial expression in brain damaged subjects. *Neuropsychologia* (1981a), **19**, 615-624.

BRUYER, R. Perception d'expressions faciales émotionnelles et lésion cérébrale: influence de la netteté du stimulus. *International Journal of Psychology* (1981b), **16**, 87-94.

BUCK, R. and DUFFY, R.J. Non-verbal communication of affect in brain damaged patients. *Cortex* (1980), **16**, 351-362.

BUTTERWORTH, B., SWALLOW, J. and GRIMSTON, M. Gestures and lexical processes in jargonaphasia. In J. Brown (ed.) *Jargonaphasia* (1981), pp. 113-124. New York/ London: Academic Press.

CAMPBELL, R. Asymmetries of facial action: Some facts and fancies of normal face movement. In R. Bruyer (ed.), *The Neuropsychology of Face Perception and Facial Expression* (1986), pp. 247-267. Hillsdale, N.J.: Lawrence Erlbaum Associates.

CARMON, A. Sequenced motor performance in patients with unilateral cerebral lesions. *Neuropsychologia* (1971), **9**, 445-449.

CHRISTOPOULOU, C. and BONVILLIAN, J.D. Sign language, pantomime, and gestural processing in aphasic persons: A review. *Journal of Communication Disorders* (1985), **18**, 1-20.

CICONE, M., WAPNER, W., FOLDI, N., ZURIF, E., and GARDNER, H. The relation between gesture and language in aphasic communication. *Brain and Language* (1979), **8**, 324-349.

CICONE, WAPNER, W. and GARDNER, H. Sensitivity to emotional expressions and situations in organic patients. *Cortex* (1980), **16**, 145-158.

COHEN, G. Theoretical interpretations of lateral asymmetries. In J.G. Beaumont(ed.), *Divided Visual Field Studies of Cerebral Organization* (1982), pp. 87-111. London/ New York: Academic Press.

COHEN, R., KELTER, S., and WOLL, G. Analytical competence and language impairment in aphasia. *Brain and Language* (1980), **10**, 331-347.

COOPER, W.E., and ZURIF, E.B. Aphasia: Information processing in language production and reception. In B. Butterworth (ed.), *Language Production, Vol. 2* (1983), pp. 225-256. London: Academic Press.

DANILOFF, J.K., NOLL, J.D., FRISTOE, M. and LLOYD, L.L. Gesture recognition in patients with aphasia. *Journal of Speech and Hearing Disorders* (1982), **47**, 43-49.

DANLY, M. and COOPER, W.E. Fundamental frequency, language processing and linguistic structure in Wernicke's aphasia. *Brain and Language* (1983), **19**, 1-24.

DAVIS, G.A. and WILCOX, M.J. Incorporating parameters of natural conversation in treatment. In R. Chapey (ed.) *Language Intervention Strategies in Adult Aphasia* (1981), pp. 169-183. Baltimore/London: Williams & Wilkins.

DAVIS, S.A., ARTES, R. and HOOPS, R. Verbal expression and expressive pantomime in aphasic patients. In Y. Lebrun and R. Hoops (eds) *Problems of Aphasia* (1979), pp. 109-123. Lisse: Swets and Zeitlinger.

DE AJURIAGUERRA, J., HÉCAEN, H. and ANGELERGUES, R. Les apraxies: Variétés cliniques et latéralisation lésionnelle. *Revue Neurologique* (1960), **102**, 566-594.

DE BLESER, R. and POECK, K. Analysis of prosody in the spontaneous speech of patients with CV-recurring utterances. *Cortex* (1985), **21**, 405-416.

DE KOSKY, S.T., HEILMAN, K.M., BOWERS, D.J. and VALENSTEIN, E. Recognition and discrimination of emotional faces and pictures. *Brain and Language* (1980), **9**, 206-214.

DENES, G., CALDOGNETTA, E., SEMENZA, C., VAGGES, K. and ZETTIN, M. Discrimination and identification of emotions in human voice by brain-damaged subjects. *Acta Neurologica Scandinavica* (1984), **69**, 154-162.

DE RENZI, E., FAGLIONI, P., LODESANI, M. and VECCHI, A. Performance of left brain damaged patients on imitation of single movements and motor sequences. Frontal and parietal-injured patients compared. *Cortex* (1983), **19**, 333-343.

DE RENZI, E., FAGLIONI, P., and SORGATO, P. Modality-specific and supramodal mechanisms of apraxia. *Brain* (1982), **105**, 301-312.

DE RENZI, E., MOTTI, F. and NICHELLI, P. Imitating gestures: A quantitative approach to ideomotor apraxia. *Archives of Neurology* (1980), **37**, 6-10.

DE RENZI, E., PIECZURO, A. and VIGNOLO, L.A. Oral apraxia and aphasia. *Cortex* (1966), **2**, 50-73.

DRUMMOND, S.S. and RENTSCHLER, G.J. The efficacy of gestural cueing in dysphasic word-retrieval responses. *Journal of Communication Disorders* (1981), **14**, 287-298.

DUFFY, J.R. and WATKINS, L.B. The effect of response choice relatedness on pantomime and verbal recognition ability in aphasic patients. *Brain and Language* (1984), **21**, 291-306.

DUFFY, R.J. and BUCK, R.W. A study of the relationship between propositional (pantomime) and subpropositional (facial expression) extraverbal behaviors in aphasics. *Folia Phoniatrica* (1979), **31**, 129-136.

DUFFY, R.J. and DUFFY, J.R. Three studies of deficits in pantomimic expression and pantomimic recognition in aphasia. *Journal of Speech and Hearing Research* (1981), **24**, 70-84.

DUFFY, R.J., DUFFY, J.R. and MERCAITIS, P.A. Comparison of the performances of a fluent and a nonfluent aphasic on a pantomimic referential task. *Brain and Language* (1984), **21**, 260-273.

DUFFY, R.J., DUFFY, J.R. and PEARSON, K.L. Pantomime recognition in aphasics. *Journal of Speech and Hearing Research* (1975), **18**, 115-132.

DUFFY, R.J. and LILES, B.Z. A translation of Finkelnburg's (1870) lecture on aphasia as 'asymbolia' with commentary. *Journal of Speech and Hearing Disorders* (1979), **44**, 156-168.

DUFFY, R.J. and MCEWEN, W.J. A study of the relationship between pantomime symbolism and pantomime recognition in aphasics. *Folia Phoniatrica* (1978), **30**, 286-292.

EHRLICHMAN, H. and WEINBERGER, A. Lateral eye movements and hemispheric asymmetry: a critical review. *Psychological Bulletin* (1978), **85**, 1080-1101.

ETCOFF, N.L. Selective attention to facial identity andf facial emotion. *Neuropsychologia* (1984a), **22**, 281-295.

ETCOFF, N.L. Perceptual and conceptual organization of facial emotions: hemispheric differences. *Brain and Cognition* (1984b), **3**, 385-412.

FERRO, J.M., MARIANO, M.G., CASTRO-CALDAS, A. and SANTOS, M.E. Gesture recognition in aphasia: A recovery study. Chianciano: Presented at the International Neuropsychological Society Meeting (1980a).

FERRO, J.M., SANTOS, M.E. CASTRO-CALDAS, A. and MARIANO, G. Gesture recognition in aphasia. *Journal of Clinical Neuropsychology* (1980b), **2**, 277-292.

FERRO, J.M., MARTINS, I.P., MARIANO, G. and CASTRO-CALDAS, A. CT scan correlates of gesture recognition. *Journal of Neurology, Neurosurgery, and Psychiatry* (1983), **46**, 943-952.

FEYEREISEN, P. Manual activity during speaking in aphasic subjects. *International Journal of Psychology* (1983), **18**, 545-556.

FEYEREISEN, P. How do aphasic patients differ in sentence production? *Linguistics* (1984), **22**, 687-710.

FEYEREISEN, P. Lateral differences in gesture production. In J.L. Nespoulous, P. Perron and A.R. Lecours (eds) *The Biological Foundation of Gesture: Motor and Semiotic Aspects* (1986a), pp. 77-94. Hillsdale, N.J.: Lawrence Erlbaum Associates.

FEYEREISEN, P. Production and comprehension of emotional facial expressions in brain-damaged subjects. In R. Bruyer (ed.), *The Neuropsychology of Face Perception and Facial Expression* (1986b), pp. 221-245. Hillsdale, N.J.: Lawrence Erlbaum Associates.

FEYEREISEN, P. and DE LANNOY, J.-D. (1985). *La Psychologie du Geste* Brussels/Liège: P. Mardaga.

FEYEREISEN, P. and LIGNIAN, A. La direction du regard chez les aphasiques en conversation: une observation pilote. *Cahiers de Psychologie Cognitive* (1981), **1**, 287-298.

FEYEREISEN, P. and SERON, X. Nonverbal communication and aphasia, a review: I. Comprehension. II. Expression. *Brain and Language* (1982), **16**, 191-212, 213-236.

FEYEREISEN, P. and SERON, X. Les troubles de la communication gestuelle. *La Recherche* (1984), **15**, 156-164.

FEYEREISEN, P., SERON, X. and DE MACAR, M.A. L'interprétation de différentes catégories de gestes chez des sujets aphasiques. *Neuropsychologia* (1981), **19**, 515-521.

FEYEREISEN, P. VERBEKE-DEWITTE, C. and SERON, X. On fluency measures in aphasic speech. *Journal of Clinical and Experimental Neuropsychology* (1986), **8**, 393-404.

FODOR, J.A. *The Modularity of Mind* (1983). Cambridge, Ma.: The MIT Press.

FOLDI, N.S., CICONE, M. and GARDNER, H. Pragmatic aspects of communication in brain-damaged patients. In S.J. Segalowitz (ed.) *Language Function and Brain Organization* (1983), pp. 51-86. New-York & London: Academic Press.

GAINOTTI, G. Some aspects of semantic-lexical impairment in aphasia. *Applied Psycholinguistics* (1982), **3**, 279-294.

GAINOTTI, G. Some methodological problems in the study of the relationships between emotion and cerebral dominance. *Journal of Clinical Neuropsychology* (1984), **6**, 111-121.

GAINOTTI, G. and LEMMO, M.A. Comprehension of symbolic gestures in aphasia. *Brain and Language* (1976), **3**, 451-460.

GARRETT, M.F. Production of speech: observations from normal and pathological language use. In A.W. Ellis (ed.) *Normality and Pathology in Cognitive Functions* (1982), pp. 19-76. London/New York: Academic Press.

GESCHWIND, N. The apraxias: Neural mechanisms of disorders of learned movement. *American Scientist* (1975), **63**, 188-195.

GLOSSER, G., WIENER, M. and KAPLAN, E. Communicative gestures in aphasia. *Brain and Language* (1986), **27**, 345-359.

GOLDBLUM, M.C. Les troubles des gestes d'accompagnement du langage au cours des lésions corticales unilatérales. In H. Hécaen and M. Jeannerod (eds) *Du contrôle moteur à l'organisation du geste* (1978) pp. 383-395. Paris: Masson.

GOLDBLUM, M.C. La reconnaissance des expressions faciales émotionnelles et conventionnelles au cours de lésions corticales. *Revue Neurologique* (1980), **136**, 711-719.

GOLPER, L.A.C., GORDON, M.E. and RAU, M.T. Coverbal behavior and perceptions of organicity. Aachen: Communication at the International Neuropsychological Society Meeting (1984).

GOODGLASS, H. and KAPLAN, E. Disturbance of gesture and pantomime in aphasia. *Brain* (1963), **86**, 703-720.

GRAVES, R. and LANDIS, T. Hemispheric control of speech expression in aphasia. A mouth asymmetry study. *Archives of Neurology* (1985), **42**, 249-251.

GRAVES, R., GOODGLASS, H. and LANDIS, T. Mouth asymmetry during spontaneous speech. *Neuropsychologia* (1982), **20**, 371-381.

GRAVES, R., LANDIS, R. and SSIMPSON, C. On the interpretation of mouth asymmetry. *Neuropsychologia* (1985), **23**, 121-122.

GROBER, E., PERECMAN, E., KELLAR, L. and BROWN, J. Lexical knowledge in anterior and posterior aphasics. *Brain and Language* (1980), **10**, 318-330.

HAALAND, K.Y. The relationship of limb apraxia severity to motor and language deficits. *Brain and Cognition* (1984), **3**, 307-316.

HAALAND, K.Y. and FLAHERTY, D. The different types of limb apraxia errors made by patients with left vs. right hemisphere damage. *Brain and Cognition* (1984), **3**, 370-384.

HAGER, J.C. and EKMAN, P. The asymmetry of facial actions is inconsistent with models of hemispheric specialization. *Psychophysiology* (1985), **22**, 307-318.

HAGER, J.C. and VAN GELDER, R.S. Asymmetry of speech actions. *Neuropsychologia* (1985), **23**, 119-120.

HAMPSON, E. and KIMURA, D. Hand movement asymmetries during verbal and nonverbal tasks. *Canadian Journal of Psychology* (1984), **38**, 102-125.

HARTJE, W., WILLMES, K. and WENIGER, D. Is there parallel and independent hemispheric processing of intonational and phonetic components of dichotic speech stimuli? *Brain and Language* (1985), **24**, 83-99.

HÉCAEN, H. Les apraxies idéomotrices: essai de dissociation. In H. Hécaen and M. Jeannerod (eds), *Du contrôle moteur à l'organisation du geste* (1978), pp. 343-358. Paris: Masson.

HEILMAN, K.M., BOWERS, D., SPEEDIE, L. and COSLETT, H.B. Comprehension of affective and nonaffective prosody. *Neurology* (1984), **34**, 917-921.

HEILMAN, K.M., GONYEA, E.F. and GESCHWIND, N. Apraxia and agraphia in a right-hander. *Cortex* (1974), **10**, 284-288.

HEILMAN, K.M., ROTHI, L. and KERTESZ, A. Localization of apraxia-producing lesions. In A. Kertesz (ed.) *Localization in Neuropsychology* (1983), pp. 371-392. New York/London: Academic Press.

HEILMAN, K.M., ROTHI, L. and VALENSTEIN, E. Two forms of ideomotor apraxia. *Neurology* (1982), **32**, 342-346.

HEILMAN, K.M. and SATZ, P. (eds) *Neuropsychology of Human Emotion* (1983). New York & London: Guildford Press.

HEILMAN, K.M., SCHOLES, R. amd WATSON, R.T. Auditory affective agnosia. Disturbed comprehension of affective speech. *Journal of Neurology, Neurosurgery, and Psychiatry* (1975), **38**, 69-72.

HEILMAN, K.M., SCHWARTZ, H.D. and GESCHWIND, N. Defective motor learning in ideomotor apraxia. *Neurology* (1975), **25**, 1018-1020.

HELM-ESTABROOKS, N., FITZPATRICK, P.M. and BARRESI, B. Visual action therapy for global aphasia. *Journal of Speech and Hearing Disorders* (1982), **47**, 385-389.

HERRMANN, M., REICHLE, Th., LUCIUS, G., WALLESCH, C. and JOHANSSEN-HORBACH, H. Analyse nonverbaler Kommunikation bei Aphasikern und deren Partnern. Bad Hersfeld: Paper presented at *The Annual Conference of the German Association for Psychosomatic Medicine* (1985).

HOLLAND, A.L. Observing functional communication in aphasic adults. *Journal of Speech and Hearing Disorders* (1982), **47**, 50-56.

JASON, G.W. Hemispheric asymmetries in motor function: I. Left-hemisphere specialization for memory but not performance. II. Ordering does not contribute to left-hemisphere specialization. *Neuropsychologia* (1983), **21**, 35-45, 47-58.

JASON, G.W. Manual sequence learning after focal cortical lesions. *Neuropsychologia* (1985) **23**, 483-496.

KADISH, J. A neuropsychological approach to the study of gesture and pantomime in aphasia. *The South African Journal of Communication Disorders* (1978), **25**, 102-117.

KATZ, R.C. Perception of facial affect in aphasia. In R.H. Brookshire (ed.) *Clinical Aphasiology. Proceedings of the Conference* (1980), pp. 78-88. Minneapolis: BRK Publishers.

KATZ, R.C., LAPOINTE, L.L. and MARKEL, N.N. Coverbal behavior and aphasic speakers. In R.H. Brookshire (ed.) *Clinical Aphasiology. Proceedings of the Conference* (1978), pp. 164-173. Minneapolis: BRK Publishers.

KELSO, J.A.S. and TULLER, B. Toward a theory of apractic syndromes. *Brain and Language* (1981), **12**, 224-245.

KELSO, J.A.S., TULLER', B., and HARRIS, K.S. A 'dynamic pattern' perspective on the control and coordination of movement. In P.F. MacNeilage (ed.) *The Production of Speech* (1983), pp. 137-173. New York/Berlin: Springer.

KENDON, A. Gesture and speech: How they interact. In J.M. Wiemann and R.P. Harrison (eds) *Nonverbal Interaction* (1983), pp. 13-45. Sage Annual Reviews of Communication Research, Vol. 11. London/Beverly Hills/New Delhi: Sage.

KERTESZ, A. and FERRO, J.M. Lesion size and location in ideomotor apraxia. *Brain* (1984), **107**, 921-933.

KERTESZ, A., FERRO, J.M. and SHEWAN, C.M. Apraxia and aphasia: The functional-anatomical basis for their dissociation. *Neurology* (1984), **34**, 40-47.

KERTESZ, A. and HOOPER, P. Praxis and language: The extent and variety of apraxia in aphasia. *Neuropsychologia* (1982), **20**, 275-286.

KIMURA, D. Manual activity during speaking. I. Right-handers. II. Left-handers. *Neuropsychologia* (1973), **11**, 45-50, 51-55.

KIMURA, D. The neural basis of language qua gesture. In H. Whitaker and H.A. Whitaker (eds), *Studies in Neurolinguistics, Vol. 2* (1976), pp. 145-156. New York/ London: Academic Press.

KIMURA, D. Acquisition of a motor skill after left-hemisphere damage. *Brain* (1977), **100**, 527-542.

KIMURA, D. Left-hemisphere control of oral and brachial movements and their relation to communication. *Philosophical Transactions of the Royal Society of London, Serie B* (1982), **298**, 135-149.

KIMURA, D. and ARCHIBALD, Y. Motor functions of the left hemisphere. *Brain* (1974), **97**, 337-350.

KIMURA, D. and HUMPHRYS, C.A. A comparison of left- and right-arm movements during speaking. *Neuropsychologia* (1981), **19**, 807-812.

KINSBOURNE, M. and HISCOCK, M. Asymmetries of dual-task performances. In J.B. Hellige (ed.) *Cerebral Hemisphere Asymmetry: Method, Theory, and Application* (1983), pp. 255-334. New York: Praeger.

KOLB, B. and MILNER, B. Performance of complex arm and facial movements after focal brain lesions. *Neuropsychologia* (1981a), **19**, 491-503.

KOLB, B. and MILNER, B. Observations of spontaneous facial expression after cerebral excisions and after intracarotid injection of sodium amytal. *Neuropsychologia* (1981b), **19**, 505-514.

KOLB, B. and TAYLOR, L. Affective behavior in patients with localized cortical excisions: role of lesion site and side. *Science* (1981), **214**, 89-91.

KREMIN, H. Recognition of faces, facial expressions and gestures in brain damaged patients. Chianciano: Communication at the International Neuropsychological Society Meeting (1980).

KURUCZ, J., SONI, A., FELDMAR, G. and SLADE, W.R. Prosopo-affective agnosia and CT findings in patients with cerebral disorders. *Journal of the American Geriatrics Society* (1980), **28**, 475-478.

LABOUREL, D. Communication non verbale et aphasie. In X. Seron and C. Laterre (eds) *Rééduquer le Cerveau* (1982) pp. 93-108. Bruxelles: Mardaga.

LAPLANE, D., ORGOGOZO, J.M., MEININGER, V. and DEGAS, J.D. Paralysie faciale avec dissociation automatico-volontaire inverse par lésion frontale. Son origine corticale. Ses relations avec l'AMS. *Revue Neurologique* (1976), **132**, 725-734.

LAPLANE, D., TALAIRACH, J., MEININGER, V., BANCAUD, J. and ORGOGOZO, J.M.

Clinical consequences of corticectomies involving the supplementary motor area in Man. *Journal of the Neurological Sciences* (1977), **34**, 301-314.

LEHMKUHL, G., POECK, K. and WILLMES, K. Ideomotor apraxia and aphasia: An examination of types and manifestations of apraxic symptom. *Neuropsychologia* (1983), **21**, 199-212.

LEVENTHAL, H. Toward a comprehensive theory of emotion. In L. Berkowitz (ed.) *Advances in Experimental Social Psychology, Vol. 13* (1980), pp. 139-207. New York/London: Academic Press.

LUFTIG, R.L. Variables influencing the learnability of individual signs and sign lexicons: A review of the literature. *Journal of Psycholinguistic Research* (1983), **12**, 361-376.

LURIA, A.R. *The Role of Speech in the Regulation of Normal and Abnormal Behaviour* (1961). New York/Oxford: Pergamon.

MCNEILL, D. So you think gestures are nonverbal? *Psychological Review* (1985), **92**, 350-371.

MAMMUCARI, A., CALTAGIRONE, C., PIZZAMIGLIO, L. and GAINOTTI, G. Spontaneous facial expressions in brain-damaged patients. Bressanone: Poster presented at *Fourth European Workshop on Cognitive Neuropsychology* (1986).

MARSHALL, J.C. The description and interpretation of aphasic language disorder. *Neuropsychologia* (1986), **24**, 5-24.

MATEER, C. and KIMURA, D. Impairment of nonverbal oral movements in aphasia. *Brain and Language* (1977), **4**, 262-276.

MONRAD-KROHN, G.H. On the dissociation of voluntary and emotional innervation in facial paresis of central origin. *Brain* (1924), **47**, 22-35.

MOODY, J.E. Sign Language acquisition by a global aphasic. *The Journal of Nervous and Mental Disease* (1982), **170**, 113-116.

MORAIS, J. The two sides of cognition. In J. Mehler, M. Garrett and E. Walkes (eds), *Perspectives on Mental Representations* (1982), pp. 277-309. Hillsdale, N.J.: Lawrence Erlbaum Associates.

NESPOULOUS, J.L. Geste et discours: Etude du comportement gestuel spontané d'un aphasique en situation de dialogue. *Etudes de Linguistique Appliquée* (1979), **2**, 100-121.

NETSU, R. and MARQUARDT, T.P. Pantomime in aphasia: effects of stimulus characteristics. *Journal of Communication Disorders* (1984), **17**, 37-46.

OMBREDANE, A. *L'aphasie et l'élaboration de la pensée explicite* (1951). Paris: Presses Universitaires de France.

PAILLARD, J. Apraxia and the neurophysiology of motor control. *Philosophical Transactions of the Royal Society of London, Serie B* (1982), **298**, 111-134.

PETERSON, L.N. and KIRSHNER, H.S. Gestural impairment and gestural ability in aphasia: A review. *Brain and Language* (1981), **14**, 333-348.

PICKETT, L.W. An assessment of gestural and pantomimic deficit in aphasic patients. *Acta Symbolica* (1974), **5**, 69-86.

POECK, K. The clinical examination for motor apraxia. *Neuropsychologia* (1986), **24**, 129-134.

POECK, K., LEHMKUHL, G. and WILLMES, K. Axial movements in ideomotor apraxia. *Journal of Neurology, Neurosurgery, and Psychiatry* (1982), **45**, 1125-1129.

POIZNER, H., BELLUGI, U. and IRAGUI, V. Apraxia and aphasia for a visual-gestural language. *American Journal of Physiology: Regulatory, Integrative and Comparative Physiology* (1984), **15**, R868-R883.

PRIGATANO, G.P. and PRIBRAM, K.H. Perception and memory of facial affect following brain injury. *Perceptual and Motor Skills* (1981), **54**, 859-869.

RATCLIFFE, G. and NEWCOMBE, F. Object recognition: some deductions from the clinical evidence. In A.W. Ellis (ed.) *Normality and Pathology in Cognitive Functions* (1982), pp. 147-171. London/New York: Academic Press.

RIMÉ, B. Nonverbal communication or nonverbal behaviour? Towards a cognitive motor-theory of nonverbal behaviour. In W. Doise and S. Moscovici (eds.) Current Issues in European Social Psychology, Vol. 1 (1983), pp. 85-135, Cambridge. Cambridge University Press.

RINN, W.E. The neuropsychology of facial expression: a review of the neurological and psychological mechanisms for producing facial expressions. *Psychological Bulletin* (1984), **95**, 52-77.

ROSS, E.D. The aprosodias: functional-anatomic organization of the affective components of language in the right hemisphere. *Archives of Neurology* (1981), **38**, 561-569.

ROSS, E.D. Right hemisphere in language, affective behavior and emotion. *Trends in Neurosciences* (1984), **7**, 342-346.

ROSS, E.D., HARNAY, J.H., DE LACOSTE-UTAMSING, C. and PURDY, P.D. How the brain integrates affective and propositional language into a unified behavioral function. Hypotheses based on clinico-anatomic evidence. *Archives of Neurology* (1981), **38**, 745-748.

ROTHI, L.J.G. and HEILMAN, K.M. Acquisition and retention of gestures by apraxic patients. *Brain and Cognition* (1984), **3**, 426-437.

ROTHI, L.J.G., HEILMAN, K.M. and WATSON, R.T. Pantomime comprehension and ideomotor apraxia. *Journal of Neurology, Neurosurgery, and Psychiatry*, (1985), **48**, 207-210.

ROTHI, L.J.G., MACK, L. and HEILMAN, K.M. Pantomime agnosia. *Journal of Neurology, Neurosurgery, and Psychiatry* (1986), **49**, 451-454.

ROY, E.A. Action sequencing and lateralized cerebral damage: Evidence for asymmetries in control. In J. Long and A. Baddeley (eds), *Attention and Performance, Vol. 9* (1981), pp. 487-500. Hillsdale, N.J.: Lawrence Erlbaum Associates.

ROY, E.A. Action and performance. In A.W. Ellis (ed.) *Normality and Pathology in Cognitive Functions* (1982) pp. 295-298. London/New York: Academic Press.

RYALLS, J.H. Intonation in Broca's aphasias. *Neuropsychologia* (1982), **20**, 355-360.

RYALLS, J.H. Some acoustic aspects of fundamental frequency of CVC utterances in aphasia. *Phonetica* (1984), **41**, 103-111.

SCHLANGER, B.B., SCHLANGER, P. and GERSTMAN, L.J. The perception of emotionally toned sentences by right-hemisphere-damaged and aphasic subjects. *Brain and Language* (1976), **3**, 396-403.

SELNES, O.A., RUBENS, A.B., RISSE, G.L. and LEVY, R.S. Transient aphasia with persistent apraxia: Uncommon sequela of massive left-hemisphere stroke. *Archives of Neurology* (1982), **39**, 122-126.

SERGENT, J. The role of the input in visual hemispheric asymmetries. *Psychological Bulletin* (1983), **93**, 481-514.

SERGENT, J. Inferences from unilateral brain damage about normal hemispheric functions in visual pattern recognition. *Psychological Bulletin* (1984), **96**, 99-115.

SERON, X., VAN DER KAA, M.A., REMITZ, A. and VAN DER LINDEN, M. Pantomime interpretation and aphasia. *Neuropsychologia* (1979), **17**, 661-668.

SERON, X., VAN DER KAA, M.A., VAN DER LINDEN, M., REMITS, A. and FEYEREISEN, P. Decoding paralinguistic signals: effect of semantic and prosodic cues on aphasic comprehension. *Journal of Communication Disorders* (1982), **15**, 223-231.

SHAPIRO, B.E. and DANLY, M. The role of the right hemisphere in the control of speech prosody in propositional and affective contexts. *Brain and Language* (1985), **25**, 19-36.

SIGNORET, J.L. and NORTH, P. *Les apraxies gestuelles* (1979). Paris: Masson.

SNODGRASS, J.G. Concepts and their surface representations. *Journal of Verbal Learning and Verbal Behavior* (1984), **23**, 3-22.

SPEEDIE, L.J., COSLETT, H.B. and HEILMAN, K.M. Repetition of affective prosody in mixed transcortical aphasia. *Archives of Neurology* (1984), **41**, 268-270.

TOGNOLA, G. and VIGNOLO, L.A. Brain lesions associated with oral apraxia in stroke patients: A clinico-neuroradiological investigation with the CT scan. *Neuropsychologia* (1980), **18**, 257-272.

TOMPKINS, C.A, and FLOWERS, C.R. Perception of emotional intonation by brain-damaged adults: the influence of task processing levels. *Journal of Speech and Hearing Research* (1985), **28**, 527-538.

TOMPKINS, C.A. and MATEER, C.A. Right hemisphere appreciation of prosodic and linguistic indications of implicit attitude. *Brain and Language* (1985), **24**, 185-203.

TUCKER, D.M., WATSON, R.T. and HEILMAN, K.M. Discrimination and evocation of affectively intoned speech in patients with right parietal disease. *Neurology* (1977), **27**, 947-950.

VARNEY, N.R. Linguistic correlates of pantomime recognition in aphasic patients. *Journal of Neurology, Neurosurgery, and Psychiatry* (1978), **41**, 564-568.

VARNEY, N.R. Pantomime recognition defect in aphasia: implications for the concept of asymbolia. *Brain and Language*, (1982), **15**, 32-39.

VARNEY, N.R. and BENTON, A.L. Qualitative aspects of pantomime recognition defect in aphasia. *Brain and Cognition*, (1982), **1**, 132-139.

WENIGER, D. Disprosody as part of the aphasic language disorder. In F.C. Rose (ed.), *Advances in Neurology, Vol. 42. Progress in Aphasiology* (1984) pp. 41-50. New York: Raven.

WYKE, M. The effects of brain lesions in the performance of an arm-hand precision task. *Neuropsychologia* (1968) **6**, 125-134.

ZAJONC, R.B. Feeling and thinking: preferences need no inferences. *American Psychologist* (1980), **35**, 151-175.

ZAJONC, R.B. On the primacy of affect. *American Psychologist* (1984), **39**, 117-123.

ZOCCOLOTTI, P., SABINI, D. and VIOLANI, C. Electrodermal responses in patients with unilateral brain damage. *Journal of Clinical Neuropsychology* (1982), **4**, 143-150.

II

Cerebral Dominance

4

The Relationship Between Brainedness and Handedness

M.J. Morgan and I.C. McManus

Introduction

> *Plato:* 'It is only the folly of nurses and mothers to whom we owe it that we are all, so to say, lame on one hand. Nature, in fact, makes the members on both sides broadly correspondent; we have introduced the difference between them for ourselves by our improper habits.' *Laws*, 794, d.

> *Aristotle* '... if we were all to practise always throwing with the left hand, we should become ambidextrous. But still by nature, left is left, and the right hand is none the less superior to the left hand, even if we do everything with the left as we do with the right. Nor because things change does it follow that they are not by nature. But if for the most part and for the greater length of time the left continues thus to be left and the right right, this is by nature.' *Magna moralia*, 1194.

The great majority of people, probably in the order of 90%, prefer to use their right hand for complex unimanual skills, notably for handwriting. At least as high a proportion have left-hemisphere dominance for speech, in the sense that left-hemisphere lesions are more likely than right-hemisphere lesions to produce aphasia. Ever since Bouillaud, on April 4th, 1865, raised the question of a possible relationship between handedness and speech lateralization (Riese, 1947), a central question in neuropsychology has been the following: is this relationship merely one of the many correlations between lateral asymmetrical organs, such as that between *situs* of the heart and digestive tract; or does it have a deeper functional and evolutionary significance?

In this chapter we shall review some of the theories that have attempted to account for the relationship between speech dominance and handedness. It will help at the outset to classify the various theories; first, according to whether individual learning or past evolution accounts for the association; and second, by the postulated order of priority between speech and handedness. *Learning theories*, not now very popular, maintain that preference for one hand biases the individual towards developing speech mechanisms in the same hemisphere that controls the preferred hand; or alternatively, that the presence of speech mechanisms in one hemisphere biases the individual towards use of the contralateral hand. *Evolutionary theories* suppose the association between speech dominance and handedness to be inherited and laid down in the evolution of the species: a critical feature of such theories is that they postulate a selective advantage to the normal arrangement of having speech and control of the preferred hand in the same hemisphere.

In either kind of theory, it is possible to have versions claiming that handedness preceded speech lateralization, or the reverse; that one pre-adapted the brain for the development of the other (Varney and Vileasky, 1980). In practice, as we shall see, the priority of handedness has been the more popular alternative in evolutionary theories, because there is evidence that hand preferences appeared very early in human evolution.

An alternative to the Learning and Evolutionary theories will be referred to rather clumsily as the *Correlational Theory*, which maintains that the association between handedness and speech dominance is accidental, or at most, dependent upon a third variable. The critical feature of this kind of theory is that the association has no particular selective advantage; nor is it learned. For example, it has been suggested (Morgan, 1977; Corballis and Morgan, 1978; Morgan and Corballis, 1978) that handedness and speech lateralization are both reflections of an underlying developmental gradient slightly favouring more rapid movement of the left hand side of the body.

We consider first the formal nature of the evidence required to distinguish between the different theories. If it is possible to classify individuals as right or left speech dominant and right or left-handed, the simplest situation to analyse is that in which an entire population is both right-handed and left-speech dominant (*Figure 1(a)*) but, while this situation is descriptively simple, it is causally intractable, since in the absence of variance there is nothing to analyse, and hence no possibility of teasing apart cause and effect; technically it is not even possible to say in such a case that handednesss and speech dominance are correlated. Consider now the situation in which the population proportions are as in *Figure 1(b)*, where we assume that 10% of the population are left handed and 10% are right-speech dominant; here the correlation between speech dominance and handedness is one. We now have variance, and this can be considered in terms of three possible causal models, shown in *Figure 1(b)* in terms of path-analytic type models, where the

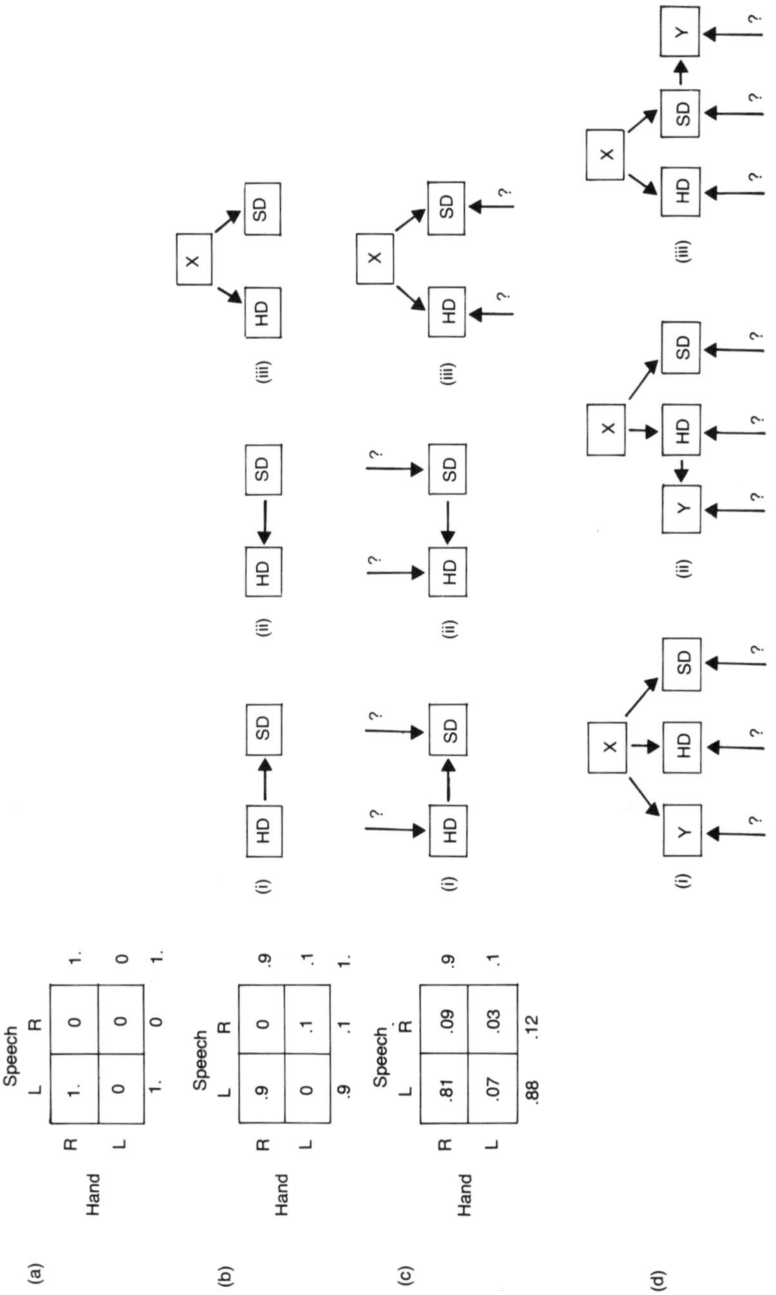
(a)
Speech
L R
Hand R 1. 0 1.
L 0 0 0
1. 0 1.
(b)
Speech
L R
Hand R .9 0 .9
L 0 .1 .1
.9 .1 1.
(c)
Speech
L R
Hand R .81 .09 .9
L .07 .03 .1
.88 .12
(i) HD SD
(ii) HD SD
(iii) X HD SD
(i) HD SD ? ?
(ii) HD SD ? ?
(iii) X HD SD ? ?
(d)
(i) X Y HD SD ? ? ?
(ii) X Y HD SD ? ? ?
(iii) X HD SD Y ? ? ?

Figure 1

arrows indicate direct causal influences (see Kenny, 1979 for an excellent introduction to path-analytic modelling). In (i) hand dominance is prior to and directly causes the speech dominance; in (ii) speech dominance is prior to and directly causes the hand dominance; and in (iii) both hand dominance and speech dominance are directly caused by some third factor (X).

All of these models predict a correlation of one between hand dominance and speech dominance. In each case some prior influence is pre-supposed which establishes the apparently 'primary' dominance. *Figure 1(c)* shows a more likely situation in which handedness and speech dominance show a more moderate correlation. Here we have three similar models to before, except that each variable has a degree of unattributable effects causing some of its variance (symbolized by '?'). By appropriate choice of parameters such models will predict the correlations shown in *Figure 1(c)*. The unattributable error may represent either errors of measurement, or other unknown causes of laterization.

Thus far we may not seem to have advanced beyond a restatement of the truism (albeit a disputed one) from elementary statistics classes, that one cannot infer causation from correlation. The advance is not in the production of new theoretical insights, but rather in the precision and clarity with which they may be stated. Consider as an example a recent suggestion by Marin, Schwartz and Saffran, (1979):

> 'The choice of the left over the right hemisphere as the locus for motor speech almost certainly had to do with an earlier established right-hand preference in the hominid line (Dart, 1949). Verbal sequencing and manual sequencing may depend on the same basic type of neural organization, a possibility that receives some support from the association between linguistic and apraxic disturbance with posterior left-hemisphere lesions (Kimura, 1976). Given that motor control for language had become established in the left hemisphere, there might then have been a tendency for other language functions to organize themselves in proximity to the motor speech cortex; thus the left hemisphere would have been the locus for the increasing specialization of auditory mechanisms that would provide the perceptual basis of verbal learning, as well as for the development of syntactic mechanisms involved in the higher-order programming of motor speech input. Aspects of lexical representation might develop, to some extent, in both hemispheres, because of their relationship to perceptual function.' (p. 208)

Without wishing to discuss at this stage whether there is evidence for these claims, we note that the model can be redrawn in the path-analytic model of *Figure 2*. Whether this model is really what the authors meant is not clear, but it is what they apparently said, and the model is now specified far more precisely. The model also raises explicitly the question of *when* the postulated causes are occurring: during the development of the individual or of the species? Unless we wish to subscribe to the strict (and probably erroneous) notion that ontogeny recapitulates phylogeny, then we must be willing to

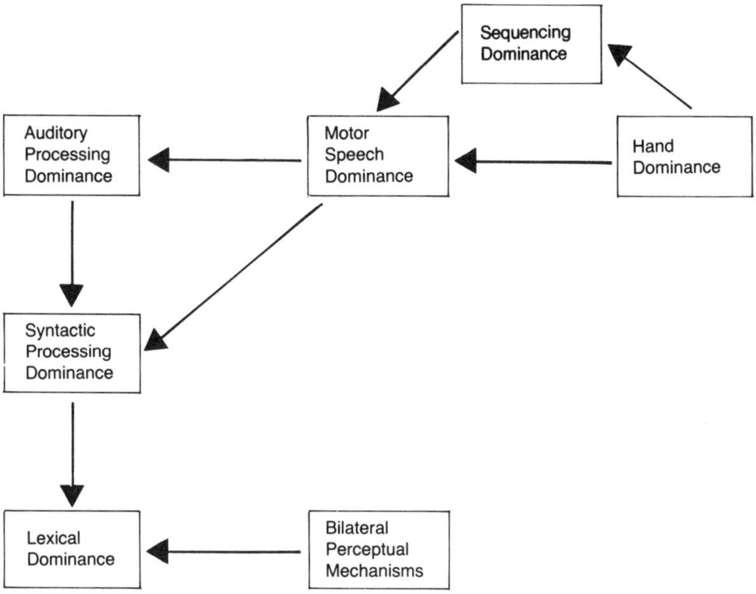

Figure 2

accept the possibility that separate causal models may be necessary for the two forms of development.

Path-analytic diagrams also force certain other conclusions. Consider model (i) of *Figure 1(b)*; it is apparent that if we wish to subscribe to this model then we must accept that in the absence of hand dominance, for whatever reason, there can be no speech dominance. The diagram also makes one realize that the hand dominance in such a case must be arising from somewhere; chance processes in general will only result in a lack of dominance and we must therefore continually look for prior causes, until we eventually arrive at some acceptable first cause (of which perhaps the only acceptable forms will be genes, asymmetry of biological molecules, or sub-atomic asymmetries).

A further question concerns the meaning of dominance. In man there is speech dominance in two very distinct senses:

1. In any individual one hemisphere is the major hemisphere and is primarily responsible for producing speech.
2. In a population, a majority of individuals have a particular hemisphere controlling that function. We may refer to these two forms (along with Denenberg, 1983) as *individual dominance* and *population dominance*. Most of the models of *Figure 1* could be conceived of in terms of either type of dominance, and once more, it is possible that different models may be responsible for each type of dominance.

A final methodological point concerns the relationships we may expect to find between handedness, speech dominance, and a third dominance variable. Consider a model of the type shown in *Figure 1(c), iii*, in which X, with some error, causes both hand dominance and speech dominance. A third dominance variable, say, Y, may be causally related to either X, HD or SD (*Figure 1(d)*). In case (ii), the correlation between Y and HD will be higher than that between Y and SD or HD and SD. In case (iii) the correlation between SD and Y will be higher than that between Y and HD or HD and SD; finally, in case (i), the correlation between Y and HD, Y and SD, and HD and SD will be identical (assuming path coefficients from X to be identical). Finally, of course, there may be independence of Y from X, HS and HD. In general we cannot easily measure SD but can measure HD, and have little hope of measuring X. The use of variables such as Y is of interest since, if the correlation of Y with HD is too high, we suspect that it is merely an alternative measure of it, while if the correlation is too low, we suspect that the variable is of no interest. If there is a moderate correlation we cannot be sure if the measure is assessing SD, or perhaps is actually a third, truly independent dominance in its own right. It thus appears that moderate correlations are of maximum theoretical interest. But perhaps the major conclusion is that without the set of all possible correlations between X, Y, HD and SD, we cannot strictly interpret the results in causal terms, and yet in general we rarely have such information.

After this preliminary analysis, we turn to consider the main classes of theory.

Learning Theories

Gowers (1878) and Bastian and Horsley (1880) reported post-mortems of individuals with a missing left-hand; in both cases the contralateral parietal lobe was apparently atrophied and vestigial. It was probably cases such as this which provided the neurological justification for theories which stated that the lateralization of language functions was entirely secondary to hand dominance, and that it was, in some sense, 'learned'. Wernicke (1906) felt that 'the left hemisphere may lose the speech functions it previously had developed if use of the left hand replaces that of the right . . . localization of the speech centre is a functional acquisition of each individual'. A similar view may be found in the writings of Jackson (1880), Paget (1887) and Bastian (1898). The theory was attractive in part because it explained the strange problem of why lateralization of function was only discovered in the mid-nineteenth century (*see* Benton and Joynt, 1960 for a review of early failures). Moxon (1886) suggested that 'the brain of educated individuals is manifestly more unsymmetrical than the brains of uneducated individuals', and

Kinnier Wilson (1926) reiterated the view of Weber (1904) that 'the dissemination of the accomplishment of writing among all classes determined the lead of the left hemisphere over the right, and at the same time finally established the localization of the speech centres in the cerebral cortex'. Thus it was only with universal literacy that Broca *could* have made his discovery. The theory also gave the possibility of therapy, or even, to use the title of a paper by Coley (1909), *The Prophylaxis of Aphasia*; 'my suggestion is that a graphic centre should be made to develop in the right side of the brain by practising writing with the left hand'. The theory also resulted in the development of the 'Ambidextral Culture Society', ambidexterity conferring upon its possessors a myriad of advantages (see Harris, 1980 for a review). The therapeutic potential was considered by Burt (1950). 'At the special schools in the Lingfield colony for epileptics a group of children who were stationary in learning were given a training in left-handedness in the hope that "additional" centres in the brain might be opened up'. The recent enthusiasm for 'two brain education' seems to support Marx's view that history repeats itself, the second time as farce.

The concept continued to have explanatory use to neurologists well into the twentieth century e.g. by Needles (1942), Zangwill (1955) and Weisenburg and McBride (1955), for whom the right brain 'is in a state of receptivity for language acquisition, the degree varying in accord with the use of the left hand for writing, Wechsler (1976) described a case of crossed aphasia in a dextral and concluded that 'the neural mechanisms involved in learning to read and write may be necessary for the complete establishment and maintenance of language dominance.'

Various objections may be found to the hypothesis that speech lateralization is acquired secondarily to hand dominance:

1. Goodglass and Quadfasel (1954) and Gloning *et al.* (1969) reported studies on brain-damaged left-handers some of whom had used their left hand for writing (n = 50), and others of whom (n = 57) had used their right hand for writing (subsequent to educational pressure). In neither case did the incidence of left-sided speech dominance relate to particular hand usage.
2. Damasio *et al.* (1976a, b) investigated the suggestion (Critchley, 1956) that illiterates rarely became aphasic since they have a more bilateral organisation of their speech centres as a result of the absence of writing. They examined 247 right-handed adults with focal brain lesions, of whom 38 were illiterate; in summary there seemed to be no difference between the illiterates and the literates in side of aphasia-producing lesion, or in quality or degree of aphasia.

A variant of the learning theory concerns the lateralization of language function in bilateral individuals. Albert and Obler (1978) concluded that:

> '[first] ... the language organisation of the average bilingual may be more ambilateral than that of a monolingual; second, that the organizational systems of the two or more languages of the bilingual are not necessarily disturbed equally with respect to cerebral language dominance ... [third] ... differential dominance patterns are not random; rather they may be influenced by such acquisition parameters as age, manner and modality of second language acquisition'. (p. 239)

Much of the evidence for such hypotheses comes from clinical cases in which bilingual patients lose just one language as a result of brain damage. The relationship to theories of illiteracy is seen in the case of the 94-year-old patient of Gorlitzer von Mundy (1959), which was retold by Paradis (1977). A 94-year-old man suffered a left hemispheric embolism which left him with a right hemiplegia and a selective aphasia. For the previous 40 years the patient had spoken German in a German environment. Until the age of 30 the patient was illiterate, ambidextrous, and spoke only Slovenian. He was then conscripted into the Austrian army for 12 years where 'he learned simultaneously to manipulate weapons with the right hand and to speak German, and thus, according to the author, German became localized in the left hemisphere. However Slovenian remained in the speech centres of both hemispheres. Consequently, when the left hemisphere was damaged, the patient lost his German and the portion of Slovenian that was stored there, but kept the Slovenian that was stored in his right hemisphere'. (Paredis, 1977, p. 93).

On the basis of such cases, Albert and Obler speculate that 'it would no longer be correct to accept the traditional dogma that the left hemisphere is necessarily dominant for language in right-handers' (p. 253).

The problem with such theories is partly that they are very imprecise (in some cases arguing that the second language should go into the right hemisphere, or in others, as Paradis above, that it will go into the left hemisphere), and partly that they are primarily based in clinical studies, from which almost every possible combination of recovery pattern has been observed (*see* Paradis, 1977). More damning, perhaps, is that in the careful study of right-handed Hebrew-English bilinguals by Gordon (1980), no evidence was found for differential lateralization of the two languages (although there was, surprisingly, a 27% incidence of left-ear advantages in these right-handed subjects, and McManus (1983) has suggested, after a statistical re-analysis of the data, that some 7% of the individuals show evidence for differential lateralization of the two languages). As a demonstration of the confusion in the literature we also note that Tzavaras *et al.* (1981) claim that illiterates are *more* left hemisphere dominant for speech (on the basis of dichotic listening tests). Sussman *et al.* (1982) have recently presented evidence that the age of acquisition of the second language affects its lateralization, early second languages (before six years of age) being left hemisphere dominant, while later acquired second languages show a more bilateral pattern.

In summary, the conclusion of Albert and Obler seems to be premature, and we may, at least for the present, assume that the monolingualism of most subjects of study has not dramatically altered their lateralization patterns.

Further Objections

Most strongly left-handed people turn out to have left hemisphere dominance for speech (Zangwill, 1960); there are also well-documented cases of 'crossed aphasia' in dextrals (Zangwill, 1979). These cases appear to be much more damaging to learning theories than to their evolutionary counterpart, because of the postulated nature of the causation. Evolutionary theories claim that the association between handedness and speech dominance has evolved because it is advantageous: but clearly such an explanation still permits genetic variability, as in the case of other desirable traits, such as having a cerebral cortex. In learning theories, however, the nature of the postulated causation is direct, in the lifetime of the individual, so exceptions are much harder to accommodate unless one postulates that the causal mechanism is only weak. Nevertheless one has to postulate only a relatively weak causal link, or alternatively the presence of several different causal processes, in order to be able to 'explain' such apparent counter-examples.

Children with congenital unilateral aplasia, or absence of one hand, should develop speech dominance contralaterally to the remaining hand if learning theories are correct. We know of no evidence to test this possibility. Loss of a hand post-natally may also be expected to have a similar effect if it occurs early enough in development. Bramwell (1899, cited by Harris, 1980) described a patient who was originally right-handed, but who shifted to use of the left-hand at the age of 17 following an accident. At the age of 57 this patient became aphasic in association with left-sided hemiplegia. Bramwell argued that speech had shifted to the right hemisphere because of the shift in handedness. A similar case is reported by Nielsen (1946). (This explanation is considerably weakened, however, by the finding of 'crossed aphasia' in dextrals who have not changed their hand preference (Zangwill, 1979)). The absence of a control group in such cases and, particularly in the case of Nielsen, the fact that the individual had left-handed relatives and hence was more likely to have right speech dominance, make the interpretation of such cases almost impossible.

There is little support from the developmental literature for the notion that handedness precedes left hemisphere specialization for language. The literature is not clear on the question of when, exactly, 'handedness' and 'speech lateralization' emerge, probably because different aspects appear at different ages. For example, infants under 1 year of age show few signs of spontaneous preference between the hands when manipulating objects, yet they may show a preference for extended reaching with the right arm (Baldwin, 1894; Wooley, 1910), and even 1–4-month-old infants have been described by Caplan and Kinsbourne (1976) as holding on to a rattle longer with the right hand. What is abundantly clear, however, is that at least some aspects of speech lateralization appear before practice of the right hand with writing and drawing. Witelson (1977) provides a number of useful tables summarizing the developmental evidence and her table 1 reveals 'a marked consistency for greater right than left [ear] scores on dichotic verbal listening tests for children as young as two or three years of age'.

Electrophysiological evidence (reviewed by Molfese, 1977) appears to support the view that there are asymmetries in response to speech sounds in infants, and even neonates. Studies with brain-damaged children, despite the widespread belief in 'equipotentiality', also indicate that speech loss is more frequent after left than right hemisphere damage, and this is true even at about 2 years of age, which is as early as language assessment can be carried out (Witelson, p. 247). These findings add weight to Kinsbourne's (1980) contention that the fundamental mechanisms of lateral asymmetry are probably present at birth. There is thus very little evidence to support the hypothesis that handedness precedes speech lateralization in development.

Evolutionary Theories

The principal ideas we shall try to examine in this section are the following: (1) the tool theory; (2) the gestural theory of language origin; (3) Brain's 'tongue muscle' theory; (4) Levy's theory of 'cognitive style'; (5) the theory of the 'leading hemisphere'; (6) Kinsbourne's attentional theory. All these attempt to provide a rationale for the strong association between right handedness and left hemisphere dominance of speech. They all make implicit assumptions about the actual evolution of handedness and speech dominance, and it is worth briefly considering the limited data on this question. It is also worth stressing that many modern accounts, written from an academic perspective in the late twentieth century, make the implicit assumption that the most crucial thing in the evolution of man is the sudden emergence of a larger brain, and that all other characteristics, in particular an upright posture, evolved secondarily to the larger brain. However, modern anthropological work (*see* for example Gould, 1980) supports the early nineteenth century view (reiterated in modified form by Freud in *Civilisation and its Discontents*) that the upright posture, with its freeing of the hands for skilled work, evolved *before* the evolution of a larger brain, bipedalism appearing by at least three million years B.C. (Leakey, 1981).

The Evolution of Handedness and Speech Dominance

(i) Handedness

Here we may consider two types of evidence — comparative and archaeological. Most studies take as their starting point that handedness is not found in animals, and the results of Collins (1968, 1969, 1970), who found that exactly 50% of mice were right pawed, and 50% were left pawed, are usually quoted here. It is important to note that these mice showed individual dominance, but they did not show population dominance: individual dominance in animals seems to be the rule. There have been repeated attempts at finding population dominance in animals, but these have generally failed to replicate, or to be studied further; examples include the rat (Tsai and Maurer, 1930; Peterson, 1931; Herren and Lindsley, 1935), and the cat (Cole, 1955). Much interest has centred on the monkeys, in view of their phylogenetic closeness to man. Despite some claims that there is a population dominance (e.g. Ettlinger, 1961; Ettlinger and Moffett, 1964; Brooker *et al.*, 1981) the consensus seems to be that there is only individual hand dominance and not population dominance in the monkeys (Finch, 1941; Cole and Glees, 1951; Warren, 1953; Lehmann, 1978, 1980), a conclusion not convincingly refuted by the most recent review (MacNeilage *et al.*, 1987).

Denenberg (1983) has emphasized that individual dominance may be selected for in lower vertebrates in order to assist in spatial perception, and he cites two studies, by Zimmerberg *et al.* (1978) and Camp *et al.* (1981), in which animals that had strong individual rotational biases performed better on spatial problems than did those without such biases. Of course the fact that individual dominance *might* be selected for does not necessarily mean that all species will show individual dominance — *see* McManus (1981b) for a negative example in *Drosophila* — although it should also be noted that Collins (1981, 1985) has recently presented evidence for selection and genetic control of degree rather than direction of asymmetry of pawedness in mice, and that Ward and Collins (1985) have shown that such mice show neuroanatomical differences from less lateralized mice.

An interesting case of population dominance may be found in the parrot; Broca himself raised this possibility at the Norwich Meeting of the British Association in 1868 (*see* Bateman, 1870, p. 165), and it had earlier been suggested by Sir Thomas Browne in his *Pseudodoxia Epidemica (IV, V)*. Given the propensity for imitation of speech in these birds, and the clear lateralization of song in some birds (Nottebohm, 1979) it is of some interest that there is good evidence for a population dominance for footedness (Friedman and Davis, 1938; Rogers, 1981). A similar phenonemon in the peacock was claimed by the Chinese Sung Dynasty Emperor, Hi Tsung (Anonymous, 1957).

The general conclusion from comparative work is that man is almost unique in possessing population dominance for handedness. When did this dominance rise? The study of works of art (e.g. Dennis, 1958; Coren and Porac, 1977) suggests that from the early Egyptian period through to the present day, approximately 7.4% of paintings have shown left-handers, but it must be borne in mind in the interpretation of such material that lateralized artistic representations in works of art are not necessarily veridical — *see* McManus, 1976 for an example. Prior to the onset of civilization there is less evidence as to handedness. The recent technique of micro-wear analysis of tools provides good evidence that between 6 and 20% of neolithic (about 4000 BC) implements were produced by left-handers (Spennemann, 1984), and that at least some individuals in a palaeolithic Belgian site (8900 BC) were left handed (van Noten *et al.*, 1980). Prior to this we have only the poor and ambiguous data to be obtained from cave paintings (*see* Uhrbrock, 1973 for a review), followed by a vast gap until the evidence of Dart (1948) that Australopithecus (one million years BC) was right-handed, killing prey with a blow to the skull from a stone held in the right hand (although the statistical evidence reported is far from totally convincing). Recently Toth (1985) has argued, on the basis of a detailed analysis of the asymmetric pattern of flaking in stone tools, that right-handedness predominated in sites from the lower Pleistocene (about 1.5 million years BC) and middle Pleistocene (about 200 000 years BC) periods, although his method does not allow any accurate estimation of rates of left-handedness. As a counter-balance to the above theories we also note the eccentric suggestion of Gooch (1977) that Neanderthal man was predominantly left-handed.

In summary, man is probably the only animal with population hand dominance for skilled activity, and this dominance probably arose sometime before the onset of civilization; little else can be said with any certainty. Specific preferences for use of the otherwise *non*-dominant hand are rare in man; Dimond and Harries (1984) have described an interesting example which has evolutionary implications. Face-touching, which is interpreted as a form of emotional expression, is more common with the *left* hand in man, and this is also the case in the great apes, but not in monkeys, suggesting a relatively recent evolutionary origin, perhaps connected with right-hemisphere function.

(ii) Cerebral Dominance

Once more we may consider comparative and archaeological evidence. As far as comparative work is concerned we may look for evidence of functional dominance, be it for language or otherwise. Warren and Nottebohm (1976) concluded that there was no evidence for functional dominance in monkeys, but several lines of evidence suggest that conclusion might be premature. Hamilton *et al.* (1974) reported evidence from seven monkeys which, for several tasks involving movement and orientation detection, suggested right hemisphere dominance; and on other tasks there was evidence of strong individual dominance in the absence of population dominance. Pohl (1982, 1983) has reported evidence for individual, but not population, dominance in processing of dichotic stimili in baboons. More excitingly, Petersen *et al.* (1978) have reported work suggesting that the left-hemisphere of the Japanese Macaque contains cells specialized for the detection of species-specific vocalizations, and Heffner and Heffner (1984) have reported that discrimination of such sounds is critically dependent upon the integrity of the left but not the right temporal cortex; if these results are replicable then they must surely be of great importance in our understanding of the evolution of language and dominance. Finally, in a recent review, Denneberg (1983) has presented evidence that might be interpreted as existence of population dominance both in chickens and in rats, especially for emotional behaviours.

A further line of evidence concerns morphological cerebral asymmetries. Since the report of Geschwind and Levitsky (1968) that the *planum temporale* of normal human brains is larger on the left side than the right, a flurry of work has investigated such asymmetries.

Nevertheless, it is worth noting that the asymmetry has not as yet been reported in relation to either handedness, or speech loss after cerebral damage, and in the absence of such data the asymmetry may just as well be interpreted as a correlate of *situs*, or some other anatomical asymmetry. The same criticism does not apply to the work of Le May (1976), where an asymmetry of cerebral blood vessels has been related to handedness. From a re-analysis of the data of Hoadley and Pearson (1929), McManus (1982) has shown that the distribution of human skull asymmetry is bimodal, and infers that this bimodality may reflect two separate types of speech dominance. Morphological asymmetries have been examined in monkeys. Yeni-Komshian and Benson (1976) demonstrated an asymmetry in chimpanzees (but not in rhesus monkeys) and Le May and Geschwind (1975) found asymmetries in the brain of orang-utans. Several studies (Abler, 1976; Le May, 1976) have reported morphological studies of prehistoric skulls and found evidence for asymmetries. Studies of cranial endocasts suggest that both *H. erectus* and *H. habilis* had well-developed Broca's and Wernicke's areas, and that these areas are relatively underdeveloped in Australopithecines and the modern apes (Tobias, 1981; Holloway, 1981).

There is some evidence for functional asymmetries, and better evidence for morphological asymmetries indicating population dominance in the higher apes, and such results are at least consistent with the prehistoric remains of man.

(1) The Tool Theory

There are recent discussions of this theory by Frost (1981), Calvin (1982), and Steklis and Harnad (1976) (although Steklis (1985) has recently withdrawn his earlier support for the theory). A volume of the Proceedings of the New York Academy of Sciences (1976) was devoted to the 'Origins and Evolution of Language and Speech', and many of the articles contain material relevant to the following discussion. The essence of the theory is this: human beings are distinguished from non-humans by their bipedal gait, by tool-using behaviour, by their preference for using the right hand in complex motor skills and, finally, by language. The Tool theory attempts to link these human characteristics together in a systematic way. To start with, the hominids are the only Primate group for which the primary functions of the forelimbs are other than for locomotion, thus freeing the forelimbs for the making and using of tools, albeit some 1½–2 million years before the first appearance of stone tools in the fossil record (Isaac, 1981). Many tools require different skills from the two hands, as in the chipping of a flint or the throwing of a spear. In many of these cases the left hand merely holds or steadies the object being manipulated, while the right hand performs the skilled action. This meant that the motor mechanisms for the more skilled actions involved in tool making and tool using evolved in the left hemisphere. There then follows the most difficult and crucial step in the argument. Why did the development of motor skills in the left hemisphere facilitate the development of language mechanisms there? We quote Frost (1980) here:

> '. . . the co-lateralization of the neural substrates mediating skilled serial motor praxis and those mediating speech in the left hemisphere is likely to be more than a coincidence. The co-occurrence of these mechanisms in the left hemisphere is very likely related to the fact that speech, like tool behaviour, involves skilled serial motor activity, but . . . it is the actions of tongue, lips and vocal chords rather than arms, hands and fingers which must be precisely timed and sequenced.' (p. 455)

Putting this more fancifully, we may say that the left hemisphere, having acquired the skills to control precise movements of the hands, finds that many of these same skills can be used to control the voice. The upright, asymmetrical, tool using, loquacious ape has evolved, to the satisfaction of theory.

(2) The Gestural Theory

This has a great deal in common with the tool theory and the two accounts have evolved in parallel. A comprehensive historical review by Hewes (1976) will be found in the New York Academy of Sciences Symposium referred to earlier. The psychological implications of the theory have been spelled out by Kimura in several publications (e.g. 1977) and it is Kimura's version of the theory that will provide the principal basis for the account we give here.

The Gestural theory of language origin maintains that '. . . the initial form of language was gestural, in the sense that the propositional, predicative, or reporting functions were based on gestural signs, with vocal sounds serving much as they do non-human mammals, for the social communication of affect' (Hewes 1976, p. 482). Manual communication thus preceded vocal communication in evolution, and it is thus in manual communication that we must seek the origins of cerebral asymmetry. The next link in the chains of reasoning is therefore that the *right* hand, and in consequence the *left* hemisphere, took on the major role in manual communication (signing). Why the right hand? Here the gestural and tool theories converge, as Kimura (1976, p. 153) explains:

> 'One may speculate, therefore, that the necessary condition for the development of the communication system we use was the freeing of the upper limbs from locomotor activity. This permitted the development of tool use and the necessary manual dexterity to handle tools. Given that such manual skills existed, it is reasonable to suggest that hand movements could readily be employed in a communication situation, perhaps initially in a manner imitative of the object described. . . .'

So the left hemisphere developed motor skills through tool use and these were subsequently transferred to manual communication. The next stage in the argument also resembles the tool theory. When speech finally arrived on the scene, it was able to make use of the pre-adapted motor skills in the left hemisphere, and hence speech became lateralized as well. Thus the more skilled hand and the speech mechanisms are controlled by the same hemisphere for definite evolutionary reasons.

(3) Brain's 'tongue-muscle' theory

Both the tool theory and the gestural theory argue that precise motor control of the hands has eventually led to speech dominance. Brain's theory specifically rejects this proposal and looks at the evolution from the other direction:

> '. . . it seems more probable that the establishment of the left hemisphere in man as the major hemisphere for speech resulted in the development of the right hand as the dominant hand. Emotional noises, both in man and in the lower animals, are simple involuntary performances, and such simple reactions can utilise symmetrical and bilateral pathways. In contrast to this, speech calls for articulation — the precise integration of the small muscles of the lips, tongue, palate and larynx, besides the respiratory muscles, so that these contract synchronously on the two sides with such delicacy that a variety of sounds can be differentiated through a range of fine gradations. This motor integration seems to require that the motor cortex of both hemispheres should be under the control of a single co-ordinating centre, 'the motor speech centre'. Speech, in other words, necessitates localization.' (Brain, 1961; pp. 25–26).

And once speech has been lateralized to one hemisphere then hand dominance would rapidly follow.

It should be noted at this point that the three theories presented are primarily theories of the correlation of hand dominance and speech dominance *within individuals.* If exactly half the population were right-handed and left-speech dominant, and the remainder were left-handed and right-speech dominant, then the above theories could remain almost unchanged. The theories therefore produce no account of population dominance for speech and handedness, beyond the trivial statement that at least one of them exists, and causes the other. This seems to be a serious defect; in each case the models confuse dexterity with right-handedness.

The following key proposals are shared by the tool and gestural theories, and our first task will be to discuss their validity:

1. Tool use in general involves greater skill and finer control on the part of the right hand.
2. As a result of evolution, the right hand (or more correctly, the left hemisphere) has acquired a greater potentiality for skilled motor control.
3. The skills developed by the left hemisphere do not transfer to the right hemisphere, because duplication of function is avoided wherever possible, in order to make the most economical use of available space; in other words, there is a selective advantage to asymmetry.
4. Manual skills and speech resemble one another sufficiently to share a common neural substrate, at least in part.

We now discuss these issues separately. In so far as these key proposals support both the tool/gesture theories and the tongue-muscle theory, then a lack of specification of the theoretical models is demonstrated.

(a) Tool use involves greater skill in the right hand

It must immediately be apparent that since the world is to a first approximation symmetric, then there is no necessary advantage in using tools with the right rather than the left hand *per se.* Nevertheless it is true that for many skills, for example, chipping a flint, throwing a spear, or scraping a bone, the right hand is usually the one carrying out the more skilled actions. Frost (1980) points out that in such examples the left hand performs merely a holding or steadying role, if it has one at all. The hypothesis may thus very well be true for early examples of tool using behaviour. In passing, however, we should like to express doubts about the over-enthusiastic application of this principle to the great variety of modern manual skilled behaviours. Once it has been decided *a priori* that the left hand is deficient in skill, it is all too easy to explain away any apparent counter-example by special pleading. For example, in the playing of many modern stringed instruments, the left hand has the difficult task of holding down the strings in the correct spatio-temporal pattern, so that the right hand can cause them to vibrate at the correct frequency. On the face of it this seems to demand greater skill by the left hand, but we have seen it suggested that this is just another example of the left hand holding an object while the right hand acts upon it! This sort of assertion makes it virtually meaningless to claim that the right hand has, in general, greater skill. We shall return to this theme below; in the meantime, we agree that the account given by Frost and others for *early* tool use is a plausible one. However, the study by Wright (1972), in which an orang-utan (probably left-handed) learned, by imitation, to produce and use stone tools, suggests that population right-handedness *per se* is not essential for the development of tool use (although there is interesting evidence that handedness concordance between teacher and pupil can facilitate the learning of manual skills (Michel and Harkins, 1985)).

(b) The right hand (left hemisphere) has evolved a greater potentiality for motor skill

It is beyond question that the right hand is much more skilful than the left at tasks that it carried out habitually, such as handwriting. (Of course, this remark applied only to right-handed people; we shall deal with the problem of left handedness later.) But does this mean that the right hand has some *intrinsic* advantage in acquiring skill? We would follow Dimond (1970) in arguing that it does not; as he points out, 'lateral preference is not the same thing as cerebral dominance': thus it may be that the only reason why the right hand is more skilful at writing and other tasks is that it has practised them more, and that this practice has failed to transfer to the left hand, just as skills acquired by the left hand may fail to transfer to the right. It may be objected that no rational account of handedness is possible unless the hands differ in their potential for skill; but such reasoning is erroneous. The origin of the skill difference might be an inherited *preference* for using the right hand, rather then skill coming first and preference second. After all, infants manifest handedness by a reaching preference long before it is possible to demonstrate differences in skill. Might not what is true of ontogeny be also true of phylogeny?

If there is indeed a preference for using the right hand, irrespective of an underlying skill difference, then a skill difference will soon result as a consequence of differential practice. In almost any task involving different functions of the two hands, we would maintain, people are less able to do with one hand what they normally do with the other, even if the original choice is idiosyncratic rather than species-specific. (The same is probably true of which side of the nose is used in pea-rolling competitions, in highly practised competitors.) Thus the superior skills of the right hand cannot be used as evidence for an inherited superiority of the left hemisphere in skilled tasks, unless differential practice can be ruled out as an explanation. In using such an argument we would argue that *preference* may be fundamental, but that this preference should not be regarded as *mere preference*. In the case of another human behavioural asymmetry (hand-clasping), which appears to be purely preferential, one of us has described significant geographical variations, and evidence of a genetic mechanism (McManus and Mascie-Taylor, 1979). It should also be remembered that in the case of vision, sighting eye dominance bears no relation to acuity dominance, which might have been suspected to be the underlying skill difference upon which the sighting dominance depended (Porac and Coren, 1976).

The clearest evidence for an innate skill difference would be a demonstration that right handers could never acquire, with the left hand, skills that are normally performed with the right hand. One might look here for acquisition of left-handed writing and drawing in right-handed patients with right hemiplegia, if it were not for certain obvious difficulties of interpretation. First, it would be unwise to make too much of a difference in fine motor skill between a brain-damaged and normal subject, or between a brain-damaged patient and their pre-traumatic performance. Second, there may very well be sensitive periods for the development of such skills as writing, and if so it would be unreasonable to expect the left hand to acquire, later in life, skills which the right hand acquired in childhood.

One possible way round these difficulties is to examine children who are born without one or other hand, and to see whether there are left–right differences *between* subjects. Weinstein *et al.* (1964) studied strength and co-ordination of children born with only one upper extremity. The principal motivation of the study was to evaluate the importance of practice in determining skill asymmetry, and it was expected that there would be some superiority of the group in which the right hand had been spared. The data apparently failed to support this hypothesis, from which it is tempting to deduce the important fact that there are no inter-subject differences in skills of the two hands when the opportunities for practice have been equalized. If valid, this argues against the hypothesis that skill differences are primary, and in favour of the alternative that they are acquired by differential practice. However, the results in the paper are published with very little statistical data, and there is a relatively small number of children with terminal arm aplasia. A more difficult problem is that any such study is necessarily a between-subject analysis, and hence the between-subjects design will be far less sensitive to relatively small differences and there is a great danger of a Type I error, particularly if one wishes to 'prove' the null hypothesis.

A further source of data on this question is that of children with limb abnormalities due to maternal thalidomide usage. The only published report of which we are aware (Smithells, 1970) is too brief to be of any help. If anecdote is of any use in such cases, then we could mention an acquaintance of one of us (ICM) who has a symmetric thalidomide deformity involving normal upper arm and elbows, with complete absence of both forearms except for the proximal inch or so, and a rudimentary 'hand', consisting of a single digit. This person states that he has never been in any doubt that he is 'right-handed' — this seeming to be the limb which he naturally prefers to use for complicated tasks. A further anecdote describes a case of a child with complete upper and lower arm absence, with a rudimentary hand attached to each shoulder. The child in question was finding great difficulty in learning to write with a pencil in the right 'hand'. When the pencil was attached to the left 'hand' then writing developed fluently: the implication is that this child was, in some sense, 'left-handed'. (A related case may be found in Poeck (1964) who reported the case of a child without forearms or hands who said that 'voluntary' movements with the phantom of the left hand were more skilful than similar movements with the phantom of the right hand.) Such cases, as with the cases of unilateral aplasia, are clearly of great potential for disentangling the origins of hand skill and hand preference, although as yet there is little substantial evidence available.

Another way of looking at the problem is to examine left-handers, who are quite frequently forced by social pressures early in life to use their initially non-preferred hand for skills such as hand-writing. If skill differences are dependent upon inherited predispositions of the hemispheres, we should expect skills acquired by the non-preferred hand to be inferior. Is there any evidence for this from left-handers who have been forced to switch hands? In other words, are such people less skilled at writing and drawing than right-handers, or than left-handers who have not been forced to switch? This is a crucial question to which there appears to be no clear answer in the literature; although there have been many claims that enforced changes produce emotional changes, we know of no direct evidence that skills as such are affected. In the case of playing musical instruments, Oldfield (1969) found no evidence to suggest that left-handers were at a disadvantage in having to play right-handed instruments and his conclusion is interesting:

> '... handedness is not a matter of superior inherent "dexterity" or the capacity for agility, precision and speed in the [preferred] hand.'

Although here it might be argued that some form of selection has resulted in only the most ambidextrous of left-handers eventually manifesting as professional musicians.

Similarly, Walker (1980) also uses the argument of musicians to support the suggestion that:

> '... human handedness is largely a matter of preference rather than a consequence of biologically programmed inadequacies of the minor hemisphere.'

It could be argued against this that the case of left-handers throws little light on the general question of the origin of skill differences, because left-handers are often claimed to be less weakly lateralized than right-handers and would not thus be expected to show strong differences in motor skill between the hemispheres. On examination, however, this argument is revealed as somewhat circular, in as much as one line of evidence that left-handers are 'less lateralized' comes from skill tests, the results of which are actually in accord with the hypothesis that skill differences result from practice. For example, Benton *et al.* (1962) (cited by Satz *et al.*, 1967) found that many self-classified left-handers showed striking superiority of the *right* hand on a manual co-ordination test. This is just what we should expect if these left-handers had been forced by social pressures to use their right hand, and if skill differences are determined by usage, not by inherited differences between the hemispheres. Similarly, Satz *et al.* (1967) found that in a manual dexterity test (picking up pins with tweezers) left-handers were no worse than right-handers with their right hands: the most striking fact was the inferiority of right-handers to left-handers when using their *left* hand. This is just what we should expect from the practice hypothesis. Left-handers are also claimed to be less lateralized and more variable in their laterality on the basis of handedness questionnaires. McManus (1979) has demonstrated that these differences are entirely due to items for which there is either social pressure (e.g. the hand used to hold a knife and fork) or mechanical pressure (e.g. in the use of items with a right-hand screw thread). Thus these left-handers are 'dextrous' in accord with the demands of society: otherwise they use their preferred hand, and show as strong a degree of asymmetry as right-handers.

At this point it would be desirable to distinguish clearly the two main senses in which the term 'handedness' has been used in the literature (*cf.* Oldfield, 1971; Annett, 1972). The first refers to the subject's preferences in carrying out everyday tasks such as hand-writing and hammering, and is usually assessed by self-report in questionnaire form. The second refers to objectively determined performance differences between the two hands in tasks such as frequency of tapping, reaction time, balancing a dowell rod, or moving pegs around a board (Annett, 1972). We shall refer to these two kinds of handedness as 'handednesss/preference' and 'handedness/skill' in order to be quite clear about which we mean in a particular context. Now, it is the essence of the class of evolutionary theory that we are considering to suppose that there is an intimate relation between 'handedness/preference' and 'handedness/skill'. It is claimed that the left hemisphere has evolved special mechanisms for the control of manual skill, which subsequently transfer to the control of speech. But the evidence that humans acquired handedness/skill early in evolution comes necessarily from preference measures, since psychologists were not around at the time with their peg-boards to test differences in skill between the hands. There is thus a rather crucial gap in the theory, and it is important that it should be bridged by convincing evidence demonstrating a clear relation between handedness/skill and handedness/preference.

Unfortunately for the tool theory and related accounts, the evidence is that preference and skill measures are related only rather loosely. As Annett

(1972, 1978) has pointed out, skill difference between the hands show an approximately normal distribution both in left and right handers, with a wide spread in both cases. For example, in Galton's data on grip strength, the distribution of difference scores follows an approximate normal distribution in which the mean is shifted from the zero point by about 0.44 SDs. This means that about 33% of the sample actually showed a *left*-hand superiority: and since this is far too high a proportion to represent left-handers as they would be classified on a preference test, it must be concluded that a number of right-handers (by preference) actually show a left-hand superiority in grip strength. Similarly, Annett's (1974) figures for peg moving show a shift from the mean of 0.5 SDs and 1.10 SDs in males and females respectively, again suggesting that quite a large proportion of right-handers (preference) show a left hand superiority in a skill test.

The National Child Development Study (*see* McManus, 1981) administered two unimanual tasks to over 12 000 11-year-old children for details of the classification of handedness and background. The first test involved using a pencil to mark as many small squares as possible on a sheet of graph paper in one minute, using first one hand and then the other. The second test required the child to pick up and transfer 20 matchsticks to the other side of the table. In each case a laterality index (R–L/R+L) was computed for each child (*see* McManus, 1985b). The overall distribution of the scores for the square-making task was bimodal with considerable overlap of the distributions of right and left handers. For the matches task the overlap was much more marked, although the means of the two distributions were still in the expected directions. In contrast to these overlapping measures of skill difference, the measures of handedness in the National Child Development Study showed a clear separation (*see* McManus, 1981a).

It is thus quite mistaken to start from the fact that about 90% of people write with the right hand, and to deduce from this that 90% of people have more skilled right hands. As Oldfield puts it:

> '. . . tasks which in the precise form presented are unfamiliar to the subject, and which he is given little or no opportunity to practice, produce a distribution of indices which, while not symmetrical, is roughly bell-shaped with an outstanding mode not far from the neutral point, and sometimes . . . another small one near the left hand end. That is to say, the right–left differences displayed by such methods are relatively small and *certainly do not correspond with* the gross disparity between the two hands which is manifest in well practised tasks.' (Oldfield, 1971, p. 97)

We are not denying that some skill tests, such as tracing, and cutting out shapes with scissors (Shankweiler and Studdert-Kennedy, 1975) will discriminate virtually perfectly between hands. But these are highly practised tasks (and in one case involve using an asymmetric tool). In the case of unpractised tasks like Crawford pegs and Crawford screws,

Shankweiler and Studdert Kennedy found virtually zero correlation between asymmetry scores and handedness as measured by tracing and scissors, in a group of self-classified right-handers. This lack of correlation contrasted with the high intercorrelation between scissors and tracing. (Although note here that handedness and skill are being assessed *within* right-handers. It is quite conceivable that there may be a strong correlation of handedness and skill between right and left handers, but no correlation within either handedness group.) Furthermore, only tracing and cutting were significant predictors of ear advantage in a dichotic CV test: the unpractised tasks showed if anything a weighting in the wrong direction. Shankweiler and Studdert-Kennedy conclude from this '... that well-practised tasks, which are nearly always carried out by the same hand, should be used for measurements of manual laterality. This would ensure that differential experience in use of hands, otherwise a potent uncontrolled variable, does not contribute to the variance'. This is one line of reasoning: another might be that cerebral lateralization correlates with preference, and only secondarily with skill, as we are suggesting here.

Shankweiler and Studdert-Kennedy seem to be suggesting that skill differences between the two hands will show themselves best in asymptotic performance. This is a reasonable position, and it may be tested by taking a relatively unfamiliar task like Crawford pegs and training both hands in short, alternating sessions until performance shows no further improvement. Four experiments have been reported which broadly fit this description. Peters (1981) has reported a study on the relatively unskilled task of finger-tapping. In general the dominant index finger has a maximum tapping speed score 10% greater than the non-dominant index finger. Peters examined the effect of long-term practice on the difference between the hands: fourteen subjects completed from 200 to 1150 trials each involving 10 seconds tapping with the right and the left hand. In thirteen of the fourteen subjects there was no evidence of a diminution of the difference in performance of the two hands, despite an improvement in performance with both hands through the experiment. Hicks (1974) asked 160 right-handed subjects to cover sheets of paper in capital letters printed inverted and reversed. Two blocks of ten trials were used, with a quarter of the subjects using the right-hand during both blocks, a quarter using the left-hand during both blocks, and the remaining subjects changing hands between blocks 1 and 2, half from right to left, and the rest vice versa. From the present viewpoint the interesting finding is that the rate of learning was greater with the right than the left-hand, and that the relative advantage of the right-hand increased as the experiment went on. It is also of some interest that in those subjects who changed hands between blocks there was a greater transfer of skill from right hand to left hand than vice versa. Similar results have been found by Taylor and Heilman (1980), and McManus and Stagg (1984).

The third experiment is that of Annett *et al.* (1974) who reported extended practice on the Annett peg moving task. This experiment differed from the previous ones in that in two out of the three subjects there was a significant diminution in the degree of manual asymmetry. Finally, Perelle *et al.* (1981) reported that practice with the Crawford Small Parts Dexterity Test reduced the degree of skill asymmetry to a non-significant amount. Several objections may be found to these experiments. However intense the practice it seems unlikely that it could reverse the habits of a lifetime, particularly in an adult with a non-plastic brain. It might also be questioned whether, in any case, the subjects were sufficiently motivated to learn with their non-dominant hand, given that such learning ran counter to all their previous intuitions of their learning abilities. It is, after all, noteworthy that the high motivation for success found in skilled pianists or typists produces much less performance asymmetry between the hands.

In summary the evidence is confused as to whether the right hand is innately more skilful or merely preferred and hence more practised at the tasks. The case for a more 'skilful' left hemisphere is thus not proved, and we turn to examine the next critical element in the tool and gestural theories.

(c) Competition for neural space has prevented unnecessary duplication of functions in the two hemispheres

This is a central and plausible proposition in both the tool and gestural theories. Once again we quote Frost:

> 'If we advance the premise that both praxic and non-praxic functioning were essential to the early hominids, it would follow that *both* of the corresponding neural substrates would have to be represented in the hominid cortex: thus neither can be extensively represented at the expense of the other. By consequence of the trade-off principle, any increase in the praxic substrates will enhance the ability to make and use tools while producing a decrement in non-praxic functioning while any increase in the non-praxic substrates will have the reverse effect. The expected evolutionary result of this competition for neural space would be a distribution of the praxic and non-praxic substrates within the cortex which would maximize tool making and using ability while minimizing the loss of non-praxic functioning.' (Frost, 1980, p. 451)

The perfect solution to this competition problem is, of course, to parcel out the different functions in opposite hemispheres. This reasoning accounts very neatly for the specialization of the right hemisphere for visuo-spatial abilities. Exactly the same line of argument has been advanced by Levy (1977) in her 'cognitive style' theory:

> 'Lateralization appears to provide for a minimization of interference effects in neural activity patterns and a maximization of the computers integrating these patterns. If two very different kinds of cognitive capacities are to be present, then joint optimization of the level of these capacities seems to require lateralization.' (p. 815)

This is a plausible retrospective account of the origin of lateralization, but is there any way to test it? On the face of it the theory seems to predict that individuals who have not adopted the optimum strategy will be at a cognitive disadvantage; and the obvious group to look at here is those left-handers who have retained left hemisphere language control, while presumably invading the right hemisphere for the control of manual skill (praxis). Such individuals should, according to Levy (1977), manifest inferior visuospatial abilities. Another reason why this should be so is that a right hemisphere contribution to language is more likely in sinistrals than in dextrals, both according to clinical findings on aphasia, and from the results of unilateral ECT and amylobarbital tests (*see* Bradshaw, 1980 for a review).

From an evolutionary point of view, the hypothesis of a cognitive deficit in sinistrals raises the intriguing question of why left-handedness has remained so common, relative to other genetically deleterious traits such as haemophilia. Possible answers might include the following:

1. Incomplete heritability of the trait.
2. Relaxation of selection pressures against cognitive deficit followed by a random drift upwards in gene frequency.
3. A rather weak selection pressure is in equilibrium with a quite high mutation pressure.
4. An unknown selective advantage of sinistrality, such as higher fertility (McManus, 1979) acts in opposition to the putative cognitive disadvantage and has resulted in a situation of balanced polymorphism (Sheppard, 1975).

The high incidence of left handedness is a general problem for evolutionary theories, because they all attempt to derive the majority state of affairs from some supposed selective advantage. However, it is time to leave this fascinating but unsolved problem on one side for the moment, and ask if there is really anything to explain: is there in fact any evidence for a cognitive disadvantage to sinistrality?

Levy (1977) reported that left-handers had significantly lower scores than dextrals on tests of spatial ability, and not on language tests. Her study was criticized by Newcombe and Ratcliffe (1973) for involving an occupationally restricted group (college students); their own more extensive study of 410 men and 410 women of various occupations found no significant difference in WAIS IQ, either verbal or performance. Heim and Watts (1976) examined this problem with test AH 2/3 and found no evidence that left-handers did less well on performance/visuospatial tasks. (A total of 2165 sinistrals were used ranging from 9-year-old children to adult students.) Curiously, the results did suggest that left-handers —especially if they were male — did better on numerical tasks, a result quite contrary to Levy's hypothesis.

In a more recent large-scale study, of a housing estate in Cambridge

(England), Mascie-Taylor (1980) found that left-handers were significantly worse than right-handers on performance but not verbal IQ. This supports Levy's findings. But in an even larger sample, of 7169 children in the National Child Development Study (NCDS), McManus and Mascie-Taylor (1983) found no significant effects of handedness on non-verbal IQ. They did, however, find that left-handers scored very slightly but significantly less well than right-handers on G, the factor that accounted for 91% of the common variance in the four tests used, Reading, Maths, Verbal Ability and Non-Verbal Ability.

It is difficult to draw firm conclusions from this mass of contradictory findings, unless it be that Levy's suggestion of a visuospatial deficit in sinistrals holds only under special conditions, at present unspecified. There is evidence from the two most extensive studies of a slight difference in favour of right-handers, although it should be emphasized that the effect is very small indeed. We tend to agree with the conclusion of Bradshaw's (1980) review, that '... Levy's hypothesis of a specific visuospatial disability amongst sinistrals is unsupported.'

Finally, we consider the idea that sinistrality, and its alleged cognitive deficit, results from otherwise undetectable left hemisphere damage resulting from 'birth stress' (Bakan, 1977). This hypothesis has been strongly contested by others (*see* McManus, 1981 for a review) and, in a large-scale study of the NCDS dataset, McManus found little evidence to support it. Incidentally, McManus and Mascie-Taylor (1983) found no evidence either to support the idea that the slightly lower G score of sinistrals was due to a severely impaired sub-group: the same effect was found if the lowest-scoring 5% was removed from the sample.

(d) Do speech and manual praxis share a common neural mechanism?

The most difficult problem for the speech and gestural theories is to bridge the gap between the evolution of the left hemisphere as a controller of skilled manual movements, and its role in the control of speech and language. This gap is bridged by the proposal that speech and manual praxis have sufficient in common for speech, when it evolved, to make use of pre-adapted neural mechanisms in the left hemisphere. Thus Kimura (1976) has proposed that 'brain regions considered to be important for symbolic language processing might better be conceived as important for the production of motor sequences which happen to lend themselves readily to communication' (p. 145). Before considering the evidence that Kimura advances for this interesting idea, we shall ask what kind of shared properties have been specified, and try to assess the general plausibility of the argument.

In point of fact, Kimura appears to have offered a variety of ideas relating speech to manual praxis, and it is not easy to know which one to consider as fundamental. Kimura (1976) argued that the special contribution of the left hemisphere both to speech and to manual praxis, is the 'running off or patterning' of smaller units: phonemes or syllables in the case of speech, single flexions in the case of movements. In support of this idea are the findings of several studies that temporal acuity is apparently greater in the left hemisphere in normals (Efron, 1963a; Hammond, 1981) and in brain-damaged populations (Efron, 1963b; Carman and Nachshon, 1961), and that the perception (Gordon, 1978) and production (Woolf *et al.* 1977; Ibbotson and Morton, 1981) of rhythms is superior in the left hemisphere. In a later article (Kimura, 1977) greater stress was laid on the presence in the left hemisphere of a spatial mechanism for the 'accurate positioning of oral and brachial musculature.' These suggestions are not necessarily incompatible, since the sequencing or patterning function could clearly depend upon accurate positional information; we do wonder, however, whether neural capacities defined in such very general terms are not in danger of explaining too much. Is there any example of a complex behaviour that could not be included *a posteriori* under such an umbrella if it were found to be affected by left hemisphere lesions? Conversely, is it possible to exclude from under the umbrella those functions that are known to have a specific contribution from the right hemisphere, such as visuospatial manipulation?

Kimura (1977, p. 539) acknowledges that the idea of a special left hemisphere involvement in spatial control of body movements may appear implausible given the neuropsychological evidence for a right hemisphere involvement in complex spatial abilities. McFie and Zangwill (1960) described severe spatial disorders following right parietal lesions. As a recent example, Kolb and Whishaw (1980, p. 249) describe Mr P, a 67-year-old man who had suffered a right parietal stroke; he was impaired at combining blocks together to form designs (constructional apraxia) and generally impaired at drawing freehand *with either hand*, copying drawings or cutting out paper figures.

Kimura attempts to circumvent this difficulty by proposing a distinction between spatial control exerted by external visual cues, and control by the internal body schema. Only the latter, she suggests, is the property of the left hemisphere. An immediate objection is that the spatial deficits associated with right parietal lesions go far beyond an inability to deal with external spatial relations: they can include neglect of the left side of the body and difficulties in dressing the left side of the body; and even in more severe cases, problems in dressing extending to the right side of the body as well. Moreover, these impairments are more common following right than left hemisphere lesions (Geschwind, 1965, p. 599).

Another problem is concerned with music production, which clearly shares many of the properties of speech, such as complex sequencing and fine motor control of the lips: and which should therefore involve the left hemisphere according to Kimura's hypothesis. However, left hemisphere lesions and left carotid sodium amytal injections can produce aphasia while leaving singing ability relatively intact (Kolb and Whishaw, 1980, p. 201). Many severely aphasic patients can hum a tune or sing the words of a previously learned song (e.g. Yamadori *et al.*, 1977). If two such closely related skills as speaking and singing have different neural substrates, perhaps even control from opposite hemispheres, it becomes a bit implausible to argue that speech and manual praxis have common neural substrates, merely because they share certain properties at a highly abstract level of description.

Kimura brings forward four lines of evidence to support the idea of an intimate relation between speech and manual activity:

1. The association between hand preference and speech lateralization.
2. The frequent association between hand movements and speaking.
3. The frequent association between limb apraxia, aphasia and left hemisphere lesions.
4. The association between disorders of manual communication (signing) and left hemisphere lesions in the deaf.

The first point reiterates the fundamental problem: why are people generally right-handed and left hemisphere dominant for speech? Preference is not necessarily the same thing as skill, and there is little evidence for an association between manual skill asymmetry and speech lateralization, once differences in practice have been taken into account. Shankweiler and Studdert-Kennedy found no correlation between dichotic asymmetry and manual asymmetry for unpractised skilled tasks, although there was a clear correlation with practised tasks. The obvious point is also worth mentioning that the association between handedness and speech lateralization is far from being invariable: many left-handers have left hemisphere speech dominance and there are cases of right-handers with right hemisphere speech (Zangwill, 1960, 1979).

Kimura's second argument is the frequent association between speech and gestures, particularly by the right hand. In an observational study (Kimura, 1976) more right- than left-hand movements were found during speaking than during either silent verbal activity or humming, and speaking was accompanied by three times more right hand movements than left. Furthermore, Kinsbourne and his collaborators (cf. Kinsbourne, 1975) have shown in a number of studies that speech interferes with skilled right-hand performance such as balancing a dowel rod, finger tapping and sequential finger movements. The left hand is less affected by vocalization. Kinsbourne uses this and other evidence to argue for 'an archaic . . . relationship between language and right-sided action'. Indeed, McNeill (1985) has argued, primarily on linguistic grounds, that gestures and speech share a common computational stage (or, in more recent terms, a 'module'), and that at a deep level they are functionally equivalent.

Oldfield (1969) made the very interesting observation about left-handed musicians that they have no apparent difficulty in playing right-handed musical instruments, but do find it unnatural and difficult to conduct with the baton in their right hands. Oldfield suggests that the preferred hand has more immediate access to the individual's intentions and conceptions than does the minor hand. Peters (1981) has reported that right-handers find it easier to tap as quickly as possible with the right hand while following a beat with their left, than to attempt the reverse arrangement. Kinsbourne has argued that there is an *attentional* bias towards the left hemisphere, which explains not only why we are right-handed and left hemisphere dominant for speech, but also why we find it difficult to divide attention between speech and right-hand activity. Some recent evidence for an attentional bias is Rabbitt's (1978) observation that reaction times are faster for the right hand when the subject's response involves choice between hands, but not when all responses are carried out with a single hand.

We have mentioned the attentional theory here because it would seem to provide a way of explaining why speech and hand movements are sometimes related, without invoking Kimura's idea that they share a common neural mechanism (except in the trivial sense that they are both in the same hemisphere). It would be interesting to have evidence from left-handers, to see if gestures during speech are made with the normally preferred hand, or with the hand controlled by the hemisphere dominant for speech.

The third line of evidence Kimura uses to support her position is the association between limb apraxia and left hemisphere lesions. The term 'Apraxia' goes back to Liepmann's description of the 'Regierungsrat' case history (*see* Geschwind, 1967 for an historical and critical review). The important observation for present purposes is that left hemisphere lesions can produce motor disturbances in the right hand, which is to be expected, but also in the *left* hand: so called 'sympathetic' dyspraxia. This suggests that the left hemisphere has some responsibility for both hands in the case of complex movements. The disturbance can be manifested in inability to respond to verbal commands, to carry out imitation movements, and to indicate the normal use of objects by handling them appropriately. Liepmann found this syndrome frequently associated with right hemiplegia and aphasia, but never with the left hemiplegia: he explained his data by the hypothesis that the left hemisphere is dominant for more than speech — in addition it contains the memory for skilled movements.

Geschwind (1967) supported Liepmann's findings and his interpretation, and argued against the obvious alternative explanation: that the failure of the left hand is simply due to comprehension difficulty. Thus one of Geschwind's own patients failed badly on verbal commands and imitation and also did poorly on object handling, but could respond appropriately with single word utterances to difficult questions such as 'What occupation were you engaged in before you became ill?' When asked 'Do you know how to use a hammer?' the patient responded 'Nails', but could not indicate how a hammer should be used. This view is disputed by Ettlinger (1969) who pointed out that, whilst he had been able to simulate human neuropsychological syndromes such as the agnosias by selective cortical removal in monkeys, he had never produced an apraxia, despite the obvious ability of these animals to carry out skilled activities. He then went on to consider the problem of patients with callosal sections who, as Dimond also points out, do not apparently suffer from sympathetic dyspraxia except in response to verbal commands: 'Not a single case was impaired at copying movements or using objects with the left hand, and yet such impairment would have been observed if these actions were always organised in the left hemisphere'. Ettlinger therefore concludes that the fundamental defect in classical apraxia is an inability to perform *verbal* commands, a conclusion supported by the finding of Kools *et al.* (1971) that apraxia in mentally retarded children is primarily related to defects of verbal comprehension.

The association of apraxia with aphasia is problematic. Most authors (e.g. Brown, 1972 (based on a re-analysis of Liepmann's patients), Benson, 1979; Geschwind, 1965; Goodglass and Kaplan, 1979; Heilman, 1979) agree that apraxia is commonly associated with aphasia, although all authors accept that it is relatively common to find aphasia without apraxia and less common to find apraxia without aphasia. This dissociation suggests that two separate functional processes are involved: indeed Geschwind (1955) suggests that 'the relationship is one of anatomical propinquity of lesions; the apraxia frequently accompanies the aphasia but is independent of it' (Geschwind, 1965, p. 609). This relative independence of apraxia and aphasia is also shown by the relative independence of ideational apraxia and ideo-motor apraxia, although the severity of both forms is related to the severity of aphasia, be it Broca's, Wernicke's or global (de Renzi *et al.*, 1968). Although the study of de Renzi *et al.* suggests no difference in the preferential association of apraxia with Broca's rather than Wernicke's aphasia, this has been suggested by Geschwind (1967), and would seem to be a necessary assumption if his disconnection model is to be accepted. However, in a careful study of the localization of cerebral lesions (by computed tomography) and their relationship to apraxia, no tendency was found for apractics to have anterior rather than posterior lesions (Basso *et al.*, 1980).

A separate problem also arises with the syndrome of facial apraxia, which seems to show a closer relationship with Broca's aphasia than Wernicke's, although it is relatively independent of limb apraxia (de Renzi *et al.* 1966). Geschwind (1967) suggests that facial apraxia is only a special form of sympathetic dyspraxia involving a lesion of a slightly different pathway, one which lies closer to Broca's area.

Another approach to apraxia has been to study motor behaviour in individuals with right- or left-sided lesions. Heilman (1975) found that amongst right-handed aphasics with right hemiparesis, tapping rate in the left-hand was reduced in the patients with a clinical apraxia. In contrast Haaland, Porch and Delaney (1980) could find no difference in tapping rate between apractic and non-apractic patients, although they did find deficits on a task of precise steadiness. Haaland and Delaney (1981) could find no differences between right and left hemisphere lesion groups in a study of a number of motor tasks. Similarly Wyke (1971) found no convincing difference between right and left hemisphere lesions in unimanual or bimanual motor tasks, although her earlier study (Wyke, 1968) had found evidence suggesting that left brain lesions impaired contralateral movements far more than did right brain lesions. There thus seems to be a major discrepancy between clinical apraxia and inability to carry out conventional laboratory tests of lateralized motor skill, suggesting that apraxia may well involve a symbolic component which is missing from our more normal description of handedness.

Kimura and Archibald (1974) required patients with vascular accidents limited to either the left or right hemisphere to perform a number of motor tasks. There were no differences between the two groups in single finger flexions or in the copying of a static hand posture, but in the copying of manual sequences the left hemisphere group was worse, whichever hand was used. Kimura (1976) argues that the deficit was not attributable to a language impairment in the left hemisphere group, on the grounds that there was no significant correlation between scores on the aphasia battery and scores on movement copying. This is a double-edged argument, because what happens in these circumstances to the claim that speech and motor control have a common neural basis?

Critchley (1953) suggested that lesions in the left parietal lobe resulted in defects of language of gesture — asemasia. Goodglass and Kaplan (1963) found that gesture and pantomime were both impaired in aphasics, although they found that the gestural ability was less impaired than the pantomiming ability; there was also a correlation between severity of aphasia and severity of gestural and pantomiming defect. De Renzi *et al.* (1980) examined gestural ability in 280 patients. In those with left-sided lesions there was a defect in imitating gestures in 80% of aphasic patients and only 50% of non-aphasic patients, but a 'non-negligible minority' of 20% of the non-aphasic patients with right-sided lesions also had gestural disturbances. Kolb and Milner (1981) examined the ability to perform complex arm and face movements in patients who had had unilateral removals of areas of cortex. For arm movements the left parietal removals were more impaired; face movements were impaired by lesions of *either* the right or the left frontal regions. Thus there is a very confused picture as to the role of asymmetric neural functions in controlling pantomime, gesture and expression. For a review see Peterson and Kirshner (1981).

A problem in all these studies and in Kimura's (1977) study is that they have been carried out almost exclusively with right-handers, so that it is difficult to decide whether the greater involvement of the left hemisphere in motor control is due to the presence of language there, or to the fact that this hemisphere controls the dominant (preferred) hand. This matter could be settled by studying a group of left-handers with left hemisphere language dominance, assessed by the sodium amytal method. If 'sympathetic apraxia' of the right hand were found after right hemisphere lesions, the view would be supported that the hemisphere dominant for handedness contains the memories of motor movements or some such: but it would argue against Kimura's hypothesis that manual praxis is closely related to speech. If the opposite result were found, that is, greater impairment of manual praxis after left hemisphere lesions, as in dextrals, Kimura's hypothesis would be supported, although it would then be something of a puzzle why these subjects should have preferred to use their left hands. Finally, the absence of a difference between left and right hemisphere effects could readily be attributed to a more bilateral representation of language, and thus of manual praxis, in the two hemispheres.

Haaland and Delaney (1981) have re-examined the problem of inter-hemispheric differences in manual praxis and have come to different conclusions from Kimura. They studied performance both of CVA and tumour groups on grip, tapping, static and vertical groove steadiness, maze co-ordination, and grooved pegboard tasks. All brain-damaged groups performed more poorly than controls on the hand contralateral to the lesion, and also on the ipsilateral hands in the case of the more complex tasks. But the pattern of results was the same in the left and right hemisphere groups. Haaland and Delaney point out that, 'The grooved pegboard task requires at least six different movements including reaching, grasping, turning and insertion . . . suggesting that Kimura's hypothesis is incorrect'.

Thus we are not entirely convinced by the evidence of a special language-related involvement of the left hemisphere in the motor control of complex sequences. Even if there were greater agreement about the facts than is the case, there would still be a problem of interpretation. Is the left hemisphere involved in both sets of function because they share some neural mechanisms, or is it just a coincidence? We have suggested that the study of left-handers is vital here, because many of them will have control of the preferred hand by the right hemisphere but speech control from the left. Another problem that has to be faced is the possible role of language loss *per se* in causing apraxic defects through comprehension deficits: Kimura's theory is on the horns of a dilemma here, because correlation of apraxia with aphasia is required to prove the sharing of neural mechanisms, but too high a correlation is undesirable, because then it is difficult to exclude the possibility that the only underlying deficit is linguistic. A more precise formulation of the degree of overlap between speech and manual praxis would be helpful.

(4) The Attentional Theory

In a highly stimulating attack upon the laterality problem, Kinsbourne has proposed (e.g. 1975) that language and the preferred hand are controlled by the same hemisphere because there is an underlying gradient of attention favouring a turning to the right side of space.

Kinsbourne points out that evidence of behavioural asymmetry in non-human animals frequently involves an asymmetrical orientating tendency. The clearest evidence for brain asymmetry in animals comes from the study of subcortical mechanisms implicated in arousal. Glick *et al.* (1977) described contralateral circling behaviour in rats with unilateral lesions in the nigrostriatal system, and postulated that rotation in normal rats reflects an intrinsic nigrostriatal asymmetry. Subsequently it was indeed found that normal rats have a 10–15% left–right difference of dopamine content in the striatum. Marshall, Berrios and Sawyer (1980) demonstrated that dopaminergic terminals in the neostriatum are critical for orientation: unilateral neostriatal lesions reduced orientation to contralateral touch, whereas similar damage to other dopamine systems did not. Giehrl and Distel (1980) found what looks like a species-specific asymmetry in the Syrian hamster, related to the caudate nucleus. When descending from a centreboard these animals turn more often to their right than to their left (79% of occasions): the tendency was reversed after small caudate lesions.

These studies are exciting because they suggest an actual mechanism for functional brain asymmetries, rather than relying upon unobservable differences in neuronal organization. It is perhaps easier to see how a relatively simple left–right chemical asymmetry could be coded embryologically than to understand how the two halves of the brain could be programmed to develop different circuitry (for a general discussion of the embryological problem see Morgan, 1977 and Corballis and Morgan, 1978); and descriptions of new chemical asymmetries in the brain are appearing at an increasing rate, as neurochemists begin to look for them. To give another example that may have behavioural significance, Gerandai *et al.* (1979) have found a 96% left–right difference in the medio-basal hypothalmus (rat) of the hypothalamic luteinizing-hormone-release hormone. Of course, chemical differences can also underlie structural differences, a rather nice model for this being the unilateral induction of limb defects in rats by the teratogenic compound, acetazolamide.

Kinsbourne suggests that people have an inherited rightwards orientating tendency, possibly dependent upon asymmetrical hemispheric activation from subcortical structures. A suggestive line of evidence for subcortical involvement in laterality comes from the work of Petrie and Peters (1980) of an asymmetry in the strength of the grasp reflex in infants of 17 days. Pointing out that the grasp reflex can also be elicited in anencephalics, Petrie and Peters note that, 'the possibility that the observed asymmetry is subcortical in origin cannot therefore be discounted.' (As an illustration of the frequent conflicts of evidence in the developmental literature on asymmetry, we should note that Petrie and Peters, in contrast to Caplan and Kinsbourne (1976) found no differences in the duration of rattle holding in their infants, either in unilateral or bimanual tests.)

Another piece of evidence begins with the observation of Gesell and Ames (1947), confirmed later by Turkewitz and Birch (*cf.* Turkewitz, 1977), that infants spend approximately 91% of their time lying with their head turned to the right of the body midline. There is also a tendency for predominant rightwards head turning in response to sensory stimulation, both aversive and non-aversive (Liederman and Kinsbourne, 1980). Coryell and Mitchell (1978) make the intriguing suggestion that the right turning posture tends to evoke the asymmetrical tonic neck reflex, i.e. the infant extends the limb on the side to which the head is turned. This could mean that the infant gets greater sensorimotor experience with the right than with the left hand, and Coryell and Mitchell claim that 'Knowledge of which hand an infant has had more visual experience of, as a result of its postural preference, reliably predicts the hand which will be used most in a visually elicited reaching test at 12 weeks.' It must be stressed that in considering work on early postural asymmetries there is little evidence that the asymmetry reliably predicts subsequent adult handedness. Thus the prospective study of Michel (1981) only considered handedness at 22 *weeks* of age. The study of Viviani *et al.* (1978) considered handedness at 7 years of age (when handedness probably correlates well with subsequent handedness; McManus, 1981a) but since only twenty-two children were followed up, of whom twenty-one were right-handed, it is clear that the significant correlation reported can only refer to degree of lateralization, and not direction. As an aside, it is of interest that neonatal head turning in response to tactile stimulation is apparently sensitive to birth stress, as assessed by the Apgar score (Turkewitz *et al.* 1968) while it is highly unlikely that handedness is related to birth stress (McManus, 1981a).

All of this supports the view that manual asymmetries may be a special case of an asymmetrical rightwards turning tendency. But where does language come into the picture? Kinsbourne offers evidence for what he terms a 'synergism' between language and right-sided motor activity:

1. While people are pondering verbal material they tend to move heads and eyes to the right.

2. When subjects think verbally while making a simple visual discrimination (gap in a line) the concurrent verbal activity biases attention in space so that accuracy is greatest in the right half visual field (Kinsbourne, 1975, Expt 1).
3. Notwithstanding the fact just described, there is interference if the subject tries to speak while engaging in skilled movements with the right hand. For instance, dowel balancing with the right hand is more affected by speaking than is the same task carried out with the left hand.

The second two points are difficult to reconcile, since one involves facilitation of right-sided activity by vocalization, and the other a decrement: but presumably the point is that speaking and visual attention do not require a common processor, while speaking and manual activity do. Once again, then, we are back to the idea that speech and skilled manual activity share the same neural substrate. The version of this hypothesis that Kinsbourne seems to favour is that speech originally represented internalized actions and still bears the mark of this archaic association (*cf.* also Reynolds, 1976). As Kinsbourne (1978) puts it:

> We emerge with a model of language origins in relation to the right hand and right-sided action. We would suppose that protoman first made utterances that were coincident with and driven by the same rhythm as the movement in question. As this skill further evolved, the utterances became internalized and detached from overt action, so that they became capable of assuming a signalling role in the absence of their referents. A vast degree of further elaboration and transformation would then ultimately result in the highly intricate language systems prevalent in most human societies. However, even in the most sophisticated speaker, verbal activity is not completely free of corollary somatic movement produced on an involuntary basis.' (p. 558)

The asymmetry of speech is explained by saying that there is no need for it to have evolved bilaterally; Kinsbourne differs from most other theorists in seeing no particular advantage or disadvantage to the present arrangement, and he expressly denies that left-handedness confers any cognitive disadvantage. Speech presumably got started in the left hemisphere because of the presence there of the praxic mechanisms (*see* above quotation). The reasoning here is slightly difficult to follow, in the light of the attentional gradient, probably of subcortical origin, presumably the neural *mechanisms* as such for the control of skilled movement are present in both hemispheres: and in these circumstances it is not clear why speech should have become lateralized, unless it is just a coincidence after all.

Many of the comments in previous sections of this chapter are relevant to Kinsbourne's theory. We tend to agree with his suggestion that handedness is in origin a matter of preference (attentional bias) rather than of preprogrammed differences in skill. The argument that speech and praxis share neural mechanisms is similar to Kimura's account, which we discussed in

Section (d). Perhaps the most unusual feature of Kinsbourne's theory is also its weakest point: we refer to the denial that lateralization of *speech* depends upon pre-programmed differences in cerebral organization. The problem here is that the theory would seem to predict that it is much easier than is fact the case for individuals to learn to speak with their right hemisphere after left hemisphere damage: why should this in fact be so difficult if all that is involved is a switch in attention? The shift should be even easier for young children to effect, yet even here it seems that claims for 'equipotentiality' have been considerably exaggerated (Witelson, 1977), a problem further discussed by Kinsbourne (1978, p. 562).

A variant of the attentional bias theory is that of Gazzaniga (1974) who suggests, along with Kinsbourne, that 'structural-genetic factors' (such as the *planum temporale* asymmetry) cause the right hand to move more, and hence to explore the world more. This then results in, and potentiates, engrams being stored in the left hemisphere; as a result the right hand is used preferentially to explore the world, and hence a positive feedback results in left cerebral dominance. Nottebohm (1979) implies that motor asymmetries are present from birth, and manifest in early speech; thus in his own son he observed that early babbling tended to be associated with shifts of the tongue towards the right side of the mouth. The problem with such models is, as Gazzaniga recognised, that left-handers do not, in general, show right hemispheric speech dominance. To explain this away by saying that 'The phenomenon of left handedness is, at best, a complicated affair . . .', is, at best, special pleading.

Correlation Theories

In relation to the theories we have discussed up to now, the correlational theories stand as a null hypothesis, for they deny that there is any functional reason for the association between speech lateralization and handedness. A convenient starting point is the observation that a partial list of lateral asymmetries in man would include: left aorta distributes oxygenated blood to body, liver displaced to right, kidneys at different heights, left testicle hangs lower than right, gut coiling, and higher incidence of breast cancer on the left (for other examples of unilateral disease presentation *see* McManus, 1979). A list in animals would include: coiling in gastropods, the single Narwhal tusk on the left, the epithalamus of amphibia, ovaries of birds, migration of the eye in flat fish (for these and many other examples *see* Neville (1976) and Morgan (1977)).

Since so many asymmetries exist, why pick on just two of them — handedness and speech lateralization — for explanation? Even if we arbitrarily confine our attention to the brain of man, it is becoming clear that speech and handedness are not the only asymmetries. In particular, there is the well-documented specialization of the right hemisphere for visuospatial processing, and possibly for music. Particularly in the tool and gestural theories, these asymmetries are considered to be secondary to speech lateralization (cf. also Corballis and Morgan, 1978) but there is no strong evidence for this, and it is motivated mainly by a philosophical prejudice that makes the possession of propositional speech the main defining attribute of mankind. If we took a more Celtic view of man as the only animal to invent new songs, or possibly a Polynesian view of man as navigator, we might come to a different opinion about which is the 'leading hemisphere'.

Thus an extreme view might be that speech lateralization and handedness are no more functionally related than, say, speech and the kidneys. On this view, the exceptional cases where they are dissociated would be like cases of isolated dextrocardia, where the heart but not the liver and gut shows reversed *situs*. A less extreme view is that the various forms of laterality may be embryologically related, without there being any particular functional reason for their association (Corballis and Morgan, 1978; Morgan and Corballis, 1978). There is indeed quite strong evidence in the case of other lateral asymmetries that they are not coded for entirely separately in development. This is illustrated by the condition of *situs inversus viscerum et cordis* in which not only the heart, but also the liver and gut, have reversed asymmetry. In amphibia there is experimental evidence that brain asymmetry correlates with that of liver and gut. Von Woellwarth (1950) studied habenular asymmetry (the habenular nucleus is larger on the left than on the right) after various treatments of the early embryo, and found that reversed *situs* of the habenular invariably correlated with reversed arrangement of the internal organs.

On the basis of this and other examples, Morgan (1977) and Corballis and Morgan (1978) argued that there may be a common source of asymmetries, possibly related to molecular chirality, and that this in general tends to favour more rapid development of the left side of the body. A considerable body of comment, much of it pointing critically to possible counter-examples, followed publication of the articles by Corballis and Morgan (1978) and Morgan and Corballis (1978) in *The Behavioural and Brain Sciences*, to which the interested reader is referred for further details.

A different correlation model has been proposed by one of us (ICM) which is related to that of Annett (1978), and in which there is more than a mere chance association of lateralities, but rather each laterality (say speech and handedness) is dependent upon a single gene. The model originates in a genetic model of handedness, in which there are two alleles, D (for Dextral) and C (for Chance). The three genotypes, DD, DC and DD produce progeny containing respectively 0, 25 and 50% of left-handers. Consider DC genotypes. One in four of these individuals are left-handed, with chance factors alone determining which one in four is left-handed. If we allow the same gene to control speech dominance, then one in four of DC genotypes will be phenotypically right-speech dominant. If these two chance processes are independent, then one in sixteen of DC genotypes will be left-handed and right-speech dominant, six in sixteen will be cross-lateralized, and nine in sixteen will be right-handed and left-speech dominant. When one takes account of the DD and CC genotypes then it can be shown that the model can predict the observed incidences of right speech dominance in right and left-handers (*see* McManus, 1984, 1985a for a more detailed account). Here no functional advantages are required for particular forms of cerebral organization, and there is no functional similarity betwen speech and manual praxis; the only similarity between the two processes is that their lateralization is determined by the same genetic mechanism.

Conclusion (General)

We have considered a number of theories that try to account for the statistical relationship between speech lateralization and handedness. The theory that the association is learned has, in our view, little evidence to support it. Evolutionary theories share several common themes: that the left hemisphere has developed special mechanisms for skilled manual control; that speech and manual control share a common neural substrate; and that there is a selective advantage to the present system of inter-hemispheric differences. These claims have been considered critically. We have questioned whether the right hand, and the left hemisphere, are really pre-programmed to acquire special skills, rather than being merely preferred. We have also found little evidence, in our view, to support the speculative idea that speech and hand control share an underlying neural substrate; likewise the claim that there is a selective advantage to the present system of asymmetry. Finally, we outline the 'null hypothesis' that the relation between speech and handedness is accidental, in that it is at most a non-functional expression of a common molecular chirality acting during early development or a necessary consequence of a single gene controlling two lateralized processes.

Our conclusion is that evolutionary theories are highly stimulating; indeed, perhaps a little too stimulating, since they necessarily force us to ask (and usually, not to succeed in answering adequately) questions about the entire gamut of human language and cerebral specialization. It is perhaps not journalistic hyperbole to claim that 'All human life is there'.

References

ABLER, W.L. Asymmetry in the skulls of fossil man; evidence of lateralised brain function? *Brain, Behaviour and Evolution* (1976), **13** 111-115.

ALBERT, M. and OLBER, L. *The Bilingual Brain: Neurophysiological and Neurolinguistic Aspects of Bilingualism* (1978), New York: Academic Press.

ANNETT, M. The distribution of manual asymmetry. *British Journal of Psychology*, (1972), **63**, 345-358.

ANNETT, M. Handedness in the children of two left-handed parents. *British Journal of Psychology* (1974), **65**, 129-131.

ANNETT, M. *A Single Gene Explanation of Right and Left Handedness and Brainedness* (1978), Coventry: Lanchester Polytechnic.

ANNETT, M., HUDSON, P.T.W. and TURNER, A. The reliability of differences between the hands in motor skills. *Neuropsychologia*, (1974), **12**, 527-531.

ANONYMOUS. *Sung Dynasty Album Paintings* (1957), Peking: Chinese Classic Art Publishing House.

BAKAN, P. Left-handedness and birth order revisited. *Neuropsychologia* (1977), **15**, 837-839.

BALDWIN, J.M. The origin of right-handedness. *Popular Science Monthly* (1894), **44**, 606-615.

BASSO, A. LUZZATTI, C. and SPINNLER, H. Is ideo-motor apraxia the outcome of damage to well-defined regions of the left hemisphere? *Journal of Neurology, Neurosurgery, and Psychiatry* (1980), **43** 118-126.

BASTIAN, H.C. *A Treatise on Aphasia and Other Speech Defects* (1898), London: H.K. Lewis.

BASTIAN, H.C. and HORSLEY, V. Arrest of development in the left upper limb, in association with an extremely small right ascending parietal convolution. *Brain* (1880), **3**, 113-116.

BATEMAN, F. *On Aphasia* (1870), London: Churchill.

BENSON, D.F. *Aphasia, Alexia and Agraphia* (1979), Edinburgh: Churchill Livingstone.

BENTON, A.L. and JOYNT, R.J. Early descriptions in aphasia. *Archives of Neurology*, (1960), **3**, 205-221.

BENTON, A.L., MEYERS, R. and POLDER, G.J. Some aspects of handedness. *Psychiatrica et Neurologia* (1962), **144**, 321-337.

BRADSHAW, J.L. Right hemisphere language: Familial and non-familial sinistrals, cognitive deficits and writing hand position in sinistrals, and concrete-abstract, imageable-dimensions in word recognition. A review of inter-related issues. *Brain and Language* (1980), **10**, 172-188.

BRAMWELL, B. On crossed aphasia . . . *Lancet* (1899), **i**, 1473-1479.

BRAIN, R. *Speech Disorders: Aphasia, Apraxia and Agnosia*, (1961), London: Butterworths.

BROOKER, R.J., LEHMAN, R.A.W., HEIMBUCH, R.C. and KIDD, K.K. Hand usage in a colony of Bonnett monkeys, *Macaca radiata. Behaviour Genetics* (1981), **11**, 49.

BROWN, J.W. *Aphasia, Apraxia and Agnosia: Clinical and Theoretical Aspects* (1972), Springfield, Ill.: C.C. Thomas.

BURT, C. *The Backward Child*, 3rd edn. (1950), London: University of London Press.

CALVIN, W.H. Did throwing stones shape hominid brain evolution? *Ethology and Sociobiology*, (1982), **3**, 115-124.

CAMP, D.M., THERRIEN, B.A. and ROBINSON, T.E. Spatial learning ability is related to an endogenous asymmetry in the nigro-striatal dopamine system in rats. *Society for Neuroscience Abstracts* (1981), **7**, 455.

CAPLAN, P.J. and KINSBOURNE, M. Baby drops the rattle: asymmetry of duration of grasp by infants. *Child Development* (1976), **47**, 532-534.

CARMAN, A. and NACHSHON, I. Effect of unilateral brain damage on perception of temporal order. *Cortex*, (1971), **7**, 410-418.

COLE, J. Paw preference in cats related to hand preference in animals and men. *Journal of Comparative Physiology and Psychology* (1955), **48**, 137-140.

COLE, J. and GLEES, P. Handedness in monkeys. *Experimentia* (1951), **7**, 224-225.

COLEY, F.C. The prophylaxis of aphasia. *The Practitioner* (1909), **2**, 238-240.

COLLINS, R.L. On the inheritance of handedness, I. *Journal of Heredity* (1968), **59**, 9-12.

COLLINS, R.L. On the inheritance of handedness, II. *Journal of Heredity* (1969), **60**, 117-119.

COLLINS, R.L. The sound of one paw clapping; an enquiry into the origin of left handedness. In G. Linzey and D.D. Thiessen (eds) *Contributions to Behaviour-Genetic Analysis; the Mouse as a Prototype* (1970). New York: Appleton-Century-Crofts.

COLLINS, R.L. A demonstration of an inheritance of the direction of asymmetry that is consistent with the notion that genetic alleles are left-right indifferent *Behaviour Genetics* (1981), **11**, 596a.

COLLINS, R.L. On the inheritance of the direction and degree of asymmetry. In S.D. Glick (ed.) *Cerebral Lateralization in Sub-human Species* (1985), pp. 41-70. New York: Academic Press.

CORBALLIS, M.C. and MORGAN, M.J. On the biological basis of human laterality; I. Evidence for a maturational left-right gradient. *The Behavioral and Brain Sciences* (1978), **1**, 261-269.

COREN, S. and PORAC, C. Fifty-centuries of right-handedness; the historical record. *Science* (1977), **198** 631-632.

CORYELL, J. and MICHEL, G. How supine postural preferences of infants can contribute towards the development of handedness. *Infant Behaviour and Development* (1978), **1**, 241-257.

CRITCHLEY, M. *The Parietal Lobes* (1953). London: Arnold.

CRITCHLEY, M. Premorbid literacy, and the pattern of subsequent aphasia *Proceedings of the Royal Society of Medicine* (1956), **49**, 335.

DAMASIO, A.R., CASTRO-CALDAS, A. GROSSO, J.T. and FERRO, J.M. Brain specialisation for language: does not depend on literacy *Archives of Neurology* (1976a), **33**, 300-301.

DAMASIO, A.R., CASTRO-CALDAS, A., GROSSO, J.T. and FERRO, J.M. Brain specialisation for language: not dependent on literacy *Archives of Neurology* (1976b), **33**, 662.

DART, R.A. The predatory implemental technique of Australopithecus. *American Journal of Physical Anthropology* (1949), **7**, 1-38.

DENENBERG, V.H. Animal studies of laterality. In K.M. Heilman and P. Satz

Neuropsychology of Human Emotion (1983), pp. 65-84. New York: Guilford Press.

DENNIS, W. Early graphic evidence of dextrality in man. *Perceptual and Motor Skills* (1958), **8**, 147-149.

DIMOND, S.J. Cerebral dominance — or lateral preference in motor control. *Acta Psychologia* (1970), **32**, 196-198.

DIMOND, S. and HARRIES, R. Face-touching in monkeys, apes and man: evolutionary origins and cerebral asymmetry *Neuropsychologia*, (1984), **22**, 227-233.

EFRON, J.R. The effect of handedness on the perception of simultaneity and temporal order, *Brain* (1963a), **86**, 261-284.

EFRON, R. Temporal perception, aphasia and deja vu. *Brain*, 1963b), **86**, 403-424.

ETTLINGER, G. Lateral preferences in monkeys. *Behaviour* (1961), **17**, 275-287.

ETTLINGER, G. Apraxia considered as a disorder of movements that are language dependent; evidence from cases of brain bisection. *Cortex* (1969), **5**, 285-289.

ETTLINGER, G. and MOFFETT, A. Lateral preferences in the monkey. *Nature (Lond.)* (1964), **204** 606.

FINCH, G. Chimpanzee's handedness. *Science* (1941), **94**, 117-118.

FRIEDMAN, H. and DAVIS, M. Left-handedness in parrots. *The Auk*, (1938), **55**, 478-480.

FROST, G.T. Tool behaviour and the origins of laterality. *Journal of Human Evolution* (1980), **9**, 447-459.

GAZZANIGA, M. Cerebral dominance viewed as a decision system. In S.J. Dimond, and J.G. Beaumont (eds) *Hemisphere Function in the Human Brain* (1974). London: Paul Elek.

GERENDAI, I., ROTSZTEJN, W. MARCHETTI, B. and SCAPAGNINI, U. LH-RH changes in the medio-basal hypothalamus after unilateral ovariectomy. In A. Polleri, and R.M. Macloed (eds) *Neuroendocrinology; Biological and Clinical Aspects* (1979), pp. 97-102, London: Academic Press.

GESCHWIND, N. Disconnexion syndromes in animals and man. *Brain*, (1965), **88** 237-294, 585-644.

GESCHWIND, N. The apraxias. In E.W. Straus and P.M. Griffith (eds) *Phenomenology of Will and Action* (1967), pp. 91-102. Pittsburgh: Duquesne University Press.

GESCHWIND, N. and LEVITSKY, W. Human brain; left-right asymmetries in temporal speech region. *Science*, (1968), **161**, 186-187.

GESELL, A. and AMES, L.B. The development of handedness. *Journal of Genetic Psychology*, (1947), **70**, 155-175.

GIEHRL, T. and DISTEL, H. Asymmetric distribution of side preference in hamsters can be reversed by lesions of the caudate nucleus. *Behavioural Brain Research* (1980), **1**, 187-196.

GLICK, S.D., JERUSSI, T.P. and ZIMMERBERG, B. Behavioural and neuropharmacological correlates of nigrostriatal asymmetry in rats. In S. Harnad, R.W. Doty, L. Goldstein, J. Jaynes and G. Krauthamer (eds) *Lateralisation in the Nervous System*, (1977), pp. 213-249. New York: Academic Press.

GLICK, S.D. and ROSS, D.A. Lateralisation of function in the rat brain. *Trends in Neurological Sciences* (1981), **4**, 196-199.

GLONING, I., GLONING, K., HAUB, G. and QUATEMBER, R. Comparison of verbal behaviour in right-handed and non-right-handed patients with anatomically verified lesion of one hemisphere. *Cortex*, (1969), **5**, 43-52.

GOOCH, S. *The Neanderthal Question* (1977), London: Wildwood Howe.

GOODGLASS, H. and KAPLAN, E. Disturbance of gesture and pantomime in aphasia. *Brain* (1963), **86**, 703-720.

GOODGLASS, H. and KAPLAN, E. Assessment of cognitive deficit in the brain-injured patient. In M.S. Gazzaniga (ed.) *Handbook of Behavioural Neurobiology, Vol. II: Neuropsychology*, (1979), New York: Plenum Press.

GOODGLASS, H. and QUADFASEL, F.A. Language laterality in left-handed aphasics. *Brain* (1954), **77**, 521-548.

GORDON, H.W. Left hemisphere dominance for rhythmic elements in dichotically presented melodies. *Cortex* (1978), **14**, 58-70.

GORDON, H.W. Brain and Language. *Cerebral organisation in bilinguals; I. Lateralisation* (1980), **9**, 255-268.

GORLITZER VON MUNDY, V. A 94 year old with one German language center and probably two Slovenian language centers. In M. Paradis (ed.) *Readings on Aphasia in Bilinguals and Polyglots* (1959), Quebec: Didier.

GOULD, S.J. *Ever Since Darwin; Reflections in Natural History* (1980), Harmondsworth: Penguin Books.

GOWERS, W.R. The brain in congenital absence of one hand. *Brain* (1878), **1**, 388-390.

HAALAND, K.Y. and DELANEY, H.D. Motor deficits after left or right hemisphere damage due to stroke or tumour. *Neuropsychologia* (1981), **19**, 17-27.

HAALAND, K.Y., PORCH, B.E. and DELANEY, H.D. Limb apraxia and motor performance. *Brain and Language* (1980), **9**, 315-323.

HAMILTON, C.R., TIEMANN, S.B. and FARRELL, W.S. Cerebral dominance in monkeys? *Neuropsychologia* (1974), **12**, 193-197.

HAMMOND, G.R. Finer temporal acuity for stimuli applied to the preferred hand. *Neuropsychologia* (1981), **1981**, 325-329.

HARRIS, L.J. Left-handedness; Early Theories, Facts and Fancies. In J. Herron (ed.) *Neuropsychology of Left-handedness* (1980), pp. 3-78. New York: Academic Press.

HEFFNER, H.E. and HEFFNER, R.S. Temporal lobe lesions and perception of species-specific vocalisations by macaques. *Science* (1984), **226** 75-76.

HEILMAN, K.M. A tapping test in apraxia. *Cortex* (1975), **11** 259-263.

HEIM, A.W. and WATTS, K.P. Handedness and cognitive bias. *Quarterly Journal of Experimental Psychology* (1976), **28**, 355-360.

HERREN, R.Y. and LINDSLEY, H.B.A note concerning cerebral dominance in the rat. *Journal of Genetic Psychology* (1935), **47**, 469-472.

HEWES, G. The current status of the gestural theory of language origin. *Annals of the New York Academy of Sciences* (1976), **280**, 482-504.

HICKS, R.E. Asymmetry of bilateral transfer. *American Journal of Psychology* (1974), **87**, 667-674.

HOADLEY, M.F. and PEARSON, K. On measurement of the internal diameters of the skull in relation (i) to the prediction of its capacity (ii) to the 'pre-eminence' of the left hemisphere. *Biometrika* (1929), **21**, 85-123.

HOLLOWAY, R.L. Exploring the dorsal surface of hominoid brain endocasts by stereo-plotter and discriminant analysis. *Philosophical Transactions of the Royal Society B* (1981), **292**, 155-166.

IBBOTSON, N.R. and MORTON, J. Rhythm and dominance. *Cognition* (1981), **9**, 125-138.

ISAAC, G.L. Archaeological tests of alternative models of early hominid behaviour; excavation and experiments. *Philosophical Transactions of the Royal Society, B* (1981), **292**, 177-188.

JACKSON, J.H. On aphasia, with left hemiplegia. *Lancet* (1880), **ii**, 637-638.

KENNY, D.A. *Correlation and Causality* (1979). New York: John Wiley & Sons.

KIMURA, D. The neural basis of language qua gesture. In H. Whitaker and H.A. Whitaker (eds) *Studies in Neurolinguistics, Vol. 2* (1976), pp. 145-156. New York: Academic Press.

KIMURA, D. Acquisition of a motor skill after left-hemisphere damage. *Brain* (1977), **100**, 527-542.

KIMURA, D. and ARCHIBALD, Y. Motor functions of the left hemisphere. *Brain* (1974), **97**, 337-350.

KINSBOURNE, M. The mechanism of hemispheric control of the lateral gradient of attention. In P.M.A. Rabbitt and S. Dornic (eds) *Attention and Performance, Vol. V* (1975), pp. 81-96. London: Academic Press.

KINSBOURNE, M. The ontogeny of cerebral dominance. In R.W. Rieber (ed.) *The Neuropsychology of Language* (1976), pp. 181-191. New York: Plenum Press.

KINSBOURNE, M. Evolution of language in relation to lateral action. In M. Kinsbourne (ed.) *Asymmetrical Function of the Brain* (1978), pp. 553-565. Cambridge: Cambridge University Press.

KINSBOURNE, M. A model for the ontogeny of cerebral organisation in non-right-handers. In J. Herron (ed.) *Neuropsychology of left-handedness* (1980), pp. 177-185. New York: Academic Press.

KOLB, B. and MILNER, B. Performance of complex arm and facial movements after focal brain lesions. *Neuropsychologia* (1981), **19**, 491-503.

KOLB, B. and WHISHAW, I.Q. *Fundamentals of Human Neuropsychology* (1980), San Francisco: W.H. Freeman.

KOOLS, J.A., WILLIAMS, A.F. VICKERS, M.J. and CAELL, A. Oral and limb apraxia in mentall retarded children with deviant articulation. *Cortex* (1971), **7**, 387-400.

LEAKEY, M.D. Tracks and tools. *Philosophical Transactions of the Royal Society of London, B* (1981), **292**, 95-102.

LEHMANN, R.A.W. The handedness of rhesus monkeys; I. Distribution. *Neuropsychologia* (1978), **16**, 33-42.

LEHMANN, R.A.W. Distribution and changes in strength of hand preference of Cynomolgus monkeys. *Brain, Behaviour and Evolution* (1980), **17**, 209-217.

LE MAY, M. and GESCHWIND, N. Hemispheric differences in the brains of great apes. *Brain, Behaviour and Evolution* (1975), **11** 48-52.

LEVY, J. Evolution of language lateralization and cognitive function. *Annals of the New York Academy of Sciences* (1976), **280**, 810-820.

LIEDERMAN, J. and KINSBOURNE, M. Rightward motor bias in newborns depends upon parental right-handedness. *Neuropsychologia* (1980), **18**, 579-584.

MCFIE, J. and ZANGWILL, O.L. Visual-constructive disabilities associated with lesions of the left hemisphere. *Brain* (1960), **83**, 243-260.

MCMANUS, I.C. Right-left and the scrotum in Greek sculpture. *Nature (Lond.)* (1976), **259**, 426.

McMANUS, I.C. *Determinants of Laterality in Man* (1979), University of Cambridge, unpublished PhD. Thesis.
McMANUS, I.C. Handedness and birth stress. *Psychological Medicine* (1981a), **11** 485-496.
McMANUS, I.C. Wing-folding in Drosophila. *Animal Behaviour* (1981b), **29**, 626-627.
McMANUS, I.C. The distribution of skull asymmetry in man. *Annals of Human Biology* (1982), **9**, 167-170.
McMANUS, I.C. The interpretation of laterality. *Cortex* (1983), **19** 187-214.
McMANUS, I.C. The genetics of handedness in relation to language disorder. In F.C. Rose (ed.) *Advances in Neurology, Vol. 42: Progress in Aphasiology* (1984), pp. 125-138. New York: Raven Press.
McMANUS, I.C. Handedness, language dominance and aphasia: a genetic model. *Psychological Medicine, Monograph Suppl. Number 8* (1985a).
McMANUS, I.C. Right- and left-hand skill: failure of the right shift model. *British Journal of Psychology* (1985b), **76** 1-16.
McMANUS, I.C. and MASCIE-TAYLOR, C.G.N. Hand clasping and arm-folding; a review and a genetic model. *Annals of Human Biology* (1979), **6**, 527-558.
McMANUS, I.C. and MASCIE-TAYLOR, C.G.N. Bio-social correlates of cognitive abilities. *Journal of Bio-social Science* (1982) **13**, 289-306.
McMANUS, I.C. and STAGG, C. Asymmetric transfer and mirror-image transfer of a motor skill. Paper presented to *The Motor Skills Research Exchange, Amsterdam, July 1984*.
McNEILAGE, P.F. STUDDERT-KENNEDY, M.G. and LINDBLOM, B. Primate handedness reconsidered. *Behavioral and Brain Sciences* (1987) (*in press*).
McNEILL, D. So you think gestures are non-verbal? *Psychological Review* (1985), **92**, 350-371.
MARIN, O.S.M., SCHWARTZ, M.F. and SAFFRAN, E.M. Origins and distribution of language. In M.S. Gazzaniga (ed.) *Handbook of Behavioural Neurobiology, Vol. II: Neuropsychology* (1979), pp. 179-213. New York: Plenum Press.
MARSHALL, J.F., BERRIOS, N. and SAWYER, S. Neostriatal dopamine and sensory inattention. *Journal of Comparative and Physiological Psychology* (1980), **94**, 833-846.
MASCIE-TAYLOR, C.G.N. Hand preference and components of IQ. *Annals of Human Biology* (1980), **7**, 235-248.
MICHEL, G.F. Right-handedness; a consequence of infant head-orientation preference? *Science* (1981), **212** 685-687.
MICHEL, G.F. and HARKINS, D.A. Concordance of handedness between teacher and student facilitates learning manual skills. *Journal of Human Evolution* (1985), **14**, 597-601.
MOLFESE, D.L. Infant cerebral asymmetry. In S.J. Segalowitz and F.A. Gruber (eds) *Language Development and Neurological Theory* (1979), pp. 21-35. New York: Academic Press.
MORGAN, M.J. Embryology and inheritance of asymmetry. In S. Harnard, R.W. Doty, L. Goldstein, J. Jaynes and G. Krauthamer (eds) *Lateralisation in the Nervous System* (1977), pp. 173-194. New York: Academic Press.
MORGAN, M.J. and CORBALLIS, M.C. On the biological basis of human laterality; II

The mechanisms of inheritance. *The Behavioral and Brain Sciences* (1978), **1** 270-277.

MOXON, W. On the connexion between loss of speech and paralysis of the right side. *British and Foreign Medico-Chirurgical Record* (1886), **37**, 481-489.

NEEDLES, W. Concerning transfer of cerebral dominance in the function of speech. *Journal of Nervous and Mental Diseases* (1942),, **95**, 270-277.

NEVILLE, A.C. *Animal Asymmetry* (1976). London: Edward and Arnold.

NEWCOMBE, F. and RATCLIFF, G. Handedness, speech lateralisation and ability. *Neuropsychologia* (1973), **11** 399-407.

NIELSON, J.M. *A Textbook of Clinical Neurology* (1946), New York: Hoeber.

VAN NOTEN, F., CAHEN, D. and KEELEY, L. A palaeolithic campsite in Belgium. *Scientific American* (1980), **242**, 44-51.

NOTTEBOHM, F. Origins and mechanisms in the establishment of cerebral dominance. In M.S. Gazzaniga (ed.) *Handbook of Behavioural Neurobiology, Vol. II: Neuropsychology* (1979), pp. 295-348. New York: Plenum Press.

OLDFIELD, R.C. Handedness in musicians. *British Journal of Psychology* (1969), **60**, 91-99.

OLDFIELD, R.C. The assessment and analysis of handedness; the Edinburgh inventory. *Neuropsychologia* (1971), **9**, 97-113.

PAGET, G.E. Notes on an exceptional case of aphasia. *British Medical Journal* (1887), **ii**, 1258-1259.

PARADIS, M. Bilingualism and aphasia. In H. Whitaker and H.A. Whitaker (eds) *Studies in Neurolinguistics, Vol. III* (1977), p. 65. New York: Academic Pess.

PERELLE, I.B., EHRMAN, L. and MANOWITZ, J.W. Human handedness; the influence of learning. *Perceptual and Motor Skills* (1981), **53**, 967-977.

PETERS, M. Handedness; effect of prolonged practice on between hand performance differences. *Neuropsychologia* (1981), **19**, 587-590.

PETERSEN, M.R., BEECHER, M.D., ZOLOTH, S.R., MOODY, D.B. and STEBBINS, W.C. Neural lateralisation of species-specific vocalisations by Japanese macaques (*Macaca fuscata*). *Science* (1978), **202**, 324-327.

PETERSON, L.N. and KIRSCHNER, H.S. Gestural impairment and gestural ability in aphasia: a review. *Brain and Language* (1981), **14**, 338-348.

PETERSON, G.M. A preliminary report on right- and left-handedness in the rat. *Journal of Comparative Psychology* (1931), **12**, 243-250.

PETRIE, B.F. and PETERS, M. Handedness; left/right differences in intensity of grasp response and duration of rattle holding in infants. *Infant Behaviour and Development* (1980), **3**, 215-221.

POECK, K. Phantoms following amputation in early childhood and in congenital absence of limbs. *Cortex,* (1964), **1**, 269-275.

POHL, P. Hemispheric lateralisation of speech perception in the baboon. *International Journal of Primatology* (1982), **20**, 323.

POHL, P. Central auditory processing. V: Ear advantages for accoustic stimuli in baboons. *Brain and Language* (1983), **20**, 44-53.

PORAC, C. and COREN, S. The dominant eye. *Psychological Bulletin* (1976), **83**, 880-897.

RABBIT, P. Hand dominance, attention and the choice between responses. *Quarterly Journal of Experimental Psychology* (1978), **30**, 407-416.

DE RENZI, E., MOTTI, F., and NICHELLI, P. Imitating gestures; a quantitative approach to ideo-motor apraxia. *Archives of Neurology* (1980), **37**, 6-10.

DE RENZI, E., PIECZURO, A. and VIGNOLO, L.A. Oral apraxia and aphasia. *Cortex* (1966), **2**, 50-73.

DE RENZI, E., PIECZURO, A. and VIGNOLO, L.A. Ideational apraxia; a quantitative study. *Neuropsychologia* (1968), **6**, 41-52.

REYNOLDS, P.C. Language and skilled activity. *Annals of the New York Academy of Sciences* (1976), **280**, 150-166.

RIESE, W. The early history of aphasia. *Bulletin of the History of Medicine* (1947), **21**, 322-334.

ROGERS, L.J. Environmental influences on brain lateralisation. *The Behavioral and Brain Sciences* (1981), **4**, 35-36.

SATZ, P., ACHENBACH, K. and FENNEL, E. Correlations between assessed manual laterality and predicted speech laterality in a normal population. *Neuropsychologia* (1967), **5**, 295-310.

SHANKWEILER, D. and STUDDERT-KENNEDY, M. A continuum of lateralisation for speech perception. *Brain and Language* (1975), **2**, 212-225.

SHEPPARD, P.M. *Natural Selection and Heredity* 4th edn. (1975). London: Hutchinson.

SMITHELLS, R.W. Hand and foot preference in thalidomide children. *Archives of Disease in Children* (1970), **45**, 224.

SPENNEMANN, D.R. Handedness data on the European Neolithic. *Neuropsychologia* (1984), **22**, 613-615.

STEKLIS, H.D. Primate communication, comparative neurology, and the origin of language re-examined. *Journal of Human Evolution* (1985), **14**, 157-173.

STEKLIS, H.D. and HARNAD, S.R. From hand to mouth; some critical stages in the evolution of language. *Annals of the New York Academy of Sciences* (1976), **280**, 445-455.

SUSSMAN, H.M., FRANKLIN, P. and SIMON, T. Bilingual speech; bilateral control? *Brain and Language* (1982), **15**, 125-142.

TAYLOR, H.G. and HEILMAN, K.M. Left-hemisphere motor dominance in right-handers. *Cortex*, (1980), **16**, 587-603.

TOBIAS, P.V. The emergence of man in Africa and beyond. *Philosophical Transactions of the Royal Society, B* (1981), *292*, 43-56.

TOTH, N. Archaeological evidence for preferential right-handedness in Lower and Middle Pleistocene and its possible implications. *Journal of Human Evolution* (1985), **14**, 607-614.

TSAI, L.S. and MAURER, S. Right-handedness in white rats. *Science* (1930), **72**, 436-438.

TURKEWITZ, G. The development of lateral differences in the human infant. In S. Harnad, R.W. Doty, L. Goldstein, J. Jaynes and G. Krauthamer (eds) *Lateralisation in the Nervous System* (1977), pp. 251-259. New York: Academic Press.

TURKEWITZ, G., MOREAU, T. and BIRCH, H.G. Relation between birth condition and neurobehavioural organisation in the neonate. *Pediatric Research* (1967), **2**, 243-249.

TZAVARAS, A. KAPRINIS, G. and GATZOYAS, A. Literacy and hemispheric specialisation for language; digit dichotic listening in illiterates. *Neuropsychologia* (1981), **19**, 565-570.

UHRBROCK, R.S. Laterality in Art. *Journal of Aesthetics and Art Criticism* (1973), **32**, 27-35.

VARNEY, N.R. and VILENSKY, J.A. Neuropsychological implications for pre-adaptation and language evolution. *Journal of Human Evolution* (1980), **9**, 223-226.

VIVIANI, J., TURKEWITZ, G. and KARP, E. A relationship between laterality of functioning at 2 days and at 7 years of age. *Bulletin of the Psychosomatic Society* (1978), **12** 189-192.

WALKER, S.F. Lateralisation of function in the vertebrate brain; a review. *British Journal of Psychology* (1980), **71**, 329-367.

WARD, R. and COLLINS, R.L. Brain size and shape in strongly and weakly lateralised mice. *Brain Research* (1985), **328**, 243-249.

WARREN, J.M. Handedness in the rhesus monkey. *Science* (1953), **118**, 622-623.

WARREN, J.M. and NOTTEBOHM, A.J. The search for cerebral dominance in monkeys. *Annals of the New York Academy of Sciences* (1976), **280**, 732–744.

WEBER, E. Eine Erkärung für die Art der Vererbung der Rechtshändigkeit. *Zentralblatt für Physiologie* (1904), **18**, 425-432.

WECHSLER, A.F. Crossed aphasia in an illiterate dextral. *Brain and Language* (1976), **3**, 164-172.

WEINSTEIN, S. and SERSEN, E.A. and VETTER, R.J. Phantoms and somatic sensation in cases of congenital aplasia. *Cortex* (1964), **1**, 276-289.

WEISENBURG, T. and MCBRIDE, K.E. *Aphasia: A Clinical and Psychological Study* (1935). New York: Hafner.

WERNICKE, C. *Wernicke's Works on Aphasia*. Translated by G.H. Eggett (1906; 1977). The Hague: Mouton.

WILSON, S.A.K. *Aphasia* (1926). London: Kegan, Paul, Trench Trubner.

WITELSON, S.F. Early hemisphere specialisation and interhemispheric plasticity: an empirical and theoretical review. In S.J. Segalowitz and F.A. Gruber (eds) *Language Development and Neurological Theory* (1977), p. 213. New York: Academic Press.

VON WOELLWARTH, C. Experimentelle Untersuchungen über dem Situs inversus der Eingeweide und der Habenula des Zwischenhirns bei Amphibien. *Wilhem Roux Archiv für Entwicklungsmechanik* (1950), **144**, 178-256.

5

Physiological Differences Between Left and Right

John F. Stein

Introduction

The prehistoric cave painters at Lascaux and Altamira depicted a few left- as well as right-handed hunters. Clearly the problem of handedness has interested people for a very long time. Man is distinguished from all other animals not only by his capacity for speech but also by usually preferring to use the right hand for precision tasks (Gardner, 1943). No other species shows such a consistent preference for using one limb rather than the other. I shall argue in this chapter that this fondness for the right hand probably evolved because highly skilled movements could be successfully developed only by confining the neural machinery required to control them to one hemisphere.

In birds it is now clear that the left half of the brain is almost entirely responsible for another example of precise motor co-ordination, the sequencing of the multitude of respiratory and vocal muscles which is necessary to produce their songs (Nottebohm, 1980). In higher primates right handedness probably evolved before the development of speech (Corballis and Morgan, 1978). But both required perfection of a mechanism for generating co-ordinated sequences of actions from widely separated muscles. Approximately 90% of humans direct from left-sided cortical centres both the precisely fractionated and co-ordinated contractions of the respiratory and vocal muscles which are required for speaking, and also the control of the muscles of the right arm for writing and other fine motor accomplishments.

In this chapter I wish to develop the idea that the differences that exist between the hemispheres are not primarily sensory, but are consequences of evolutionary pressures which lead to each hemisphere becoming specialized for a particular style of sensorimotor control. I will suggest that the left hemisphere is responsible for the precise sequencing in space and time of the actions of widely separated muscles, for the purpose of communication by gesturing, speaking or writing. These interactions may have developed originally to meet the requirements of the shared use of tools. In contrast I will argue that the right hemisphere generates a more 'holistic' style of control, less fractionated in time, and is probably responsible for guiding the movements of the whole animal in relation to the outside world, and for the expression of emotions. The differences which have been emphasized by many investigators between the sensory, perceptual and cognitive functions of each hemisphere (Sperry, 1968) are less significant than the differences that we can observe between the styles of motor control for which they are responsible. Probably, the differences in sensory processing have evolved secondarily, in order to meet the specialized control requirements dictated by the motor style of each hemisphere.

In the last decade research interest in hemispheric specialization has experienced explosive growth which has swollen the literature to almost unmanageable proportions (Mountcastle, 1962; Dimond, 1972; Kinsbourne, 1974; Corballis and Beale, 1976; Harnad, 1977; Gazzaniga and Ledoux, 1978; Steel-Russell *et al.* 1979; Porac and Coren, 1981; Bradshaw and Nettleton, 1983; Mesulam, 1983; Geschwind and Galaburda, 1985; Springer and Deutsch, 1985). The great majority of this work has been concerned with attempting to localize specialized perceptual systems which are supposed to be located in one or other hemisphere and has particularly concentrated on mechanisms judged to underly language comprehension. Many have devoted their energies to the question of the lateralization of sensory mechanisms because in this area there is considerable controversy, and not everyone is convinced that lateralization of such processing exists at all. But nobody is in any doubt that differential hemispheric specialization underlies speech production and handedness. Indeed in order to justify claims that various components of a specialized sensory system for processing language reside in the left hemisphere it is usually considered necessary to relate them to the site of speech production in the same subjects. Localization of this control system by techniques such as the Wada test (Wada, 1949) is agreed to be the surest indicator of the side in which language is located in any individual.

In order to produce speech the contractions of a large number of different muscles situated on both sides of the body, in abdomen, chest, larynx, pharynx, tongue and lips must be precisely timed and finely fractionated. The motoneurones controlling these muscles are widely distributed on both sides of the middle of the brainstem and spinal cord. The upper motoneurones controlling them form part of the diffuse, medially descending, bilateral motor systems, which originate in both the left and right frontal lobes. Conducting this orchestra probably cannot be achieved successfully by linking the primary motor representations of these muscles. Communication via the lengthy intracortical and commissural connections between these areas would consume too much time. Moreover, it is unlikely that there are any direct interconnections at all between some of these regions. For example, the motorcortical representations of the left side of the abdomen and the right side of the lip are not linked with each other. Therefore in order to evolve the ability to speak, primates probably first had to establish a specialized region in one hemisphere which was capable of taking over the sequencing and co-ordination of all these muscles when they are employed for vocalization. This is Broca's area, a region of cortex which is able to make use of the direct connections which exist between the premotor region of the frontal lobe (of which it is part) and motoneurones on both sides of the midline which supply axial muscles in the abdomen, diaphragm, chest, larynx and pharynx. Broca's area also enjoys indirect connections to the representations of other muscles involved in speech production which are situated in the primary motor cortex. For writing, a similar specialization was required, but the problem was already neatly solved by the convenient localization of the representation of all the muscles of the right arm in the left motor cortex close behind Broca's area.

For several reasons emphasis on the motor control basis of hemispheric specialization makes the whole subject more tractable for physiologists. First, it is easier to study complex motor accomplishments in experimental animals than it is to analyse complicated sensory abilities, for animals' movements can be conveniently observed, but they cannot report their perceptual experiences. Secondly, motor attributes in animals are often wholly lateralized naturally; as examples we may consider birdsong (Nottebohm, 1980) or paw preference (Warren, 1958). Thirdly, motor output can be lateralized artificially by surgical or other manipulations, and then studied in animals (Myers and Sperry, 1958). Finally in humans hemispheric specialization in the motor sphere, for speech and handedness, is unambiguous; incontrovertibly it exists in over 95% of human beings (Annett, 1964). Hence relating physiological measurements to motor output is likely to be rewarding. Accordingly this chapter will be divided into sections on animal work, then various physiological measures that have been employed in humans, followed by a more speculative section on the mechanisms which may be responsible for developing and maintaining hemispheric differences.

Lateral Asymmetries in the Invertebrate Nervous System

A perfectly symmetric animal would be entirely unable to tell left from right (Corballis and Morgan, 1978) so it would find it impossible to tell which side stimuli were coming from or to make appropriate responses to them. Even amoebae observed over several hours are found to have a tendency to circle in only one direction, as do most single-celled animals (Schaeffer, 1928). In practice, animals are not usually perfectly symmetrical, but large morphological asymmetries are relatively rare in the animal world. There are only two major groups of invertebrates, gastropods and crustaceans, in which obvious anatomical asymmetries are commonly found.

The most numerous and arguably the most successful group of animals, the insects, appear bilaterally symmetrical, but many species demonstrate clear functional asymmetries, which probably reflect subtle physiological differences between their two sides. As mentioned earlier these are essential if the animal is to tell left from right. For example, in the motoneurones which supply the leg muscles of the milkweed bug (*Oncopeltus fasciatus*) (Chapple, 1966) and in those which innervate the flight muscles of the flying locust (Wilson, 1968), discharge frequencies differ on the two sides, so that each individual has a tendency to turn to one or the other side. But there is no consistency about the direction of turning across individuals; veering to the left or right is equally common in the population. So although the tendency to turn may be hereditary, the direction of turning is not apparently specified genetically. This theme, that the degree but not the direction of asymmetries is inherited, will recur frequently in this chapter.

Interestingly the tendency of locusts to turn to one side is checked in the normal animal only by reference to visual feedback from the passing world. It seems that a turning tendency is artificially imposed on the animal in order to ensure that a left/right polarization is continuously drummed into its nervous system; presumably this is necessary to reinforce the polarity of its 'internal map'.

The delights of the gastropod nervous system for the electrophysiologist are well known; they have large, anatomically constant, readily identifiable neurones which are easy to impale; but the habit of many gastropods to rotate 180° to the left during larval development is completely unexplained. It is often complicated by a secondary reversion to symmetry, so that attempts to study the fundamental asymmetry neurophysiologically are fraught with difficulty (Chapple, 1977).

The bilateral asymmetry of decapod crustaceans has yielded much interesting information. The lobster has one large claw, which is called the 'crusher', although in fact it is mainly used for sexual display. The smaller claw on the other side is used for cutting and feeding. The muscles controlling each claw are physiologically distinct; only the crusher has a significant number of slow, powerful muscle fibres (Jahromi and Atwood,

1971). These differences between the muscles on the two sides are associated with differences in their innervation. The fast muscles on the cutter side are controlled by a small number of large motoneurones which discharge infrequently, whilst the slow muscles on the crusher side are supplied with a larger number of small motoneurones, which discharge regularly and rapidly. The motor supply to these muscles not only controls their contractions, but also imposes on them, by trophic action, their biochemical and physiological characteristics. The crusher can develop on the right or the left side in different animals; so there is no overall population bias to either the right or the left. But which side develops the larger claw is determined by its innervation. If the nerve to the crusher is cut its development is arrested. In fact cutting the nerve to the 'snapper' in another crustacean, the snapping shrimp (Mellon and Stevens, 1978), causes the smaller 'pincer' claw to develop into a second snapper; this implies that normally the snapper nerve inhibits growth of the pincer into a snapper.

The abdomen of another crustacean, the hermit crab, coils to the right, probably because it lives in the cast-off shells of right curling gastropods. This torsion gives rise to asymmetries in the muscles of the abdomen and of the motoneurones supplying them (Thompson, 1903). Those on the left have higher firing frequencies and are smaller; those on the right are large and discharge less rapidly. The functional significance of this is not yet known. In this instance, however, these specializations are on the same side in all individuals; so the hermit crab may yet prove a useful species for studying at a cellular level the neuronal mechanisms underlying bilateral asymmetries, which are the same for the whole population — 'population stable'.

This brief excursion into the field of invertebrate asymmetries has been undertaken to emphasise two points. First, bilateral asymmetry may exist in individuals without all members of the species choosing the same side. The tendency to develop asymmetries may be inherited without prescribing whether their direction is to the left or right side. This seems to be true in most animals, except birds and higher primates; in these the left side is always favoured for fine, temporally sequenced, motor control. The second lesson to be learnt from studying invertebrates is that the asymmetries found in these simple animals primarily involve specializations of their motor apparatus and its control.

Birds

Some of the strongest evidence that cerebral asymmetry has a motoric basis has emerged from study of the lateralization of song production in birds (Nottebohm, 1980). Birds are one of the few species of animal to make, like man, comprehensive use of vocalizations for the purpose of communication. The adult male canary may use up to 30 different syllables in his song (Nottebohm, 1970); his voice approaches the sophistication of that of humans. Accordingly it is of exceptional interest to find that canaries have not only evolved completely lateralized control of this complex motor accomplishment, but that the specialized areas responsible are invariably found on the left hand side of the brain (Nottebohm, 1980).

The vocal system of song birds consists of the abdominal and thoracic air sacs, which are controlled by respiratory muscles, and the syrinx, which is a muscular organ situated at the union of the right and left bronchi. At the head of each main bronchus, there are two sound sources, each of which is controlled by the lavish syringeal musculature. Further variations in air flow can be effected by movements of the larynx which is situated above it. Motor innervation is provided chiefly by tracheosyringal branches of the hypoglossal nerve.

Canaries develop adult song patterns during their first year of life, but the details and many of the syllables employed alter season by season (Marler and Waser, 1977). Nevertheless the basic pattern of their songs appears to be inherited; canaries brought up in isolation produce a recognizable, although primitive, song. But young birds usually imitate the songs of adults with whom they are in contact so that, if reared as a group, they all develop similar shared song patterns (Nottebohm, 1970). If an adult canary is deafened its singing will regress, and eventually revert to the standard of a beginner. If young canaries are deprived of auditory feedback before contact with other canaries they develop even more abnormal song repertoires which include many unusual noises such as clicks and hisses.

Thus it is evident that canary song has many points of similarity to our own speech. The vocalizations are complex; there is a basic structure to the song which is inherited; but important details of the song are dependent on vocal learning. The birds need auditory feedback of their voices and motoric feedback from their own song production systems in order to develop normal singing. They also need to be able to imitate the songs of other birds.

Two differences from human speech are both of supreme interest and experimentally advantageous. Only male canaries sing: moreover their singing is seasonal, lasting from spring to mid-August. Each year each bird develops a new set of songs. The question whether sex differences in cerebral lateralization exist in humans is at present a hotly debated issue (Mcglone, 1980), as is the development and plasticity of vocalization mechanisms in humans. Both these problems could perhaps be studied now using canary song as a model.

Fernando Nottebohm's most dramatic finding was that section of the left hypoglossal nerve almost completely abolishes a canary's ability to sing, whereas cutting the right hypoglossal nerve has hardly any effect (Nottebohm, 1980). After the left nerve had been cut the birds were able to make only three of the 200 odd frequency changes which constitute normal singing. It seems that Nottebohm was fortunate in selecting canaries to study. Parrots, for example, employ both the left and right hypoglosssal nerves to control their potentially magnificent array of vocalizations (Nottebohm, 1976), as do humans. Nevertheless in all three, canaries, parrots and humans, ultimate control over the vocal musculature probably resides in the left side of the brain.

Nottebohm went on to show that left hypoglossal control over the syrinx in the canary is vested entirely in left sided structures in the brain. Lesions in a small area of the left hyperstriatum ventrale, pars caudale (HVc — this area may be homologous to the temporal cerebral cortex in mammals) disturbed the quality of singing in much the same way as cutting the left hypoglossal nerve (Nottebohm, 1977). Similarly ablation of another nucleus in the left half of the brain, the left nucleus robustus archistriatalis (NRA — the mammalian equivalent of this is not yet clear) has profoundly deleterious effects on song production, but lesioning the right HVc or the right NRA had no noticeable effects on song production.

Contrary to expectation, if canaries were studied in the year following left-sided cerebral ablations, their singing was found to have made a remarkable recovery, although still demonstrably inferior to that of canaries subjected to right sided or no lesions a year earlier. This plasticity results from the fact that during autumn and winter months both the left HVc and NRA of normal canaries regress to the same size as those on the right. Regrowth occurs at the beginning of the following song season (Nottebohm, 1981). No such changes are seen in other parts of the male canary brain, or in females.

The size of left HVc and NRA is closely correlated with testicular weight and blood androgen levels (Nottebohm, 1981). Moreover the change in the size of these nuclei appears to be the result not only of increases in the length of dendrites and in the number of their branches, but also of division and growth of new neurones. Similar changes can be induced out of season in males or in ovariectomised females, by injecting androgens. These females then begin singing their hearts out like males.

It is likely therefore that the recovery of singing, which follows in the year after ablation of left HVc and NRA, is mediated by the same rejuvenation process which underlies the normal yearly cycle of growth and regression in these nuclei. After left-sided ablations the right HVc and NRA grow and can take over singing, under the influence of circulating androgens. Hence, destruction of the right hypoglossal nerve thereafter permanently eliminates the birds' ability to sing.

Clearly the neural mechanisms which mediate canary singing deserve further close scrutiny, as they bear such striking resemblances to so many features of our own vocalization system. In concluding this section, again the point to be emphasized is that the lateralization of singing in the canary in structures on the left side of the brain is a sensorimotor control phenomenon. No differences between the two sides have been observed for simple auditory analysis, for example.

Mammals

The brain of a more conventional laboratory animal, the rat, is, on the face of it, entirely bilaterally symmetrical. Frequently unilateral lesions are made and bilateral tests designed on the assumption that the unlesioned side may be used as a control. However Glick has made a virtue of an observation that must have been made many times and overlooked by previous students of the rotating rat, namely that even normal rats have a consistent tendency to veer always to the same side (Glick *et al.* 1976). In different individuals, turning to the right or left is almost equally common. Similarly rats consistently choose one paw rather than the other with which to remove food from a tube. Individual rats use the same paw on different occasions, but it is equally common for rats to be right or left pawed.

A large body of evidence has now accumulated to show that unilateral lesions of the nigrostriatal pathway causes rats to rotate away from the side which releases more dopamine (DA) or has developed more DA receptors (Ungerstedt, 1974). Thus after 6-hydroxydopamine lesions of the nigro-striatal system on one side, administration of amphetamine causes the rats to rotate towards the lesioned side (ipsiversively). Amphetamine causes release of dopamine from the intact side. It is presumed that the released dopamine somehow activates postural and locomotor programmes on the intact side more effectively; so the rats veer towards the side of the lesion. If on the other hand dopamine, or one of its agonists such as apomorphine, is administered, the rats circle away from the lesion (contraversively). This is probably because previous removal of the dopaminergic nigrostriatal pathway on one side causes increased growth of dopamine receptors on that side, in an attempt to compensate for the decrease in the amount of dopamine they have experienced. Hence these receptors subsequently become hyperactive compared with those on the intact side; and when stimulated by apomorphine they cause the animals to circle away from the lesion.

Glick and his colleagues have extended these findings to the normal rat (Glick, 1985). Their results suggest that the tendency of most rats to turn to one side, even without nigrostriatal lesions, may also relate to differences in dopamine release on the two sides. They found that the DA content of the left and right substantia nigrae of normal rats differs by up to 15%; after amphetamine administration this difference may increase to 25%. After injections of amphetamine, rats rotate in the direction contralateral to the side containing the higher level of dopamine; this suggests that this pharmacological asymmetry in intact rats may be important to the animals' normal behaviour.

The fact that rats rotate in only one direction in a specially designed rotometer may not seem very important but, if it could be shown that they exhibit the same turning tendencies when exploring their natural environment, this could have great functional significance. Webster introduced the interesting idea that an animal with asymmetric locomotor and postural behaviour might be better able to remember its spatial location (Webster, 1977), because this neurological asymmetry ought to assist it in laying down a reliable cognitive map. This would enable the animal to remember the layout of its environment and its position in it more accurately. Thus, the degree of polarization, rather than the direction of any asymmetry, is what would confer selective advantage on the animal when defending its territory, finding a mate or choosing safe pathways for retreat from enemies.

Glick has produced some evidence in favour of this idea (Glick, 1973). Turning tendencies seem to be advantageous to the animal that owns them. Rats with strong and consistent circling in a rotometer took many fewer trials in a quite different situation, when learning to escape shock or find food in a T maze, where the only cues were spatial. In other words when the animals had to remember on which side the food or shock were located, those with stronger turning tendencies appeared to be at an advantage. Furthermore, these animals showed much higher retention of the memory of which arm of a T maze was likely to shock them than their less asymmetric colleagues.

A more controversial claim is that a higher proportion of any given population of rats favours the right side, by tending to circle clockwise; using their right paw to extract food from a well; or running initially to the right in a T maze. The differences are never large, and barely attain significance; e.g. Cowey found that in a sample of 14 rats on 59% of occasions they chose to run down the right side of a T maze (Cowey and Bozeck, 1974); nevertheless this was significantly different from chance. Such a preference for the right side may be related to biochemical and/or anatomical differences between the right and left basal ganglia and cerebral hemispheres. Diamond and her colleagues have shown that in male rats some areas of the cerebral cortex of the right hemisphere are thicker than on the left (Diamond, 1980). Interestingly, these differences may be influenced by testosterone levels. Kolb has also found that the right frontal cortex is more bulky in cats (Kolb *et al.*, 1983), but the exact mechanisms are bound to be complex as there appear to be species and sex differences. Moreover, motor cortical control over the limbs operates via crossed connections, whereas the premotor cortex and basal ganglia make mainly ipsilateral connections with postural and locomotor muscles.

In summary, the work with mammals other than primates has demonstrated that lateral preferences related to posture and locomotion probably do exist. But even though a slight population preference for the right rather than the left hand side may be confirmed, neither the trend nor the evidence is strong. None the less it seems possible that the right hemisphere first became specialized for controlling postural, locomotor and emotional behaviour in relation to territory, leaving to the left hemisphere the specialized tasks of manual skill and communication. Left hemispheric dominance is only clearly found in birds and higher primates; these are the species in which the most complex forms of communication have evolved.

Non-human Primates

Most studies in primates lower than humans have failed to find any consistent population trend in favour of right handedness (Warren and Nonneman, 1976). Individual monkeys clearly prefer to use one hand rather than the other for precise, complex, manipulative tasks. This preference is particularly evident when the monkey has to perform bimanual operations in which one hand has to perform a delicate action whilst the other is engaged in something simpler, such as holding a door open (Warren, 1977). However, such preferences are weaker than in humans, and show no particular bias for the right hand. Even when firmly established they tend to be task specific, only generalizing to other manipulative tasks if the motor problems are similar. Thus a monkey may prefer to use his right hand for opening boxes but his left hand for grabbing food from a tray.

Roger Sperry and colleagues (Sperry, 1974) first showed that when normal monkeys are trained in visual discrimination tasks, involving simple motor responses, memory engrams for the tasks are normally laid down in both hemispheres. If the splenium of the corpus callosum and anterior commissure are intact, this is true even if training is directed to only one hemisphere. This is achieved by patching the contralateral eye after cutting the optic chiasm. Thus even with strongly lateralized visual input there is no evidence that memory traces are laid down in just one hemisphere in normal animals. There is therefore no evidence of hemispheric specialization for this type of simple task in normal rhesus monkeys. But lateralization for these tasks can be imposed on the animals if both the splenium of the corpus callosum and anterior commisure are cut (Hamilton, (1977).

Investigators may have chosen the wrong sort of task to study, however. If we expect the left hemisphere to be specialized for communication by means of vocalization or gesture, and the right to be responsible for whole-body orientation in relation to the environment, then clearly, with respect to both the sensory modalities and the motor responses employed, it is inappropriate to study simple visual discriminations. Since the repertoire of vocalizations produced by rhesus monkeys is quite meagre compared with those of birds or humans, it might be most sensible to consider a function which may have evolved earlier in the right hemisphere of primates, namely the sensory control of locomotor and postural mechanisms in relation to laying down a 'cognitive map'. Unfortunately this approach has not yet been tried.

However, audiomotor control has been investigated. Dewson and Cowey (1969) found in rhesus monkeys that unilateral damage to the superior temporal gyrus on either side results in persistent deficits in auditory controlled behaviour, and it appears that a monkey requires both cortices to perform most auditory tasks efficiently. Although there was no suggestion from this work that either side was superior in this role, Dewson then went on to show (1979) that the left cerebral hemisphere may play a crucial role in successfully mastering an audiovisual matching task. He trained monkeys to press a red button after a delay if they had previously heard a pure tone or a green button if they had heard a noise. Monkeys with left superior temporal ablations were apparently unable to remember which tone they had heard after only 2 seconds delay, whereas animals tested before lesions, or those which were lesioned in the right temporal lobe, could reliably recall the tones 20 seconds or more afterwards. Further investigation showed that animals with left-sided lesions performed poorly only if the delay between sound and lighting up the response panels was varied from trial to trial, so that it is unlikely that the deficit found in these monkeys was the result of a simple failure to remember which sound they had heard. Rather it is likely that the animals with left-sided lesions performed poorly when the delay was varied because they were unable to associate the correct tone with the appropriate motor response. To perform the task properly the animals had first to identify which sound had occurred, prepare themselves to hit the correct button, and then wait until it was illuminated. Although the motor act required was simple, triggering the correct responses required the monkey to learn a sequence of cues with variable timing. Hence the faculty in the monkey which only the left superior temporal auditory association area appears to possess, seems to be the ability to organize correctly cued motor responses, when there are variable temporal relationships between a sequence of cues. It would seem likely, therefore, that the perfection of a reliable mechanism for the timing and sequencing of fractionated muscle contractions is a fundamental function of the left hemisphere. Likewise in humans the left hemisphere appears to be specialized for this kind of motor co-ordination.

The effects of lesioning the auditory association cortex might be expected to be even more illuminating, if the complex vocalizations that monkeys themselves use to communicate with each other are studied, rather than irrelevant simple sounds (Marler, 1978). This approach has been successfully followed by Stebbins and his group (1978). Japanese macaque monkeys make two different sorts of 'coo' sound when seeking contacts with other animals. In the first a smooth vowel sound occurs early in the 'word'; in the second the smooth sound occurs late. This subtle difference, which is almost imperceptible to the human observer, is the only distinction between the two calls. Nevertheless, Japanese macaques can be easily trained to make different responses to the two sounds when they are played in either ear from a tape recorder. Rhesus monkeys on the other hand, like humans, find it much more difficult to make the discrimination, though they can eventually learn it.

Stebbins then investigated whether there is any evidence for a special role for the left hemisphere in this discrimination. He compared the rate of learning and the number of errors made by the monkeys when the sounds were presented via the right or the left ear (Rosenzweig, 1951). All the Japanese macaques learnt the discrimination more quickly and with fewer errors if the sounds were played into the right ear; the rhesus monkeys also showed evidence of a right ear advantage. Neither species showed any ear advantage for making a simpler discrimination between high- and low-pitched calls. Since the right ear enjoys preferential access to the left hemisphere, these findings were interpreted to favour the idea that the left hemisphere in these monkeys is specialized to detect fine temporal distinctions, particularly those found in species specific vocalizations. The finding that rhesus monkeys also had a right ear advantage when discriminating the calls of another species, the Japanese macaque, suggests that this attribute of the left hemisphere may generalize to all vocalizations intended for communication. Indeed it has even been claimed that using their right ears monkeys can discriminate human speech sounds as well as human infants can (Petersen *et al.*, 1978).

However, in neither monkeys nor humans has it ever been shown that such fine auditory discriminations are an exclusive function of the left hemisphere (Tallal and Schwartz, 1980). In fact it is clear that for most purely auditory discriminations both right and left hemispheres participate to some extent. Ploog found (1981) that unilateral lesions of the auditory cortex, whether in the left or right temporal lobe, never produced a significant effect on a squirrel monkey's ability to recognize the vocalizations of other squirrel monkeys. Even though Stebbins' evidence implies that the left hemisphere may be superior for this task Ploog found that it required large lesions of the superior temporal gyrus on both sides to abolish the animals' ability to recognize species specific vocalizations altogether.

This result is reminscent of auditory agnosia in humans, first described by Sigmund Freud. In this condition patients cannot discriminate any complex sounds, whether animal noises, melodies, musical instruments or speech itself. Post mortem large bilateral lesions of both temporal lobes are almost invariably found. Thus although the left hemisphere may be superior at analysing vocalizations, in both monkeys and men it certainly has no monopoly over this function. The right hemisphere appears to be able to perform many types of auditory discrimination almost as well as the left.

It might be argued that Wernicke's 'sensory' aphasia rather than auditory agnosia is the condition with which we should be comparing animal models. Sensory aphasia is specific for language; the patients can usually discriminate other complex sounds normally. If we could define a lesion which prevented an animal from identifying the calls of its own species, but still allowed it to discriminate other complex sounds we would perhaps have found a better model for Wernicke's aphasia.

Such a model has not been developed for two main reasons. In the first place investigators have concentrated on the problem of auditory processing rather than speech production in aphasia. It is significant that pure word deafness, i.e. an isolated disorder of comprehension with normal speech and writing, is extremely rare. Much more common is syntactic and nominal aphasia where expression of an idea in speech or writing by means of the correct use of words and their correct syntactical ordering in grammatical sentences is disturbed. Recognition and comprehension of words is commonly unaffected. Though Wernicke's aphasia is usually considered to be primarily a disorder of comprehension, it usually reveals itself as a disorder in the generation of speech, an inability to choose the right words in the right order. On the other hand, it is agreed that Broca's expressive aphasia is the result of a patient not being able to put together elementary articulatory gestures correctly, in order to formulate proper words and sentences. Unlike in dysarthria, the actual execution of articulatory movements is unaffected.

Both Wernicke's and Broca's aphasias reveal the breakdown of stages in the construction of the motor programme for normal speech. The former disturbs choice of appropriate words and the correct grammatical structures for them to go in; Broca's aphasia prevents the patient from selecting the correct vocal gestures necessary to produce the chosen words. The final stage revealed by dysarthria is the failure to be able to pronounce the words properly because the detailed motor execution of the vocal gestures which pass to the muscles themselves is deficient.

A fruitful way of trying to develop an animal model for dysphasia might be to concentrate not solely on the receptive aspects of monkey vocalizations, but to consider the motor pathways from cortical areas which are known to be responsible for the auditory control of vocalization. Much is known about a bilaterally symmetrical system responsible for spontaneous vocalizations in monkeys (Jurgens and Ploog, 1970), which arises in the cingulate gyrus on both sides, but very little is known about whether the control which the auditory system exercises over this bilateral vocalization pathway in monkeys is lateralized, as it is in birds and humans.

A second reason why a successful primate model for Wernicke's and Broca's aphasia has so far failed to see the light of day is that the monkeys commonly used in the laboratory may not have the essential anatomical prerequisites to enable marked hemispheric specialization to develop at all. Geschwind's group has produced much evidence (Geschwind, 1974) to show that consistent structural differences between the cerebral hemispheres are present in higher primates, but not in monkeys. In humans the sylvian fissure in the left hemisphere is significantly longer and more horizontal posteriorly than that in the right hemisphere, because the left planum temporale below and the parietal operculum above are both expanded more on the left than right hand side in the human brain, a difference found not only in modern adult man, but in the human fetus, Peking man, and in all great apes (orang-utans, chimpanzees and gorillas). It is not found in monkeys and lesser apes, the primates which are commonly studied in laboratories, so that attempts to study functional lateralization in the lower primates are that much less likely to succeed.

Ape Language

Recently there has been a surge of interest in whether great apes can master the rudiments of language (Lemay and Geschwind, 1975; Seuren, 1978). If they definitely can, then, after all, the great apes may possess the fundamental cerebral attributes required for a degree of linguistic competence. A number of attempts have been made to perform such a 'language transplant' on non-human primates. But most have foundered on account of the modality employed; the phonic character of our language defeats non-human primates. Because the monkey larynx is incapable of producing 'human' sounds, monkeys are probably unable to decode human speech though their own repertoire of squeals and shrieks is extensive. However, when the Gardners (1971), Premack (1971) and Rumbaugh's group (1977) began using sensory modalities other than the auditory, their ape subjects managed to learn fairly complex forms of communication. This convinced many that some form of true linguistic communication had been established with these animals but others are still not convinced, and believe the communication to be no more than a sophisticated example of the 'clever Hans' phenomenon (Wade, 1980). This is a debate that will continue, partly because even professional linguistic philosophers and psychologists cannot really agree on what constitutes true language and what 'mere' communication. The important point is that teaching some form of language to chimpanzees has come through concentrating on the motor accomplishments in which they excel, i.e. the use of their hands, not their voices. It has been necessary to discard much of what is known or suspected about their capacities for decoding complex sounds, and concentrate on their motor accomplishments. Significantly, Washoe, the chimpanzee taught sign language by the Gardners, preferred to use her right hand to make signals. It seems therefore that a fruitful area of research might be to look for more signs of lateralization of manipulative abilities such as these in primates.

Summary

By considering the results of studies using animals, the theme has been developed that specialization of the cerebral hemispheres is primarily a sensorimotor control phenomenon. In contrast to studies with humans, the majority of investigators have concentrated on motor signs of lateralization. In invertebrates the motor nerve supply to limb muscles controls their contractions, and also exerts trophic effects which determine which side shall grow larger. Although many exhibit lateral asymmetries, right- or left-sided specialization is equally common. In birds there is now strong evidence that singing is controlled exclusively by left-sided structures in the brain, and that these grow and regress cyclically under hormonal control. Lower mammals are more like invertebrates; the more that subtle lateral specializations are searched for the more common they appear to be. But left- or right-sided structures may be almost equally favoured by different individuals. In higher primates it seems that the trend towards right handedness and left brainedness for communication made its first appearance; this culminated in the unequivocal specialization in most humans of the left hemisphere for speech and writing, and of the right for visuospatial orientation.

Physiological Measures in Humans

The EEG

Many investigators have attempted to make use of the EEG to identify processing differences between the hemispheres in humans (Donchin *et al.* 1977), since the measurements are non-invasive and relatively easy to perform. Also analysis of the EEG gives millisecond by millisecond time resolution, so that in theory it is possible to follow changes in sensory input, cognitive activity or motor output exactly when they occur. But the greatest advantage claimed for the EEG is that it gives an objective measure of what is actually going on inside a subject's head; the investigator does not need to rely on verbal reports or upon the accuracy of subjective responses.

It is not yet clear, however, that gross electrical changes taking place in the cerebral cortex do give much useful information bearing on the question of hemispheric specialization. For what dominates the EEG is rhythmic activity in the long surface dendrites of neurones, most of whose cell bodies lie in the deeper layers of the cortex. When rhythmic activity is detected in scalp electrodes, even after the attenuation effected by the CSF, cranium and skin, this probably indicates that many thousands of dendrites beneath the electrodes are doing much the same thing at the same time. When such rhythmic activity is marked, the individual processing functions of the neurones are probably completely submerged; common mode activity dominates. When all these neurones are behaving synchronously, they are probably not indulging in the kind of differentiated activity which presumably underlies hemispheric specialization.

Over 50 years ago Adrian and Matthews discovered that the alpha rhythm recorded in the EEG over the occipital cortex is blocked by visual stimulation (Adrian and Matthews, 1934). In other words, as suggested above, when the alpha rhythm in the EEG is prominent it probably denotes inactivity of the underlying cortex, rather than the reverse. Unfortunately it has turned out to be unsafe to assume that the corollary holds true, namely that reduction in alpha activity is a reliable indication of specialized processing by an area of cortex. Alpha block is a very rough and non-specific measure of the involvement of the cerebral cortex in any specific processing activity; it is almost as non-specific as the alpha rhythm itself. Hence it tells us little in detail about underlying cerebral processing. Both the alpha rhythm and alpha block are mainly the result of the activity of the non-specific thalamic nuclei (Brazier, 1975); hence they probably indicate little about operations peculiar to each hemisphere.

Nevertheless, if a crude measure is the only one we have available we must try to make the best of it. Comparison of alpha power in EEG recordings taken from homologous sites in the two hemispheres whilst subjects are engaged in verbal or non-verbal tasks should at least enable us to tell whether one hemisphere is more active than the other during the task. Many such studies have now been undertaken; and most agree that there are indeed small differences between the two hemispheres (Donchin *et al.*, 1977). These are usually expressed as the ratio of alpha power in right/left hemisphere, so that a larger number indicates dominance of the left hemisphere for the task under consideration. But there is no agreement as to whether the handedness of the subject, or the type of task which he is currently performing has the more important effect on hemispheric activation. The only secure conclusion that has emerged so far is that alpha power is usually lower in the left hemisphere of right handers relative to that in their right hemisphere (Butler and Glass, 1974). This attenuation is particularly marked when subjects are engaged in verbal pursuits, especially speaking, writing, or mentally composing speech or letters (Galin and Ornstein, 1972). However, the majority of studies have found that in general alpha power is lower in the left hemisphere whatever the task a subject is engaged in (Galin and Ellis, 1975). Hence evidence for the expected corollary of the verbal result, namely that alpha power should be lower in the right hemisphere during a spatial task, is weak (Galin and Ornstein, 1972).

In part these modest results are the result of methodological difficulties and differences between studies, since it is difficult to define and validate a reliable resting state measure with which EEG changes during task performance can be compared. The analyses which have been employed have been many and various (Donchin *et al.*, 1977): total EEG power, power within the alpha frequency range, power outside the alpha frequency range (probably only minor changes occur outside the alpha range in fact); total duration of alpha rhythm, alpha control ratio (the latency by which alpha block follows a visual stimulus which is itself triggered by the appearance of alpha rhythm — Goodman *et al.*, 1980), or various measures of alpha synchrony. The variety of the methods employed shows how unreliable EEG measures of hemispheric differences have turned out to be.

Similarly, an astonishing variety of tasks presumed to utilize the left hemisphere differentially have been employed (Doyle *et al.*, 1974; Dumas and Morgan, 1975; Gordon, 1980). They have included composing or writing letters, searching for words, mental arithmetic, verbal listening and even verbal descriptions of the components of chords, a task which could only be given to professional musicians. Those alleged to involve the right hemisphere (Young, 1982) have included spatial manipulation of blocks, tonal memory, drawing, spatial imagery, listening to music, imagining emotions and even hypnosis (Morgan *et al.* 1971). These very different tasks reflect investigators' disparate intuitions about what the left or right hemispheres might be specialized for. If we couple this variety with the unsatisfactory nature of EEG measures available, and recall also that investigators often have great difficulty in checking whether their subjects were indeed carrying out what they were asked to do, it is actually surprising that the results have been as consistent as they have.

A potentially more promising approach has been to investigate the degree of 'coupling' between adjacent cortical areas in one hemisphere (Callaway and Harris, 1974). The assumption here is that increased coupling indicates preferential usage of those areas for the task that the subject is currently performing. This is not an unreasonable idea since the measure of coupling employed reflects the degree to which one area affects its neighbours more than others during particular tasks, i.e. how specialized those areas are for the task. Callaway and Harris have shown convincingly that when subjects are asked to perform even silent verbal analysis of written material the coupling between occipital and parietal lobes increases, but this occurs only in the left hemisphere. On the other hand, when subjects perform spatial analyses of pictorial stimuli, coupling increases more in the right hemisphere. The non-parametric statistical method employed for analysing these results had the great advantage that analysis of EEG was not confined to the alpha rhythm. All frequencies below 125Hz were considered, so that higher frequency signals in the EEG which may have represented specific processing mechanisms were probably given fair weight.

Apart from the difficulties with using the EEG to quantify hemispheric differences which have been outlined above, a major weakness of most studies attempting to assess cerebral lateralization by means of EEG measures is that they have taken little account of the potential importance of the way in which each hemisphere is specialized for particular types of motor control. Indeed it is often quoted as a positive advantage of EEG methods that no motor responses are necessary to determine what each hemisphere is doing. But, if in fact each hemisphere is primarily specialized to control different kinds of motor output, preventing the subject making overt motor responses may be a great mistake. It is significant that the studies which show the greatest magnitude and reproducibility of hemispheric differences are those in which the subjects were required to perform overt actions — speaking, writing or making designs with blocks. Unfortunately no studies have been carried out in which the EEG was measured during the performance of the sort of operations for which the right hemisphere is likely to be most specialized, such as orientation of the whole body in relation to the environment (route finding) or the expression of emotions.

Event Related Potentials

A major problem for those who wish to use the EEG for detecting subtle differences in electrical activity of the hemispheres, which might reveal their separate processing functions, is that it is non-specific. By itself the EEG can tell us little about which sensory inputs, which sensorimotor processes, or which motor pathways, are engaged during any particular task. When techniques for averaging EEG potentials specifically evoked by controlled sensory input or in advance of motor output were introduced (Regan, 1972), they seemed to offer a way out of this difficulty. For in principle the averaging technique enables any small signals, specifically related to whatever trigger is employed, to be separated from the noise in which they are normally embedded in the raw EEG. Any electrical activity locked in time to the trigger sums over trials, whereas the rest of the EEG is treated as 'noise' and reduced in proportion to the square root of the number of averages.

As is so often the case, the actual outcome has been disappointing. Even though the signals, disembedded from a scalp electrode record by the averaging process, are indeed locked in time to the stimulus, they are not anatomically specific, as they still derive from many thousands of neurones both underlying and distant from the electrode, so that only the average properties of the surface dendrites of that mass are revealed, not the details of each one's processing. Furthermore, short and discrete triggers or accurately periodic stimuli are required for the averaging process, so that it is impossible, when using evoked potentials (EPs), to study cortical activity directly over a longer time scale in order to investigate lengthy operations such as verbal processing or spatial orientation. Recently, indirect techniques using a short sensory stimulus, such as a flash (Papanicolaou, 1978) or click (Shucard *et al.*, 1978) as a 'probe' for the degree of engagement of each hemisphere in concurrent tasks, have been introduced in an attempt to overcome this problem.

Averaged event related potentials which follow or precede the trigger at short latencies are often termed 'exogenous' (Donchin *et al.*, 1977), because they are highly dependent on the parameters of the stimulus, but they exhibit little intrinsic variability and are hardly affected by the mental state of the subject. Later waves which are called 'endogenous' are much more variable, because they are dependent upon a subject's cognitive state, direction of attention, emotional condition, etc. As the major sensory and motor pathways decussate, the earliest exogenous EP waves tend to be slightly larger contralateral to the half of the body stimulated (Beaumont, 1982) or the limb which is moved. Unfortunately it is usually only in the later, endogenous, waves, which already display great variability, that differences between the processing styles of the two hemispheres may be demonstrable.

Motor-event Related Potentials

The largest and most consistent asymmetries in event related potentials (ERP) have been obtained for the slow potentials which may precede movement by up to 10 seconds. These are associated with preparation for action and are termed contingent negative variations (CNV) (Walter *et al.*, 1964) or Readiness Potentials (RP) (Deecke *et al.*, 1969). The negative readiness potential is bilateral, but is usually several microvolts larger over the left frontal cortex if subjects use their right hand, whether they are right or left handers (Deecke et al., 1969). This difference is particularly marked if the task to be performed demands precise, finely fractionated, sequential control, and if it is associated with a verbal command (Jarvilehto and Fruhstorfer, 1970). When using their left hands neither left or right handers show any significant differences between the readiness potentials recorded over the right hemisphere compared with the left. Thus there is probably something special about the right hand and the left frontal cortex (maybe the location of Broca's area) in almost everybody, not just right handers.

This clear result tells us nothing directly about the lateralization of speech production, but it does confirm the suggestion made earlier that frontal control of speech production and handedness are closely related. Even in left handers (more than half of whom nevertheless have a left-sided 'speech centre'), the readiness potential is still largest in the left hemisphere following a verbal command, when they prepare to use their right hands. Such enhancement is not found in the right hemisphere of left handers before they move their preferred left hand.

It was confidently expected that analysis of motor potentials preceding speech would be even more conclusive, and perhaps provide a reliable, easy and non-invasive technique to replace the Wada procedure for establishing the side of the speech centres in patients facing surgery, cortical excisions, or in experimental subjects. Unfortunately these hopes have not been realized, and recording of speech related evoked potentials has turned out to be much more difficult than expected for a number of reasons (Grozinger *et al.*, 1977).

First, speech is always tied to expiration, so that normal variations in the EEG which are also tied to respiration can easily be mistaken for speech related potentials. Secondly, the airburst which leads to phonation has often been used to trigger averaging of the EEG; but it lags by a considerable time both the onset of activity in articulatory muscles and sometimes even the commencement of audible sound. Hence many of the EP waves which were formerly ascribed to motor activity preceding speech have now been shown to be contaminated by early auditory potentials evoked by the subject already hearing his own voice. Thirdly, extracranial potentials which are caused by scalp muscle activity and eye and tongue movements may also precede vocalization by tens of milliseconds (Szirtes and Vaughan, 1977); these are picked up by the recording electrodes and are difficult to eliminate without complex signal processing, and they may easily be misinterpreted as specific prespeech EEG potentials.

Such problems are not insurmountable, and one clear fact has already emerged from this discouraging battle with artefacts. Despite the involvement of muscles located on both sides of the body, in all vocal activity there is a clear bilateral asymmetry in the readiness potential (RP) and the contingent negative variation (CNV) preceding speech. As expected, this favours the left hemisphere, and starts earlier in the left hemisphere than the RP or CNV for other movements (Szirtes and Vaughan, 1977). The difference between the hemispheres is larger than that for movements of the right hand, and is greatest over Broca's area in the left prefrontal region. If proper attention is paid to avoiding artefacts the difference is probably stable within, and robust across, subjects; and when completely standardized may yet prove as reliable as the Wada technique.

The brevity of this section on motor potentials suggests two things. First it indicates how little work has been devoted to motor event related potentials, presumably because people are put off by the technical problems. Secondly, the small number of studies implies paradoxically that the results are already sufficiently clear cut that they do not need to be repeated, an implication that echoes the motor theme of this chapter. Attempts to quantify the specialization of the hemispheres for controlling different types of movement are likely to be more successful than looking for sensory, perceptual or cognitive indices. Differences between the hemispheres' conduct of sensory processes are probably secondary to their primary specialization for more control.

Electrodermal Responses

An intriguing motor response, much studied by psychophysiologists, is the autonomic component of the orientation response to a novel stimulus. This may provide a biological index of attention, as revealed by the reactions of the autonomic nervous system (Gruzellier, 1982). A convenient way to measure these is to record changes in the electrical conductivity of palmar or plantar skin surfaces. Skin conductivity level (SCL) or transient skin conductance changes (SCR) reflect mainly the activity of eccrine sweat glands; in the hands or feet these appear to respond almost entirely to emotional stimuli, and not to participate primarily in thermoregulatory reactions.

Although unilateral stimulation of the prefrontal cortex causes autonomic reactions throughout the whole body, and bilateral changes in skin conductance levels are observed (Wang, 1964), the results of lesions in the prefrontal cortex suggest that cortical regulation of the eccrine glands in the hands and feet is primarily ipsilateral (Livanov *et al.*, 1973). This ipsilateral control may, however, be masked by stronger contralateral influences, when the hand or foot are engaged in active or even passive responses. Hence electrodermal responses to unexpected stimuli are symmetrical in 75% of normals, and inconsistently lateralized in the rest.

Nevertheless consistent lateral asymmetries in electrodermal responses may occur in a high proportion of psychotic patients (Mackay, 1984). When, for example, schizophrenics are subjected to unexpected and loud 1000 Hz tone bursts lasting several seconds (Gruzellier, 1982), there are clear differences in electrodermal responses between their left and right sides. The abnormal degree of lateralization in these patients may be the result of a pathological alteration in the way in which the right hemisphere controls emotional expression (Morison, 1979). An overactive right hemisphere may characterise schizophrenics, and submission to the left is found in depressives. However, the magnitude of these effects is small; the validity of these claims would be much strengthened if there were more direct and independent measures of hemispheric activation during emotional reactions in normal subjects. For the moment we muct conclude that asymmetric electrodermal responses may reveal the hemisphere which is controlling emotional responses, but that this is not yet proven.

Sensory Evoked Potentials

The shortest latency exogenous cortical potentials are evoked by sensory stimuli applied to one half of the body, and are lateralized in the primary receiving areas of the opposite hemisphere (Regan, 1972). However, the largest of the early waves found in most sensory evoked responses (hence the one most favoured in clinical practice) is usually bilateral and symmetrical, even after unilateral stimulation. This first large negative wave principally reflects activity in sensorimotor association cortex, rather than in the primary receiving areas, commissural transfer between the two sides having already taken place. It was argued above that only the waves occurring still later, in association with the control of appropriate motor responses, fully reflect the different processing styles of each hemisphere (Donchin *et al.*, 1977).

Visual Evoked Potential (VEP) — Simple Stimuli

Differences in the earliest waves of the VEP may be estimated by comparing potentials recorded using electrodes placed over the left and right occipital cortices, but these can be entirely explained by the anatomy of the visual pathways, and individual differences in the disposition of the calcarine cortex (Blumhardt *et al.*, 1977). The effect of these anatomical factors is most clearly seen when the two halves of the visual field are stimulated separately (Beaumont, 1982). However, when subjects are asked deliberately not to attend to the stimuli, left/right asymmetries tend to disappear, and all components become smaller (Buchsbaum and Drago, 1977). This emphasizes the importance of controlling the direction of subjects' attention, and their cognitive 'set', if reliable results are to be obtained with any of the EP measures which are to be discussed. When subjects act merely as passive observers, hemispheric asymmetries seem always less likely to be found.

VEP — Complex Stimuli

Most investigators agree that in most right handers if attention, cognitive state and eye position are suitably controlled, verbal stimuli projected in the right visual hemifield elicit larger mid and late latency VEP waves in the left hemisphere, compared with those in the right hemisphere following left visual hemifield presentations (McKeever and Huling, 1970; Buchsbaum and Fedio, 1970). Beyond this limited finding agreement breaks down (Rugg, 1982). In particular no consistent differences in the VEP response to linguistic or non-linguistic stimuli in the left or right hemisphere are consistently observed, unless the stimuli are presented in the contralateral hemifield. In other words complex stimuli have to be lateralized already for VEP differences between verbal and non-verbal processing to become clearly apparent. Even then the differences are small, often amounting to no more than 2 μV.

In fact, despite theoretical arguments suggesting the contrary, VEP indices of hemispheric asymmetry turn out often to be inferior to EEG ones. This is not surprising when it is remembered that most activities involve both hemispheres, at least in their early stages, since both visual hemifields are necessarily employed. Hence symmetrical engagement of both hemispheres dominates the evoked potential. Any subtle signs of specialization of the left for language or the right for spatial processing which may appear later in the VEP are easily submerged.

Although it is encouraging that some studies have produced evidence suggesting that VEP asymmetries follow verbal or non-verbal visual stimuli, and that these are consistent with expectations about hemispheric specialization derived from psychological and neurological studies, there is much disagreement, and claimed differences are very small. On the face of it vision does not seem to be the best modality to choose to attempt to detect clear evoked potential differences anyway; but it would be premature to dismiss the VEP technique entirely as a means of investigating cerebral asymmetries, since most of the studies so far reported have suffered from methodological deficiencies. Nevertheless, it seems unlikely that the VEP technique will by itself make a great contribution to our understanding of the lateralization of hemispheric function.

Auditory Evoked Potentials (AEP)

Although it was widely expected that recording the averaged auditory potentials evoked by verbal or non-verbal stimuli would demonstrate clearer hemispheric differences than using visual stimuli, the same kinds of problem have emerged. It is generally agreed that each ear, despite its bilateral connections, projects predominantly to the contralateral temporal lobe (Rosenzweig, 1951). It has been found that the right ear enjoys a slight advantage in comprehension over the left when different words are played into both ears simultaneously (Broadbent, 1954), which is usually attributed to input from the right ear passing directly to the left hemisphere, and then managing to suppress in some way the competing input from the left ear, which arrives there later in time, because it has to travel indirectly via the right hemisphere and corpus callosum. Hence it was natural to expect that verbal stimuli would yield larger auditory evoked potentials in the left compared to the right hemisphere.

The outcome, of course, has been much more complicated (Friedman *et al.*, 1975). Most investigators agree that stimulation of the right ear produces a different distribution of AEPs over the scalp from stimulating the left ear. Usually larger responses are found contralaterally (Kimura and Archibald, 1974) but, whether speech or non-speech sound stimuli are used, many investigators still find left hemisphere preponderance (Tallal and Schwartz, 1980). Thus there is no agreement that speech always yields larger AEPs in the left hemisphere if the ears are equally stimulated. As with visual stimulation , the most consistent result seems to be that AEPs recorded over the left hemisphere are usually larger for speech than non-speech sounds if they are played into the right ear of right-handed people. The result is even stronger if subjects with no left-handed close relatives are chosen (Morais and Gott, 1972). Again, therefore the most favourable combination of circumstances must be selected to obtain consistent AEP results.

The difficulty of demonstrating larger AEPs over the left hemisphere following speech sounds has recently become less surprising, as it has now become doubtful that the left hemisphere really does contain a detection system which is specific for speech as opposed to other complex sounds (Kay, 1982). It may be superior to the right hemisphere for discriminating certain of the amplitude and frequency modulations (Kay and Mayers, 1982) characteristically found in speech, but these also occur in non-speech sounds. Hence to maximize differences between the AEPs of the left and right hemispheres it would probably be better to employ low (2–4 Hz) amplitude and frequency modulations to stimulate the right hemisphere, and higher frequency (10–50 Hz) modulations to stimulate the left hemisphere.

Linguistic Processing

It now appears unlikely that the left hemisphere is primarily specialized for language comprehension as such, although it is clearly specialized for speech production. A more promising use of the auditory evoked potential method has been to employ it to 'probe' the level of activity in each hemisphere, whilst a subject is involved in a linguistic or semantic processing task (Brown *et al.*, 1976), preferably if it is preparatory to speech. This approach has been more successful. A number of studies have appeared in which various combinations of phonemes and words were used to elicit EPs whilst the subject was engaged in analysing them. Most have supported the view that the linguistic processing required for controlling speech takes place mainly in the left hemisphere (Donchin *et al.*, 1977). The evidence in favour of the idea that the processing of non-verbal auditory stimuli, such as musical chords, takes place mainly in the right hemisphere is weaker (Damasio and Damasio, 1980), and often amounts to no more than the conclusion that it does not specifically take place in the left hemisphere.

Attempts to detect AEP waves signifying that a subject has understood the meaning of a sentence have also been quite successful (Chapman, 1973). Such comprehension always involves active participation by the subject; it is sometimes known as 'conceptual motor activity'. It can often lead to signs in the EMG that the vocal musculature is subliminally engaged. In a study where subjects had to distinguish between the homophone 'led' (the verb) or 'lead' (the metal), AEPs elicited by the key words differed in the left hemisphere alone (Brown *et al.*, 1976), but the differences were not found in the temporal lobe. The largest were recorded between Broca's motor speech area and its homologue in the right frontal lobe. Similarly in a study reported by Hillyard, N400 in AEPs following the first six words of a sentence were always larger over the left frontal lobe (Hillyard and Kutas, 1982), and when the seventh word was made semantically anomolous (The black cat sat on the —big) N400 was smaller over Broca's area. The importance of the frontal speech regions, in what may at first seem purely passive language comprehension tasks, is also one of the main lessons of cerebral blood flow studies, as will be demonstrated later.

In summary, passive listening to speech gives inconsistent and small differences between left and right hemispheres, but active participation, particularly when that culminates in vocalization, gives rise to larger and more reliable differences. These are found in frontal, motor, regions of the cerebral cortex, rather than in occipital or temporal areas. Such findings are what we would expect from the hypothesis that hemispheric specialization has developed to control different types of motor activity.

Cerebral Blood Flow

Recently methods have been developed for measuring the flow of blood through particular regions of the brain either by injecting xenon 133 into the carotid artery or by means of positron emission tomography (PET scan), or using P^{31} nuclear magnetic resonance (NMR). With the latter techniques separate measures of blood flow and neuronal metabolism can theoretically be obtained. Very small changes in cellular activity may be reflected in changes in cerebral blood flow; hence regional blood flow measures are now ofen used as an alternative to electrophysiological recording methods, when attempting to assess the degree of activation of a particular cortical region.

The advantage of blood flow measures is that theoretically the activity of extremely small regions may be measured; the resolution of the techniques, particularly the PET scan, is improving year by year, but some of the disadvantages are similar to those of EEG based methods. It is not at all clear to what particular analytic functions of neurones a change in the blood flow supplying them relates. For example, the methods probably lump together excitatory and inhibitory actions of cells. Yet there is some evidence from the visual cortex to suggest that inhibitory actions may in fact be associated with higher levels of metabolic activity than excitatory ones. A further problem with blood flow measurements is that their time resolution is poor, of the order of minutes, rather than the millisecond time scale that EEG based methods can achieve.

Disappointingly, most investigators report that they have been most impressed, not by hemispheric differences during tasks such as speech (Ingvar and Schwartz, 1974; Larsen *et al.*, 1978), or spatial activities, such as block design (Lassen *et al.*, 1978), but by the similarities between the regional blood flows of the two hemispheres. During passive sensory testing, differences between the two hemspiheres seldom amount to more than a few per cent; and are often barely significant statistically. Even during activities expected to be mediated mainly by the dominant hemisphere, such as verbally recalling from visual memory the contents of a subject's bedroom (Roland *et al.*, 1980), increases in regional cerebral blood flow occur bilaterally in most cortical regions, including Broca's area and its homologue on the right, and also in the auditory areas on both sides. Only in the anterior part of the inferior frontal region and in the middle and inferior temporal regions (i.e. regions that are well below the classical auditory areas, and probably relate more to visual memory) were selective increases in the left hemisphere seen.

The fullest reports to have appeared describing results using the PET scan have come from the UCLA group (Phelps *et al.*, 1982). Unfortunately these investigators did not usually ask their subjects to respond actively during the tests; so they had little control over what the subjects actually were doing or thinking. During monaural verbal stimulation they found that blood flow in both temporal cortices increased markedly. In left frontal and lateral occipital areas the blood flow increased more than in the homologous regions of the right hemisphere, although blood flow always tended to be higher in the left than the right hemisphere, even at rest. During subjects' attempts to picture the scene described in a Sherlock Holmes story, whether it was played into either ear, blood flow in the left hemisphere increased most markedly over the left lateral occipital region (by 15%) but, when the subjects listened to music, blood flow increased most in the right parieto-occipital region. Thus recent results from blood flow measures present a mildly convincing picture of left hemisphere dominance for speech reception, and support the idea that the right hemisphere is particularly involved in musical perception. However, blood flow measures are probably not yet sensitive enough to detect the subtle changes in neuronal activity that underly hemispheric specialization.

Action Theories of Speech Processing

A motor hypothesis for hemispheric lateralization has recently been provided with further impetus, because the 'motor' theory of speech decoding has gained wide acceptance (Liberman *et al.*, 1967). In essence it is argued that perceptual distinctions between different speech sounds are not achieved by detecting the differences in their acoustic content alone. Because speech sounds that are categorized as perceptually identical can nevertheless contain widely different acoustic components, a subject probably needs to use knowledge about the motor programmes which he has to employ to produce such sounds himself in order to categorize them. Humans understand different sounds as the same words even though their acoustic structure may vary greatly. This 'linguistic constancy' is probably achieved partly by the subject being able to compare the auditory input generated by speech with the stored motor programmes which he would have to use in order to produce the words himself (Kuhl, 1979).

It was originally suggested that all speech comprehension depends upon the hearer actually generating the motor patterns which he would have to use to produce similar words at the time of hearing them. Then after testing a number of 'hypotheses' about what is being said against the template of how the subject himself would say them, the best match to any articulatory motor pattern would be accepted as identifying what had been in fact said. In this 'strong' motor form, the hypothesis now has few adherents, for several reasons (Harvey and Howell, 1983). In the first place, if many stages of such hypothesis testing were necessary, speech comprehension would be far slower than the lightning pace observed. Furthermore there is now ample evidence that there is nothing about speech sounds that is 'special'. In principle at least, man's ability to decode speech can be explained in terms of the sensory processes which have been shown to underly his ability to analyse simpler amplitude and frequency modulated sounds (Kay, 1982). Also the motor theory cannot explain how it is that we can comprehend speech that we could not possibly produce. Most people can instantly understand the speech of those who have suffered laryngectomies, or of someone exhaling helium; but these are articulatory motor experiences that most of us have never experienced before. Finally the 'strong' motor theory cannot account for the fact that speech may be understood by the congenitally mute (Lenneberg, 1962). In contrast the congenitally deaf are often also rendered mute because they lack the assistance of the auditory feedback which is essential for anyone to learn to speak. If speech were entirely decoded by reference to the motor patterns required to produce it, the state of affairs should be the other way about. Mute people ought not to be able to comprehend spoken language, but there would be no reason why deaf people should be mute.

Nevertheless a motor contribution to speech processing is highly likely (McNeilage, 1970). A weaker form of the motor theory is now widely accepted. It has recently been buttressed by the finding in song birds by Williams and Nottebohm (1985) that the motor neurones of the left hypoglossal nucleus which innervate the syrinx (*see* earlier) show a selective response to specific song syllables, probably the same syllables that each produces when it discharges. Thus each vocalization may be perceived as an individual member of a set of vocal gestures each of which is represented by specific motor neurones with vocalization specific auditory inputs. This is therefore an avian parallel to the motor theory of human speech production.

How we decode the highly complex acoustic structure of speech still remains a largely unsolved problem. It seems likely that normal children develop their abilities to produce and comprehend speech simultaneously. They probably learn to generate templates in the left hemisphere which serve both to generate motor programmes for producing speech sounds and to assist in categorizing the content of other people's speech. Learning the motor patterns required for speaking appears to inform the auditory system about the acoustic structure of speech, whilst the invariants of acoustic structure that must be recognized in order to decode speech sounds as particular phonemes are recognized as the same invariants that the articulatory system must learn to generate in order to produce them. Eventually precise and reliable associations are made between the patterns of sound which each produces. Thus recognizing a word probably requires recognition of the same sensorimotor set as speaking that word; what is invariant about the sound of a word is also invariant in the pattern of motor activity required to produce it. The motor contribution to speech decoding is therefore probably most important and most vulnerable during childhood, when speaking and understanding language are being developed.

Rarely children have disorders of the executive control of their articulatory muscles; they are dysarthric rather than mute. Eventually such children usually learn to recognise speech, but they experience much greater difficulty than normals. Probably they only learn to understand speech if they can still lay down central associations between the motor commands for speech patterns generated in Broca's area with auditory feedback from other people. They learn to speak with such difficulty because they suffer the disadvantage of frequently hearing the peculiar modulations characteristic of their own speech. Also they lack the normal reinforcement provided by proprioceptive feedback from their own articulatory muscles. In normal children interactions between acoustic input, vocal motor outflow and proprioceptive feedback from articulatory muscles facilitate the rapid development of speech and language comprehension. Nevertheless the fact that congenitally deaf children learn to speak with much greater difficulty than the congenitally mute suggests that auditory feedback is the most important element in this mix. This, it will be recalled, was also one of the lessons from experiments with the development of birdsong.

Mechanisms of Hemispheric Specialization

So far I have concentrated upon evidence that hemispheric asymmetries exist. Though the physiological evidence from humans is patchy, the results in general provide support for the interpretation emphasized here that each hemisphere is primarily specialized to mediate a particular type of motor control. We ought therefore briefly to consider how these specializations might develop, and then how the two hemispheres are nevertheless able to work together so successfully.

Development

At birth the infant brain is only one quarter the size of that in adults. By the age of 2 it has more than tripled in size, and has approached its final dimensions. As we have seen, even in the fetus, anatomical signs of hemispheric asymmetry are already apparent. Paediatric neurologists are well aware that, up to the age of 2, damage to the left hemisphere hardly impedes the development of speech at all (Basser, 1962), and it seems that if necessary the right hemisphere can entirely take over language functions. Presumably no irreversible specialization of either the left or right side occurs before then. Between the age of 2 and puberty, left-hemispheric dominance for speech appears to become increasingly strong (Kinsbourne, 1975) so that, after puberty, aphasia almost always follows damage to the left hemisphere, whilst foreign languages can no longer be learnt without a tell-tale accent (Lenneberg, 1967). Differences in the amounts of choline acetyl transferase in the temporal lobes on the two sides seem to develop in parallel with the maturation of hemispheric specialization, and the process is not complete until puberty.

Despite this conclusion, as mentioned previously, morphological signs of lateral specialization can be found much earlier even in the fetus. Ingenious methods have demonstrated that in newborn infants there are probably functional differences between the right and left hemispheres, for example, a lower threshold for verbal sound stimuli in their right ears. Conditioned suck rate or the direction of eye movements (Gur, 1975) following verbal or noise stimuli applied to left or right ear have been measured. Similar results have been reported by investigators using evoked potentials to measure infants' responses to speech, compared with musical sounds (Molfese and Radtke, 1982). As is the case for the same techniques used in adults, these claims have not gone unchallenged. It is still not certain how left hemispheric specialization increases as a child grows older: indeed it has even been claimed that both morphological and functional specialization is fully developed at birth.

Even if differences in the processing abilities of the cerebral hemispheres of a newborn child dependent upon the morphological differences between them are real, the infant brain has tremendous ability to reorganize itself. This plasticity is what makes it possible to remove the left hemisphere before the age of 2 with every prospect of the child developing normal speech (Basser, 1962). Even up to the age of 5 only minor problems result from left hemispherectomy.

Function of the Corpus Callosum

How do the two hemispheres share control of behaviour in normal situations? How do they avoid interfering with each other? A popular idea is that of left hemispheric 'dominance'. This was derived from Sperry's finding that in split brain patients the left hemisphere seems to assume control over all the patients' responses in situations where the two hemispheres are presented with simultaneous but conflicting inputs (Sperry, 1974). However, such dominance is observed only when the subject is required to provide verbal responses to stimulation; the left hemisphere is dominant only for speech. If non-verbal output is allowed, the right hemisphere can produce powerful responses to its own input (LeDoux *et al.*, 1977).

A more attractive theory is that there is continuous competition between the hemispheres for the levers of control (Semmes, 1968). Hence the main function of the corpus callosum, it is postulated, is not so much to inform one hemisphere what the other is doing, but rather to keep the other under control. According to this hypothesis the hemisphere that is better at performing any particular function will automatically inhibit the other, and take over control of the whole body. It is therefore able to make use of any relevant information that the other hemisphere may be able to provide. This makes sense of the oft-reported finding that two hemispheres are usually better than one, whether for understanding language or for route finding (Galaburda and Geschwind, 1984).

Neither theory really explains why severing the corpus callosum in adults has, in general, so little effect. The answer may well be that the corpus callosum plays a more important role in the development of hemispheric specialization in children than it does in adults. For example, in animals there is now a great deal of evidence to show that activity in the corpus callosum is one of the main agents by which 'exuberant' connections which are characteristic of the immature visual system are deleted, leaving behind only the precise retinotopic projections found in the adult (Innocenti, 1979). An intact corpus callosum is particularly important in assisting to establish correct binocularity (Cynader *et al.*, 1981), so that only congruent inputs from the two eyes, representing the same point in space rather than non-corresponding regions, come to influence single neurones in the visual cortex. The corpus callosum itself becomes asymmetric if it does not receive equal inputs from the two visual hemifields. This state of affairs may be achieved experimentally by cutting the optic chiasm and suturing one eye, when only the hemisphere ipsilateral to the open eye receives structured visual input. The 'seeing' hemisphere comes to dominate the visual traffic in the corpus callosum, so that its influence over the non-seeing hemisphere becomes more pronounced than normal. The representation of the contralateral hemifield in the non-seeing hemisphere is now entirely provided by the good eye and the corpus callosum. The non-seeing hemisphere ceases to have any effect on the seeing hemisphere via the corpus callosum; so all cells there are driven only by the open eye.

Though these results have not yet been repeated for other sensory modalities or for motor areas, we can speculate that competition between homologous cortical regions on the two sides, mediated by bilateral traffic in the corpus callosum, is essential for normal establishment of hemispheric specialization. Humans with congenital agenesis of the corpus callosum display much more serious defects than adult commissurotomy patients. They show reduced hemispheric asymmetry (Jeeves, 1979). They tend to have low IQ. They are unable to cross-match visual or tactile stimuli applied to one half of the body with inputs to the other half. They are therefore significantly impaired in motor co-ordination and skill. The surviving signs of hemispheric specialization which these subjects nevertheless do exhibit are probably the result of the fact that they usually develop a very large anterior commissure, which can presumably compensate to some extent for their lack of a functioning corpus callosum.

The time that it takes for myelination of the corpus callosum to be completed is probably significant; in humans this is not until about the age of 5. If there is brain damage on one side early in life when the callosal connections are immature, proper hemispheric specialization probably cannot develop later on (Denenberg, 1981). There can be no balanced competition between homologous regions if one side is already damaged. Hence the developmental lag in the maturation of the corpus callosum is probably designed to ensure that early in development neural plasticity in both hemispheres is retained, as a hedge against brain injury; such damage is particularly common at birth. Later in development the corpus callosum can assist in maximizing differences between homologous cortical areas, in order to specialize them for different roles. This ensures that homotopic areas of cortex are not wasted trying to perform identical functions.

Probably competitive interhemispheric effects are mainly inhibitory. Many lines of evidence converge to suggest that the 'dominance' commonly ascribed to the left hemisphere for speech related behaviours is associated with inhibition of emotional output from the right hemisphere (Denenberg, 1981). Likewise there are many instances, particularly in psychopathology, of emotional activity, perhaps mediated by the right hemisphere, effectively inhibiting speech (Denenberg, 1981). But it must be admitted that at present we possess only a very sketchy understanding about the role of inhibitory mechanisms in interhemispheric communications. The electrical responses in the corpus callosum following stimulation of the parietal lobe on one side, consist of trains up to five negative/positive waves whose precise form varies with the position of the stimulating and recording electrodes (Mountcastle, 1962). Thus complex patterns of excitation and inhibition, distributed in time and space, characterize interhemispheric transfer; but about the nature of the information they transmit we have only the vaguest of ideas.

Summary and Conclusions

This survey of the differences between the hemispheres in humans, which it has been possible to reveal using physiological techniques, may seem disappointing. In general the physiological methods applicable to humans lack sufficient resolution to demonstrate reliable differences between the hemispheres. It is not at all clear how physiological indices of cortical function relate to the different ways in which each hemisphere processes sensory input in order to control the motor functions for which it is responsible. Measuring the amplitude of the alpha-wave over each half of the scalp seems not to be a reliable way of determining the degree of involvement of one or other hemisphere in speech or self-orientation. Neither visual, auditory, or motor evoked potentials reveal unambiguously which hemisphere is most involved in communication, visual orientation or emotional expression. Not even the recent introduction of methods for measuring cerebral metabolism and blood flow in different cortical areas has yet been able to contribute significantly to a solution of these problems.

The major positive contribution of physiologists to the problem of hemispheric specialization has come from a traditional source — experiments using animals. Even though few animals can speak, precisely localized ablation, stimulation and recording experiments have produced clear evidence for lateralized control of many communicative functions in animals. The outcome of these studies is to suggest that it would probably be more fruitful to concentrate effort upon relating physiological measures of regional cortical activity in humans to the style of motor control exercised by each hemisphere, rather than attempting to detect small differences in sensory processing. It seems likely that the fundamental dichotomy between the hemispheres concerns the kind of sensorimotor control which each exercises. The right hemisphere probably became specialized early in evolution to control an animal's orientation with respect to its territory. Hence it is also concerned with the holistic visuospatial analysis of scenes and the animal's relation to them. Perhaps it is also involved in the expression of emotions. The left hemisphere probably became specialized later in time to take charge of serial analysis in space and time for the control of communication by voice and gesture.

References

ADRIAN, E.D. and MATTHEWS, B.H.C. The Berger rhythm: Potential changes recorded from the occipital lobes in man. *Brain* (1934), **37**, 355–385.

ANNETT, M. The inheritance of handedness and cerebral dominance. *Nature (Lond.)* (1964), **204**, 59–60.

BASSER, L.S. Hemiplegia of early onset and the faculty of speech with special reference to the effects of hemispherectomy. *Brain* (1962), **85**, 427–460.

BEAUMONT, J.G. (ed.) *Divided Visual Field Studies* (1982). London: Academic Press.

BLUMHARDT, L.D., BARRETT, G. and HALLIDAY, A.M. The asymmetrical visual evoked potential to pattern reversal in one half field and its significance for the analysis of visual field defects. *British Journal of Ophthalmology* (1977), **61**, 454–461.

BRADSHAW, J.L. and NETTLETON, N.C. The nature of hemispheric specialization in man. *Behavioural and Brain Sciences* (1981), **4**, 51–93.

BRADSHAW, J.L. and NETTLETON, N.C. *Human Cerebral Asymmetry* (1983). New Jersey: Prentice Hall.

BRAZIER, M. *The Electrical Activity of the Nervous System* (1975). London: Pitman.

BROADBENT, D.E. The role of auditory localization in attenuation and memory span. *Journal of Experimental Psychology* (1954), **47**, 191–196.

BROWN, W.S., MARSH, J.T. and SMITH, J.C. Evoked potential waveform differences produced by the perception of different meanings of an ambiguous phrase. *Electroencephalography and Clinical Neurophysiology* (1976), **41**, 113–123.

BUCHSBAUM, M. and FEDIO, P. Hemispheric differences in evoked potentials to verbal and non-verbal stimuli in the left and right visual fields. *Physiology and Behaviour* (1970), **5**, 207–210.

BUCHSBAUM, M. and DRAGO, D. Hemispheric asymmetry and the effects of attention on visual evoked potentials. *Progress in Clinical Neurophysiology* (1977), **3**, 243–253.

BUTLER, S.R. and GLASS, A. Asymmetries in the EEG associated with cerebral dominance. *Electroencephalography and Clinical Neurophysiology* (1974), **36**, 481–491.

CALLAWAY, E. and HARRIS, P.R. Coupling between cortical potentials from different areas. *Science* (1974), **183**, 873–875.

CHAPMAN, R.M. Evoked potentials of the brain related to thinking. In F.J. McGuigan and R.A. Schoonover (eds) *The Psychophysiology of Thinking: Studies of Covert Processes* (1973), pp. 69–108. New York: Academic Press.

CHAPPLE, W.D. Motoneuron responses to visual stimuli in *Oncopeltus fasciatus. Journal of Experimental Biology* (1966), **45**, 401–410.

CHAPPLE, W.D. Asymmetry in invertebrate nervous systems. In S. Hernad (ed.) *Lateralization in The Nervous System* (1977), pp. 3–18. New York: Academic Press.

CORBALLIS, M.C. and MORGAN, M.J. On the biological basis of human laterality. Evidence for a maturation of the left-right gradient. *Behavioral and Brain Sciences* (1978), **1**, 261–269.

CORBALLIS, M.C. and BEALE, I.L. *The Psychology of Left and Right* (1976). New Jersey: Erlbaum.

COWEY, A. and BOZECK, T. Contralateral 'neglect' after unilateral dorsomedial prefrontal lesions in rats. *Brain Research* (1974), **72**, 53–63.

CYNADER, M., LEPORE, F. and GUILLEMOT, J. Interhemispheric competition during postnatal development. *Nature (Lond.)* (1981), **290**, 139–140.

DAMASIO, A.R. and GESCHWIND, N. *Annual Review of Neuroscience* (1984), **7**, 127–144.

DAMASIO, A.R. and DAMASIO, H. Musical faculty and cerebral dominance. In M. Critchley and R.A. Henson (eds) *Music and the Brain* (1980), pp. 141–155. London: Heinemann.

DEECKE, L., SCHEID, P. and KORNHUBER, H.H. Distribution of readiness potential, pre-motion positivity and motor potentials in the human cerebral cortex preceding voluntary finger movements. *Experimental Brain Research* (1969), **7**, 158–168.

DENENBERG, V.H. Hemispheric laterality in animals and the effects of early experience. *Behavioural and Brain Sciences* (1981), **4**, 1–49.

DEWSON, J.H. and COWEY, A. Discrimination of auditory sequences by monkeys. *Nature (Lond.)* (1969), **222**, 695–697.

DEWSON, J.H. Preliminary evidence of hemispheric asymmetry of auditory function in monkeys. In S. Harnad, R.W. Doty, L. Goldstein, J. Jaynes and G. Krauthamer (eds) *Lateralization in the Nervous System* (1977), pp. 63–71. New York: Academic Press.

DEWSON, J.H. Toward an animal model of auditory cognitive function. In C.L. Ludlow and M.E. Doran-Quine (eds) *The Neurological Bases of Language Disorders in Children: Methods and Directions for Research*. NINCDS Monograph No. 22, (1979), pp. 19–24. Washington, D.C.: Government Printing Office.

DIAMOND, M.C. New data supporting cortical asymmetry differences in males and females. *Behavioural and Brain Sciences* (1980), **3**, 233–234.

DIMOND, S.J. and BEAUMONT, J.G. (eds) *Hemisphere Function in the Human Brain* (1974). London: Paul Elek.

DIMOND, S.J. *The Double Brain* (1972). London: Churchill.

DONCHIN, E., KUTAS, M. and MCCARTHY, G. Electrocortical indices of hemispheric lateralization. In S. Harnad (ed.) *Lateralization in the Nervous System* (1977). New York: Academic Press.

DOYLE, J.C., ORNSTEIN, R. and GALIN, D. Lateral specialization of cognitive modes. II. EEG frequency analysis. *Psychophysiology* (1974), **11**, 567–578.

DUMAS, R. and MORGAN, A. EEG asymmetry as a function of occupation, task and task difficulty. *Neuropsychologia* (1975), **13**, 219–228.

FRIEDMAN, D., SIMSON, R., RITTER, W. and RAPIN, I. Cortical evoked potentials elicited by real speech words and human sounds. *Electroencephalography and Clinical Neurophysiology* (1975), **38**, 13–19.

GALABURDA, A.M. and GESCHWIND, N. *The Biological Foundations of Cerebral Dominance* (1984). Cambridge Ma.: MIT Press.

GALIN, D. and ELLIS, R.R. Asymmetry in evoked potentials as an index of lateralized cognitive processes: relation to EEG alpha asymmetry. *Psychophysiology* (1975), **13** 45–50.

GALIN, D. and ORNSTEIN, R. Lateral specialization of cognitive mode: An EEG study. *Psychophysiology* (1972), **9**, 412–418.

GARDNER, B.T. and GARDNER, R.A. Two-way communication with an infant chimpanzee. In Schrier and Stollinitz (eds) *Behaviour of Non-Human Primates* (1971), Vol. 4, pp. 117–184. New York: Academic Press.

GARDNER, A.D. Motolateral dominance in feet and hands. *Psychological Record* (1943), **5**, 2–63.

GAZZANIGA, M.S. and LEDOUX, J.E. *The Integrated Mind* (1978). New York: Plenum.

GESCHWIND, N. *Selected Papers on Language and The Brain* (1974). Dordrecht: Reidel.

GESCHWIND, N. and GALABURDA, A.M. *Archives of Neurology* (1985), **42**, 428–552.

GLICK, S.J., JERUSSI, T.P. and FLEISHER, L.N. Turning in circles: the neuropharmacology of rotation. *Life Sciences* (1976), **18**, 889–896.

GLICK, S.D., MEIBACH, R.C., COX, R.D. and MAAYANI, S. Multiple and interrelated functional asymmetries in rat brain. *Life Sciences* (1979), **25**, 395–400.

GLICK, S.D. Enhancement of spatial preferences by amphetamine. *Neuropharmacology* (1973), **12**, 43–47.

GLICK, S.D. *Cerebral Lateralization in Non-human Species* (1985). New York: Academic Press.

GOODMAN, D.M., BEATTY, J. and MULHOLLAND,, T.B. Detection of cerebral lateralization using contingent visual stimulation. *Electroencephalography and Clinical Neurophysiology* (1980), **48**, 418–431.

GORDON, H.W. Degree of ear asymmetry for perception of dichotic chords and for illusory chord localization in musicians of different levels of competence. *Journal of Experimental Psychology, Human Perception and Performance* (1980), **6**, 517–527.

GROZINGER, B., KORNHUBER, H.H. and KRIEBEL, J. Human cerebral potentials preceding speech production, phonation and movements of the mouth and tongue, with reference to respiratory and extracerebral potentials. *Progress in Clinical Neurophysiology* (1977), **3**, 87–103.

GRUZELLIER, J. Lateral asymmetries in electrodermal activity and psychosis. In Gruzellier (ed.) *Hemispheric Asymmetries in Psychopathology* (1982). Oxford: Elsevier.

HAMILTON, C.R. Investigations of perceptual and mnemonic lateralisation in monkeys. In S. Harnad (ed.) *Lateralisation in the Nervous System* (1977). New York: Academic Press.

HARNAD, S.R., DOTY, R.W., GOLDSTEIN, L., JAYNES, J. and KRAUTHAMER, G. (eds) *Lateralization in the Nervous System* (1977). New York: Academic Press.

HARVEY, N. and HOWELL, P. Perceptual and motor equivalents in speech. In *Language Production* (1983), Vol. 2 London: Academic Press.

HILLYARD, S.A. and KUTAS, M. The lateral distribution of event related potentials during sentence processing. *Neuropsychologia* (1982), **20**, 579–592.

INGVAR, D.H. and SCHWARTZ, M.S. Cerebral blood flow in speech and reading. *Brain* (1974), **96**, 274–288.

INNOCENTI, G.M. Adult and neonatal characteristics of the callosal zone at the boundary between areas 17 and 18 in the cat. In I. Steele-Russell (ed.) *Structure and Function of the Cerebral Commissures* (1979). London: Macmillan.

JAHROMI, S.S. and ATWOOD, H.L. Structural and contractile properties of lobster leg-muscle fibers. *Journal of Experimental Zoology* (1971), **176**, 475–486.

JARVILEHTO, T. and FRUHSTORFER, H. Differentiation between slow cortical potentials asociated with motor and mental acts in man. *Experimental Brain Research* (1970), **11**, 309–317.

JEEVES, M.A. Some limits to hemispheric integration in cases of callosal agenesis and partial commissurotomy. In I.S. Russell, H.W. van Hoff and G. Berlucchi (eds) *Structure and Function of Cerebral Commissures* (1979), pp. 449–474. London: Macmillan.

JURGENS, U. and PLOOG, D. Cerebral representation of vocalisation in the squirrel monkey. *Experimental Brain Research* (1970), **29**, 75–83.

KAY, R.H. and MAYERS, R. Ear advantages for detecting frequency changes in sounds. *Journal of Physiology* (1982), **328**, 40–41P.

KAY, R.H. Hearing modulation in sounds. *Physiological Review* (1982), **62**, 894–975.

KIMURA, D. and ARCHIBALD, Y. Motor functions of the left hemisphere. *Brain* (1974), **97**, 337–350.

KINSBOURNE, M. *Hemispheric Disconnection and Cerebral Function* (1974). Illinois: C. Thomas.

KINSBOURNE, M. The ontogeny of cerebral dominance. In D. Aaronson (ed.) *Developmental Psycholinguistics and Communication Disorders* (1975). New York: New York Academy of Science.

KOLB, B., SUTHERLAND, R.J., NONNEMAM, A.J. and WHISHAW, I.Q. Asymmetry in the cerebral hemispheres of the rat, mouse, rabbit and cat. The right hemisphere is larger. *Experimental Neurology* (1983), **78 (2)** 348–359.

KUHL, P.K. Models and mechanisms in speech perception. *Brain, Behaviour and Evolution* (1979), **16**, 291–292.

LARSEN, B., SKINHO, E. and LASSEN, N.A. Regional cortical blood flow in right and left hemisphere during automatic speech. *Brain* (1978), **101**, 193–211.

LASSEN, N.A., INGVAR, D.H. and SKINHO, E. Brain function and blood flow. *Scientific American* (1978), **239**, 62–71.

LEDOUX, J.E., WILSON, D.H. and GAZZANIGA, M.S. A divided mind: observations on the conscious properties of the separated hemispheres. *Annals of Neurology* (1977), **2**, 417–421.

LEMAY, M. and GESCHWIND, N. Hemispheric differences in the brains of great apes. *Brain, Behaviour and Evolution* (1975), **11**, 48–52.

LENNEBERG, E.H. Understanding language without the ability to speak. A case report. *Journal of Abnormal Psychology* (1962), **65**, 419–425.

LENNEBERG, E.H. *Biological Foundations of Language* (1967), New York: Wiley.

LIBERMAN, A.M., COOPER, F.S., SHANKWEILER, D. and STUDDART-KENNEDY, M. Perception of the speech code. *Psychological Reviews* (1967), **74**, 431–461.

LIVANOV, M.N., GAVRILOVA, N.A. and ASLANOV, A.S. Correlations between biopotentials in the frontal parts of the human brain. In K.H. Pribram and A.R. Luria (eds) *Psychophysiology of the Frontal Lobes* (1973), pp. 91–107. New York: Academic Press.

MCGLONE, J. Sex differences in human brain asymmetry. *Behavioural and Brain Sciences* (1980), **1**, 215–263.

MACKAY, A.V.P. Sinistral findings in Schizophrenia. *Trends in Neuroscience* (1984), **7**, 107–109.

MCKEEVER, W.F. and HULING, M. Left hemispheric superiority in tachistoscopic word recognition performance. *Perception & Motor Skills* (1970), **30**, 763–766.

MCNEILAGE, P.F. Motor control of serial order in speech. *Psychological Review* (1970), **77**, 182–196.

MARLER, P. Vocal ethology of primates. In Chivers (ed.) *Advances in Primatology* Vol. 1, (1978), pp. 745–801. New York: Academic Press.

MARLER, P. and WASER, M.S. Development of canary song. *Journal of Comprehensive Physiological Psychology* (1977), **91**, 8–16.

MELLON, DE. F. and STEVENS, P.J. Transformation of claws in the snapping shrimp. *Nature (Lond.)* (1978), **272**, 246–248.

MESULAM, M.M. Hemispheric specialisation for directed attention. *Trends in Neuroscience* (1983), **6**, 384–387.

MOLFESE, D.L. and RADTKE, R.C. Statistical and methodological problems with auditory evoked potentials and sex related problems in brain development. *Brain and Language* (1982), **16** 338–341.

MORAIS, L. and GOTT, P.S. The relation of cerebral dominance and handedness to visual evoked potentials. *Journal of Neurobiology* (1972), **3**, 65–77.

MORGAN, A.H., MCDONALD, P.J. and MCDONALD, H. Differences in bilateral alpha activity as a function of lateral eye movements and hyponotizability. *Neuropsychologie* (1971), **9** 459–469.

MORISON, D. Cortical localisation of affect. *Science* (1979), **205**, 313.

MOUNTCASTLE, V.P. (ed.) *Interhemispheric relations and cerebral Dominance* (1962). Baltimore: Johns Hopkins Press.

MYERS, R.E. and SPERRY, R.W. Interhemispheric communication through the corpus callosum. *Archives of Neurology and Psychology* (1958) **80**, 298–303.

NOTTEBOHM, F. Ontogony of bird song. *Science* (1970), **167**, 950–956.

NOTTEBOHM, F. Phonation in the parrot. *Journal of Comprehensive Physiology* (1976), **108**, 157–170.

NOTTEBOHM, F. Asymmetries in neural control of canary vocalisation. In S. Harnad (ed.) *Lateralization in the Nervous System* (1977). New York: Academic Press.

NOTTEBOHM, F. Brain pathways for vocal learning in birds. In J. Sprague (ed.) *Progress in Psychobiology*, Vol. 9 (1980). New York: Academic Press.

NOTTEBOHM, F. Laterality and seasons in song control. *Trends in Neuroscience* (1981), **4**, 104–106.

PAPANICOLAOU, N. Cerebral excitation profiles in language processing. The photic probe techniques. *Brain and Language* (1978), **9**, 269–280.

PETERSEN, M.R., BEECHER, M.D., ZOLOTH, S.R., MOODY, D.B. and STEBBINS, W.C. Neural lateralisation of species specific vocalisations in Japanese macaques. *Science* (1978), **202**, 324–327.

PHELPS, M.E., MAZZIOTA, J.C., CARSON, R.E. and KUHL, D.E. Changes in cerebral metabolism following auditory stimulation. *Neurology* (1982), **32**, 921–938.

PLOOG, D. Neurobiology of primate audio vocal behaviour. *Brain Research Reviews* (1981), **3**, 35–61.

PORAC, C. and COREN, S. *Lateral Preferences and Human Behaviour* (1981). Berlin: Springer.

PREMACK, D. In Schrier (ed.) *Behaviour of Non-human Primates*, Vol. 4, (1971). New York: Academic Press.

REGAN, D. *Evoked Potentials in Psychology, Sensory Physiology and Clinical Medicine* (1972). London: Chapman & Hall.

ROLAND, P.E., VERNET, K.E. and LASSEN, N.A. Verbal report from visual memory. *Neuroscience Letters* (1980), **55**, 478.

ROSENZWEIG, M.R. Representation of the two ears in the auditory cortex. *American Journal of Physiology* (1951), **167**, 147–158.

RUGG, M.D. Electrophysiological studies. In J.G. Beaumont (ed.) *Divided Visual Field Studies* (1982). London: Academic Press.

RUMBAUGH, D.M.E. (ed.) *Language and Learning by Chimpanzees — The LANA Project* (1977). New York: Academic Press.

SCHAEFFER, A.A. *Journal of Morphology* (1928), **95**, 293–398.

SEMMES, J. Hemispheric specialisation. A possible clue to mechanism. *Neurophysiologia* (1968), **6**, 11–26.

SEUREN, P.A.M. Language and communication in primates. In Chivers (ed.) *Advances in Primatology*, Vol. 1, (1978), pp. 909–919. London: Academic Press.

SHUCARD, D., SHUCARD, J., CUMMINS, K. and THOMAS, D. The two tone probe technique. *Psychophysiology* (1978), **16**, 189.

SPERRY, R.W. Hemisphere disconnection and writing in conscious awareness. *American Psychologist* (1968), **23**, 723–733.

SPERRY, R.W. Lateral specialisation in the surgically separated hemispheres. In F.O. Schmidt (ed.) *Neurosciences Third Study Program* (1974). Cambridge, Ma.: MIT Press.

SPRINGER, S.P. and DEUTSCH, G. *Left Brain, Right Brain* (1985). San Francisco: W.H. Freeman.

STEBBINS, W.C. Hearing in primates. In Chivers (ed.) *Advances in Primatology*, Vol. 1, (1978), pp. 705–720. London: Academic Press.

STEELE-RUSSELL, I., VAN HOFF, M.W. and BERLUCCHI, G. *Structure and Function of The Cerebral Commissures* (1979). London: Macmillan.

SZIRTES, J. and VAUGHAN, H.G. Characteristics of cranial and facial potentials associated with speech production. In J. Desmedt (ed.) *Language and Hemispheric Specialisation in Man. Progress in Clinical Neurophysiology*, Vol. 3 (1977). Basel: Kargar.

TALLAL, P. and SCHWARTZ, J. Temporal processing, speech perception and hemispheric asymmetry. *Trends in Neuroscience* (1980), **3**, 309–311.

THOMPSON, M.T. The metamorphosis of the hermit crab. *Proceedings of the Boston Society of Natural Science* (1903), **31**, 147–209.

UNGERSTEDT, U. Brain dopamine and behaviour. In F. Schmidt (ed.) *The Neurosciences; 3rd Study Proceedings* (1974), pp. 695–704. Cambridge Ma.: MIT Press.

WADA, J.A. A new method for the determination of the side of cerebral speech dominance by the intracarotid injection of Na amytal in man. *Medical Biology* (1949), **4**, 221–222.

WADE, N. Ape language — self-deception? *Trends in Neuroscience* (1980), **3**, IX.

WALTER, W.G. *et al. Nature (Lond.)* (1964), **203**, 380–384.

WANG, G.H. *The Neural Control of Sweating* (1964). University of Wisconsin Press.

WARREN, J.M. The development of paw preferences in cats and monkeys. *Journal of Geriatric Psychology* (1958), **93**, 229–236.

WARREN, J.M. Handedness and cerebral dominance. In S. Harnad (ed.) *Lateralization in The Nervous System* (1977). New York: Academic Press.

WARREN, J.M. and NOTTEBOHM, A.J. The search for cerebral dominance in the rhesus monkey. *Annals of The New York Academy of Science* (1976),**298**, 176–194.

WEBSTER, W. Hemispheric asymmetry in cats. In S. Harnad (ed.) *Lateralisation in The Nervous System* (1977), pp. 446–479. New York: Academic Press.

WILSON, D.M. Asymmetry and reflex modulation of locust flight. *Journal of Experimental Biology* (1968), **48**, 631–641.
YOUNG, A.W. *Functions of the Right Cerebral Hemisphere* (1982). London: Academic Press.

6

Observations on Right Hemisphere Language Function

Dahlia W. Zaidel

Introduction

It is well known that many aphasics partially recover speech, comprehension, writing or reading eventually. Rate and extent of recovery vary depending not only on the size of the lesion and its aetiology (tumour versus stroke, for example) but also on the sex of the patient (Kertesz and Sheppard, 1981), familial handedness (Luria, 1947; Subirana, 1958), and the age at onset (Hecaen, 1976). A common suggestion is that the intact right hemisphere in the majority of right-handed aphasic patients may be involved in the compensatory process. The evidence from neurological patients with different aetiologies confirms the involvement of the right hemisphere in linguistic skills (Smith, 1966; Gazzaniga and Sperry, 1967; Zaidel, E., 1976; Cummings *et al.*, 1979; Cavalli *et al.*, 1981), but the underlying mechanisms responsible for the functional reorganization are not known. It is not clear, for example, how much of the recovered language can be attributed to partial recovery in the left hemisphere, to both hemispheres working together, or to the right hemisphere exclusively. To complicate matters, the very notion of right hemisphere language has recently been questioned (Gazzaniga, 1983; Zaidel, E., 1983). To help resolve the issue, it is necessary to assess further the extent of right hemisphere capabilities, especially in respect to the production of language, in order to gauge the possibility of language take-over by this hemisphere.

I present here a case of a patient who underwent commissurotomy, not because he ever suffered from aphasia or had sustained injury to brain regions in the left hemisphere commonly associated with language specialization, but rather because his case may help illuminate some of the mechanisms of linguistic changes that takes place during recovery from aphasia. This case is informative because some of the analysis of linguistic functions observed here may serve to highlight discrete stages of language recovery which would otherwise be masked by extensive brain damage as well as provide definitive evidence for right hemisphere expressive language capability. Specifically, the emphasis in the experimental approach is to use some of the upper limits of language acquisition by the right hemisphere following disconnection from the left as a model for related compensatory changes in the central or peripheral nervous system.

Commissurotomy

Surgical section of the forebrain commissures in higher mammals including man has been shown reliably to result in multiple deficits of interhemispheric integration (Sperry, 1968; 1974). Following disconnection, the cerebral hemispheres display differential functional abilities of most cognitive skills but these hemispheric differences are observable only under special conditions in a neurological examination or in the laboratory. In testing not aimed at teasing hemispheric differences apart, impairments have been found for memory (Zaidel, D.W. and Sperry, 1974) and for motor functions (Zaidel and Sperry, 1977). Otherwise the surgery appears to have left the basic physiological processes and personality traits unimpaired.

From the start, patients of P.J. Vogel and J.E. Bogen who had undergone complete commissurotomy, i.e. section of the corpus callosum, anterior and hippocampal commissures, have displayed what has come to be known as the syndrome of hemispheric disconnection (Sperry, Gazzaniga, and Bogen, 1969), including an inability to name verbally, or in writing, while blindfolded the names of objects felt in the left hand, and of figures projected tachistocopically to the left visual half-field (LVF). In short, the patients showed absence of transfer of information from one hemisphere to the other, symptoms which are still largely present some 20 or so years after surgery.

At the same time, a few persistent changes in the above picture were noted a few years after surgery in a young patient (LB) and are presented in this chapter. The changes that are relevant to the present discussion include the correct naming of certain objects felt (blindly) in the left hand or of figures appearing in the LVF, all of which were not reported during the early period following surgery (Gazzaniga and Sperry, 1967). The tests to be described here were administered during a 2-year period, 5–7 years postoperatively and the initial results were reported informally by Zaidel, D.W. and Sperry (1972). Subsequent studies using the visual tachistoscopic method have confirmed the general picture of a functional reorganization of sensory and/

or cognitive capabilities in this patient and to some limited extent in a few of the other commissurotomy patients of the Bogen and Vogel series (Teng and Sperry, 1973; Kumar, Bogen, and Bogen, 1977; Johnson, 1980, 1984a, b; Myers and Sperry, 1985).

The aim of this study was to search for language production in speech and writing instead of for language comprehension because the latter had been studied separately, and extensively, by Zaidel, E. (1973, 1978, 1980). In brief, the bulk of the findings on auditory comprehension were based on repeated use of a special scleral lens technique which allows free scanning of input in one visual half-field at a time without discomfort (Zaidel, E., 1975). Right hemisphere auditory language comprehension for single words was found to be equivalent to a vocabulary of an average 17-year-old (at the time he was 20–23 years of age) and with a rich lexical semantic system. The visual vocabulary was inferior to his auditory vocabulary and he seemed to read ideographically, i.e. obtaining meaning directly from the orthography, without intermediate translation into an auditory representation. In addition, LB's right hemisphere was found to not understand nonredundant phrases more than three words long and to have some grammar and limited syntax.

It is important to stress at this point that LB, as with most of the patients in the Bogen–Vogel series, is assumed to have sustained some right hemisphere damage as a result of surgical retraction of that hemisphere. The retraction was a necessary procedure during the operation. Thus, the observed right hemisphere capabilities become more significant in light of the presence of some damage.

Case Report

LB is a right-handed male who was born in May, 1952, with the aid of a Caesarean section. His weight at birth was 5 lb (2270 g). Because of his weight and because he was cyanotic he was placed in an incubator for 8 days. Later, his development appeared normal but, at age 3, epileptic seizures began and those became worse with time. When he was examined, no neurological abnormality was found, skull X-ray, brain scan, pneumoencephalogram and bilateral carotid angiogram were all normal. EEG records indicated that there were diffuse abnormalities. Since his seizures became progressively worse (despite heavy medication), and reportedly interfered with his school work, it was decided to perform complete commissurotomy.

In April, 1965 (age 12 years and 11 months) he underwent surgery. During the operation the right hemisphere was retracted slightly, no bridging veins were interrupted, the fornices were not sectioned, and the operation was considered uneventful. The corpus callosum, anterior and hippocampal commissures were sectioned. His postoperative progress was smooth and unusually rapid compared with other patients undergoing the same surgery. Following surgery, seizures were alleviated (medication was continued but at a reduced level). Eight left-sided Jacksonian episodes in the 3 years after surgery suggested right hemisphere abnormality. Prior to surgery there was no clear indication of right-hemisphere epileptic focus (Gazzaniga and Sperry, 1967; Sperry, Gazzaniga and Bogen, 1969; Bogen and Vogel, 1975).

Testing Procedures and Results

Somesthesis

The general procedure consisted of blind palpation of 2-inch high letters or numbers by the left or right hands. These stimuli were placed on a thick towel to minimize auditory cues and were shielded from sight behind a screen. Right-hand performance was found to be 100% accurate and is not reported here in detail.

Spelling and Reading

Under the conditions outlined above, two tests which were originally administered to LB approximately 4 years postoperatively by Levy, Nebes and Sperry (1971) were readministered 7 years postoperatively. In the first task, he was asked to arrange scrambled letters into single words. Following each arrangement he was asked to name aloud the word spelled. Theoretically he should not have been able to produce correct naming responses since speech functions are lateralized to the left hemisphere in this right-handed subject. However, this was not the case. *Table 1* summarizes the findings and clearly shows a high level of accuracy ($p<0.0006$) in the follow-up test.

Table 1 **Letter arrangement by the left hand out of view**

	*4 years postoperatively**		*7 years postoperatively*	
Stimulus	*Word spelled*	*Word said*	*Word spelled*	*Word said*
I,F	IF	-	IF	IF
A,C,N	CAN	-	CAN	AIL
B,O,Y	BOY	-	BOY	BOY
E,P,T	PET	-	PET	PET
B,Y	BY	-	BY	BY
O,S	SO	-	SO	SO

- = Couldn't say.

* Reported by Levy, Nebes and Sperry (1971)

Table 2 Reading words presented out of view to the left hand

	*4 years postoperatively**	*7 years postoperatively*
Stimulus		
IF	Don't know	IF
SO	Don't know	SO
BY	Don't know	BY
CAN	TO	CAN
HAT	NT	HAT
BOY	Don't know	BOY
PET	Don't know	PET
FAT	NT	FAT
DAY	NT	DAY
SOON	NT	SOON
WALK	NT	WALK
YEAR	NT	YEAR
ACID	NT	ACID
EARTH	NT	EARTH
TIGHT	NT	TIGHT

NT = Not tested.
* Reported by Levy, Nebes and Sperry (1971).

In the second follow-up test, unscrambled letters were placed behind the screen and the task was simply to name the entire word after all the letters were palpated in order. *Table 2* summarizes the findings. Again, we see a remarkable improvement in performance. Of the 14 correctly named words, 6 were not named in the 4-year postoperative test whereas they were named 7 years postoperatively. It is noteworthy that two irregular words, namely 'walk' and 'tight', were read correctly.

At the same time, some qualitative aspects of LB's performance suggests the use of unusual reading strategies; for example, compared with reading with the right hand, reading with the left was far slower. He often took up to 45 seconds to read one word, which would suggest the use of cross-cueing strategies proposed earlier by Gazzaniga and Sperry (1967).

Speaking or writing with the left hand

Two tests were given to assess LB's right hemisphere speech and writing capabilities. In both, separate series of single numbers, letters, geometrical shapes, common objects familiar from previous experiments, and common objects not used in any of the previous asessment involving LB, were all presented out of view. The task in the first test consisted of identifying each item verbally. In the second test (administered 1 week later), the task

Table 3 **Spoken and written identification of stimuli presented to the left hand out of view. Writing was with the left hand, also out of view**

	% Correct	
Stimuli	*Speaking*	*Writing*
Numerals	100	100
Letters	50	95
Geometric shapes	75	83
Familiar common objects	16	NT
Non-familiar common objects	10	33
Non-familiar common objects with pre-trial exposure	70	NT

NT = Not tested.

consisted of writing the name of the item with the left hand. Immediately following a few, randomly selected, written responses, verbal confirmation was requested. The results of these tests are summarized in *Table 3*.

Two main findings emerge:

1. Familiarity is an important factor in correct naming. The best example is seen in the results with pretrial exposure. The fact that one-digit numerals have a small set of alternatives, namely, 10, may parly explain why their naming were twice as accurate as those of single letters, which have 26 possible alternatives. Geometrical shapes were named correctly four times better than familiar common objects and seven times better than the non-familiar common objects.
2. Correct written responses appear consistently more frequently than in the series involving verbal answers. This could be interpreted as another form of familarity since these trials followed by 1 week the trials in which verbal responses were requested.

Qualitatively, differences among the various stimuli were noticeable during the tactual manipulation stage. While LB's identification of numbers appeared confident, the responses to the shapes or common household objects were frequently hesitant or protracted. It was clear that he considered various features in the stimulus — e.g., length, weight, size, texture, or function — before responding. In some trials he appeared to be whispering one or two characteristics; in other trials he silently balanced an item or placed it between his thumb and index finger. Strategies of this kind proved useful in approximately one-third of the trials. But they were not a necessary condition for correct naming because in trials where these strategies were not overtly adopted some answers were none the less correct.

Table 4 **Percentage of correct responses on tactual cross-retrieval trials**

Stimuli	*Left hand (input) right hand (output)*	*Right hand (input) left hand (output)*
Familiar common objects	50	83
Nonsense wire shapes	10	20
Non-familiar common objects	20	80

Chance = 20% correct.

The fact that he was able to consider specific stimulus characteristics suggests the use of the ipsilateral sensory projection systems (Levy, Nebes, and Sperry, 1971). Only crude information is assumed to be relayed via uncrossed somesthetic pathways but it is possible that repeated testing can lead to change and improvement in discrimination. Yet, in this case, due to the limitations inherent in the ipsilateral system much of the hemispheric disconnection syndrome remains unaltered. In summary, LB's performance in tests of speech and writing was better 5 years postoperatively than when tested shortly after surgery (Gazzaniga, Sperry, and Bogen, 1967).

Cross-transfer of Tactual Information

In view of the correct high naming rate it became necessary to determine the extent to which the left hemisphere was aware of stimuli presented to the right hemisphere. Consequently, a series of tests measuring the cross-transfer of somesthetic information was administered. After perceiving tactually one object presented to only one hand, LB had to retrieve the same object with the other hand from among an array of 6 or 7 similar objects. The different types of objects administered and the results are presented in *Table 4*. Perusal of this table shows that there was some ability to cross-transfer certain types of information but more so in one direction than in the other. Thus if initial input was to the right hand (left hemisphere) then a substantial amount of information was transmitted to the right hemisphere, whereas the reverse was not the case. Furthermore, we see, again, the role of familiarity in performance. Thus, when comparing the transfer of nonsense wire shapes in either direction with the transfer of familiar or non-familiar common objects, the latter led to an increase in accuracy. At the same time, the presence of hemispheric disconnection despite his highly skilled performance is highly visible.

Vision

Stimuli (2 × 2 slides) were projected onto a translucent screen for a duration of 100 ms which is less than the 180 ms taken to initiate a saccade in the direction of the flash. As a precaution against eye movements, the stimuli were presented randomly to the left (LVF) or right (RVF) visual half-fields. In addition, eye movements were monitored by means of two non-polarizing Beckman electrodes placed lateral to each eye, and a third ground electrode on the forehead between the two eyebrows. Eye movements were measured to an accuracy of 1 degree (Trevarthen and Tursky, 1969; Levy, Trevarthen and Sperry, 1972). Those trials on which eye movements were recorded were discounted. It was noted, however, that lateral eye movements during testing were rare, occurring approximately once per 100 trial presentations.

The centre of the projected lateralized images was offset 3–4 degrees of visual angle to the left or right of the fixation point. Each stimulus subtended an angular width of approximately 3 degrees and angular length of approximately 4 degrees. The experimental set-up included two Kodak carousel slide projectors attached to electromechanical shutters (Gerbrands G1167). LB sat in front of the screen at a distance of 18 inches (46 cm) with his gaze fixated on a central point. The distance was kept constant with the use of a head-and-chin-rest. Onset of the stimuli triggered a digital millisecond clock/counter (Monsanto 101B) which measured reaction time (RT) to the nearest millisecond. A spoken response into a unidirectional microphone terminated the count and responses were printed on a high-speed printer (Monsanto 512A).

Speaking or Writing (with the left hand)

Two separate tests were conducted. In the first, separate series of digit numerals (0–9), single letters, two-letter words, words with pre-trial exposure, geometrical shapes, or pictures of familiar objects, were presented to the LVF or RVF. The task was to name each stimulus as it appeared. The results of this test are presented in *Table 5*. This table shows clearly an identical pattern to that shown in *Table 2*. Again, the best performance is with numbers and the worst with pictures of objects. Previous exposure contributed to good performance as can be seen in the series with pretrial exposure of the stimuli. The naming of geometric shapes was limited to the simplest shapes, such as, circle, square, or triangle.

Qualitatively, LB's performance revealed frequent head movements following LVF trials. When asked to explain the reason for such movements he reported to be pretending that his nose was a pencil with which he could reconstruct the projected image. Such 'sketches' reportedly aided his efforts to name the image. In fact, only on a few such occasions was the verbal response correct.

The second test, administered a month later, consisted of projecting the same series of words, geometric shapes, and pictures, alternatively to the LVF or RVF. The task was to write with the left hand the names of stimuli seen in the LVF; writing with the write hand was requested for RVF presentations. Since the latter combination proved to be 100% accurate the results are not included in *Table 5*.

Table 5 **Percentage of correct verbal identification of separate series of stimuli presented to left (LVF) or right (RVF) visual half-fields**

	% Correct	
Stimuli	*LVF*	*RVF*
Numerals	100	100
Letters	92	100
Geometric shapes	43	100
Words (2 letters)	15	100
Words (3 or 4 letters) with pre-trial exposure	80	100
Pictures	0	100

On a random sample of intermittent trials in the LVF a verbal report of the written answer was requested. *Table 6* summarizes the findings. With writing, we see the emergence of high level linguistic performance. Without spoken confirmation the source of the correct written responses with the left hand is unclear. Correct verbal confirmation is usually taken to mean left hemisphere control of the response. The reverse implies right hemisphere control. The fact that a substantial number of written responses appeared to be controlled by the right hemisphere is significant. In comparison, in a previous study, Levy *et al.* (1971) reported the case of commissurotomy patient, AA, who was able to write the names of two pictures out of 54 trials. Also, unlike AA, in the present case all written answers were executed spontaneously in script. This was true even when, in the case of stimulus words, the projected words were all in capital letters. *Figure 1* shows examples of six written names followed by incorrect verbal reports (*see Table 6*).

Table 6 **Percentage of correct left-hand written identification of stimuli presented in the LVF (all RVF right-hand responses were 100% accurate)**

	% Correct	
Stimuli	*Words written*	*Verbal confirmation*
Words	75	50
Geometric shapes	86	67
Pictures	73	55

LVF = left visual half-field.
RVF = right visual half-field.

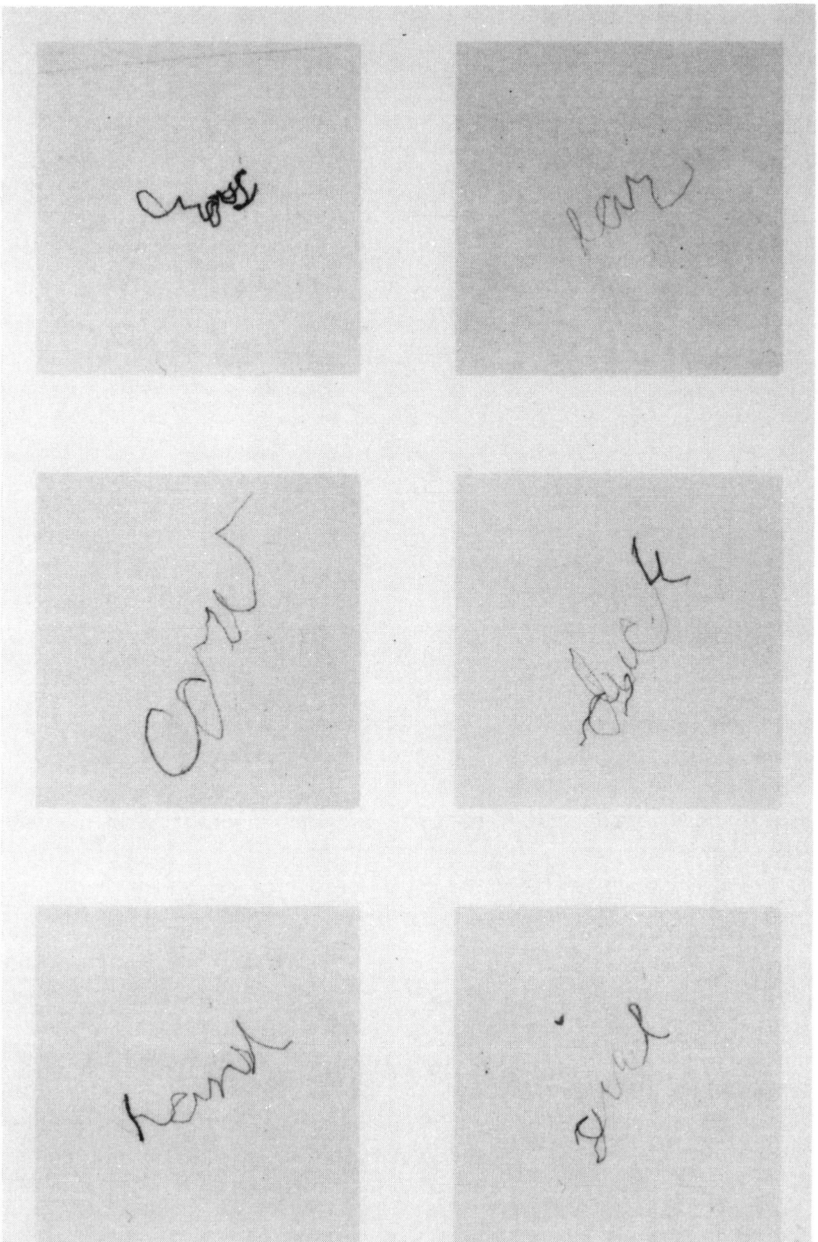

Figure 1 Examples of responses written with the left hand following left visual half-field presentations, (cross, ear, cow, duck, hand, girl).

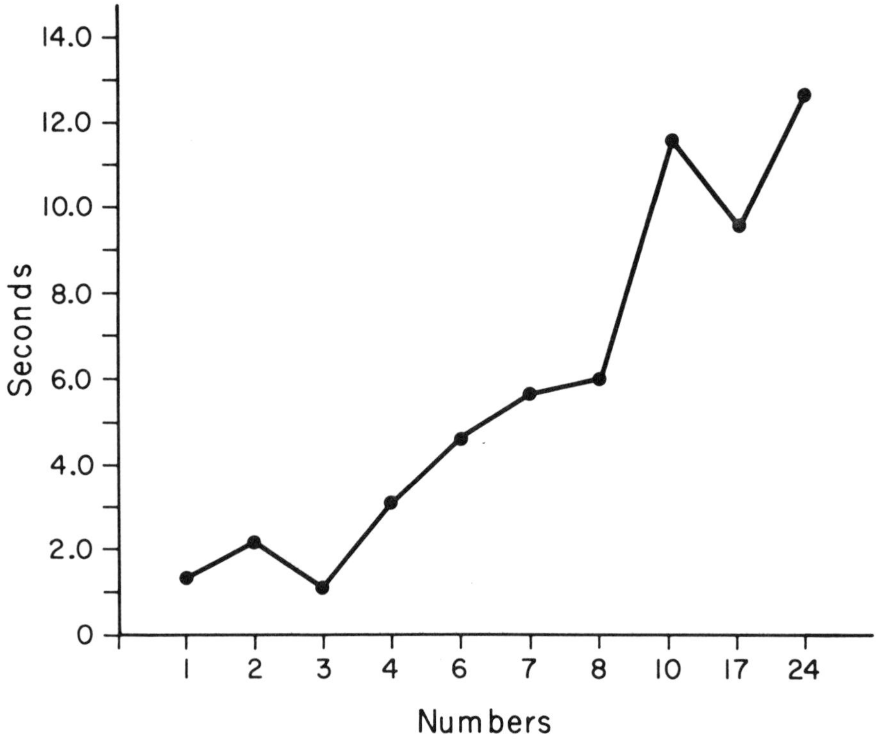

Figure 2. Verbal reaction-time to numerals presented to left or right visual half-fields.

Verbal Reaction Time (RT)

In order to delineate further the characteristics of language capacity of the right hemisphere, speed of verbal response was also measured. The identical series of single numbers, letters, or geometrical shapes was projected tachistoscopically under the conditions described above. We did not use the picture stimuli because of the high error rate seen previously. The task here was to name about each stimulus by speaking into a unidirectional microphone. The results for the correct responses are summarized in *Table 7.*

Three major patterns emerge:

1. RVF responses are significantly faster ($p<0.05$) than LVF responses.
2. The order from fastest to slowest is different within each hemisphere.
3. Low numbers in the conventional sequence presented in the LVF are reported faster than high numbers.

Table 7 **Comparison of mean verbal reaction time (correct responses) to separate series of stimuli**

	Stimuli		
Visual half-field	*Numerals*	*Letters*	*Geometric shapes*
Left	4.55 sec	10.16	4.352
Right	2.96	1.05	1.66

It is important to stress the fact that numbers were not presented sequentially. The order of presentations is crucial in eliciting the effects reported here, and sequential presentation would have washed out the observed results. A graphic summary which best illustrates this result is presented in *Figure 2.*

Upon request, LB described his naming strategies as consisting of a re-visualization, i.e. mental recreation of a horizontal row of numerals similar to that displayed in his elementary school. A mental scan proceeded from left to right, ending when a match was made between the stimulus and the appropriate mental number. From his description, it is not possible to say whether one or both hemispheres were involved in the process but given the RT his account appears credible.

Discussion

The results of several tests administered to LB appear to demonstrate right hemisphere support of a wide range of linguistic capabilities, including language production. Evidence for right hemisphere expressive language is limited but clearly present. It is best seen in written responses with the left hand following the presentation of pictorial stimuli in the LVF. Had the written responses been named correctly we would have had to conclude that the information became available, somehow, to the left hemisphere as well.

With these results in mind, how can right hemisphere language be characterized? First, during right hemisphere writing it is important to note that letters were not printed; they were written in cursive script using a deliberate manual style. Spontaneous cursive writing is consistent with the notion of a mature linguistic knowledge in the right hemisphere. Further, it would appear that within the right hemisphere writing may be strongly dissociated from, and superior to, speaking. This would imply that, as long as production does not involve control of the speech musculature, the right hemisphere is capable of some expressive linguistic skill. From an ontogenetic/phylogenetic perspective this is a reasonable explanation: the use of one hand during writing precludes the need for competition for control of the hand whereas the existence of only one speech apparatus demands the control of only one hemisphere at a time.

At the same time, even though correct speaking responses were obtained for both the left hand and LVF, we cannot be certain, for reasons outlined below, that they were produced solely by the right hemisphere. The correct spoken responses following left hand or LVF input did not appear identical with those produced following right hand or RVF input. Instead, responses were slow or protracted and involved elaborate overt strategies. RT in the LVF was nearly 10 times longer than in the RVF under one testing condition. If the right hemisphere was in fact mainly responsible for producing the responses, why did it take so long? There are three possible interpretations:

1. The information was transferred subcallosally to the left hemisphere from whence the verbal response emanated. According to this interpretation the RT reflects time lost during the transfer.
2. The information reached both hemispheres but in a degraded form in the left hemisphere. This condition could occur if the extrageniculate visual system was used to relay some aspects of the information to the left hemisphere. It has already been suggested (Schneider, 1969) that crude visual information about both half-fields is transmitted to each hemisphere via midbrain centres. Behavioral evidence suggesting the increased role of such a pathway following commissurotomy has been reported (Trevarthen and Sperry, 1973). The same system may mediate residual vision in patients with 'blind sight' (Poppel, Held, and Frost, 1974; Perenin and Jeannerod, 1978; Torjusses, 1978; Weiskrantz *et al.*, 1974; Weiskrantz, 1986). A delayed speech response in LB's case may then be attributed to the time taken for reconstruction of a degraded image in the left hemisphere.
3. 'Sluggish speech' in the right hemisphere (Butler and Norsell, 1969). Since speech would be a function that is newly practised by the right hemisphere, it can be argued that it still lacks the fine tuning present in the speech-specializing hemisphere.

Considering LB's young age when the surgery was performed as well as possible functional reorganization due to the early onset of his epilepsy, it is not entirely surprising that so much linguistic skill is exhibited by his right hemisphere. The presence of long-standing epileptic seizures is generally believed to promote the formation of compensatory processes. One way in which this can be accomplished according to one view (Geschwind, 1974) is when paralysis of language areas due to repeated seizures triggers the onset of recovery in other areas. Seen in this way, the range of latent or dormant linguistic abilities observed in LB may all have started developing long before the surgery. With intact forebrain commissures such bilateral development could take place, albeit asymmetrically. Disconnection can then be considered to have removed certain physiological constraints on overt multiple language functions. In any case, the long-term improvement or changes reported here have not been reported for the earlier post-surgical period. By the same token, the postoperative left-sided Jacksonian episodes suggest the presence of some damage in the right hemisphere (Bogen, 1976) which we would expect to work against language take-over in that hemisphere. That recovery occurred, despite extracallosal damage, may be considered significant. Furthermore, had early damage occurred to the primary language centres we should have expected abnormal language functions in the disconnected left hemisphere of LB. No such evidence was found here. From this it is more reasonable to conclude that LB's right hemisphere represents approximately the language competence of the normal right hemisphere.

In order to assess the extent to which the level of LB's right hemisphere expressive skill represents the typical potential of that hemisphere to gain control over language it is necessary to draw analogies to the performance of aphasic patients. A few points should be considered. First, it cannot be said with certainty that LB can speak with his right hemisphere, for the reasons already outlined. But it can be said reliably that his right hemisphere can control writing. Even so, the extent of the writing skill is very limited. Secondly, some patients are known to recover speech eventually and, at least in some cases, the evidence points to exclusive control of that skill by the right hemisphere (Crocket and Estridge, 1951; Hillier, 1954; Smith, 1966; Kinsbourne, 1971; Smith and Sugar, 1975; Cummings *et al.*, 1979). The most compelling direct evidence for the assumption of speech production by the right hemisphere in patients rendered aphasic after left hemisphere infarcts was published by Kinsbourne (1971). He reported that in two such cases an injection of amobarbital into the right carotid artery abolished speech whereas injection into the left carotid artery left language virtually unchanged. Thirdly, patients who underwent left hemispherectomy for the removal of glioma (Smith and Sugar, 1975) have been reported to regain speech, although compared with comprehension, at a reduced level.

Since there is no strong evidence from the present set of experiments for speech production by the right hemisphere and in view of the considerations listed above, it would appear that a disconnected right hemisphere represents an intermediate level of linguistic expressive skill. From the point of view of recovery, the potential is greater for two callosally connected hemispheres, even if unilaterally damaged, or for a single right hemisphere. We can assume that LB represents the upper limit of speech capacity in the disconnection syndrome, free of reorganization due to early significant neurological history. Instead, the linguistic skills acquired by his right hemisphere may be thought of as being more representative of the right hemisphere under a state of intact callosal connections to the left hemisphere in the normal brain, than of either a unilaterally damaged hemisphere or an isolated one where pathological inhibition of the right hemisphere may be quite prevalent.

From the foregoing we may speculate that there exists a hierarchy of right hemisphere language functions. Those functions that are lateralized to the right hemisphere in the presence of an intact left hemisphere are auditory language comprehension, some reading (Zaidel, E. 1978), and some writing. Functions that can develop in the right hemisphere when the left is substantially damaged or is removed include the previous ones plus speech. And, considering functional recovery, different retraining strategies may well apply to these two different classes of functions.

Some of the strategies observed in commissurotomy patients during attempts to name LVF or left-hand stimuli may have general clinical implications. For example, the rehearsal or subvocal sequential enumeration of alternatives, especially during automatized sequences (alphanumeric, for example) where there is an awareness in the left hemisphere of right hemisphere recognition, is also reported in several cases of total visual–verbal disconnection as early as the last century (e.g. Broadbent, 1872). In such cases, a general deficit of object naming is a prominent symptom. And there, too, success on the task depends on the number of alternatives in the choice set (Oxbury *et al.*, 1969; Zaidel, D. and Sperry, 1973). This strategy may be a useful clinical tool in appropriate aphasic syndromes. It should be noted that the strategy involves the co-ordination of two isolated but intact functional units by an intact control process whose integrity is necessary for successful compensation of the verbal deficit.

Acknowledgements

The research reported here was supported by USPHS Grant no. 03372 and the F.P. Hixon Fund awarded to R.W. Sperry. The work was carried out in R.W. Sperry's Psychobiology Laboratory at Caltech. Writing this chapter was made possible through USPHS Grant no. 18973 awarded to DWZ.

References

BOGEN, J.E. Linguistic performance in the short-term following cerebral commissurotomy. Studies in Neurolinguistics, Vol. 2, (1976). New York:Academic Press.

BOGEN, J.E. and VOGEL, P.J. Neurologic status in the long term following complete cerebral commissurotomy. In F. Michel and B. Schott *Les Syndromes de Desconnexion Calleuse Chez L'Homme* (1975). Lyon: Hopital Neurologie.

BROADBENT, W.H. On the cerebral mechanism of speech and thought. *Medico-Chirurgical Transactions* (1872), **55**, 145–194.

CAVALLI, E., DE RENZI, E., FAGLIONI, P. and VITALE, A. Impairment of right brain-damaged patients on a linguistic cognitive task. *Cortex* (1981), **17**, 545–555.

CROCKET, H.G. and ESTRIDGE, N.M. Cerebral hemispherectomy. *Bulletin of the Los Angeles Neurological Society* (1951), **16**, 71–87.

CUMMINGS, J.L., BENSON, D.F., WALSH, M.J. and LEVINE, H.L. Left-to-right transfer of language dominance: A case study. *Neurology* (1979), **29**, 1547–1550.

GAZZANIGA, M.S. and SPERRY, R.W. Language after section of the cerebral commissures. *Brain* (1967), **90**, 131–148.

GAZZANIGA, M.S. Right hemispheric language following brain bisection — a 20 year perspective. *American Psychologist* (1983), **38**, 525–537.

GESCHWIND, N. Late changes in the nervous system: an overview. In D.G. Stein, J.J. Rosen and N. Butters (eds) Plasticity and Recovery of Function in the Central Nervous System (1974). New York: Academic Press.

HECAEN, H. Acquired aphasia in children and the ontogenesis of hemispheric functional specialization. *Brain and Language* (1976), **3**, 114–134.

HILLIER, W.F. Total left cerebral hemispherectomy for malignant glioma. *Neurology* (1954), **4**, 718–721.

JACKSON, J.M. Remarks on the diagnosis and treatment of diseases of the brain. *British Medical Journal* (1888), **ii** 59–63; 111–117.

JOHNSON, L.E. *Interhemispheric Visual Communication in Human Commissurotomy Subjects*. Unpublished Doctoral Dissertation, California Institute of Technology (1980).

JOHNSON, L.E. Vocal responses to left visual stimuli following forebrain commissurotomy. *Neuropsychologia* (1984a), **22**, 153–166.

JOHNSON, L.E. Bilateral visual cross-integration by human forebrain commissurotomy subjects. *Neuropsychologia* (1984b), **22**, 167–175.

KERTESZ, A. and SHEPPARD, A. The epidemiology of aphasic and cognitive impairment in stroke. *Brain* (1981), **104**, 117–128.

KINSBOURNE, M. The minor cerebral hemisphere as a source of aphasic speech. *Archives of Neurology* (1971), **25**, 302–306.

KUMAR, S., BOGEN, G.M. and BOGEN, J.E. Verbal cross-clueing following cerebral commissurotomy. *Neuroscience Abstracts* (1977), **8**, 69.

LEVY, J., NEBES, R.D. and SPERRY, R.W. Expressive language in the surgically separated minor hemisphere. *Cortex* (1971), **7**, 49–58.

LEVY, J., TREVARTHEN, C.B. and SPERRY, R.W. Perception of bilateral chimeric figures following hemispheric deconnexion. *Brain* (1972), **95**, 61–68.

LURIA, A.R. *Traumatic Aphasia: It's Syndromes, Psychopathology and Treatment* (1947). Moscow: Academy of Medical Sciences.

MYERS, J.J. and SPERRY, R.W. Interhemispheric communication after section of the forebrain commissures. *Cortex* (1985), **21**, 249–260.

OXBURY, J.M., OXBURY, S.M. and HUMPHREY, N.K. Varieties of color anomia. *Brain* (1969), **92**, 847–860.

PERENING, M.J. and JEANNEROD, M. Visual function within the hemianopic field following early cerebral hemidecortication in man — I. Spatial localization. *Neuropsychologia* (1978), **16**, 1–13.

POPPEL, E., HELD, R. and FROST, D. Residual visual function after brain wounds involving the central visual pathways in man. *Nature (Lond.)* (1973), **243**, 295–196.

SCHNEIDER, G. Two Visual Systems. *Science* (1969), NY 163, 895–902.

SMITH, A. Speech and other functions after left (dominant) hemispherectomy. *Journal of Neurology, Neurosurgery and Psychiatry* (1966), **29**, 467–471.

SMITH, A. and SUGAR, O. Development of above normal language and intelligence 21 years after left hemispherectomy. *Neurology* (1975), **25**, 813–818.

SPERRY, R.W. Hemisphere deconnection and unity in conscious awareness. *American Psychologist* (1968), **23**, 723–733.

SPERRY, R.W. Lateral specialization in the surgically separated hemispheres. In P.J. Vinken and G.W. Bruyn (eds) *The Neurosciences Third Study Program* (1974). Cambridge: MIT Press.

SPERRY, R.W., GAZZANIGA, M.S. and BOGEN, J.E. Interhemispheric relations: The neocortical commissures; syndromes of hemisphere disconnection. In P.J. Vinken and G.W. Bruyn (eds) *Handbook of Clinical Neurology* (1969). Amsterdam: North Holland.

SUBIRANA, A. The prognosis in aphasia in relation to cerebral dominance and handedness. *Brain* (1958), **81**, 415–425.

TENG, E.L. and SPERRY, R.W. Interhemispheric interaction during simultaneous bilateral presentation of letters or digits in commissurotomized patients. *Neuropsychologia* (1973), **11** 131–140.

TORJUSSEN, T. Visual processing in cortically blind hemifields. *Neuropsychologia* (1978), **16** 15–21.

TREVARTHEN, C.B. and TURSKY, B. Recording horizontal rotations of head and eyes in spontaneous shifts of gaze. *Behavioral Research Methods and Instrumentation* (1969), **1**, 291–293.

TREVARTHEN, C.B. and SPERRY, R.W. Perceptual unity in the ambient visual field in humancommissurotomy patients. *Brains* (1973), **96** 547–570.

WEISKRANTZ, L. *Blindsight: A case study and its implications* (1986), Oxford: Oxford University Press.

WEISKRANTZ, L., WARRINGTON, E.K., SANDERS, M.D. and MARSHALL, J. Visual capacity in the hemianopic field following a restricted occipital ablation. *Brain* (1974), **97**, 709–726.

ZAIDEL, D. and SPERRY, R.W. *Functional Compensation and Re-education Following Commissurotomy*. Caltech Biology Annual Report, No. 87 (1972).

ZAIDEL, D. and SPERRY, R.W. Performance on the Raven colored progressive matrices test by subjects with cerebral commissurotomy. *Cortex* (1973), **9** 34–39.

ZAIDEL, E. Auditory vocabulary of the right hemisphere following brain bisection or hemidecortication. *Cortex* (1976), **12** 191–211.

ZAIDEL, E. *Linguistic Competence and Related Functions in th Right Cerebral Hemisphere of Man Following Commissurotomy and Hemispherectomy*. Doctoral Dissertation, California Institute of Technology. Dissertation Abstracts International, 34, 2350B. University Microfilms No. 73-26, 48 (1973).

ZAIDEL, E. Concepts of cerebral dominance in the split brain. In M. Buser and G. Rougeul-Buser (eds) *Cerebral Correlates of Conscious Experiences* (1978). Amsterdam: Elsevier/North Holland.

ZAIDEL, E. Language in the right hemisphere, convergent perspectives —response. *American Psychologist* (1983), **83**, 542–548.

7

Language-related Functions of the Right Cerebral Hemisphere

Elliott D. Ross

Introduction

Until recently, most clinical inquiries into human language and behaviour have been directed toward understanding left hemisphere functions and the aphasias. Right hemisphere contributions to language have been considered minimal when judged by left hemisphere standards. This particular bias can be traced to the fundamental discoveries of Broca (Broca, 1865, 1960) and Wernicke (Wernicke, 1977) that lesions in the left hemisphere cause spectacular deficits in the verbal components of language which are not encountered with focal right brain lesions. Subsequently, vast numbers of studies have been done to delineate the linguistic and related functions of the left hemisphere which has led to the widely held view that the 'dominant' or 'major' hemisphere is the left while the right is relegated to a 'minor' or 'non-dominant' role (Ross and Mesulam, 1979). Nevertheless, neurological (De Kosky *et al.*, 1980; Gorelick and Ross, 1987; Heilman, Scholes and Watson, 1975; Hughes, Chan and Su, 1983; Ross, 1981; Ross, Edmondson and Seibert, 1986; Ross *et al.*, 1981; Ross, Holzapfel and Freeman, 1983; Ross and Mesulam, 1983; Ross and Rush, 1981; Tucker, Watson and Heilman, 1977), neuropsychological (Benowitz *et al.*, 1983; Dimond, Farrington and Johnson, 1976; Sackeim and Gur, 1978; Schwartz, Davidson and Maer, 1975; Wexler, 1980), acoustical (Blumstein and Cooper, 1974; Edmondson, Chan, Seibert and Ross, 1987; Ross, Holzapfel and Freeman, 1983; Shapiro and Danly, 1985; Van Lancker, 1980; Zurif, 1974) and physiological (Larsen, Skinhoj and Lassen, 1978; Ross, 1981), evidence has been gathered in the last decade to show that the right hemisphere actively contributes to language and behaviour through its major role in modulating attitudes and emotions via affective prosody and gesturing. This chapter will introduce the reader to the emerging data supporting the concept that the right hemisphere is dominant for organizing the non-verbal aspects of language and behaviour.

Prosody

Prosody represents a complex component of the acoustical signal that communicates linguistic, attitudinal, emotional, pragmatic, dialectical and idiosyncratic information through the use of pitch, loudness, timbre, tempo, stress, accent, pauses and intonation. These particular aspects of language are considered *suprasegmental* as opposed to the *segmental* components. The smallest phonological unit of language is called the *segment* which in non-technical terms is most akin to the syllable. Segments are the building blocks for words (lexicon) in non-tone languages[1], such as English. Words, in turn, are temporally concatenated into *syntactical* relationships to form phrases, sentences, and discourse which then convey meanings and concepts beyond the single word (Van Lancker, 1980). These particular features of language — segments, words and syntax — are the substrates for the *propositional* components of language which are disrupted in the aphasic deficits that follow left brain injury. However, suprasegmental features are also present in language which, in addition to enhancing the linguistic aspects of speech by modifying meaning through syntactical disambiguation (*see* below), also convey attitudes and emotions (Crystal, 1969, 1975; Monrad-Krohn, 1963; Van Lancker, 1980). These particular features are best embraced under the term *prosody* which refers to the melody, pauses, intonation, stresses and accents applied to the *articulatory-line.*

The prosodic features of language are graded phenomena making them more difficult to study than the discretely organized linguistic features (Crystal, 1969, 1975; Van Lancker, 1980). Nevertheless, since prosody adds such complexity and richness to language, it must be considered as a crucial

[1] In tone languages, such as Taiwanese, Mandarin Chinese and other east-Asian languages, most sub-Saharan African languages and many Papuan and Amerindian languages, the building blocks of words are formed from both segments and segmentally bound, short-term, intonation contours called *tones*. For example, in Mandarin Chinese articulating the word 'ma' with a high-flat intonation contour (tone) means mother, whereas 'ma' articulated with a low-falling followed by a rising intonation contour means horse! In English, however, varying intonation across a syllable or even a word does not alter meaning although it may impact intent through affective prosody. Because of this fundamental difference between tone and non-tone languages, contrasting the effect of brain lesions on speech in these two language-types can be very insightful when asking questions about universal organization and lateralization of brain-behavioural relationships (*see* Aprosodias in Tone Languages).

part of communication. In fact, studies of infants have shown that the fundamental building blocks for speech and language acquisition are the prosodic, not the linguistic, elements (Crystal, 1969, 1975; Lewis, 1936). Furthermore, it has been amply demonstrated that if the non-verbal intent of an utterance is at variance with its literal meaning then the non-verbal intent will take precedent (De Groot, 1949), i.e. if the sentence 'I had a great day' is spoken using ironic prosody it will be interpreted as a negation.

The first systematic inquiry into the neurology of prosody was initiated by Monrad-Krohn (1947) who, during World War II, observed a patient with a shrapnel wound to the left frontal area causing a Broca's aphasia. This woman made a rather remarkable recovery except for a lingering Germanic-like accent even though she was a native Norwegian. This caused her great emotional distress during the Nazi occupation because she was constantly mistaken for a German and socially ostracized. She was reported to have preserved overall speech melody, as evidenced by her ability to sing, intonate and emote. Her abnormal dialectical accent was the result of the inappropriate application of stresses and pauses to the articulatory-line.

On the basis of this patient and others, Monrad-Krohn (1947a, b, 1963) divided prosody into four components: *intrinsic, intellectual, emotional* and *inarticulate*. Intrinsic prosody serves specific linguistic purposes and also gives rise to dialectical and idiosyncratic differences in speech quality. The patient described above illustrates a disturbance of this particular component of prosody. Examples of linguistic uses of prosody are: raising intonation at the end of a statement to indicate a question; changing the stress on certain segments of a word to clarify its grammatical class (Blumstein and Goodglass, 1972), i.e. con' vict (noun) versus con vict' (verb); or changing the stress on certain words and altering the pause structure to disambiguate potentially ambiguous syntax (Crystal, 1975; Van Lancker, Canter and Terbeek, 1981), i.e. — 'The man'... and wo'man dressed in black... came to visit', implying that only the woman was dressed in black versus 'The man and woman dressed in black'... came to see us', implying that both were dressed black. Intellectual prosody adds attitudinal components to language. For example, if the sentence 'He is clever' is emphatically stressed on 'is', it becomes a resounding acknowledgement of the person's ability. If the emphatic stress resides on 'clever' with a slight terminal rise in intonation, sarcasm becomes apparent. If 'he' is emphatically stressed, then the sentence again acknowledges the person's ability but also implies that perhaps his associates are not very clever. Emotional prosody is used for imparting emotions into speech and inarticulate prosody is the use of para-linguistic elements, such as grunts and sighs.

Monrad-Krohn also described and categorized various clinical disorders of prosody. *Dysprosody* may occur in patients with fairly good recovery from motor-types of aphasia causing a change in dialectical voice quality that gives rise to a 'foreign accent', such as in the patient described above. Dysprosody, therefore, is primarily a disorder associated with left hemisphere lesions that alter intrinsic prosody. *Aprosody* is the general lack of prosody encountered in Parkinson's disease as part of the akinesia and masked facies. *Hyperprosody* is the excessive use of prosody that is often observed in manic patients or in Broca's aphasics who have very few words at their disposal but use them to their utmost to convey attitudes and emotions. Although Monrad-Krohn did not describe disorders of prosody from focal right brain damage, he did surmise that there should be disorders of prosodic comprehension that are complementary to disorders of prosodic production.

Recent studies in patients with focal brain lesions, to be detailed below, have shown that right brain damage may seriously impair both production and comprehension of the affective components of language, encompassing attitudinal and emotional prosody and gestures, without disturbing propositional language (Gorelick and Ross, 1987; Heilman, Scholes and Watson, 1975; Ross, 1981; Ross *et al.*, 1981; Ross, Holzapfel and Freeman, 1983; Ross and Mesulam, 1979; Tucker, Watson and Heilman, 1977). These prosodic components coupled with gestures impart vitality to discourse and communicate important social, pragmatic and emotional messages, that in many instances are far more important than the actual words chosen (De Groot, 1949).

Kinesics

Gestural behaviour can be considered a non-verbal paralinguistic component of communication that is closely aligned with the prosodic features of speech (Crystal, 1969, 1975). The study of limb, body, and facial movements associated with non-verbal communication is called *kinesics,* (Critchley, 1970). Movements that are used for semiotic or referential purposes should be classified as pantomime, according to Hughlings-Jackson (1932) and Critchley (1939), since they convey specific semantic information, whereas movements used to colour, emphasize, and embellish speech are best classified as gestures. It should be noted, however, that this classification is not universally adhered to in the literature which may help explain some of the 'contradictory' observations and conclusions that have been published. Since most kinesic activity blends gestures and pantomime into a single movement, any analysis of kinesics should always pay attention both to its semantic (pantomimal) content as well as to its emotional and attitudinal (gestural) content.

Despite an extensive non-clinical literature on kinesic behaviour, beginning with Darwin (1955), only a few contemporary studies have addressed the neurology of pantomime and gestures. Disturbances in the performance and comprehension of pantomine in patients have been firmly linked to aphasia and left brain damage (De Renzi, Motti and Nichelli, 1980; Gainotti and Lemmo, 1976). Pantomimal disorders in the presence of comprehension deficits has been attributed to the patient's general inability to comprehend symbols. In aphasics who do not have comprehension problems, loss of pantomimal production is best correlated with the presence of ideomotor apraxia, according to Goodglass and Kaplan (Goodglass and Kaplan, 1963). Other studies, however, have not shown such tight correlation of the specific kinesic disturbance to the comparable linguistic disturbance (Cicone *et al.*, 1979; Delis *et al.* 1979; Feyereisen and Seron, 1982), although all studies to date have found that disorders of pantomime are almost always the result of left hemisphere damage resulting in aphasic deficits (Feyereisen and Seron, 1982; Goodglass and Kaplan, 1963; Seron *et al.* 1979).

Gestural kinesics has not been well studied neurologically although it has been noted occasionally in the literature that gestural activity is often preserved in aphasic patients (Critchley, 1939; Hughlings-Jackson, 1879). The first paper to address the possible relationship of gestures to right brain damage and loss of affective prosody was published in 1979 by Ross and Mesulam (1979) They observed that lesions of the right frontal operculum may cause complete loss of spontaneous gestural activity without disturbances in praxis. The suggestion was made, therefore, that gestural behaviour was a dominant function of the right hemisphere, in keeping with its putative role in the modulation of affective behaviour. Since then a number of studies have lent further support to this hypothesis.

Utilizing a bedside examination technique, Ross (1981) and also Gorelick and Ross (1987) found that patients with right frontal damage who acutely lost the ability to gesture retained their ability to comprehend gestures. In contrast, patients with right parieto-temporal opercula lesions were unable to comprehend the meaning of gestures even though they could gesture spontaneously and had no difficulty with praxis. DeKosky *et al.* (1980) found that right brain damaged patients were severely impaired when asked to recognize the emotional content of facial expressions whereas left brain damaged patients performed almost as well as normals. Utilizing the Profile Of Non-verbal Sensitivity (PONS) test which evaluates a subject's ability to comprehend facial, limb and body kinesics and intonational aspects of the voice, Benowitz *et al.* (1983) were able to quantify non-verbal communication in brain damaged patients. They found that right hemisphere damage severely impaired the ability of patients to comprehend gestural kinesics, in particular those involving facial expressions. Left brain damage, even of considerable extent, led to only very mild deficits. Thus the right hemisphere appears specialized not only for producing gestures but also for comprehending their meaning.

Right Hemisphere and Affective Behaviour

Until very recently our knowledge concerning the right hemisphere's contribution to both language and behaviour has been very rudimentary even though Hughlings-Jackson (1932) pointed out, as early as 1879, that densely aphasic patients were usually capable of communicating their emotions despite profound verbal deficits. Jackson even hypothesized that the emotional aspects of communication might be a function of the right hemisphere. Nevertheless, almost 100 years were to pass before the first neurological studies were published which corroborated his hypothesis.

In the 1970s a series of neuro-linguistic studies, utilizing dichotic auditory testing techniques, by Blumstein and Cooper (1974) and others (Van Lancker, 1980) showed that the left ear was better (right hemisphere advantage) at discerning the intonational aspects of speech whereas the right ear was better (left hemisphere advantage) at discerning the segmental aspects of speech. The first clinical study to formally demonstrate that right hemisphere damage severely disrupted affective language was published by Heilman, Scholes and Watson (1975). They tested the ability of patients with focal brain damage to recognize the affective content of neutral statements spoken with various emotional intonations and found that right brain damaged patients were markedly impaired on the task when compared with normals and aphasic controls. In a follow-up study, Tucker, Watson and Heilman (1977), showed that right brain damaged patients also had great difficulty producing affective renditions of neutral statements on request and imitation. Although the patients did not have CT scans, it was felt clinically and by isotope scans that most of the lesions associated with loss of affective processing involved the right superior-posterior temporal and inferior parietal lobes.

In 1979 Ross and Mesulam reported on the behaviour of two patients with CT verified infarctions of the right inferior frontal and anterior-inferior parietal regions. Neither patient was aphasic or apraxic but both complained bitterly of their almost total inability to insert affective and attitudinal variation into their speech and gestural behaviour. One patient was a school teacher, who despite her persistent left arm monoplegia, was able to return to the classroom. Her main difficulty was that she could no longer control the classroom because (said in a monotone voice) 'I cannot put any emotion into my voice or actions and the pupils do not know when I am angry and mean business'. The other patient was a surgeon who had tremendous problems interacting with his wife and family because of his inability to modulate his tone of voice to make it socially acceptable. Thus when he asked his wife to do something, it always came out as a flat commanding statement rather than a pleasant request for a favour. Neither of these patients seemed to have difficulty perceiving the display of affect in others and they both insisted that they could feel and experience emotions inwardly.

Based on these patients and the previous publications by Heilman and associates (Heilman, Scholes and Watson, 1975; Tucker, Watson and Heilman, 1977), Ross and Mesulam (1979) hypothesized that: (1) the right hemisphere was dominant for organizing the affective–prosodic components of language and gestural behaviour; and (2) the functional/anatomic organization of affective language in the right hemisphere mirrored the organization of propositional language in the left hemisphere. An issue not resolved by the Ross and Mesulam paper, however, was whether the prosodic deficits from right brain damage were just relegated to the attitudinal and emotional aspects of prosody or if the deficits also involved the more linguistic (intrinsic) aspects of prosody. The studies by Weintraub, Mesulam and Kramer (1981) and Heilman *et al.* (1983) and publications by Danly, Cooper and Shapiro (1983) and Danly and Shapiro (1982) and Blumstein and Goodglass (1972) have looked more carefully at this issue in both right and left brain damaged patients. The composite data from these publications indicates that the linguistic components of prosody may be impaired by either right (Heilman *et al.*, 1983; Weintraub, Mesulam and Kramer, 1981) or left (Blumstein and Goodglass, 1972; Danly, Cooper and Shapiro, 1983; Danly and Shapiro, 1982) brain damage but that the affective components are disrupted almost exclusively by right brain damage (Heilman *et al.*, 1983).

In 1981, Ross approached the issue of whether the anatomical organization of the affective components of language in the right hemisphere was, in fact, similar to the organization of the linguistic components in the left hemisphere. He published a series of ten patients with focal right brain damage from infarction, localized by CT scan, who were assessed at the bedside in a manner similar to the method utilized for propositional language. Thus, the patients were examined qualitatively for (1) their spontaneous use of affective prosody and gesturing during conversation; (2) their ability to repeat, through imitation, verbally neutral sentences with affective prosody; (3) their ability to auditorily comprehend affective prosody; and (4) their ability to comprehend visually the gestural components of kinesic behaviour. The patients were collected consecutively and it was found that all patients who had lesions bordering the right Sylvian fissure had some disorder of affective language. Because the clustering of affective-prosodic deficits appeared similar to the clustering of linguistic deficits seen in left brain damage (Benson, 1979), these particular syndromes were called *aprosodias* and the same modifiers were applied for classification purposes as those used in the aphasias (*Figure 1, Table 1*). The aprosodias, therefore, should be viewed as encoding/decoding disorders of affective behaviour. In a recent follow-up study using blinded evaluations, Gorelick and Ross (1987) found that 12 of 14 consecutive patients admitted to a stroke service with a focal right-brain lesion had combinations of affective deficits that corresponded with the aprosodic classifications and localizations published previously. They also reported encountering 12 patients with aphasia in their series of 15 consecutive patients with left hemisphere strokes, thus supporting the hypothesis that the aprosodias are as common as the aphasias if these deficits in affective language are sought by clinicians.

Aprosodias

Some practice is required to test patients at the bedside for deficits in affective language but, once the clinician familiarizes himself with the analysis, it can readily be incorporated into the routine neurological examination much the same way one conventionally tests for propositional language. The tasks described below are easily and flawlessly done by normals regardless of educational level.

Spontaneous affective prosody and gesturing

During the interview observations should be made whether there is affective prosody in the patient's voice, especially when he is asked emotionally loaded questions, such as, how he feels about his neurological deficits, if he has experienced a loss of a loved one, or if he has had any close calls with death or serious injury. One should ignore the overall loudness or softness of speech and pay strict attention to the finer aspects of prosodic variation and gesturing to see if they convey emotional or attitudinal information and whether or not it is appropriate to the situation under discussion.

Repetition of affective prosody

In this evaluation a declaration sentence, void of emotional words, should be used. The patient is then asked to repeat the sentence with exactly the same affective tone used by the examiner. Thus, the statement 'I am going to the other movies' is said in a happy, sad, tearful, disinterested, angry or surprised voice. Repetition ability should be judged on how well the patient imitates the affective prosody of the examiner. Merely raising or lowering the overall loudness of voice without other prosodic variation or raising the voice at the end of a statement to indicate a question should not be interpreted as constituting good affective-prosodic repetition.

Comprehension of affective prosody

To examine comprehension of affective prosody a declarative statement, void of emotional words, should be produced by the examiner with differing affective tones. Standing behind the patient during this assessment will

Table 1 The Aprosodias

	Spontaneous affective prosody and gesturing	*Affective-prosodic repetition*	*Affective-prosodic comprehension*	*Comprehension of emotional gesturing*
Motor	Poor	Poor	Good	Good
Sensory	Good	Poor	Poor	Poor
Global	Poor	Poor	Poor	Poor
Conduction	Good	Poor	Good	Good
Transcortical Motor	Poor	Good	Good	Good
Transcortical Sensory	Good	Good	Poor	Poor
Mixed Transcortical	Poor	Good	Poor	Poor
(anomic)	(good)	(good)	(good)	(poor)

The existence of anomic aprosodia has been hypothesized. Motor, sensory, global, and transcortical sensory aprosodias have good anatomical correlation with lesions in the left hemisphere known to cause homologous aphasia. Conduction aprosodia has been encountered in the recovery phases from other motor-types of aprosodias and also following a large temporoparietal infarction (*see* text for discussion).

avoid giving the patient visual clues (*see* below). The patient is then asked to identify what kind of affect was injected into the statements. Sometimes a multiple choice format is necessary to initially orient the patient to the requested task.

Comprehension of gestural kinesics

This is done by the examiner standing in front of the patient conveying a particular affective state using gestural activity involving the face and limbs. As with affective-prosodic comprehension, the patient is requested to identify the emotion by name or description. Occasionally, a multiple choice format is needed during initial testing to help orient the patient to the task.

Functional–Anatomical Correlates

Using the bedside evaluation outlined above, disorders of affective behaviour following right brain damage can be classified into the subtypes shown in *Table 1*. The CT correlates of the aprosodias are present in *Figure 1*, which is a composite based on the published cases of aprosodias with lesions involving predominantly a cortical–subcortical distribution (Gorelick and Ross, 1987; Ross, 1981). The technique for mapping the CT lesion on to the right hemisphere template in *Figure 1* is described in Gorelick and Ross (1987).

Motor aprosodia (Figure 1)

Patients with motor aprosodia (Gorelick and Ross, 1987; Ross, 1981; Ross *et al.*, 1981) usually present with a moderate to severe left hemiplegia and variable left sided sensory loss. On CT, the lesions have involved predominantly the right frontal and anterior parietal opercula that is homologous in distribution to lesions in the left hemisphere known to cause persistent Broca (motor) aphasia (Benson, 1979; Kertesz, 1979; Mohr, 1976). Patients have also been encountered with motor aprosodia from subcortical lesions, two with right basal ganglia intracerebral haemorrhages (unpublished observations) and one with an infarction of the right internal capsule confirmed at autopsy (Ross *et al.* 1981). Most patients with motor aprosodia will have transient anosognosia and dysarthria early in their course, but their persistent language deficit is characterized by flat monotone speech with loss of spontaneous gesturing in the non-paralysed limbs and face. Repetition of affective prosody is severely compromised but comprehension of affective prosody and visual comprehension of emotional gesturing remains intact. Some patients who have been followed up to 1 year have shown remarkable improvement in their gestural ability but only incomplete improvement of spontaneous affective prosody. This observation suggests that the neurology of gestures and affective prosody share a common anatomical substrate but that the overlap is not total.

Two patients became severely depressed following their stroke, but never displayed a depressive affect in speech or gestures (Ross, 1981; Ross and Rush, 1981). Their motor aprosodia remained unchanged even after the depression was treated. Thus, the flattening of spontaneous affective behaviour in motor aprosodia is a true neurological deficit that cannot be accounted for by either psychiatric or psychological explanations. Another interesting finding in these patients is that, under extreme emotional conditions, patients with motor aprosodia are often able to laugh or cry in a fleeting all or none fashion reminiscent of the pathological affect

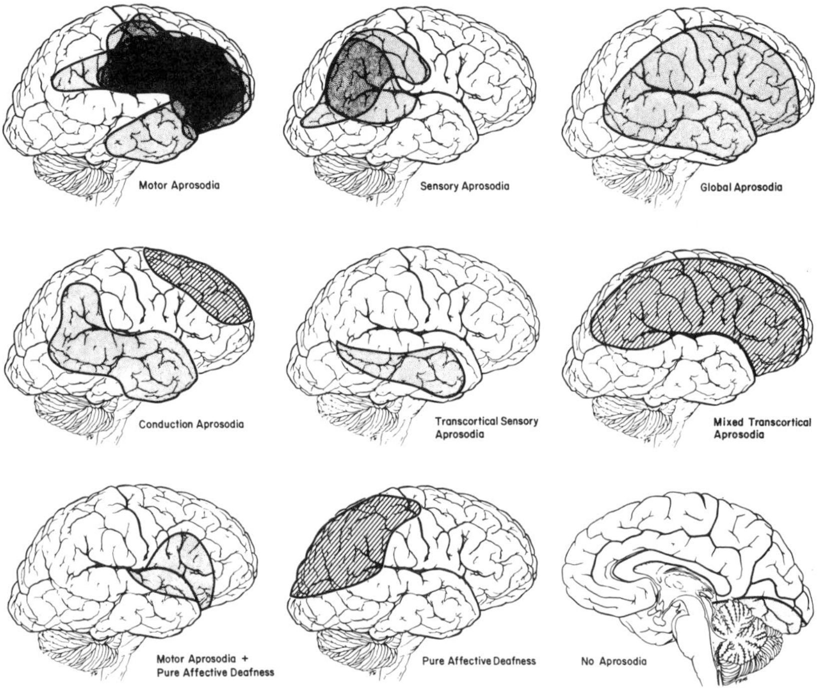

Figure 1 The composite distribution of published (Gorelick and Ross, 1987; Ross, 1981), predominantly cortical, lesions associated with various aprosodias is displayed on a right lateral template of the brain. Stippled lesions represent ischaemic strokes or, in the patient with transcortical sensory aprosodia, a discrete haemorrhage without oedema by CT examination. The case of conduction aprosodia indicated by hatch-marks represents a recovery phase from an initial motor-type aprosodia. The patient with pure affective deafness had a large haemorrhage with tracking oedema making functional–anatomic correlation impossible. The case of mixed transcortical aphasia was evaluated many months post-stroke and, therefore, probably represents a recovery-type of prosodia (*see* text).

encountered in pseudobulbar palsy. Thus the ability to display extremes of emotional motoric behaviour appears to be available to these patients despite their flattened affect which strongly suggests that these displays are organized by motor systems that are separate from the right frontal neocortex (*see* below).

Sensory Aprosodia (Figure 1)

Patients with sensory aprosodia (Gorelick and Ross, 1987; Ross, 1981) are characterized by having excellent affective prosody in speech and active spontaneous gesturing. Auditory comprehension of affective prosody, visual comprehension of emotional gesturing, and repetition of affective prosody are severely impaired. Some of the patients will have moderate deficits in vibratory and position sense and stereognosis on the left side and a dense left hemianopsia. Hemiplegia has not been encountered. The CT lesions, so far, have involved the right posterior temporal and posterior parietal opercula. This particular distribution is consistent with left hemisphere lesions known to cause Wernicke (sensory) aphasia (Benson, 1979; Kertesz, 1979; Kertesz and Benson, 1970). During the interview, the patients often appear somewhat euphoric and overly happy even when they talk about their stroke and the possibility of losing their job.

Global Aprosodia (Figure 1)

Patients with global aprosodia (Ross, 1981) usually demonstrate large right peri-Sylvian lesions involving the frontal, parietal, and temporal lobes on CT or occasionally a deep right intracerebral haemorrhage (unpublished observations). A severe left hemiplegia with hemisensory loss and hemianopsia is usually present. Since the patients lack the ability to display affect through prosody and gestures they give the impression of a flattened affect. Comprehension and repetition of affective prosody and visual comprehension of emotional gesturing are severely compromised. Over time, affective–prosodic comprehension and gesturing may improve but spontaneous affective prosody usually remains severely curtailed. The lesions encountered so far have been consistent with the left peri-Sylvian distribution of brain damage known to produce global aphasia (Benson, 1979; Kertesz, 1979). The improvement in affective–prosodic comprehension is also consistent with Kertesz's observations (1979) that the most likely parameter to improve in global aphasics is comprehension.

Conduction aprosodia (Figure 1)

Gorelick and Ross (1987) reported two patients with conduction aprosodia. One of the cases was examined many months after stroke which involved the right anterior cerebral artery territory and, therefore, most likely represented a recovery deficit from an acute motor-type aprosodia. To this point, the original patient (case 1) reported by Ross and Mesulam (1979) was recently re-examined in August of 1986, nearly 8 years post-stroke. She had recovered a good deal of spontaneous gesturing and affective prosody but still had very poor affective repetition. Comprehension of affective language was completely normal and unchanged. Thus her motor aprosodia had evolved into a conduction aprosodia. The other patient reported by Gorelick and Ross (1987) sustained an ischaemic infarction involving the lateral temporal and inferior parietal cortices. Although one would have predicted that the patient should have had a sensory aprosodia this was not the case. However, this finding is consistent with some of the lesion distributions in the left hemisphere found to correlate with conduction aphasia even though conduction aphasia is classically associated with focal inferior parietal lobe damage (Benson, 1979).

Transcortical motor aprosodia

Patients with transcortical motor aprosodia (Ross, 1981) have emotionally flat and agestural speech with preserved repetition and comprehension of affective prosody and emotional gesturing. The reported patients with this condition had a left hemiparesis without sensory loss. One of the patients had a metastatic tumor with tracking edema involving the right frontal, parietal and temporal lobes, thus, negating any precise functional-anatomical correlations. The other had a right striatal infarction by CT. Interestingly, her transcortical motor aprosodia rapidly resolved over a two week period which would be consistent with some of the transient motor-type aphasias that have been observed following left striatal lesions (Benson, 1979; Hermann *et al.*, 1966; Naeser *et al.* 1982).

Transcortical sensory aprosodia (Figure 1)

Transcortical sensory aprosodia has been described in two patients. Spontaneous affective prosody and repetition as well as emotional gesturing were preserved. However, comprehension of affective prosody was severely impaired. Comprehension of emotional gesturing could not be tested in one patient (Ross, 1981) because he was blind secondary to severe cataracts but the other patient (Gorelick and Ross, 1987) demonstrated a marked deficit. The CT scan of the former showed a large superficial intracerebral haemorrhage, involving the right anterior-inferior temporal lobe with sparing of its posterior-superior aspect (Ross, 1981). This particular distribution, with sparing of the posterior-superior temporal lobe, is consistent with left hemisphere lesions that are associated with transcortical sensory aphasia (Benson 1979; Kertesz, 1979). Except for transient coma and left hemiplegia, which completely resolved within 6 hours, the patient did not sustain any elementary neurological deficits from the haemorrhage. The other patient (Gorelick and Ross, 1987) had a right basal ganglia bleed involving the neostriatum and posterior limb of the internal capsule. This subcortical location is consistent with sites of injury reported recently for analogous transcortical aphasias.

Mixed transcortical aprosodia (Figure 1)

One patient has been reported to have a mixed transcortical aprosodia (Ross,

1981). The lesion, by CT scan, involved the right supra-Sylvian region and a small portion of the posterior temporal operculum. She had a severe left hemiplegia with hemisensory loss. The patient's affective language was first evaluated six months after the stroke, at which time she had markedly attenuated gesturing and spontaneous affective prosody. Repetition of affective prosody, however, was excellent but not fully normal whereas comprehension of affective prosody and emotional gesturing was very poor. Although repetition of affective prosody was not perfectly normal, it was so much better than her spontaenous affective prosody that she was classified as having a mixed transcortical aprosodia even though her lesion seemed to be most consistent with a global aprosodia. Perhaps, if she had been evaluated closer to her ictus, she would have demonstrated a global aprosodia. Interestingly, Kertesz (1979) has reported that patients with large supra-Sylvian lesions with minimal involvement of the superior temporal lobe may initially present with a global aphasia that subsequently evolves into a mixed transcortical or even a transcortical aphasia. These observations are pertinent to this patient since her mixed transcortical aprosodia eventually evolved into a transcortical motor aprosodia.

Pure affective deafness (Figure 1)

A single patient has been reported with the syndrome of pure affective deafness (Gorelick and Ross, 1987) which is analogous to the left hemisphere syndrome of pure word deafness (*see* below). Although the patient had an intracerebral haemorrhage involving the occipital lobe with extensive tracking oedema making functional–anatomic correlations tenuous, from a strictly phenomenological point of view it confirmed the existence of pure affective deafness. The syndrome is characterized by intact spontaneous affective prosody and gesturing, affective repetition and (visual) comprehension of gesturing with loss of affective–prosodic comprehension.

Pure affective deafness + motor aprosodia (Figure 1)

One patient has been encountered with a syndrome best described as pure affective deafness (in the original paper (Ross, 1981) the term pure prosodic deafness was used) and motor aprosodia. The patient was admitted to the hospital with a severe left hemiplegia without sensory loss or aphasia. His voice was flat and devoid of affective variation and his gesturing was very blunted. Repetition and comprehension of affective prosody were poor, but comprehension of emotional gesturing was flawless. The CT scan showed an enhancing lesion consistent with an acute infarction, involving the right frontal operculum, anterior insula and the anterior temporal operculum with sparing of the posterior temporal and parietal operculum. This case was interpreted as an example of motor aprosodia in combination with pure affective deafness since the constellation of deficits is similar to left brain damaged patients who have been reported to have 'global aphasia without alexia' (Heilman *et al.*, 1979). The right frontal opercular lesion easily accounted for the patient's flat and agestural speech and poor affective-prosodic repetition. The auditory comprehension difficulty for affective prosody could be attributed to the anterior temporal lesion assuming it isolated the right posterior–superior temporal lobe from ipsilateral and contralateral auditory inputs, much like the mechanism postulated to explain pure word deafness arising from a unilateral lesion in the left temporal lobe (Gazzaniga *et al.*, 1973). If the visual connections to the right posterior temporal operculum remained intact, as suggested by the CT scan, then it is not surprising that this patient was able to comprehend visually emotional gesturing even though he was uanble to auditorily comprehend affective prosody.

Aprosodias in Tone Languages

The clinical research outlined above applies to speakers of English, a non-tone language. An important issue to address is whether the aprosodias are encountered universally, thus implying a fundamental principle of brain organization. A good litmus test would be to assess affective prosody in tone language speakers with brain damage. Such a clinical study was carried out by Hughes, Chan and Su in 1983 in patients who spoke Mandarin Chinese. They found, using a qualitative assessment of affective prosody, that aprosodias occurred following focal right brain damage in a similar fashion described previously in English speakers (Ross, 1981). Furthermore, the patients had no alterations in tone production and comprehension and, thus, did not display deficits in linguistic processing, e.g. tone aphasias, which is an expected occurrence following left focal brain damage (Gandour and Dardarananda, 1983; Naeser and Chan, 1983).

A similar study was undertaken by Edmondson and Ross (unpublished observations) in Taiwanese speakers with the same results. However, when they attempted to measure the acoustical consequences of affective flattening in the voices of their right brain damaged patients using techniques that easily detect loss of affective prosody in English speakers (Ross, Holzapfel and Freeman, 1983; Shapiro and Danly, 1985), they were unable to distinguish patients from controls. This led to the development of a more elaborate computer-assisted method of analyzing prosody employing 12 acoustical parameters measuring different aspects of timing, pausing, fundamental frequency and intensity. When the more elaborate procedures were applied to quantitate the acoustical concomitants of affective prosody in normal speakers of English, Mandarin, Taiwanese and Thai (Ross, Edmondson and Seibert, 1986), marked differences in the acoustic profiles were found between English and the other three tone languages. These differences readily explained why the initial attempts to acoustically quantify affective prosody in Taiwanese patients were unsuccessful; specifically tone language speakers do not manipulate, for the most part, intonation-related acoustic parameters for affective signalling in contrast to English speakers. The more elaborate computer-assisted methods were applied recently to quantifying loss of affective prosody in right brain-damaged Taiwanese speakers (Edmondson *et al.*, 1987). This time, marked changes in the acoustical profiles were found that easily distinguished patients from controls. Interestingly, as one would expect, the acoustic profile in Taiwanese patients with motor-type aprosodias when compared to English patients was distinctly different.

Based on Van Lancker's hypothesis (Van Lancker, 1980) that the modulation of pitch-related cues in languages are distributed between the hemispheres in regards to their linguistic vs. paralinguistic functions, Ross, Edmondson and Seibert (1986) have proposed a more general corollary: 'if the modulation of a specific acoustical parameter is lateralized in the brain to either the right or left hemisphere, the lateralization is dependent on the behavioral properties of the parameter and not on its acoustical properties'. Thus human language appears to show the universal feature of a composite that is the product not only of the specific imperatives of the inter- and intra-hemispheric organization of brain tissue but also the brain's ability to react to the acoustical properties peculiar to a language, i.e. tone *vs.* non-tone, during the experience of language acquisition (Edmondson *et al.*, 1987).

Conclusion

The existence of various aprosodias following focal right brain damage in both tone and non-tone languages supports powerfully the suggestion that the right hemisphere dominantly modulates the affective components of language and behavior. This modulation is organized much like the left hemisphere's contribution to the phonological, lexical, grammatical and cognitive aspects of language and behavior. In addition, some of the recovery patterns observed in patients with aprosodia are similar to those described with aphasia (Benson, 1979; Kertesz, 1979). Subcortical lesions in the right hemisphere may produce aprosodias (Gorelick and Ross, 1987; Ross, 1981; Ross *et al.*, 1981), just as subcortical lesions in the left hemisphere may produce aphasic deficits (Benson, 1979; Damasio *et al.*, 1982; Naeser *et al.*, 1982). It has also been postulated that appropriate lesions in the right hemisphere, involving the parietal operculum or the angular gyrus, might produce aprosodias that are homologous to conduction and anomic aphasia but to date these syndromes have not yet been encountered (*Table 1*) (Ross, 1981).

An important issue needing further clarification concerns the relationship of the right neocortex to emotions, in general. Although the right neocortex appears to dominantly modulate the formal decoding and encoding of graded affective behaviours, it does not appear to be responsible for generating extreme emotional displays, such as laughing, crying or anger, or the experiential aspects of emotions as evidenced by the following. Patients who have motor or global aprosodia, producing a loss of spontaneous affective behaviours, have been reported to be able to display the extremes of emotions during very sad, happy, or angry situations (Gorelick and Ross, 1987; Ross, 1981; Ross and Rush, 1981). These displays tend to be all or none, uncontrollable, and socially embarrassing, giving them the quality of pathological displays of affect (Benson, 1979; Poeck, 1969; Wilson, 1924). Unlike true pathological affect, however, the displays are generally mood congruent. Thus, one must conclude that the motoric organization of extreme emotional displays are modulated by areas of the brain outside the right neocortex (Ross and Stewart, 1987). Most likely these areas reside in the temporal limbic system, basal forebrain and diencephalon since lesions and epileptic discharges in these regions may induce extreme displays of emotion that usually take the form of pathological affect regulation (Malamud, 1967; Poeck, 1969; Pribnam and Melges, 1969; Reeves and Plum, 1969; Wilson, 1924).

Although patients with motor aprosodia lose their ability to encode affective behaviour, except for extreme emotional displays, they may continue to experience the entire range of emotional feeling states, including severe melancholic depression (Ross, 1981; Ross and Mesulam, 1979; Ross and Rush, 1981). This suggests, therefore, that emotional experience and affective behaviours are dissociable from each other with each having a different neuroanatomical substrate. Current evidence has implicated the temporal limbic system as the crucial anatomical structure for the experiential aspects of both emotions and other mental phenomena (Gloor *et al.*, 1982; Halgren *et al.* 1978). This particular dissociation between affective display and emotional experience is also well known to occur in patients who have pathological regulation of affect from either bilateral lesions involving the descending neocortical motor pathways emanating from areas 4 and 6 which results in pseudo-bulbar palsy (Benson, 1979) or unilateral lesions involving diencephalic or limbic structures (Poeck, 1969; Wilson, 1924). These patients are characterized as having uncontrollable bursts of laughing and crying that are usually precipitated by trivial environmental stimuli. Their emotional displays generally occur in the absence of a corresponding emotional experience.

From the above observations, it is clear that clinicians must be exceedingly careful about assessing the internal emotional state of patients who suffer brain damage. Merely observing overt affective behaviours or relying solely on the patient's verbal reports can lead to faulty impressions and conclusions. For instance, although many right brain damaged patients are traditionally described as being indifferent (Gianotti, 1972), they may actually harbour a full component of concern (Ross, 1981; Ross and Rush, 1981) even to the extent of a suicidal depression (Ross and Rush, 1981). Conversely, even in the absence of underlying sadness and dysphoria, the flat affect caused by right brain damage may give the erroneous impression that the patient is depressed (Ross and Rush, 1981). These considerations clearly show that special attention to both the content and associations of affective behaviour, verbal reports and also vegetative functions are necessary in order to accurately assess the internal emotional state of patients with brain damage (Ross and Rush, 1981). This becomes even more crucial with the recent realization that major depression is a common late sequelae of stroke not accounted for by bereavement mechanisms (Robinson, Starr and Price, 1984). If one uses DSM-III based psychiatric diagnostic criteria, Robinson, Starr and Price (1984) have reported a 25% incidence of post-stroke depression. However, using a non-DSM-III approach, based on the guidelines suggested by Ross and Rush (1981), Gordon and co-workers (1985; Ross *et al.*, 1987) have reported an incidence of post-stroke depression as high as 65%! Thus, the ability of a clinician to identify and treat post-stroke depression should have an enormous impact on the rehabilitation management of patients with not only right but also left brain injury.

The pathophysiological correlations in patients with aprosodia have, so far, only indicated that the right hemisphere may play a dominant role in the modulation of graded affective behaviours. Additional evidence suggests that this may reflect a more general specialization of the right hemisphere for all non-verbal and paralinguistic aspects of communication (Benowitz *et al.*, 1983). However, we do not yet know if the right hemisphere is specialized for processing the entire range of emotional experience. Although several authors believe in this global-type of right hemisphere function (Dimond, Farrington and Johnson, 1976; Gianotti, 1972; Schwartz, Davidson and Maer, 1975; Suberi and McKeever, 1977; Terzian, 1964; Wexler, 1980), others stress that both hemispheres may participate in the experience of emotion with each hemisphere having its greatest impact on a different type of emotion (Ross and Rush, 1981; Sackeim *et al.* 1982; Sackeim and Gur, 1978). Clinical research over the next several decades should help to further clarify some of the unanswered issues concerning the right hemisphere's pivotal role in affect, emotions, language and behaviour.

References

Benowitz, L.L., Bear, D.M., Rosenthal, R. Mesulam, M.M. Zaidel, E. and Sperry, R.W. Hemispheric specialization in nonverbal communication. *Cortex* (1983), **19**, 5.

BENSON, D.F. *Aphasia, Alexia, and Apraphia* (1979). New York: Churchill Livingstone.

BLUMSTEIN, S. and COOPER, W. Hemispheric processing of intonation contours. *Cortex* (1974), **10**, 146.

BLUMSTEIN, S. and GOODGLASS, H. The perception of stress as a semantic cue in aphasia. *Journal of Speech and Hearing Research* (1972), **15**, 800.

BROCA, P. Remarqes sur le siege de la faculte du langage articule, suives d'une observation d'aphemie. In G. von Bonin (trans) *The Cerebral Cortex* (1960). Springfield: C.C. Thomas.

BROCA, P. Sur le siege de la faculte du language articule. *Bulletin d'Anthropologie* (1865), 6, 377.

CICONE, M., WAPNER, W., FOLDI, N., ZURIF, E. and GARDNER, H. The relationship between gesture and language in aphasic communication. *Brain and Language* (1979), **8**, 324.

CRITCHLEY, M. *The Language of Gesture* (1939). London: Edward Arnold.

CRITCHLEY, M. *Aphasiology and Other Aspects of Language* (1970. London: Edward Arnold, Chapter 15.

CRYSTAL, D. *Prosodic Systems and Intonation in English* (1969). Cambridge University Press.

CRYSTAL, D. *The English Tone of Voice* (1975). New York: St Martin's Press.

DAMASIO, A.R., DAMASIO, H., RIZZO, M., VARNEY, N. and GERSCH, F. Aphasia with nonhaemorrhage lesions in the basal ganglia and internal capsule. *Archives of Neurology* (1982), **39**, 15.

DANLY, M., COOPER, W.E. and SHAPIRO, B. Fundamental frequency, language processing, and linguistic structure in Wernicke's aphasia. *Brain and Language* (1983), **19**, 1.

DANLY, M. and SHAPIRO, B. Speech prosody in Broca's aphasia. *Brain and Language* (1982), **16** 171.

DARWIN, C. *The Expressions of the Emotions in Man and Animals* (1955). New York: Philosophical Library.

DEGROOT, A. Structural linguistics and syntactic laws. *Word* (1949), **5**, 1.

DEKOSKY, S.T., HEILMAN, K.M., BOWERS, D. and VALENSTEIN, E. Recognition and discrimination of emotional faces and pictures. *Brain and Language* (1980), **9**, 206.

DELIS, D., FOLDI, N.S., HAMBE, S., GARDNER, H. and ZURIF, E. A note on temporal relations between language and gestures. *Brain and Language* (1979), **8**, 350.

DE RENZI, E., MOTTI, F. and NICHELLI, P. Imitating gestures: a quantitative approach to ideomotor aproxia. *Archives of Neurology* (1980), **37**, 6.

DIMOND, S.J., FARRINGTON, L. and JOHNSON, P. Differing emotional responses from right and left hemispheres. *Nature (Lond.)* (1976), **261**, 690.

EDMONDSON, J.A., CHAN, J-L., SEIBERT, G.B. and ROSS, E.D. The effect of right-brain damage on acoustical measures of affective prosody in Taiwanese patients. *Journal of Phonetics* (1987), (in press).

FEYEREISEN, P. and SERON, X. Nonverbal communication and aphasia: a review. I. Comprehension, II. Expression. *Brain and Language* (1982), **16**, 191 and 213.

GANDOUR, J. and DARDARANANDA, R. Identification of tonal contrasts in Thai aphasic patients. *Brain and Language* (1983), **18**, 98.

GAINOTTI, G. Emotional behavior and hemispheric side of the lesion. *Cortex* (1972), **8**, 41.

GAINOTTI, G. The relationships between emotions and cerebral dominance: A review of clinical and experimental evidence. In J. Gruzelier and P. Flor-Henry (eds) *Hemisphere Asymmetries of Function in Psychopathology* (1979). Amsterdam: Elsevier/North-Holland Biomedical Press.

GAINOTTI, G. and LEMMO, M. Comprehension of symbolic gestures in aphasia. *Brain and Language* (1976), **3**, 451.

GAZZANIGA, M.S., GLASS, A.V., SARNO, M.T. *et al.* Pure word deafness and hemispheric dynamics: A case history. *Cortex* (1973), **9** 136.

GLOOR, P., OLIVER, A., QUESNEY, L.F., ANDERMANN, F. and HOROWITZ, S. The role of the limbic system in experiential phenomena of temporal lobe epilepsy. *Annals of Neurology* (1982), **12**, 129.

GOODGLASS, H. and KAPLAN, E. Disturbance of gesture and pantomime in aphasia. *Brain* (1963), **86**, 703.

GORDON, W.A. (principle investigator). *Treatment of affective deficits in stroke rehabilitation*. Grant #NS-22471, NINCDS, funded as of 9/23/85.

GORELICK, P.B. and ROSS, E.D. The aprosodias: Further functional-anatomic evidence for the organization of affective language in the right hemisphere. *Journal of Neurology, Neurosurgery and Psychiatry* (1987), **50**, 553.

HALGREN, E., WALTER, R.D., CHERLOW, D.G. and CRANDALL, P.H. Mental phenomena evoked by electrical stimulation of the human hippocampal formation and amygdala. *Brain* (1978), **101**, 83.

HEILMAN, K.M., BOWERS, D., SPEEDIE, L. and COSLETT, H.B. The comprehension of emotional and nonemotional prosody. *Neurology (Supplement 2)* (1983), **33**, 241.

HEILMAN, K.M., ROTHI, L., CAMPANELLA, D. *et al.* Wernicke's and global aphasia with alexia. *Archives of Neurology* (1979), **36**, 129.

HEILMAN, K.M. SCHOLES, R. and WATSON, R.T. Auditory affective agnosia: Disturbed comprehension of affective speech. *Journal of Neurology, Neurosurgery and Psychiatry* (1975), **38** 69.

HERMANN, K., TURNER, J.W., GILLINGHAM, F.J. and GAZE, R.M. The effects of destructive lesions and stimulation of the basal ganglia on speech mechanisms. *Confinia Neurology* (1966), **27**, 197.

HUGHES, C.P., CHAN, J-L. and SU, M.S. Aprosodia in Chinese patients with right cerebral hemisphere lesions. *Archives of Neurology* (1983), **40**, 732.

HUGHLINGS-JACKSON, J. On affections of speech from disease of the brain. *Brain* (1879), **2**, 202.

HUGHLINGS-JACKSON, J. Words and other symbols. In J. Taylor (ed.) *Selected Writings of John Hughlings Jackson* (1932), p. 205. London: Hodder & Stoughton.

KERTESZ, A. *Aphasia and Associated Disorders* (1979). New York: Grune & Stratton Inc.

KERTESZ, A. and BENSON, D.F. Neologistic jargon: A clinicopathological study. *Cortex* (1970), **6** 362.

LARSEN, B., SKINHOJ, E. and LASSEN, N.A. Variations in regional cortical blood flow in the right and left hemispheres during automatic speech. *Brain* (1978), **101**, 193.

LASSEN, N.A., INGVAR, D.H. and SKINHOJ, E. Brain function and blood flow. *Scientific American* (1978), **239**, 62.

LEWIS, A. *Infant Speech: A Study of the Beginnings of Language* (1936). New York: Harcourt, Brace, and World.

MALAMUD, N. Psychiatric disorder with intracranial tumors of limbic system. *Archives of Neurology* (1967), **17** 113.

MOHR, J.P. Broca's area and Broca's aphasia. In H. Whitaker and H.A. Whitaker (eds) *Studies in Neurolinguistics* (1976), Vol. 1, p. 201. New York: Academic Press.

MONRAD-KROHN, G.H. Dysprosody or altered 'melody of language'. *Brain* (1947), **70** 405.

MONRAD-KROHN, G.H. The prosodic quality of speech and its disorders. *Acta Psychiatrica Neurologica* (1947), **22**, 255.

MONRAD-KROHN, G.H. Altered melody of language ('Dysprosody') as an element of aphasia. *Acta Psych Neurol Supp.* (1947), **46** 204.

MONRAD-KROHN, G.H. The third element of speech: Prosody and its disorders. In L. Halpern (ed.) *Problems of Dynamic Neurology* (1963), p. 101. Jerusalem: Hebrew University Press.

NAESER, M.A., ALEXANDER, M.P., HELM-ESATBROOKS, N., LEVINE, H.L., LAUGHLIN, S.A. and GESCHWIND, N. Aphasia with predominantly subcortical lesion sites: Description of three capsular/putaminal aphasia syndromes. *Archives of Neurology* (1982), **39**, 2.

NAESER, M. and CHAN, S.W.C. Case study of a Chinese aphasic with the Boston Diagnostic exam. *Neuropsychologia* (1983), **18**, 389.

POECK, K. Pathophysiology of emotional disorders associated with brain damage. In P.J. Vinken and G.W. Bruyn (eds) *Handbook of Clinical Neurology* (1969), Vol. 3, p. 343. Amsterdam: North-Holland.

PRIBRAM, K.H. and MELGES, F.T. Psychophysiological basis of emotion. In P.J. Vinken and G.W. Bruyn (eds) *Handbook of Clinical Neurology* (1969), Vol. 3, p. 316. Amsterdam: North-Holland.

REEVES, A.G. and PLUM, F. Hyperphagia, rage and dementia accompanying a ventromedial hypothalamic neoplasm. *Archives of Neurology* (1969), **20**, 616.

ROBINSON, R.G., STARR, L.B. and PRICE, T.R. A two year longitudinal study of mood disorders following stroke: Prevalence and duration at six months follow-up. *British Journal of Psychiatry* (1984), **144**, 256.

ROSS, E.D. The aprosodias: Functional-anatomic organization of the affective components of language in the right hemisphere. *Archives of Neurology* (1981), **38**, 561.

ROSS, E.D., EDMONDSON, J.A. and SEIBERT, G.B. The effect of affect on various acoustic measures of prosody in tone and non-tone languages: A comparison based on computer analysis of voice. *Journal of Phonetics* (1986), **14**, 283.

ROSS, E.D., GORDON, W.A., HIBBARD, M. and EGELKO, S. Dexamethasone suppression test, post-stroke depression and validity of DSM-III based diagnostic criteria. *American Journal of Psychiatry* (1987, in press).

ROSS, E.D., HARNEY, J.H., DELACOSTE, C. and PURDY, P. How the brain integrates affective and propositional language into a unified brain function. Hypotheses based on clinicopathological correlations. *Archives of Neurology* (1981), **38**, 745.

ROSS, E.D., HOLZAPFEL, D. and FREEMAN, F. Assessment of affective behavior in brain damaged patients using quantitative acoustical–phonetic and gestural measurements. *Neurology (Supplement 2)* (1983), **33** 219.

ROSS, E.D. and MESULAM, M-M. Dominant language functions of the right hemisphere?: Prosody and emotional gesturing. *Archives of Neurology* (1979), **36** 144.

ROSS, E.D. and RUSH, A.J. Diagnosis and neuroanatomical correlates of depression in brain-damaged patients: Implications for a neurology of depression. *Archives of General Psychiatry* (1981) **38**, 1344.

ROSS, E.D. and STEWART, R., Pathological display of affect in patients with depression and right focal brain damage: An alternate mechanism. *Journal of Nervous and Mental Disease* (1987), **175**, 165.

SACKEIM, H.A., GREENBERG, M.S., WEIMAN, A.L., GUR, R.C., HUNGERBUHLER, J.P. and GESCHWIND, N. Hemispheric asymmetry in the expression of positive and negative emotions: Neurologic evidence. *Archives of Neurology* (1982), **39**, 210.

SACKEIM, H.A. and GUR, R.C. Lateral asymmetry in intensity of emotional expression. *Neuropsychologia* (1978), **16** 473.

SCHWARTZ, G.E., DAVIDSON, R.J. and MAER, F. Right hemisphere lateralization for emotion in the human brain: Interactions with cognition. *Science* (1975), **190**, 286.

SERON, X., VAN DER KAA, M.A., REMITZ, A. and VAN DER LINDEN, M. Pantomime interpretation and aphasia. *Neuropsychologia* (1979), **17**, 661.

SHAPIRO, B., DANLY, M. The role of the right hemisphere in the control of speech prosody in propositional and affective contexts. *Brain and Language* (1985), **25** 19.

SUBERI, M. and MCKEEVER, W.F. Differential right hemispheric memory storage of emotional and non-emotional faces. *Neuropsychologia* (1977), **15**, 757.

TERZIAN, H. Behavioral and EEG effects of intracarotid sodium amytal injection. *Acta Neurochirurgica* (1964), **12**, 230.

TUCKER, D.M., WATSON, R.T. and HEILMAN, K.M. Discrimination and evocation of affectively intoned speech in patients with right parietal disease. *Neurology* (1977), **27**, 947.

VAN LANCKER, D. Cerebral lateralization of pitch cues in the linguistic signal. *International Journal of Human Communication* (1980), **13**, 201.

VAN LANCKER, D. CANTER, G.J. and TERBEEK, D. Disambiguation of ditropic sentences: Acoustic and phonetic cues. *Journal of Speech and Hearing Research* (1981), **24**, 330.

WEINTRAUB, S., MESULAM, M-M. and KRAMER, L. Disturbances in prosody: A right-hemisphere contribution to language. *Archives of Neurology* (1981), **38**, 742.

WERNICKE, C. Der aphasische Symptomencomplex. Eine psychologische Studie auf anatomischer Basis. In G.H. Eggert (trans) *Wernicke's Works on Aphasia. Sourcebook and Review* (1977). Paris: Mouton.

WEXLER, B.E. Cerebral laterality and psychiatry: A review of the literature. *American Journal of Psychiatry* (1980), **137**, 279.

WILSON, S.A.K. Pathological laughing and crying. *Journal of Neurology and Psychopathology* (1924), **4**, 299.

ZURIF, E.B. Auditory lateralization: Prosodic and syntactical factos. *Brain and Language* (1974), **1**, 391.

III

Clinical Neurology

8

Aphasia: New Directions in Clinical Theory

Jason W. Brown

This chapter reviews some aspects of the microgenetic theory of aphasia in relation to studies that have appeared since the initial description. Those interested in the pertinent clinical observations, in specifics of the theory and its application to other cognitive domains and implications for the philosophy of mind are referred to Brown (1987). According to the model, language develops in relation to anterior (action) and posterior (perception) structures. There are a series of levels of perceptual representation that emerge together with levels in articulatory realization.

The Anterior Component

The motor component of the utterance develops from depth to surface over stages in the evolution of the forebrain. Initial stages bound up with respiratory timing — breath groups — and locomotor and postural rhythms are linked to axial motor systems and archaic strata in perceptual space. Upper brainstem and basal ganglia mediate an early stage of motor planning in which vocal, limb and body actions appear *in statu nascendi*, part of a motor envelope which fractionates to part acts at subsequent stages. Oscillatory or kinetic rhythms in the 'motor envelope' anticipate the appearance of discrete vocal, limb and axial motility.

The action develops through mesial limbic cortex with progressive individuation of vocal, limb and body gestures. Damage at this point gives disorders of vocal and limb initiation, transcortical motor aphasia and the alien hand syndrome. Vocal and somatic automatisms may also occur. Conceivably, an oscillator mediating the preliminary tonal or breath group of the utterance is derived to one that elaborates the speech melody, a cognitive rhythm laying down the prosodic contour or rhythmic structure of the phrase. Damage at this point gives the impression of a loss of grammatical knowledge — agrammatism — though the condition can be explained, so it is argued, through variables of motor timing, parsing, prosody and stress rather than damage to a module for the rules of grammar.

The continued microgenesis of the vocal act leads through dominant premotor (Broca) and precentral cortices which elaborate the fine temporal programmation of sound sequences and, finally, to the motor implementation of the utterance through the articulatory musculature. Damage at this point in the sequence gives rise to phonetic/articulatory defects and then to the syndrome of phonetic disintegration.

From the pathological case material one can infer the motor structure of an utterance to consist of an hierarchic series of rhythmic levels or oscillators. This series, which may arise out of periodic or circadian rhythms elaborated through hypothalamic mechanisms, begins with a fundamental frequency bound up with low level automatisms, respiration and axial motility and is hypothesized to derive to a ?harmonic of this rhythm at successive levels, laying down sequentially the speech melody or prosodic contour of the utterance and a phonetic program leading to a motor keyboard for the articulators. The utterance unfolds over layers of progressive specification, comparable with levels of selection or analysis in percept formation.

The Posterior Component

In parallel with the motor series, a posterior hierarchic system lays down levels in lexical representation. The perceptual component of the utterance evolves from a spatial construct arising most likely through upper brainstem mechanisms, with initial stages in language representation bound up with early levels in object development. From this stage there arises — through limbic-derived neocortex — a conceptual (symbolic, experiential) and affective layer out of which the forming lexical item is selected. The lexical item begins with a traversal of this stage regardless of whether the process leads to speech or speech perception. Damage at this point gives rise to unusual (at times even schizophrenic-like) word substitution and confabulatory responses. Cases of so-called nonaphasic misnaming and some forms of semantic jargon refer to disruption at this point.

The subsequent microgenesis of the emerging representation involves the specification of the lexical item through layered semantic fields, with a gradual 'honing in' on the lexical target. The word is not retrieved but realized or derived and all of the stages in this derivational process — experiential, affective, semantic category — persist as a background of personal and lexical meaning. Lexical representation occurs by way of auditory belt or posterior integration cortex of dominant hemisphere. Damage to this area gives rise to word finding difficulty or semantic paraphasia where category relations are prominent.

From this stage the perceptual (lexical) representation is derived through mechanisms in auditory and para-auditory cortex to a phonetic representation of the selected item. This involves the analysis or segmentation of abstract lexical frames analogous to the realization of articulatory or fine digital movements in the motor hierarchy. Damage at this point gives rise to phonemic errors in otherwise correctly selected lexical targets.

In speech *production* there is a simultaneous unfolding over anterior and posterior microgenetic trees. In both anterior and posterior components this leads from bilaterally organized (mesial or lateral) limbic-derived cortex, through asymmetric 'integration' (frontal or temporo-parietal) neocortex to focal left frontal (Broca) and temporal (Wernicke) regions. The various aphasic syndromes represent moments in this unfolding process, with brain damage viewed as disrupting levels in a continuum rather than centres in an interactive or functional system.

In speech *perception* the described series of posterior levels is constrained at successive levels by auditory sensation to model the physical stimulus. The autonomous system of cognitive representation active in speech production is given over to speech perception. The anterior (action) component is attenuated so that the phonemic representation derived through this system is apprehended as external or perceptual in origin. In other words, the same series of posterior hierarchic levels elaborates language production and perception, but it is the relative activity of the anterior system that determines whether the subject apprehends the achieved lexical representation as self-generated or perceived. Intermediate stages in this process are bound up with imagery and elaborate inner speech or auditory hallucination, again depending on the degree of completion of the action microgeny. In either case, whether the process leads to speech or perception, the progression is from internal representation to an exteriorized and ostensibly independent source, or object.

Put differently, it is the unfolding of the motor component that provides the feeling of intention or agency that enables the subject to distinguish an active, self-initiated representation from one that is 'passive' or perceptual. In speech production, a phonemic representation is realized together with a phonetic program and the latter carries the representation outward from speaker to external world. In perception, the action development is attenuated and the perceptual series is carried outward. Inner speech and auditory verbal hallucination — intertwined in pathology, normal in the hypnagogic state — are linked to the relative degree of act and percept development over these systems.

This model is but an outline for a theory of language organization in the brain. The pathological material is unclear as to structures involved in syntax, and other complex aspects of language — especially language at the sentence and intersentential level — cannot yet be approached from the neurological standpoint. What the theory can do is map some elements of language to brain structure and establish links between language processing and more fundamental components of cognition, account for a range of associated phenomena — e.g. problems of affect, imagery and awareness — not dealt with in linguistic models and motivate studies of transitions from lower organisms.

For example, the concept that lexical items are not looked up or retrieved from a store but selected through a layered net of word-meaning relationships, a process that involves a kind of zeroing in on target items, one that is disrupted by lesions of temporal lobe, has points of contact with observations in monkey that temporal lobe lesions impair the selection of object targets in an array of objects. On the microgenetic account, object naming is not mere labelling or association. Lexical items are selected like objects as central elements in language representation, developing from preliminary levels in object and space perception. Along these lines, the frame-content theory advanced by McNeilage *et al.* (1987) also appears consistent with the evolutionary thrust of microgenetic theory.

The predictions of this theory are very different from traditional accounts. Just to mention a few, the theory obligates that the recognition of an object — a word — occurs before its conscious perception, that is, meaning is extracted prior to awareness. Similarly, the primary cortex — e.g. auditory cortex — is assumed to mediate an endpoint in the microgeny of objects, not the initial stage of registration. Another prediction is that rather than back to front transmission, anterior and posterior language areas unfold simultaneously into the utterance. Moreover, processing is unidirectional, 'bottom-up' over the described hierarchy of levels.

Clinical Evidence

Gradually, evidence has accumulated to support the idea of semantic prior to phonological processing. Studies of deep dyslexia (Coltheart *et al.*, 1980), where patients with generally large left hemisphere lesions are unable to derive phonology from print, show semantic errors in reading, especially for concrete nouns. Such patients extract meaning from the word form even though they cannot process the word phonetically, suggesting a pre-phonological stage of lexical meaning. Similar phenomena in the auditory modality have been reported (Morton, 1980). There are reports of ability to point to semantic associates of an orally presented target on a forced choice paradigm in patients with cortical or word deafness who are otherwise unable to point to the correct object (Michel, personal communication).

Not only is word meaning extracted prior to phonology, it may be extracted prior to the conscious perception of the word. One well known study showing semantic priming for backward-masked (and not consciously perceived) words provided important early support (Marcel, 1983; *see* Holender, 1986). There are also reports of cross-field semantic priming in cases of callosal section (Gazzaniga, 1980). In our lab, we have noted that semantic priming is most pronounced in cases of severe aphasia, even when the subject has difficulty reading the target words, again suggesting that semantic processing is a preliminary stage in cognition prior to phonological analysis, prior even to conscious object or word perception.

Converging information comes from studies of pure alexia, letter-by-letter reading associated with a left occipital and, usually, splenial lesion. Recent studies suggest depressed function in the mirror right occipital area. Word evoked potentials may be flattened over the right posterior region — in spite of normal late potentials associated with meaning — suggesting mirror diaschisis (Neville *et al.*, 1979). In a related study of non-alexic patients with left and right hemisphere lesions, elevated thresholds for the identification of geometric shape were found in the ipsilateral field. This was present only in cases with hemianopia regardless of lesion side, and again points to mirror depression (Brown, 1980). Patients with pure alexia have elevated tachistoscopic thresholds for object recognition. Reading errors tend to reflect the visual complexity of the stimulus. These observations, and many others, suggest that the perception of word-form is impaired. In spite of this, patients with pure alexia show occasional semantic paralexias, may demonstrate semantic priming effects and show access to semantic information on words they are unable to read (Landis *et al.* 1980; Coslett and Saffran, 1983). These observations provide further support for the idea that meaning can be extracted from a word (an object, etc.) prior to its conscious perception.

The microgenetic model predicts that language representation unfolds from a lexical-semantic to a phonological stage. The surface of the posterior language system consists in a core zone in posterior superior temporal area for phonological processing with a lexical-semantic surround, a pattern largely confirmed by CT studies of posterior aphasia (Cappa *et al.*, 1981) and electrocortical stimulation of the posterior language zone (Ojemann, 1983). In fact, the dissection of phonological processing into a posterior phonemic and anterior phonetic component (Messerli *et al.*, 1983) was inherent in the earliest form of the microgenetic model. The concept that processing leads from a bilaterally represented lexical-semantic phase to a lateralized core phonological zone developed, in part, from the interpretation of neology as a two level (lexical, phonological) defect (Brown, 1972), an idea that is finding increasing support (Buckingham, 1981; Howard *et al.*, 1984). Studies of posterior aphasia, especially jargon, suggest that the transition through layered semantic fields toward a target lexical item, its isolation and eventual phonemic representation, occur on a continuum which can be sliced more or less arbitrarily at innumerable points (Perecman and Brown, 1985).

With regard to some aphasic disorders:

1. The model predicts that functions do not resolve in isolation but together with other performances as part of the same language level or processing stage. Thus, conduction aphasia was viewed as a disruption of phonological representation co-extensive with a stage of cognitive analysis rather than a deficit of repetition (*see* Kohn, 1984). Evidence in support of the microgenetic interpretation of conduction aphasia has been reported by Selnes *et al.* (1985). These authors document that repetition is related to Wernicke's area, not to a connecting pathway, and that repetition is involved in relation to alterations in other language behaviours, especially naming and reading aloud; i.e. it is not damaged with the degree of anatomical or functional specificity required by a pathway theory.
2. The description of word deafness as the disruption of an endpoint in phonological realization, a type of perceptual dysarthria, rather than an input disorder (Brown, 1972) finds support in various recent papers, notably that of Carramazza *et al.* (1983), demonstrating a phonological disorder in word-deaf patients. Evidence for a pre-phonological stage of semantic processing is also consistent with the microgenetic account.
3. The depiction of word finding errors as moments in a process of lexical specification, and thereby the integration of anomia with other aphasic syndromes, agrees with recent interpretations of posterior aphasia, especially by the British school, claiming that errors correspond to stages in lexical differentiation.
4. The concept that awareness of errors depends on error type, i.e. processing stage, and the implication that awareness develops with, or is elaborated by, language microgenesis finds some support in studies of error awareness in deep dyslexia (Newcombe and Marshall, 1980) and other conditions (Marshall *et al.*, 1985) where awareness and self-correction accompany phonemic but not semantic errors.
5. The account of motor and conduction aphasia as disruptions of phonological processing (Brown, 1972), and the implication that the step from ape to man depended on the evolution of linked phonological (phonetic, phonemic) devices in the Broca and Wernicke area, is supported by much current work (e.g. Messerli *et al.*, 1983).

6. The description of transcortical motor aphasia as a motoric rather than linguistic or propositional disturbance is supported by recent physiological studies in human subjects (Chauvel *et al.*, 1985). Of interest, Jurgens (1985) reports that monkeys with bilateral SMA lesions show a disruption of the isolation call, a self-generated vocalization, while other stimulus-dependent vocalizations are intact. This speaks for a problem in TMA in generating a vocal action (spontaneous speech) when it is independent of specific perceptual cues (repetition, reading aloud, naming) as predicted in early microgenetic accounts of this disorder.
7. A still more dramatic illustration of evolutionary levels in action comes from studies of patients with severe aphasia, unable to communicate orally or with their intact left hand, who can write (to dictation) with their hemiplegic right arm with the aid of a prosthesis (Brown *et al.*, 1983). The extent of preserved language ability in these cases has not yet been established, but we have studied one patient with severe non-fluent aphasia who produced grammatical sentences on picture description (Brown, 1985). This phenomenon has been interpreted as the ability to access submerged or 'buried' levels in language representation through the use of the older proximal motor system.
8. Studies of agrammatism have not consistently documented a disorder of grammatical knowledge in anterior aphasics differing from that in posteriors (Heeschen, 1985). This implies that an impairment in mental grammar is not the cause of the agrammatism in production. This conclusion is consistent with the microgenetic account, as well as with several studies in our lab which have failed to support the usual interpretation of this disorder. Thus, motor aphasics do well on reversible sentences when the sentences are controlled for real world plausbility, i.e. are equally implausible (Leslie, 1980), their sortings are aided by word stress (Kellar, 1985) and on a silent letter cancellation task they show sensitivity to functors (Ross, 1983).
9. The idea that error type reflects cognitive level finds support in studies by Gainotti *et al.* (1986) documenting a thought disorder in posterior aphasics with semantic but not phonemic errors. Early papers on microgenetic theory (Brown, 1972, 1977) are quite explicit as to this prediction.

The Nature of the Symptom

A central hypothesis concerns the nature of pathological symptoms. Traditional neuropsychology assumes that the symptoms of brain damage result from the partial or complete destruction of an area housing certain operations, representations, processes or strategies. On this view, errors represent degraded functions and omissions point to deficiency states. Thus, agrammatism signifies a loss or impoverishment in a mental grammar; paraphasia indicates a defective semantic or phonemic component.

However, there is reason to doubt the accuracy of this 'common sense' interpretation. Errors which are typical of aphasic states are found in normal speakers, particularly in learning a second language as well as in normal sleeptalking (Brown, 1972). A study of a polyglot aphasic (Perecman, 1985) disclosed translation errors similar to those in normal bilinguals. Studies of phonemic jargon indicate that phoneme frequencies do not differ from the normal (Perecman and Brown, 1981). Similar findings have been reported in other jargon cases (Lecours *et al.*, 1981). Butterworth (1985) has interpreted errors in fluent aphasics as blends related to normal language processes.

Thus there is an increasing body of data to indicate that the concept of the symptom as a normal pre-processing stage — first, by the way, advanced by Freud for the interpretation of psychopathological symptoms — is not as peculiar as it might appear. Moreover, this view, which is the very heart of the microgenetic model, adds meaning to the study of symptom formation. A symptom is no longer an aberration which serves only to localize a damaged mechanism but can be used to reconstruct the organization of normal language and cognition in the brain.

Neural Correlates

One of the earliest predictions of the microgenetic model (Brown, 1972) was that the primary cortical sensory areas were endpoints in perceptual microgenesis rather than initial stages in the building up of perceptions. This prediction, which appeared so eccentric in view of work on feature detection theory, has been supported by studies rediscovering the so-called 'blindsight' phenomena, the presence of residual vision in hemianopic fields, work that dates back to Bard (1905) and Bender and Krieger (1951). The argument that these effects are artifacts of light scatter (Campion *et al.*, 1983) does not account for the occurrence of the phenomenon in cases with cortical blindness due to bilateral striate damage. Such patients can often walk confidently around obstacles without bumping into them (Brown, 1972), a behaviour reminiscent of that in the destriate monkey, (Humphrey, 1974). There is also the fact that comparable phenomena have been described in the auditory (Michel *et al.*, 1980) and tactile (Paillard *et al.*, 1983) modalities. Scatter does not explain denial of blindness, a phenomenon presumably reflecting a visual experience at sub-surface levels, nor does it account for semantic priming in blind fields (Marcel, 1983), a finding which indicates that more than just sensory primitives are involved.

Further support for the idea that V1 represents a late stage in object formation would be provided by PET studies demonstrating metabolic activation of circumstriate cortex (V2) without activation of striate cortex. There are preliminary reports that this effect has been obtained. Of still greater interest is the report by Deacon (1988) in studies of the laminar distribution of cortico-cortical fibres in primate that the pattern of distribution from pre-frontal to pre-motor to motor cortex parallels that from inferotemporal cortex to V3 to V2 to V1 suggesting that the direction of processing in visual perception may well be the reverse of the standard theory and conform instead to predictions of the microgenetic account.

A longstanding dogma in aphasia study concerns the idea of posterior to anterior flow mediated by intervening parietal neocortex, insula or the arcuate fasciculus. However, the microgenetic concept is that of a simultaneous unfolding over anterior and posterior systems. Although there is still little data on this question, recent work in owl monkey (Merzenich and Kaas, 1980) indicates simultaneous processing in multiple visual areas and Ojemann (1984) has not found posterior to anterior conduction in two craniotomy cases in which Wernicke area stimulation and Broca area recording was carried out. In fact, the study of Fried *et al.* (1981) seems to suggest simultaneous processing in the two language areas.

On the microgenetic account, mesial frontal cortex (cingulate gyrus, supplementary motor area) was postulated to be entrained in the pre-processing of a vocal or limb action. Specifically, cingulate and SMA mediate preparatory stages in action generation prior to conscious awareness. This was inferred from the results of focal lesions (Brown, 1977). The argument that SMA lesion involves early stages in action generation is supported by studies of regional cerebral blood flow (Orgogozo and Larsen, 1979). Kornhuber's (1974, 1985) description of the readiness potential, a bilateral surface negative potential the end of which begins about 90 ms before simple finger movement, and the correlation of this potential in 1980 with a paralimbic midline source, are also consistent with the microgenetic account and confirm that SMA is involved in the programming of an action at the earlier stages. The microgenetic model of action, and specifically the role of SMA is the topic of a recent review (Goldberg, 1985).

We have studied PET maps in subjects at rest and during language stimulation (phoneme monitoring). During the latter procedure, the resting pattern of mirror cortical and thalamic correlations tends to shift to one of correlations between cortical language areas within the left hemisphere (Bartlett *et al.*, 1987). The strong positive correlations between left Broca and Wernicke areas (and right Wernicke but not right Broca areas) only during language activation suggests that these areas are entrained in a task-dependent manner out of a resting pattern of metabolic symmetry. The finding of coupled activity in left Broca and Wernicke areas is, of course, consistent with a number of hypotheses about how they are interrelated. The concept of simultaneous activation is in accord with the finding that the coupling is positively correlated, while the finding that asymmetric activation develops out of a symmetrical background is consistent with a microgenetic account of dominance establishment.

According to microgenetic theory, language dominance arises through a lifespan growth process of regional specification (Brown and Jaffe, 1975), probably linked to changes in synaptic protein. Initial right hemisphere growth was postulated, with left hemisphere acceleration at the onset of language. This process was inferred from changes in aphasia type over the lifespan (*see* Brown and Grober, 1983; Joanette *et al.*, 1983). The theory predicts greater focality of language representation in left than right hemisphere, and has implications for sex differences in degree of lateral asymmetry. Specifically, the claim is that the rate of lateralization is dependent on the sex hormones. The androgens cause an increase in (cerebral) protein synthesis and thus an accelerated rate of brain growth, with increased left hemisphere specification in males. The androgens do not have a differential effect on the hemispheres. The increase in protein synthesis accentuates the embedded trend toward left specification, which is an expression of a growth process. This theory, first proposed by Brown and Grober (1983), conflicts with that recently developed by Geschwind claiming unilateral (left) hemisphere suppression by fetal testosterone.

The microgenetic model of the maturation of language areas is in general agreement with findings that gender and IQ correlate with focality of left language representation (Mateer, 1983). Additional support comes from Buell and Coleman (1979) who document sustained dendritic growth into late life, from studies suggesting parcellation — growth through inhibition — of left hemisphere in maturation, and from studies by Scheibel *et al.* (1985). who report differences in dendritic structure in adult left and right Broca areas reflecting growth asymmetries. As predicted, a different pattern was found in the Scheibel study in two non-dextrals suggesting an accentuation of right hemisphere growth early in life.

Conclusions

The history of neuropsychological study has been characterized by a longstanding debate between unitary or holistic and association or localization models of aphasia and, by implication, other cognitive functions, a debate which has usually taken the form of choice between focal and diffuse representation of function. Over the past 20 years, however, the influence of work in behavioral neurophysiology, the appearance of modularity theory and the presumed heuristic value of componential accounts have brought about a gradual shift in neuropsychology to localization models. Ironically, AI or componential models which are theoretically linked to localization concepts tend to disclaim the relevance of brain anatomy, while in traditional localization theory, functions are frozen in static brain areas and the dynamic of processing that is central to many componential accounts is lost.

The other side of this, of course, is the failure of holistic or regression models to incorporate advances in neuropsychological study and thus provide a satisfactory framework for contemporary behavioral research. Such theories as Lashley's mass action and equipotentiality, the Jacksonian concept of re-representational levels, Jakobson's idea of linguistic regression, Goldstein's 'abstract attitude' or a process of gestalt formation, have at best a limited application for they do not address the facts of brain specialization, nor the problem of the diversity of behaviour and pathological change. Here, componential theories have an advantage, for it is easier to add an extra arrow and box to a flow diagram than to integrate new phenomena to a unitary concept. Unitary models have to deal with both the unity and the diversity of mental life, local models only with diversity.

In contrast, the microgenetic account, the first anatomical theory of aphasia since Wernicke, is a unitary model that is sensitive to neurological and behavioral complexity. The model is coherent across different cognitive domains — language, perception, action and other functions are interpretable in fundamentally the same way — and there is a coupling between patterns of cognitive processing and patterns of anatomical growth. There is a deep inner relationship between the process of microgeny and the building up of anatomical structure. Brain and cognition are interpreted from an equally dynamic standpoint. To date, however, microgenetic theory is just that, a theory of cognitive processing built up on intuitions from clinical case study. As yet there are only a few experimental studies which can be said to support the theory, and there is a good deal of conceptual baggage that needs removing before real progress can be made. Still, I look forward to the future with optimism as continued efforts are made to confirm or refute some of these new ideas.

References

BARD, L. De la persistance des sensations lumineuses dans le champ aveugle des hemianopsiques. *Semaine Medicale* (1905), **25**, 253–255.

BARTLETT, E., BROWN, J.W., BRODY, J., RUSSELL, J. and WOLF, A. Metabolic correlates of language processing. *Brain and Language* (1987, in press).

BENDER, M. and KRIEGER, H. Visual functions in perimetrically blind fields. *Archives of Neurology and Psychiatry* (1951), **65**, 72–99.

BROWN, J.W. *Aphasia, Apraxia and Agnosia* (1972). Springfield: Thomas.

BROWN, J.W. *The Life of the Mind: Collected Papers* (1987). LER, Hillsdale, N.J.

BROWN, J.W. *Mind, Brain and Consciousness* (1977). New York: Academic Press.

BROWN, J.W. Visual discrimination after lesion of the posterior corpus callosum (Letter). *Neurology* (1980), **30**, 1251.

BROWN, J.W. A Prosthesis for Writing in Severe Aphasia (1985). Washington D.C.: Presentation, ASHA.

BROWN, J.W. and GROBER, E. Age, sex and aphasia type. *Journal of Nervous and Mental Disease* (1983), **171** 431–434.

BROWN, J.W. and JAFFE, J. Hypothesis on cerebral dominance. *Neuropsychologia* (1975), **13** 107–110.

BROWN, J.W., LEADER, B. and BLUM, C. Hemiplegic writing in severe aphasia. *Brain and Language* (1983), **19**, 204–215.

BUCKINGHAM, H. Where do neologisms come from? In J.W. Brown (ed.) *Jargonaphasia* (1981). New York: Academic Press.

BUELL, S. and COLEMAN, P. Dendritic growth in the aged brain and failure of growth in senile dementia. *Science* (1979), **206** 854–856.

BUTTERWORTH, B. Jargon aphasia: processes and strategies. In S. Newman and R. Epstein (Eds.) *Current Perspectives in Dysphasia* (1985) Churchill Livingstone, Edinburgh, 61-96.

CAMPION, J., LATTO, R. and SMITH, Y. Is blindsight an effect of scattered light, spared cortex and near-threshold vision? *Behavioral and Brain Sciences* (1983), **6** 423-486.

CAPPA, S., CAVALOTTI, G. and VIGNOLO, L. Phonemic and lexical errors in fluent aphasia: correlation with lesion site. *Neuropsychologia* (1981), **19**, 171–177.

CARRAMAZZA, A., BERNDT, R. and BASILI, A. The selective impairment of phonological procesing: a case study. *Brain and Language* (1983), **18** 128–174.

CHAUVEL, P., BANCAUD, J. and BUSER, P. Participation of the supplementary motor area in speech. *Experimental Brain Research* (1985) **58**, A14.

COLTHEART, M., PATTERSON, K. and MARSHALL, J. (eds.) *Deep Dyslexia* (1980). London: Routledge & Kegan Paul.

COSLETT, H. and SAFFRAN, E. Preservation of lexical access in a patient with alexia without agraphia. Presentation, INS, (1983).

DEACON, T. Neuroanatomy applied to neuropsychology. In E. Perecman (Ed.) *Integrating theory and practice in Clinical Neuropsychology* (1988) NY. IRBN Press (in press).

FRIED, I., OJEMANN, G. and FETZ, E. Language related potentials specific to human language cortex. *Science* (1981), **212**, 353–356.

GAINOTTI, G., CARLOMAGNO, S., CRACA, A. and SILVERI, M. Disorders of classificatory activity in aphasia. *Brain and Language* (1986), **28**, 181–195.

GAZZANIGA, M. *Presentation, Cognitive Processing in the Right Hemisphere* (1980). New York: Conference of IRBN.

GOLDBERG, G. Supplementary motor area structure and function: review and hypotheses. *Behavioral and Brain Sciences* (1985), **8**, 567-616.

HEESCHEN, C. Agrammatism versus paragrammatism: a fictitious opposition. In M-L. Kean (ed.) *Agrammatism* (1985). New York: Academic Press.

HOLENDER, D. Semantic activation without conscious identification. *Behavioral Brain Sciences* (1986), **9**, 1–66.

HOWARD, D., PATTERSON, K., FRANKLIN, S., MORTON, J. and ORCHARD-LISLE, V.

Variability and consistency in picture naming by aphasic patients. In F.C. Rose (ed.) *Progress in Aphasiology* (1984). New York: Raven Press.

HUMPHREY, N. Vision in monkey without striate cortex. *Perception* (1974), **3**, 241–255.

JOANETTE, Y., ALI-CHERIF, A., DELPUECH, F., HABIB, M., PELLISSIER, J. and PONCET, M. Evolution de la semiologie aphasique avec l'age. *Revue Neurologique* (1983), **139** 657–664.

JURGENS, U. Implications of the SMA in phonation. *Experimental Brain Research* (1985), **58**, A12–A14.

KELLAR, L. Stress and syntax in aphasia. Presentation (1978). Chicago: Academy of Aphasia.

KOHN, S. The nature of the phonological disorder in conduction aphasia. *Brain and Language* (1984), **23**, 97–115.

KORNHUBER, H. Cerebral cortex, cerebellum and basal ganglia. In F. Schmitt and F. Worden (eds) *The Neurosciences* (1974). 3rd Study Program. Cambridge: MIT Press.

KORNHUBER, H. Bereitschaftspotential and the activity of the supplementary motor area preceding voluntary movement. *Experimental Brain Research* (1985), **58**, A10–A11.

LANDIS, T., REGARD, M. and SERRAT, A. Iconic reading in a case of alexia without agraphia caused by a brain tumor: a tachistoscopic study. *Brain and Language* (1980), **11**, 45–53.

LECOURS, A., OSBORN, E., TRAVIS, L., ROUILLON, F. and LAVALLEE-HUYNH, G. Jargons. In J. Brown (ed.) *Jargonaphasia* (1981). New York: Academic Press.

LESLIE, C. The interactive effects of syntax, pragmatics and task difficulty in aphasic language comprehension. Unpublished Ph.D. dissertation (1980). Columbia University.

MCNEILAGE, P., STUDDERT-KENNEDY, M. and LINDBLOM, B. (1987). Primate handedness reconsidered. *Behavioural Brain Sciences* (in press).

MARCEL, T. Conscious and unconscious perception. *Cognitive Psychology* (1983), **15** 197–237.

MARCEL, T. Presentation INS (1983). Deauville.

MARSHALL, R., RAPPAPORT, B. and GARCIA-BUNUEL, L. Self-monitoring behavior in a case of severe auditory agnosia with aphasia. *Brain and Language* (1985), **24**, 297–313.

MATEER, C. Localization of language and visuospatial functions by electrical stimulation mapping. In A. Kertesz (ed.) *Localization in Neuropsychology* (1983). New York: Academic Press.

MERZENICH, and KAAS, J. Principles of organization of sensory perceptual systems in mammals. *Progress in Psychobiology, Physiology and Psychology* (1980), **9**, 1–42.

MESSERLI, P., LAVOREL, P. and NESPOULOS, J-L. *Neuropsychologie de l'Expression Orale* 1983 Ed. Paris: CNRS.

MICHEL, F. Personal communication (1984).

MICHEL, F., PERONNET, F. and SCHOTT, B. A case of cortical deafness. *Brain and Language* (1980), **10** 367–377.

MORTON, J. Two auditory parallels to deep dyslexia. In M. Coltheart *et al.* (eds) *Deep Dyslexia* (1980). London: Routledge & Kegan Paul.

NEVILLE, H., SNYDER, E., KNIGHT, R. and GALAMBOS, R. Event related potentials in language and nonlanguage tasks in patients with alexia without aphasia. In D. Lehmann and Callaway (eds) *Human Evoked Potentials* (1979). New York: Plenum.

NEWCOMBE, F. and MARSHALL, J. Response monitoring and response blocking in deep dyslexia. In M. Coltheart, K. Patterson and J. Marshall (eds) *Deep Dyslexia* (1980). London: Routledge & Kegan Paul.

OJEMANN, G. Brain organization for language from the perspective of electrical stimulation mapping. *Behavioral Brain Sciences* (1983), **6**, 189–230.

OJEMANN, G. Personal communication (1984).

ORGOGOZO, J. and LARSEN, B. Activation of the supplementary motor area during voluntary movement suggests it works as a supramotor area. *Science* (1979), **206**, 847–850.

PAILLARD, J., MICHEL, F. and STELMACH, G. Localization without content: a tactile analogue of 'blind sight'. *Archives of Neurology* (1983), **40**, 548–557.

PERECMAN, E. Language mixing in polyglot aphasia: conscious strategy or preconscious necessity? A reply to Grosjean, *Brain and Language* (1985), **26** 356–359.

PERECMAN, E. and BROWN, J.W. Ukeleles, condessors and fosetch: varieties of aphasic jargon. *Language Sciences* (1985), **7**, 177–214.

PERECMAN, E. and BROWN, J.W. Phonemic jargon: a case report. In J.W. Brown (ed.) *Jargonaphasia* (1981). New York: Academic Press.

ROSS, E.D., Phonological processing during silent reading in aphasic patients, *Brain and Language* (1983), **19**, 191–203.

SCHEIBEL, A., PAUL, L., FRIED, I., FORSYTHE, A., TOMIYASU, U., WECHSLER, A., KAO,, A. and SLOTNICK, J. Dendritic organization of the anterior speech area. *Experimental Neurology* (1985), **87**, 109–117.

SELNES, P., KNOPMAN, D., NICCUM, N and RUBENS, A. The critical role of Wernicke's area in sentence repetition. *Annals of Neurology* (1985), **17** 549–557.

9

The Anatomical and Pathological Basis of Aphasia

Luigi A. Vignolo

The bulk of the findings discussed in this chapter derives from a study carried out on a first random series of 90 right-handed, adult patients with present or past evidence of aphasia following a cerebrovascular accident, studied in our Aphasia Unit for language assessment (Mazzocchi and Vignolo, 1979). A comparison will be made between the expected lesions according to the classic anatomo-clinical tradition and the lesions actually shown by computerized tomography (CT scan), and complemented, when possible, by further evidence obtained by pathological correlations. Aphasia due to pathology other than cerebrovascular disease will be dealt with separately.

All generalisations made are provisional since the field of anatomo-clinical correlations in aphasia is currently in full expansion. CT scan findings give a purely morphological, not functional, description of brain damage and, even within this limited scope, are fraught with limitations (to be discussed later). The introduction of more refined technical tools in the study of the functional and metabolic correlates of aphasic language, such as assessment of regional cortical blood flow (see Lassen and Roland, 1983) and positron emission computed tomography (Metter, Wasterlain, Kuhl, Hanson and Phelps, 1981) is providing new information which may well revolutionize knowledge in this field. For this reason, while keeping the notions of traditional neurology and CT scan findings as anchors, we have adopted a critical approach, with an open mind to possible new developments

Materials and Methods

The findings described have been obtained by studying adult subjects harbouring cerebrovascular lesions, usually infarcts and only rarely intracerebral haemorrhages.

The *evaluation of aphasia* has been carried out by quantitative tests, including a detailed standard language examination which allows both a qualitative assessment of disordered verbal behaviour and a quantitative measure of the patient's performance in several aspects of language: oral expression, auditory verbal comprehension, repetition, writing (to command, dictation and copying) and reading (aloud and for comprehension).

The *assessment of the site and extent of the lesion* has been done mostly by EMI scanners 1000 and 1010. A routine CT scan examination yields eight 14 mm. horizontal sections from the base of the skull to the vertex. These are then projected onto the screen of a Diagnostic Display Console and photographed using a polaroid camera. In these photographic reproductions of the sections, the vascular lesions show up as areas of abnormal hypo- or hyper-density within the brain (*see*, for example, Figures 1 and 2). The contour of the lesion is identified on each section. Whenever it is necessary to draw comparison of lesions belonging to *groups* of patients showing different clinical pictures — as is commonly the case in neuropsychological research — a further step is undertaken i.e., the contour of the lesion is transferred to a standard lateral diagram of the damaged cerebral hemisphere. The procedure followed is described in detail by Mazzocchi and Vignolo, 1978 but basically consists of two simple operations: the angle of the CT sections with respect to the orbitomeatal (OML) line is established by taking the bone structures of the base of the skull as points of references (*Figure 1*) and secondly, the contour of the lesion is traced on each section and then transferred onto the standard lateral diagram by simple computation (*Figure 2*). Finally, the use of a standard lateral diagram as a frame of reference for several cases, in spite of shortcomings to be discussed later, permits the construction of composite maps of lesions for any given group of cases, thus allowing for a quick comparison among groups (*see*, for example, *Figure 3*).

The following terms are employed to indicate the site of lesion with respect to the surface of the hemisphere: 'Cortical' lesions involve the cortex, but often encroach upon the white matter immediately underlying it. 'Superficial-and-deep' lesions damage the cortex of the hemispheric surface as well as underlying subcortical structures. 'Deep' lesions appear deep in the hemisphere, far from the convexity, but may damage those portions of the cortex that are buried in *sulci* (e.g., the insular cortex), in addition to subcortical structures; as such, they should be distinguished from 'subcortical' lesions, which entirely spare the cortex. Most aphasia-producing lesions detected by CT scan are 'superficial-and-deep' and are relatively easy to map; by contrast, it is sometimes difficult to draw the needed sharp distinction between 'deep' and truly 'subcortical' lesions on sections — a technical problem which contributes to the current differences of opinion regarding the role of sub-cortical structures in language.

The *establishment of correlation* has been made with particularly careful consideration of the time factor. Unless otherwise stated, we shall report here only those correlations established in patients who underwent the CT scan at least 21 days after the stroke and a neuropsychological examination during the 21–60 day period after the stroke. These strict criteria, albeit excluding about half the available cases, have been followed because:

1. About 21 days post-onset, oedema and possible haemodynamic alterations are reduced, and the lesion can be considered to be relatively stable, at least as far as its boundaries with the surrounding cerebral tissue are concerned;
2. In the 21–60 day period following the stroke two important factors, which can increase or diminish the effects of the lesion *per se* on the neuropsychological condition of the subject, are most probably reduced to minimum: one is 'diaschisis' (von Monakow, 1914) and the other is 'compensation'.

Diaschisis, which can be defined as the inhibition or 'shock' which paralyzes activity of areas functionally connected with those damaged, is likely to be reduced within this period, while compensation, i.e., the taking over of disrupted function by areas that are either adjacent or contralateral to the damaged areas, probably has not had time to take effect. For these reasons, the language disorder assessed within these time limits reflects the actual morphology of the lesion more accurately than the language disorder observed during preceding or subsequent periods; three to eight weeks post-stroke is the optimal period for correlation, as it minimizes non-morphological factors and hence simplifies reasoning. This by no means implies that earlier or later assessments may not offer precious localizing information, which will also be further discussed.

Some *remarks on the method* are in order. Our procedure differs from that used in other published works (Noel *et al.*, 1977; Hayward *et al.*, 1977; Naeser and Hayward, 1978; Barat *et al.*, 1978) and from that used in our own pilot study (Basso, Salvolini and Vignolo, 1979), with respect to a number of points: (1) In these studies it was assumed that all sections made a constant angle of 20° or 25° (varying with the author) to the orbitomeatal line, thus neglecting the wide variations of this angle, which ranged from 12° to 42° in 100 of our unselected cases. (2) The cortical language areas were identified only in relation to the ventricles, i.e., to reference points which are variable and, in the case of high CT sections, actually absent. (3) Most important, the fact that both the lesion and clinical picture change with time was not given the full consideration it deserves.

Even avoiding these pitfalls, the use of the CT scan as a localizing device is

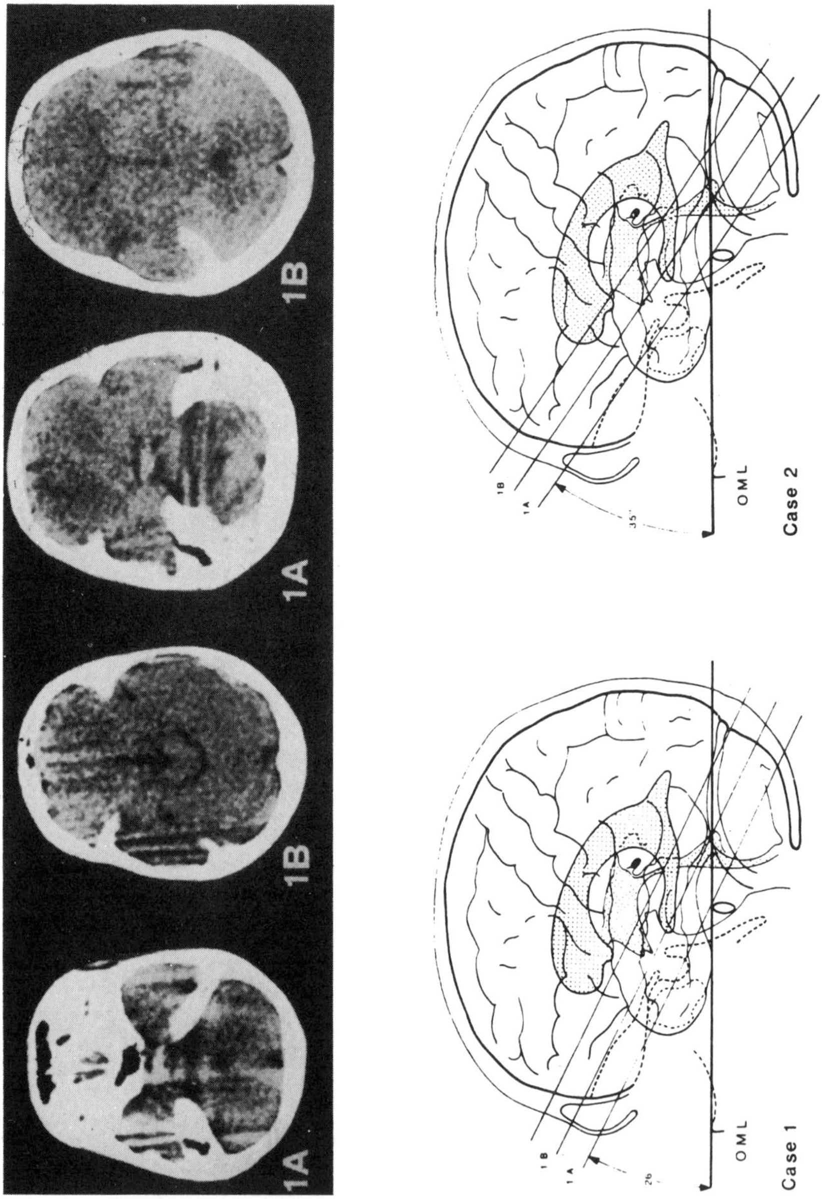

Figure 1 Identification of the angle of CT scan sections (1A, 1B) with respect to the orbitomeatal line (OML) in two cases (Case 1 = 25° and Case 2 = 35°). The landmarks (such as orbital roofs, clinoids, fourth ventricle, etc.) which appear in the scans (above) are identified on the standard lateral diagram (below) and included between two parallel lines 13mm apart (from Mazzocchi and Vignolo, 1978).

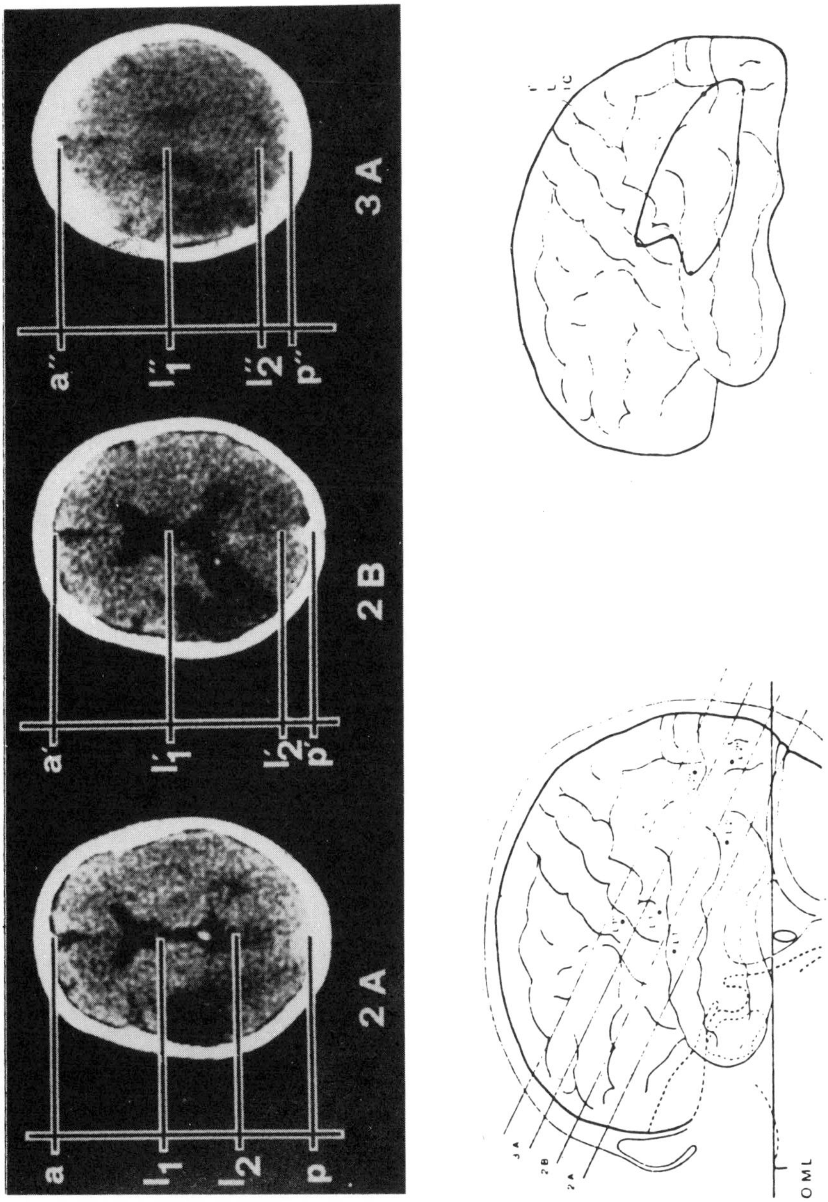

Figure 2 Mapping the lesions from CT scans on the standard lateral diagram. The anterior and posterior boundaries of the lesion in each section are first transferred upon the diagram and then connected with a continuous line (from Mazzocchi and Vignolo, 1978).

still hampered by great obstacles, especially in systematic neurological research studies where the aim is principally to *compare groups of cases*. The sources of error are numerous, either because of the equipment e.g., an EMI scanner 1000 CT may miss a small lesion (Haughton *et al.*, 1979) or be imprecise (to an extent of 5–10 mm) in locating the site of damage (Kistler *et al.*, 1975; Mort *et al.*, 1977); *or* because the patient may, during the examination, move his head, thus causing partial overlapping and changes in the inclinations of the sections. Of particular interest are those errors which occur during the 'mapping' stage. Methods similar to ours permit the transfer of the image of the calcified pineal gland on to a lateral X-ray film of the skull of an individual subject with a margin of error which varies from 3 to 10 mm (Cail and Lorris, 1979; Luzzatti *et al.*, 1979).

For our purposes, it is often necessary to transfer the images dealing with the lesions not of one, but of *several* subjects on to a *single* frame of reference, consisting of a standard lateral diagram of the brain. This obviously increases the possibility of error because, by its very nature, a diagram only shows the general pattern of fissures and convolutions, neglecting the wide range of individual variations. For example, the diagram of New and Scott (1975) employed by us reveals that the angle formed by the rolandic and sylvian fissures is about 45°, while over a random series of 22 adult brains we observed that, although the mean angle was 48°, the values ranged from 70° to 36°. In addition, the lower extremity of the rolandic cleft in the standard diagram is situated 5 mm caudally to the position of the rolandic cleft observed in 20 of the 22 brains in our series (Falzi, Perrone and Vignolo, unpublished findings). Similar objections can be raised for other aspects of this diagram, for example, the shape of the skull and position of the main landmarks.

These incomplete criticisms indicate the degree of caution necessary to evaluate clinical-CT scan correlations.

Results and Discussion

Aphasia and Side of Hemispheric Lesion

Right-handed aphasics with a lesion in the left hemisphere are the usual occurrence, while the existence, frequency and characteristics of so-called 'crossed' aphasia, i.e. aphasia resulting from lesions in the right hemisphere in right handed subjects without left handed or ambidextrous relatives, are still under discussion. The frequency of the latter depends, to a certain extent, upon the criteria used to assess (and exclude) left-handedness. When strict criteria were adopted, i.e., a score of 12/12 on Oldfield's Edinburgh Inventory, only one case was found in over 1400 aphasic patients examined by the Aphasia Unit of Milan from 1970 to 1978 (Rottoli, unpublished MD Thesis). When less stringent criteria were used, i.e. a score of 10/12 on Oldfield's Inventory, seven cases were singled out of 1439 records of patients examined between January 1976 and February 1984 (Basso *et al.*, 1985).

In both studies, the correlation between type of aphasia and site of lesion was virtually identical to that generally found in left hemisphere-damaged aphasics.

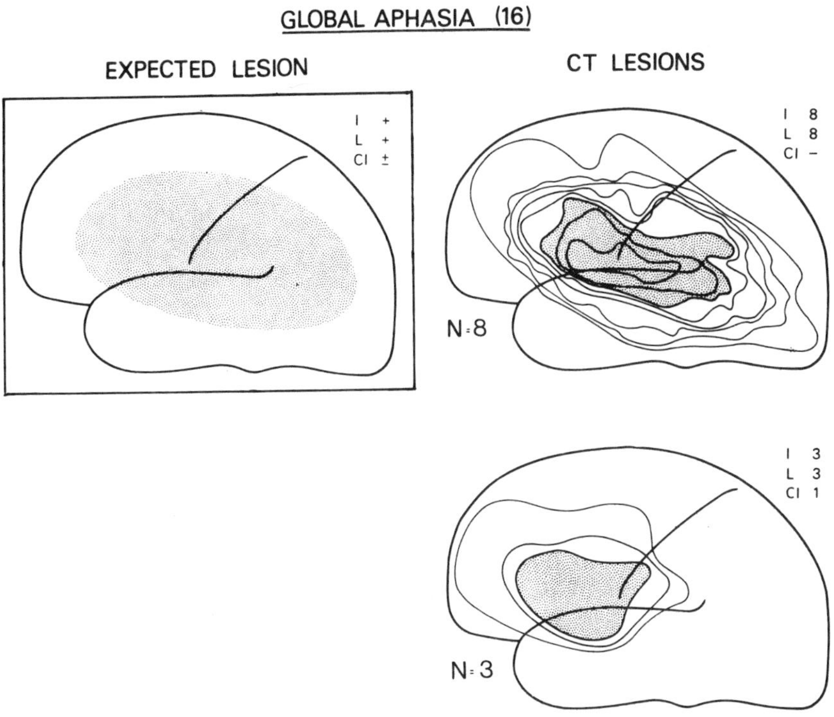

Figure 3 Global aphasia: expected lesion and composite maps of CT scan superficial-and-deep lesions. Contours do not indicate individual lesions but the degree of overlapping of lesions in a given area; they represent the boundaries of areas damaged by one lesion only (outer area), by two or by three lesions, etc. Dots cover the areas of maximum overlap. The number of lesions damaging the insula (I), the lenticular nucleus (L) and the internal capsule (C1) is shown in the upper right corner of each diagram. Purely deep and bilateral cases are not shown. N = number of cases (from Vignolo, 1981).

Aphasia and Intrahemispheric Localization

Global aphasia

It is generally accepted that this severe syndrome (speech reduced to syllabic fragments or to short recurring utterances, and severely defective auditory verbal comprehension) corresponds to the destruction of the entire language area, including both Broca's area (in the posterior part of F3) and Wernicke's area (in the posterior third of T1) and extends in depth to the insula and lenticular nucleus and even to the internal capsule. The current understanding of global (or total) aphasia implies such massive damage to the language zone as to compare with the effects of total left hemispherectomy in adults (as described by Smith, 1966). In the light of recent evidence (*Figure 3*), this view may need re-thinking. In our series, global aphasia was present in 16 out of 44 cases, but only in 8 did the CT scan show the expected vast areas of hypodensity; in one case, the lesion was large and bilateral; in the 7 unilateral cases, the lesions were unexpectedly strictly confined to the anterior language zones (excluding Wernicke's area) in 3 cases, and to the deep structures of the left hemisphere in the remaining 4 cases. In these 4 patients, the damage, while sparing the cortex of the hemispheric convexity, consistently involved the insular cortex, the lenticular nucleus and contiguous zones, extending to the internal capsule. Comparable lesions, centred on the putamen but with insular involvement, were described in 3 cases of global aphasia by Naeser *et al.* (1982). A subsequent study of 37 global aphasics examined in the optimal period for correlation (Vignolo, Frediani, Boccardi and Caverni, 1986) confirmed the possibility of lesions other than the expected large ones: while these were found in 22 patients, there were still 8 patients with exclusively anterior lesions and 4 patients with deep lesions (all of which included the insular cortex). An additional surprise was found in patients with exclusively post-rolandic lesions, involving the parieto-occipital lobes, but barely encroaching upon Wernicke's area and sparing the insula.

All these cases with lesions in unexpected sites pose further problems. The effect of small deep lesions on oral expression can be accounted for by the fact that they were never purely subcortical, but always involved the anterior insula which, as shall be seen, should be considered part of the anterior (Broca's) language area. Classic interpretation seems unable to explain the severe comprehension defect associated with the apparent integrity of Wernicke's area — a feature that the deep cases have in common with those showing either purely prerolandic or posterior occipito-parietal damage. It is perplexing that such damage, however extensive, should cause comprehension disorders as serious as those resulting from the total destruction of the language zone. There are several possible explanations. The inability of the CT scan to detect very small lesions has already been mentioned, e.g. closer scrutiny of one case with an exclusively posterior lesion showed diffuse areas of slight hypodensity in the centrum semiovale and anterior white matter of both hemispheres. This suggests that a large but partial (posterior, but perhaps also anterior) infarct of the left hemisphere, combined with several *lacunae* spread over the remaining language zone, but too small to be individually detected by the CT scan, may be responsible for global aphasia, at least in a minority of cases. On the other hand, if our findings are accepted at face value, a mass effect may be invoked for the sizeable superficial and deep lesions, either anterior or far posterior; as to the deep lesions, the classic hypothesis (Nielsen, 1946) may be advanced that they also involve acoustic pathways, both direct and crossed, thereby de-afferenting Wernicke's area. Finally, an alternative speculation is that, in our series, all cases with exclusively anterior lesions were women, and all those with exclusively posterior lesions were men (while both sexes were almost equally represented in the other subgroups). This suggests the possibility that global aphasia in the frontal patients may be due to a sex difference of language representation within the left hemisphere, as maintained by Kimura (1980):

'some of the functions dependent on the left posterior speech system in males are perhaps subserved in females by the left anterior region'. Indeed, in a further CT scan study of 37 stroke patients with global aphasia, Vignolo *et al.* (1986) found that, while 22 patients harboured the expected large lesions including Broca's and Wernicke's areas, 8 had anterior lesions sparing Wernicke's area all of whom were females, while 3 had posterior lesions sparing Broca's area and were males. (Four patients had deep lesions.) Since the whole issue of sex differences in cerebral language representation is still highly controversial, further evidence in support of Kimura's hypothesis is needed.

Whatever the explanation, the fact is that even a clear-cut syndrome such as global aphasia, entailing a virtually total loss of language, may not depend upon an equally massive destruction of the language area; indeed, this happens only in little more than half the cases.

Non-fluent Aphasia: Broca's and Transcortical Motor Aphasia

There is still disagreement as to the site of the lesion responsible for *Broca's aphasia* (non-fluent speech, usually rendered even more difficult by accompanying articulatory impediments, poor repetition and good comprehension). From the beginning of the century, two extreme, seemingly irreconciliable views, confront each other; the traditional thesis, which maintains that the destruction of the posterior part of F3 is indispensable, and that of Marie (1906) who denies any importance to this zone, upholding that the lesion should include both the posterior (temporo-parietal) language area, and an insulo-lenticular zone (the so-called 'quadrilateral'), comprising the insula, the lenticular nucleus and the structures between them. A lesion limited to the 'quadrilateral' would result not in aphasia, but in a peculiar defect of articulation known as *anarthria* (*see* above).

The possibility that Broca's aphasia appears following the destruction of the supplementary motor language area on the medial surface of the first frontal convolution has also been mentioned (Penfield and Roberts, 1959), although recent CT scan findings indicate that damage of this region is responsible, rather, for transcortical motor aphasia (*see* below). The lesions of the 9 Broca's aphasics examined in the optimal correlation period had different locations. In 5 of them, it (*Figure 4B*) did actually damage the foot of F3, sometimes encroaching upon the contiguous areas and always damaging the underlying insula. In other cases (not shown in the figure) the lesion was placed elsewhere. In one case the lesion was in frontal parasagittal location near the supplementary language area, which was presumably damaged and disconnected from Broca's area in F1. In three cases the lesion spread from the hemispheric surface and centred upon the insulo-lenticular area; the depth of the lesion differed from one case to the next, but the anterior insular cortex was consistently damaged. These cases of fully fledged Broca's aphasia with exclusively deep lesions are similar to those

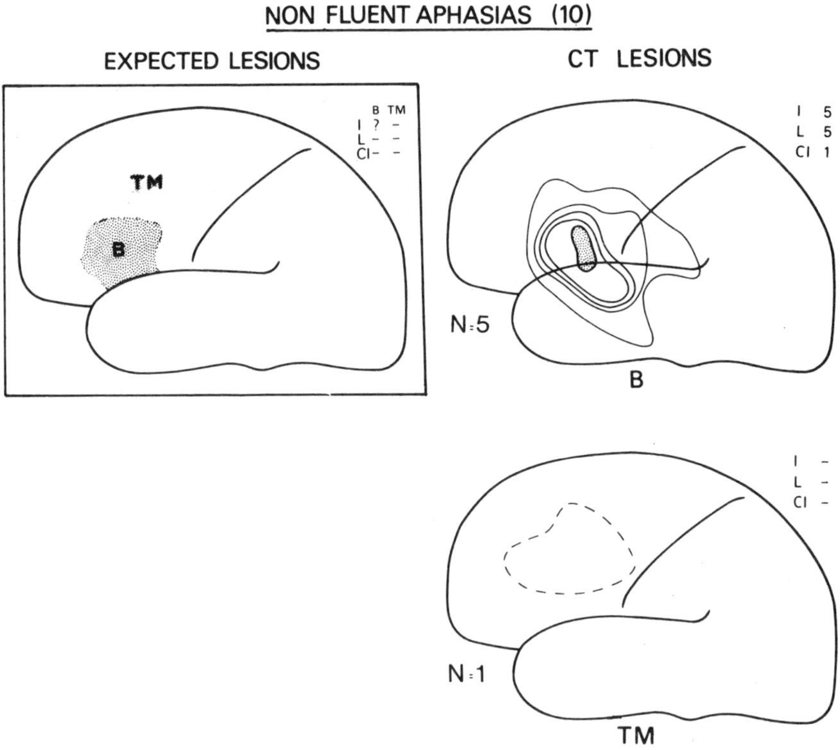

Figure 4 Broca's (B) and transcortical motor (TM) aphasia: expected lesions and composite maps of CT scan superficial-and-deep lesions. Deep and parasagittal cases are not shown. N = number of cases (from Vignolo, 1981).

with CT documentation published by Mohr *et al.* (1978). At first sight, they would appear to contradict the traditional view, since the foot of F3 is spared; but neither do they uphold the opposite theory (Marie, 1906), since the cortex of the retro-rolandic areas is not damaged. We feel that the traditional view may still offer a reasonable explanation for these findings, provided that the wider and more comprehensive formulation of the theory, expressed by Dejerine in 1914, is adopted, e.g. *Broca's area is not limited to the posterior portion of F3, but also includes the anterior insula.*

A number of recently described cases with small lesions, documented by either autopsy or CT scan or both (Mohr, 1976; Tonkonogy and Goodglass, 1981), suggest that ischemic damage strictly confined to the posterior part of F3 (Broca's area *sensu strictiore*) produces partial and transient defects of speech (such as word-finding difficulties) rather than a fully fledged and relatively stable Broca's aphasia. Therefore, it is now believed that this classic syndrome is usually associated with larger superficial-and-deep lesions, including the posterior part of F3, the central operculum, and the adjacent parietal, temporal and deeper areas. The fact that *none* of our CT scan cases of Broca's aphasia had a lesion strictly limited to the posterior part of F3 lends support to this view, but the possibility that a complete and relatively long-standing Broca's aphasia may be due to deep lesions involving the anterior insular cortex should also be stressed. As to *oral apraxia*, which is a well-known non verbal accompaniment of global, Broca's and even of some fluent aphasias with considerable phonemic disorders of speech, the underlying lesions are located mainly in the left frontal and rolandic opercula and the adjacent T1 and anterior insula (Tognola and Vignolo, 1981).

Transcortical motor aphasia

Reduced speech without articulatory disorders, good repetition and good comprehension is a rare syndrome. The damage, which is sometimes bilateral, is said to affect the marginal frontal language areas, which are located above and in front of Broca's area and include the mesial premotor area (Rubens, 1975; Masdeu *et al.*, 1978). Broca's area may in this syndrome remain untouched or be only slightly damaged. The only case of transcortical motor aphasia in our series had a typical clinical picture, and the site of the lesion was, as expected, one with the CT scan showing bilateral damage to the centrum semiovale, undermining the anterior marginal areas of language, as illustrated in *Figure 4*. The same syndrome may follow discrete subcortical lesions interrupting the thalamic–frontal connections (*see* below).

The Fluent Aphasias: Wernicke's, Conduction, Amnestic and Transcortical Sensory Aphasia

These syndromes, characterized by a fluent, though abnormal, verbal expression, result from lesions located in a large retro-rolandic region of the left hemisphere. Within this posterior language zone (*Figure 5*) *Wernicke's aphasia* (fluent speech with predominantly phonemic paraphasias and neologisms, poor repetition and poor comprehension) is said to result from the destruction of the posterior third of T1 (Wernicke's area). *Conduction aphasia* (fluent, but sometimes halting, speech and predominantly phonemic defects with phonemic groping behaviour, poor repetition and good comprehension) is believed to be caused by lesions of the posterior perisylvian areas, especially of the parietal operculum and the underlying arcuate fasciculus, i.e. lesions of structures connecting Wernicke's area to Broca's area.

Amnestic or anomic aphasias (fluent speech with frequent wordfinding difficulties, good repetition and comprehension) results from lesions of the posterior marginal areas surrounding Wernicke's zone from behind and

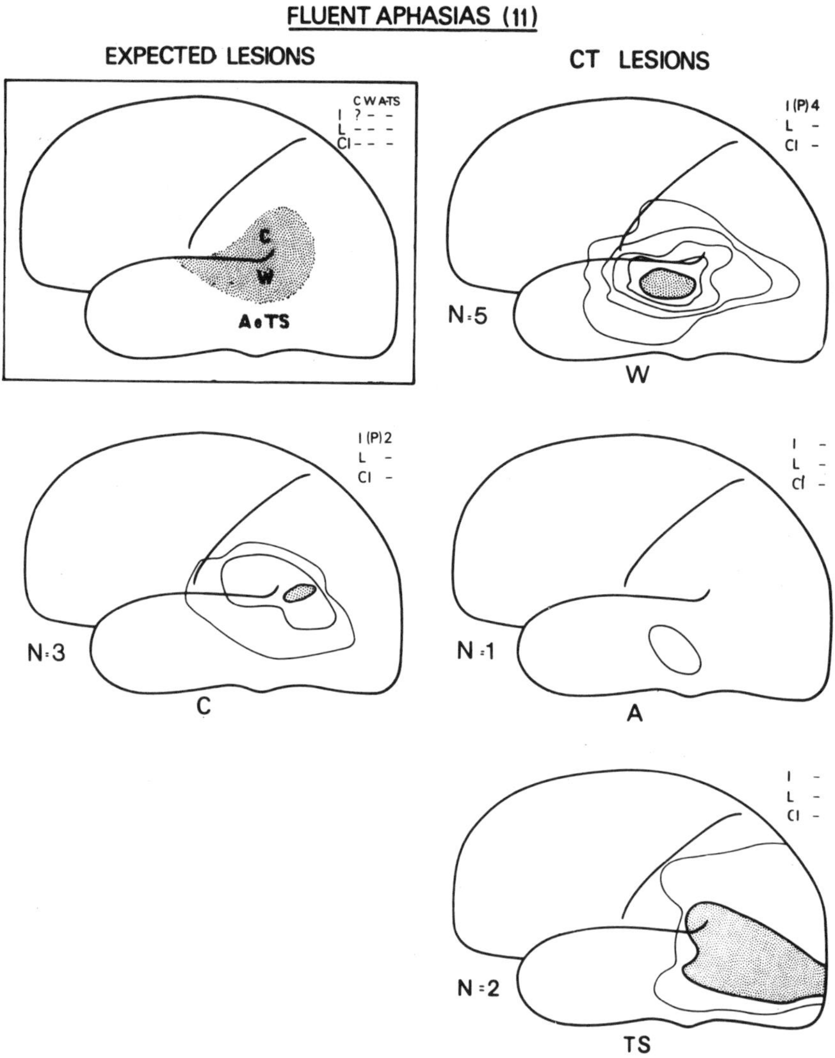

Figure 5 Wernicke's (W), conduction (C), anomic (A) and transcortical sensory (TS) aphasia: expected lesions and composite maps of CT scan superficial-and-deep lesions. N = number of cases P = posterior insula.

below. Anomic aphasia is usually associated with damage which is either abrupt, but small and well circumscribed, or slowly diffusing to larger cortical areas. Instead, when damage to the same zone is massive and complete, *transcortical sensory aphasia* ensues (fluent speech with predominantly lexical-semantic paraphasias, and strikingly good repetition, in contrast with poor comprehension with semantic confusions).

In all fluent aphasics examined in the optimal period for correlation, the lesion was found to be in the retro-rolandic areas, as expected. Within this region, the damage corresponding to Wernicke's aphasia (*Figure 5, W*) consistently affected Wernicke's area but, in addition, often extended to contiguous areas of the parietal and/or temporal lobe and, in most cases, went deeply to touch the posterior insula. As to conduction aphasia (*Figure 5, C*), only in one case was the lesion in the expected position; of the remaining two cases, one lesion was displaced posteriorly and the other, much larger, had destroyed the whole of Wernicke's area. The possibility of conduction aphasia following a lesion of Wernicke's area, rather than of structures connecting it to Broca's area, has been documented by the case with post-mortem findings described by Benson *et al.* (1973). On the other hand, the study of Damasio and Damasio (1980) confirms the classic localization. These disparities suggest that the current clinical definition of conduction aphasia is perhaps too broad to encompass disorders due to different underlying mechanisms (disruption of phonemic encoding, of short-term verbal memory, etc.) and hence to different lesion sites. In the amnestic aphasia case (*Figure 5,A*), a small zone of the posterior part of T2 was damaged, somewhat marginally located with respect to Wernicke's area — as could be predicted. Finally, the lesions underlying transcortical sensory aphasia (*Figure 5, TS*) in two recent cases (studied after completion of Mazzocchi's and Vignolo's paper) were well in agreement with expectations, as they destroyed a large part of the posterior marginal region, encroaching only a little upon Wernicke's area. When good repetition is associated with both comprehension and severe inertia, a *mixed sensory and motor transcortical aphasia* obtains. This is often referred to, after Goldstein (1917), as 'isolation of the speech area' syndrome, since the lesion describes a wide parasagittal arc, damaging, in particular, both the parieto-occipital and the frontal marginal language areas, as documented by a case of Geschwind *et al.* (1968). CT scan and autopsy evidence of lesions in mixed transcortical aphasia indicate that the posterior marginal areas include the medial aspect of the left parietal lobe (Ross, 1980).

Less severe clinical pictures, with several features resembling trans-cortical aphasias (selectively preserved repetition, in particular) may be due to subcortical vascular lesions confined to the thalamus and, in a few cases, centred on the putamen (*see* below).

Phonemic vs. Lexical–Semantic Errors in Fluent Aphasia

The distinction between phonemic and lexical–semantic errors in the speech of fluent aphasics is important in language examination. Phonemic defects are usually associated with poor repetition and indicate a defect of phonemic

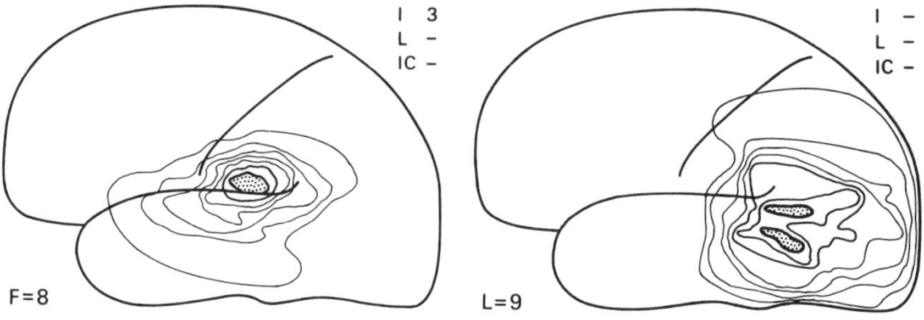

Figure 6 Composite maps of CT scan superficial-and-deep fluent aphasic patients whose speech errors on a naming task were predominantly phonemic (F = 8 cases) and predominantly lexical-semantic (L = 9 cases) (from Cappa *et al.*, 1981).

or phonological encoding (Alajouanine *et al.*, 1964; Vignolo, 1968), whilst lexical–semantic errors appear in association with strikingly good repetition, even in otherwise severe forms of fluent aphasia, such as the transcortical sensory aphasia, and seem to point, rather, to the inability to select the appropriate lexical item in the language's vocabulary.

The hypothesis that the two types of error may be associated with different lesion sites has been investigated by Cappa *et al.*, (1981), who compared CT scan findings in two matched groups of fluent aphasics, 10 with predominantly phonemic speech errors on a naming task and 11 with predominantly lexical errors. The phonemic disorders of speech were found to be associated with convexity lesions further from the sylvian fissure, i.e., more marginally located, as a group (*Figure 6*). These findings support the hypothesis that, within the posterior language zone in the convexity of the left hemisphere, the perisylvian areas, around the sylvian fissure, are more important for processing phonemes than the marginal areas; these, in turn, seem to be more important for processing entire words as meaningful units.

Pure Forms of Aphasia

Patients with so-called pure aphasia (i.e., defect is virtually confined to only one aspect of language) are rare. In the few patients in Mazzocchi's and Vignolo's series, the lesion corresponded to a surprising degree to that expected on the basis of traditional views on localization preceding the introduction of the CT scan.

Alexia without agraphia was associated with the destruction of a large portion of the left occipital lobe. Analogous correlation has been found in a study carried out since in five more cases showing the same disorders. Whatever the interpretation of the syndrome, the anatomically crucial finding seems to consist of the destruction of the posterior callosal pathways coursing leftwards from the intact right occipital lobe. These were consistently interrupted, not by a separate infarct of the splenium (Dejerine, 1892) but, more simply, by the anterior extension of the large occipital lesion, which encroached upon the incoming callosal radiations. Indeed, in the one case whose left occipital lesion lay too posteriorly to involve the callosal pathways, no alexia was found. While a large occipital infarct in the territory of the left posterior cerebral artery seems the most frequent cause of this syndrome (see also the CT scan cases of Orgogozo *et al.* 1979), the occurrence of a deep parietal hematoma undercutting the left angular gyrus (and thereby preventing access from both occipital lobes to it) has been shown to produce a somewhat different type of pure alexia without agraphia ('subangular alexia': Greenblatt, 1976, 1983; Ducarne *et al.*, in press). The syndrome rarely follows a left occipital tumour (four cases on record); in one such case the symptoms were due to compression and resolved after extirpation of the growth (Turgman *et al.*, 1979).

In *isolated agraphia* two small lesions were present, one in the upper half of the central region, the other in the upper part of the posterior parietal lobule. This localization was already specified by Russell and Espir (1961) and confirmed by our own work with Basso and Taborelli (1978). Although small lesions in the left parasagittal or medial parietal areas should be considered crucial in determining this rare syndrome, the possibility that slight damage in other language zones, such as the left perisylvian area, may bring about isolated writing disturbances of long standing has been suggested by the CT scan report of Rosati and De Bastiani (1979), who also provide a useful set of references on this subject.

The site of lesion in pure *anarthria*, defined as a disorder strictly confined to oral expression, which is disrupted in its phonemic and articulatory aspects, is controversial: while the cases observed by Marie (1906) and Moutier (1908) pointed to damage confined to a deep zone referred to as Marie's 'quadrilatère', other investigators, notably Bay (1957) maintained that the lesion could be located in the left prerolandic 'face' area. The syndrome is rarer than claimed by most investigators (notably Tissot *et al.*, 1970, who found it in 4% of aphasics). No case of pure anarthria was present in our series. The recent evidence seems to suggest that damage to the deep and subcortical structures included in Marie's 'quadrilatère' brings about fully fledged, though often atypical, aphasias, rather than the pure dissociated form in question. By contrast, true anarthria with post-mortem findings has been observed following a small superficial lesion of the inferior precentral gyrus producing either a transient syndrome (Tonkonogy and Goodglass, 1981), or a long-standing one (Lecours and Lhermitte, 1979); a transient mutism has been observed following superficial infarction confined to Broca's area alone (Mohr, 1976). These findings agree with a case of mutism evolving into typical pure anarthria after excision of a bleeding arteriovenous malformation, in which the CT scan showed damage extending from Broca's area to the inferior precentral operculum (Ruff and Arbit, 1981).

Typical and Atypical Syndromes Associated with Subcortical Lesions

The occurrence of rather typical aphasic syndromes (such as Broca's etc.) in patients whose CT scans disclosed deep lesions, presumably reaching the insular cortex, has been discussed in preceding paragraphs. In addition to these, however, the recent CT scan literature has laid more stress upon the existence of truly subcortical lesions associated with language disorders (e.g. Alexander and Lo Verme, 1980). The corresponding aphasic pictures may sometimes resemble those due to typical superficial-and-deep lesions of the convexity, but more often they are atypical and difficult to fit into a traditional classification. We shall briefly mention the aphasias due to lesions of (A) the left thalamus and (B) the left basal ganglia and neighbouring white matter.

(A) — A systematic study of all the intracerebral haemorrhages observed in a consecutive series of CT scans performed during almost 2 years (Cappa and Vignolo, 1979) disclosed 10.6% of thalamic haemorrhages — a figure that agrees with those observed by Miller Fisher (1959) and others in the period preceding the use of the CT scan. Aphasia was present in 7 of 8 cases of left thalamic bleeding (*see* example in Figure 7) and in none of 6 cases of right thalamic haemorrhages.

All these cases were examined during the acute period, i.e., within 3 weeks post-stroke; whenever detailed language examination was performed, aphasia was characterized by semantic paraphasias and word-finding defects in spontaneous speech and partially defective comprehension, in

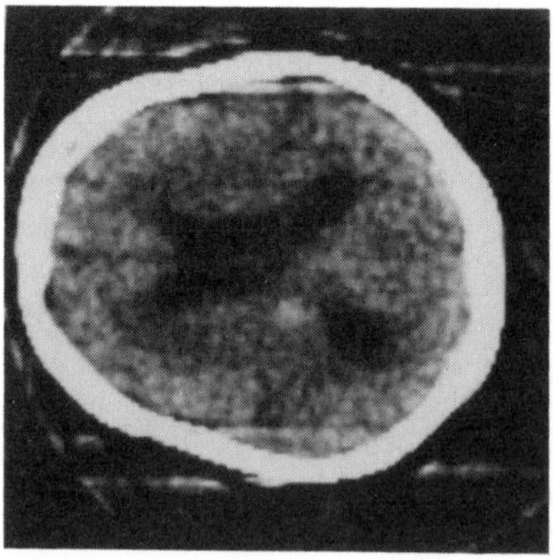

Figure 7 Left thalamic haemorrhage (white, hyperdense area) associated with fluent aphasia (from Cappa and Vignolo, 1979).

sharp contrast to singularly undamaged repetition. This dissociation is similar to that of 'transcortical' aphasias and is present in other case reports of left thalamic haemorrhages and infarcts studied by means of the CT scan (*see* McFarling *et al.* 1982, and Mohr, 1983, for recent sets of references) which strongly suggests that the function of the thalamus is related to that of the so-called marginal language zone, as it concerns principally the use of complete meaningful words rather than that of phonemes. Most thalamic aphasias are transient, which indicates that the function of the thalamus in language, however relevant, is perhaps not as crucial as believed by some authors (notably Penfield and Roberts, 1959).

(B) — The findings concerning the lesions of purely subcortical structures other than the thalamus, i.e., basal ganglia and internal capsule, are less homogeneous, and it is possible that small differences of localisation entail quite different pictures.

Few convincing cases of mild, nonfluent aphasias with some dysarthria have been described (Damasio *et al.*, 1982) following small infarcts of the anterior limb of the internal capsule, encroaching upon the caudate nucleus. Aphasic pictures reportedly similar to those due to thalamic haemorrhages have been observed in association with putaminal haemorrhages. In our experience (Cappa *et al.*, 1983) the language disorders following strictly subcortical lesions confined to the basal ganglia and adjacent structures (excluding the thalamus) are rare (about 1 out of 4 cases with such lesions seen on CT scan), generally mild and presumably transient. More extensive lesions, centred upon the putamen but involving the insula and the adjacent areas of multifiber connections, may lead to more severe and lasting deficits, similar to (though not identical with) Broca's, Wernicke's and global aphasia, depending on the site of the lesion (Naeser *et al.*, 1982). Two cases of logorrhoeic jargonaphasia with intact repetition have been observed following a small caudate haemorrhage (Cambier *et al.*, 1979) and an anatomically verified putaminal infarction (Barat *et al.*, 1981). A typical transcortical motor aphasia has been described in association with internal capsule-putaminal infarct, probably disconnecting the dorsomedial thalamic nucleus from the frontal cortex (Sterzi and Vallar, 1978). A provisional hypothesis advanced at the end of our recent studies (Cappa *et al.*, 1983) is that a crude distinction can be drawn between the *anterior* subcortical lesions (damaging the putamen and the anterior limb of the internal capsule) and the *posterior* subcortical lesions (damaging the putamen and the posterior limb of the internal capsule). The former are sometimes associated with atypical nonfluent aphasias, the latter with mild fluent aphasias (*see* Figure 8). Partial confirmation of this finding came from a subsequent paper by Tanridag and Kirschner in 1985, while other authors, such as Puel *et al.* (1984), failed to find the above-mentioned dichotomy.

In conclusion, while the discovery of subcortical lesions *in vivo* is one of the merits of the CT scan, their semeiologial counterparts are still too inhomogeneous to permit a reliable systematisation, and the possible meaning of the damaged anatomical structures in the cerebral machinery of language deserves further studies.

The Pathology of the Aphasia-producing Lesions

This chapter has dealt exclusively with the aphasias due to circumscribed cerebrovascular lesions, such as infarcts and haemorrhages, for two main reasons. Firstly, these are the most frequent cause of language disorders (up to 70% in a language rehabilitation setting that draws aphasic patients from neurological, neurosurgical, and internal medicine wards of a large university hospital). Secondly, in this kind of pathology the correlation between the clinical picture and the morphology of the stabilized lesion can be made quite reliably, provided that the time from onset is taken into account and the recommendations (set forth in the Materials and Methods) are followed. Other pathologies, however, should be considered. With head trauma, penetrating injuries may entail any form of aphasia (*see* Kleist, 1934; Russell and Espir, 1961) while closed head injuries tend to involve only the hemispheric convexity and, in particular, the marginal areas of the language zone (*see* Luria, 1970) bringing about amnestic (if mild), or transcortical (if severe), aphasias.

Gliomas, malignant cerebral tumours involving glia but largely sparing

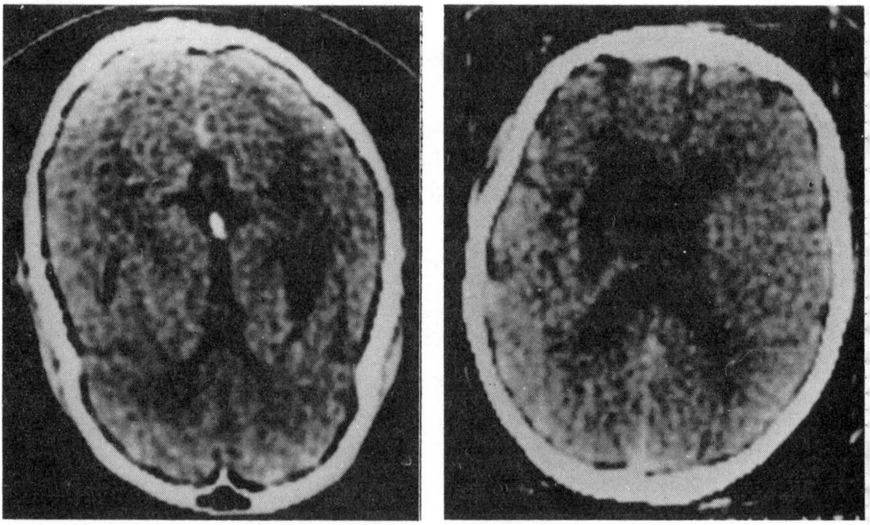

Figure 8 (A) Infarct (black, hypodense area) of anterior limb of left internal capsule and putamen, associated with atypical non-fluent aphasia.
(B) Infarct of posterior limb of left internal capsule and putamen, associated with atypical fluent aphasia (from Cappa *et al.*, 1983).

the neurons as such, may reach considerable size (for example, in the temporal lobe) with surprisingly little language impairment. This can in fact be so slight as to manifest itself merely with occasional anomias; poor auditory comprehension can be detected only by sensitive tests, such as the Token Test (De Renzi and Vignolo, 1962). Excision of such tumours, which entails removal of the neurons as well as the glia, usually brings about a fully fledged aphasia.

This is usually severe, except when the slow rate of growth of the tumour has allowed some compensation of language function to take place. Compensation by healthy cerebral tissue may also be credited for the striking 'tolerance' to long-standing compressive damage due to other slowly growing space-occupying lesions, involving language areas in young adults, such as the hydatid cysts described by Dimitri (1933). Amnestic aphasia, which is the commonest symptom of brain concussion (Heilman *et al.*, 1971) and of infiltrating tumour, is often the first symptom of other progressive diseases involving the posterior marginal areas, such as cortical atrophy and otogenic abscess (an especially frequent occurrence in the pre-antibiotic era: *see* Bonvicini, 1929).

Aphasias of different types have also been described as symptoms of encephalitis and meningo-encephalitis (Linck, 1973). Among these, herpes zoster encephalitis, which tends to selectively involve the temporal lobe, constitutes a particularly severe cause of fluent aphasia.

Conclusions

In spite of its limitations, the CT scan has confirmed the following traditional views on localisation of the language disorders: the anterior (prerolandic) site of lesions in non-fluent aphasias with good comprehension, the posterior site in fluent aphasias, as well as the locus of the damage in pure alexia and pure word deafness. The site of lesions of pure agraphia seems to be left parasagittal, either parietal or frontal. Pure anarthria is more likely to be due to a lesion of the frontal operculum than deeper structures. The expected localisation of lesions in global and conduction aphasia have been confirmed only partially. As far as Broca's aphasia is concerned, an insulo-lenticular lesion would appear to be at least as important as a lesion restricted to the posterior part of the third frontal convolution.

Several fully fledged aphasias, both typical and atypical, are associated with comparatively small lesions, both deep and even purely subcortical, the presence of which *in vivo* can be shown only by the CT scan. This is perhaps the most interesting unexpected finding of recent research in this field.

References

ALAJOUANINE, T., LHERMITTE, F., LEDOUX, M., RENAUD, D. and VIGNOLO, L.A. Les composantes phonémiques et sémantiques de la jargonaphasie. *Revue Neurologique* (1964), **110**, 5-20.

ALEXANDER, M.P. and LO VERME, S.R. Aphasia after left hemispheric intracerebral haemorrhage. *Neurology* (1980), **30**, 1193-1202.

BARAT, M., CONSTANT, P., MAZAUX, J.M., CAILLÉ, J.M. and ARNÉ, L. Corrélations anatomo-cliniques dans l'aphasie. *Revue Neurologique* (1978), **134**, 611-617.

BARAT, M., MAZAUX, J.M., BIOULAC, B., GIROIRE, J.M., VITAL, C. and ARNÉ, L. Troubles du langage de type aphasique et lésions putamino-caudées. *Revue Neurologique* (1981), **137**, 343-356.

BASSO, A., TABORELLI, A. and VIGNOLO, L.A. Dissociated disorders of speaking and writing in aphasia. *Journal of Neurology, Neurosurgery and Psychiatry* (1978), **41**, 556-563.

BASSO, A., SALVOLINI, U. and VIGNOLO, L.A. Localizzazione dei sintomi afasici: osservazioni preliminari con la Tomografia Assiale Computerizzata. *Rivista di Patologia Nervosa e Mentale* (1979), **100**, 93-102.

BASSO, A., CAPITANI, E., LAIACONA, M. and ZENOBIO, M.E. Crossed aphasia: one or more syndromes? *Cortex* (1985), **21**, 25-45.

BAY, E. Die corticale Dysarthrie un ihre Bezeihungen zur sogen motorischen Aphasie. *Deutsche Zeitschrift für Nervenheilkunden* (1957), **176**, 553-594.

BENSON, D.F., SHEREMATA, V.A., BOUCHARD, R., SEGARRA, J., PRICE, D. and GESCHWIND, N. Conduction aphasia. *Archives of Neurology* (1973), **28**, 339-346.

BONVICINI, G. Die Störungen der Lautsprache bei Temporallappenläsionen. In G. Alexander and O. Marburg (eds) *Handbuch der Neurologie des Ohres*, Vol. 2 (1929). Berlin and Vienna: Urban and Schwarzenberg.

CAIL, S.W. and LORRIS, J.L. Localization of intracranial lesions from CT scan. *Surgical Neurology* (1979), **11**, 35-37.

CAMBIER, J., ELGHOZI, and STRUBE, E. Hémorragie de la tête du noyau caudé gauche. *Revue Neurologique* (1979), **135**, 763-774.

CAPPA, S. and VIGNOLO, L.A. 'Transcortical' features of aphasia following left thalamic haemorrhage. *Cortex* (1979), **15**, 121-130.

CAPPA, S., CAVALLOTTI, G. and VIGNOLO, L.A. Phonemic and lexical errors in fluent aphasia: correlation with lesion site, *Neuropsychologia* (1981), **19**, 171-177.

CAPPA, S., CAVALLOTTI, G., GUIDOTTI, M. PAPAGNO, C. and VIGNOLO, L.A. Subcortical aphasias: two clinical CT scan correlation studies. *Cortex* (1983), **19**, 227-242.

DAMASIO, H. and DAMASIO, A.R. The anatomical bases of conduction aphasia. *Brain* (1980), **103**, 337-350.

DAMASIO, A.R., DAMASIO, H.D., RIZZO, M., VARNEY, N and GERSCH, F. Aphasia with non haemorhagic lesions in the basal ganglia and internal capsule. *Archives of Neurology* (1982), **39**, 15-20.

DEJERINE, J. Contributions à l'étude anatomopathologique et clinique des différentes variétés de cécité verbale. *Mémoires de la Société de Biologie* (1892), **4**, 61-90.

DEJERINE, J. *Sémiologie des Affections du Système Nerveux* (1914). Paris: Masson.

DE RENZI, E. and VIGNOLO, L.A. The Token Test: a sensitive test to detect receptive

disturbances in aphasics. *Brain* (1962), **85**, 556–678.
DIMITRI, V. *Aphasias* (1933). Buenos Aires: El Ateneo.
GESCHWIND, N. Aphasia with predominantly subcortical lesion sites: description of three capsular/putaminal aphasia syndromes. *Archives of Neurology* (1982), **39**, 2–14.
GESCHWIND, N., QUADFASEL, F. and SEGARRA, J. Isolation of the speech area. *Neuropsychologia* (1968), **6**, 327–340.
GOLDSTEIN, K. *Die Transkorticalen Aphasien* (1917). Jena: Fischer.
GREENBLATT, S.H. Subangular alexia without agraphia or hemianopia. *Brain and Language* (1976), **3**, 229–245.
GREENBLATT, S.H. Localization of lesions in alexia. In A. Kertesz (ed.) *Localizations in Neuropsychology* (1983). New York: Academic Press.
HAUGHTON, V.M., KHANG-CHENG HO, WILLIAMS, A.L. and ELDEVIK, O.P. CT detection of demielinated plaques in multiple sclerosis. *American Journal of Röntgenology* (1979), **132**, 213–215.
HAYWARD, R.W., NAESER, M.A. and ZARZ, L.M. Cranial computed tomography in aphasia. *Radiology*, (1977), **123,** 653–660.
HEILMAN, K.M., SAFRAN, A. and GESCHWIND, N. Closed head trauma and aphasia. *Journal of Neurology, Neurosurgery and Psychiatry* (1971), **34**, 265–269.
KIMURA, D. Sex differences in intrahemispheric organization of speech. *Behavioral and Brain Sciences* (1980), **3**, 240–241.
KISTLER, J.P., HOCHBERG, F.H., BROOKS, B.R., RICHARDSON, E.P., NEW, P.F.J. and SCHNUR, J. Computerized Axial Tomography: clinicopathologic correlation. *Neurology* (1975), **25**, 201–209.
KLEIST, K. *Gehirnpathologie* (1934). Berlin: Springer.
LASSEN, N.A. and ROLAND, P.E. Localization of cognitive function with cerebral blood flow. In A. Kertesz (ed.) *Localization in Neuropsychology* (1983). New York: Academic Press.
LECOURS, A.R. and LHERMITTE, F. *L'aphasie* (1979). Paris: Flammarion.
LINCK, H.A. Ätiologie und Arten der Aphasie. *Beschäftigungstherapie und Rehabilitation* (1973), **3**, 22–32.
LURIA, A.R. Traumatic aphasia (1970). The Hague: Mouton.
LUZZATTI, C., SCOTTI, G. and GATTONI, A. Further suggestions for cerebral-CT localization. *Cortex* (1979), **15**, 483–490.
MARIE, P. La troisième circonvolution frontale gauche ne joue aucun rôle spécial dans la fonction du langage. *Semaire Médicale* (1906), **26**, 241–247.
MASDEU, J.C., SHOENE, W.C. and FUNKESTEIN, H. Aphasia following infarction of the left supplementary motor area: a clinicopathologic study. *Neurology* (1978), **28**, 1220–1223.
MAZZOCCHI, F. and VIGNOLO, L.A. Computer Assisted Tomography in neuro-psychological research: a simple procedure for lesion mapping. *Cortex* (1978), **14**, 136–144.
MAZZOCCHI, F. and VIGNOLO, L.A. Localization of lesions in aphasia: clinical-CT scan correlations in stroke patients. *Cortex* (1979), **15**, 627–654.
MCFARLING, D., ROTHI, L.J. and HEILMAN, M. Transcortical aphasia from ischaemic infarct of the thalamus: a report of two cases. *Journal of Neurology, Neurosurgery and Psychiatry* (1982), **45**, 107–112.

METTER, E.J., WASTERLAIN, C., KUHL, D.E., HANSON, W.R. and PHELPS, M.E. 18 FDG positron emission computed tomography in a study of aphasia. *Annals of Neurology* (1981), **10**, 173–183.

MILLER FISHER, C. The pathological and clinical aspects of thalamic haemorrhage. *Transactions of the American Neurological Association* (1959), **84**, 56–59.

MOHR, J.P. Broca's area and Broca's aphasia. In H. Whitaker and H. Whitaker (eds) *Studies in Neurolinguistics* I, (1976), pp. 201–236. New York: Academic Press.

MOHR, J.P., PESSIN, M.S., FINKELSTEIN, S., FUNKENSTEIN, H.H., DUNCAN, G.W. and DAVIS, K.R. Broca aphasia: pathologic and clinical. *Neurology* (1978), **28,** 311-324.

MOHR, J.P. Thalamic lesions and syndromes. In A. Kertesz (ed.) *Localization in Neuropsychology* (1983). New York: Academic Press.

MORT, H., LU, C.H., CHUI, L.C., CANCILLA, P.A. and CHRISTIE, J.H. Reliability of computed tomography: correlation with neuropathologic finding. *American Journal of Röntgenology* (1977), **128**, 795–798.

MOUTIER, F. *L'aphasie de Broca* (1908). Paris: Steinheil.

NAESER, M.A. and HAYWARD, R.W. Lesion localization in aphasia with cranial computed tomography and the Boston diagnostic aphasia exam. *Neurology* (1978), **28**, 545–551.

NAESER, M.A., ALEXANDER, M.P., HELM-ESTABROOKS, N., LEVINE, S.A. and

NEW, P.E.G. and SCOTT, W.R. *Computed tomography of the Brain and Orbit* (*EMI scanning*) (1975).Baltimore Md.: Williams and Wilkins.

NIELSEN, J. *Agnosia, Apraxia, Aphasia* (1946, reprinted in 1965). New York: Hafner.

NOEL, G., COLLARD, M., DUPONT, H. and HUVELLE, R. Nouvelles possibilités de corrélations anatomo-cliniques en aphasiologie grâce à la tomodensitometrie cérébrale. *Acta Neurologica Belgica* (1977), **77**, 351–362.

ORGOGOZO, J.M., PERE, J.J. and STRUBE, E. Alexie sans agraphie, 'agnosie' des couleurs et atteinte de l'hémichamp visuel droit: un syndrome de l'artère cérébrale postérieure. *Semaine des Hôpitaux* (1979), **55**, 1389–1394.

PENFIELD, W. and ROBERTS, L. *Speech and Brain Mechanisms* (1959). Princeton, N.J.: Princeton University Press.

PUEL, M., DEMONET, J.F., CARDEBAT, D., BONAFÉ, A., GAZOUNAUD, Y., GUIRAUD-CHAUMEIL, B. and RASCOL, A. Aphasies subcorticales. *Revue Neurologique* (1984), **140**, 695–710.

ROSATI, G. and DE BASTIANI, P. Pure agraphia: a discrete form of aphasia. *Journal of Neurology, Neurosurgery and Psychiatry* (1979), **42**, 266–269.

ROSS, E.D. Left medial parietal lobe and receptive language function: mixed transcortical aphasia after left anterior cerebral artery infarction. *Neurology* (1980), **30**, 144–151.

RUBENS, A.B. Aphasia with infarction in the territory of the anterior cerebral artery. *Cortex* (1975), **11**, 239–250.

RUFF, R.L. and ARBIT, E. Aphemia resulting from left frontal hematoma. *Neurology* (1981), **31**, 353–356.

RUSSELL, W.R. and ESPIR, M.L.E. *Traumatic Aphasia* (1961), London: Butterworths.

SMITH, A. Speech and other functions after left (dominant) hemispherectomy. *Journal of Neurology, Neurosurgery and Psychiatry* (1966), **29**, 467–471.

STERZI, R. and VALLAR, G. Frontal lobe syndrome as a disconnection syndrome: report of a case. *Acta Neurologica* (1978), **33**, 419–425.

TANRIDAG, O. and KIRSHNER, H.S. Aphasia and agraphia in lesions of the posterior internal capsule and putamen. *Neurology* (1985), **35**, 1797–1801.

TISSOT, A., RODRIGUEZ, J. and TISSOT, R. Die prognose der Anarthrie im Sinne von Pierre Marie. In A. Leisehner (ed.) *Die Rehabilitation der Aphasie in den romanischen Ländern* (1970). Stuttgart: Thieme.

TOGNOLA, G. and VIGNOLO, L.A. Brain lesions associated with oral apraxia in stroke patients: a clinico-neuroradiological investigation with the CT scan. *Neuropsychologia* (1980), **18**, 257-272.

TONKONOGY, J. and GOODGLASS, H. Language function, foot of the third frontal gyrus and rolandic operculum. *Archives of Neurology* (1981), **38**, 486–490.

TURGMAN, J., GOLDHAMMER, Y. and BRAHAM, J. Alexia without agraphia, due to brain tumor: a reversible syndrome. *Annals of Neurology* (1979), **6**, 265–268.

VIGNOLO, L.A. The relationship between the repetition defect and the type of speech errors in fluent aphasia: cross sectional and longitudinal findings. In *Proceedings of the Conference of Language Retraining for Aphasics* (1968). Columbus: Ohio State University, Ohio State University Press.

VIGNOLO, L.A. TC: utilità e limité nella correlazione tia sede delle lesione e deficit neuropsicologici. In Parserini, A., Bergamini, L. and Loeb, C. (Eds.) *La Tomografia Computerizzatá nella Diagnostica Neurologica* (1918). Milano. Masson Italia Edition.

VIGNOLO, L.A., FREDIANI, F., BOCCARDI, E. and CAVERNI, L. Unexpected CT scan findings in global aphasia. *Cortex* (1986), **22**, 55–70.

VON MONAKOW, K. *Die Lokalisation im Grosshirn und der Abbau der Functionen durch cortikale Herde.* (1914). Wiesbaden: Bergmann.

10

The Clinical Neurology of Aphasia

M.E.L. Espir and F. Clifford Rose

It is perhaps ironic that the remarkable upsurge of interest in aphasia in recent years was concomitant with an increasing estrangement from this field of study by clinical neurologists, with the expropriation of many aspects in aphasia research from the domain of clinical neurology. Linguists now offer analyses of aphasic speech patterns and psychologists deal with cognitive processes in ways which most neurologists are not trained. This development is due not only to the increasing sophistication and diversity of aphasia research, both empirical and theoretical, but also to the conceptual simplicity, or indeed, oversimplicity, that underlines clinical relevance. The number of publications on aphasiology since the end of the second World War far exceeds that of the preceding eight decades since Broca's seminal reports but, despite enormous developments in brain imaging techniques, basic concepts in this field are still based on those of the early neurologists, notably Wernicke and Hughlings-Jackson. This paradox suggests that there is something singular to the clinical neurology of aphasia which justifies an attempt to define its domain. The first aim of the clinical neurologist is diagnosis so that he needs to know the cerebral localization of function which in aphasia is the anatomical substrate of language.

The attempt by Gall to localize mental function according to the shape of the skull marks the beginning of modern neurology, whilst Broca's pathological finding of a cavity 'the size of a hen's egg' in the left second and third frontal convolutions was the beginning of modern aphasiology. Wernicke's classification of aphasic syndromes, neatly propagated by Lichtheim in 1885, was based on the concept of localized speech centres which, despite numerous controversies, probably underlies the great attractiveness of his ideas to date. Although the consequences of modern brain imaging are reviewed elsewhere in this volume, there is one fundamental issue in the study of brain function that should be briefly considered here viz, the controversy between holistic and localization approaches. From Hughlings-Jackson to Critchley, the holistic approach dominated British aphasiology, whereas most continental neurologists preferred localizationist models, notwithstanding prominent exceptions such as Marie, Pick and Goldstein. In the two decades following the second World War, holistic views predominated in the United States with workers such as Lashley, Wepman and Sperry, but this has now given away to localizationist views despite, again, a few notable exceptions (*see* chapter by Jason Brown). Typical of the swing of the pendulum between these opposing views is the conclusion to a recent study of the impact of brain imaging on localization:

> 'it can no longer be doubted that Gall was right when he suggested in 1825 that the human brain is not a functionally homogeneous organ distributing 'vital energy' with sovereign indifference. It also can no longer be doubted that the anatomo-clinical method has been and will long remain productive, and that one of the notions it has yielded — that of the 'speech area' — is valid. Nonetheless, it is now getting more and more obvious that the biological, psychological and social determinants of functional specialisation interact . . . in a most complex fashion, and that standard contemporary teaching about the speech area and the mutual relationships of brain and language does not apply uniformly to the whole of mankind. Cheer up. A lot of work remains to be done in our field'. (Lecours *et al.*, 1984; p. 238).

A similar proposition can be put in more holistic terms, namely, that, for the localizationist approach to survive the recent findings of brain imaging techniques, the concept of 'locus' should be replaced with the less used topological notion of 'neighbourhood' as a more flexible unbounded region and, further, that variations of such neighbourhoods occur not only between, but also within, individuals, depending on both physiological and cognitive determinants. Even with this formulation, lesions in different neighbourhoods can produce similar or even identical deficits, denying the specific mapping of cognitive function to anatomical structures.

Another aspect of aphasiology that concerns the clinical neurologist is the behavioural impact of language disturbance, especially in its effects on action (praxis). Again, the most notable contributions were made by neurologists, for example, Benson's (1979) study of neurological aspects of anomia, Weinstein's (1981) study of behavioural aspects of jargonaphasia etc. Whilst this focus bears more on the issue of 'management', i.e. communicating with, and rehabilitating, the aphasic patient, that of praxis bears more on the theoretical relationship between motor and symbolic function. Here again, some of the most prominent contributions are made by neurologists (*see* chapter by Poeck) because of their clinical experience. Despite the attraction of concentrating on 'dissociation' of function, e.g., the conceptual separability of cognitive functions and the theoretical elegance of modular psychology, although some deficits of language performance can be very focused, impairment results usually favour a disturbance of more than one unitary function. This point has been demonstrated most convincingly with regard to language and motor function, which may be a methodological coincidence since production deficits are usually easier to detect than reception deficits. This suggests that, localization notwithstanding, the neurons that encode and decode language may be involved in other functions as well (*see* chapter by Feyereisen). In the words of a recent study, 'In contrast to the model of a simple machine or reflex action, we need to pay attention to the potential plurality of capabilities of the same anatomic "hardware"' (Martin and Gordon, 1979; p. 308).

Another concern that requires the experience and observation of clinical neurology is the effects of pharmacological treatment. Many drugs prescribed for specific purposes, be they hypotensives, psychotropics, antidepressants or tranquillisers, affect speech, with far-reaching implications. For example, whilst clinical experience is almost the only way these may be uncovered, some neurological disorders, e.g. Parkinsonian speech problems, can be directly investigated by pharmacological effects.

Traditionally, the clinical description of typical cases establishes the 'essence' or 'core' of the different syndromes, an ever controversial subject, whilst rare cases sketch the 'periphery', range and potential diversity of such syndromes. The most recent contributions from clinical neurology closely interact with anatomical perspectives, e.g., the documenting of 'crossed' and 'subcortical' aphasias, which emphasises that aphasiology is inherently an interdisciplinary subject, so that most case studies require the concerted input from neurologist, language pathologist and neuropsychologist.

Epidemiological considerations are also of supreme importance e.g. the incidence of aphasia following brain damage, the likelihood and extent of recovery in relation to severity, treatment and aphasia type, etc. Epidemiological data provide a good idea of prognosis and, remembering that aphasia is a social phenomenon in more than one respect, offer simple and accessible information to general practitioners and relatives without recourse to complex considerations. Differences between aphasias of varying etiologies (head injury, neurosurgery, stroke, etc.) are ascertained more easily by epidemiological, rather than neurological or neuropsychological, investigations. This may change with the advent of dynamic brain imaging techniques (e.g., PET scanning, rCBF and to some extent MRI), where more direct evidence on pathophysiology can be obtained but, until then, epidemiological studies offer invaluable information (*see* also Wade *et al.*, 1986).

The clinical neurologist can contribute to aphasiology first and foremost an experience with a wide range of neurological patients and the ability to compare and associate (rather than dissociate) deficits to which other specialists, be they language pathologists or neuropsychologists, are only seldom exposed. Secondly, and in close relation to the first, the neurologist must observe and keep alert to the rare case or drug effect that may provide novel insight. Thirdly, the neurologist offers a knowledge of anatomy and physiology of both the central and the peripheral motor systems, which again may not always be available to other specialists in the field.

The Clinical Approach

In attempting to unravel a case of aphasia or, for that matter, any neurological problem the clinician must answer two important questions: What is the lesion? and where is the lesion? Although the location and extent of the lesion determine the type and severity of the dysphasia, the mode of onset and course depend on the pathology. Sometimes the anatomical location provides helpful clues to the disease mechanism, since different pathological processes have predilections for different loci within the nervous system. The pathological cause is best sought by analysing the history, e.g. the age of onset, particularly as the effect of disorders during the development of speech will have different features from those with disruption of the fully developed function. A relentlessly progressive course without remissions suggests a degenerative or neophasic process, whilst a late age of onset argues against a congenital or inherited metabolic disorder, which would be favoured by the presence of a family history or genetic pattern.

A long duration, lack of systemic symptoms or signs, and the normality of spinal fluid, serological tests and radiological investigatons would tend to exclude toxic, traumatic, neoplastic, infectious and inflammatory disorders.

Because the left cerebral hemisphere is dominant for language in over 99% of right-handers and in 60–70% of left-handers, dysphasia will result only rarely from right hemisphere lesions and, when it does, the patient is likely to be left-handed. It is therefore always worth inquiring about handedness, bearing in mind the possibility of right cerebral dominance.

Although disorders of speech function can be described only in psychological terms, and development of speech is dependent on the integrity of all its parts, nevertheless specific disorders of speech function do occasionally occur, as evidenced by the cases of 'pure' word blindness, word deafness, motor aphasia and agraphia. Controversy continues as to whether various parts of the cerebral cortex are solely concerned with specific functions and, although speech is clearly linked with memory and other mental faculties, localized lesions of the speech area, particularly at its periphery, have resulted in the recognition of specific syndromes, each corresponding with small areas of cortical damage.

Traditionally, speech mechanisms have been considered in their setting in the hierarchy of higher cerebral function which have been regarded as residing within the cerebral cortex and the so-called association regions. These regions of the cortex were related to complex linguistic, visual-spatial and other cognitive functions.

Since Broca, aphasia has been attributed to the specialized language area in the dominant cerebral hemisphere, and relatively recently detailed anatomical studies have shown structural differences between the left and right temporal gyri, the temporo-parietal area being larger in the dominant hemisphere. Even more recently, advances in neurochemistry and positron-emission tomographic scanning has shown that the deeper gray structures, the basal ganglia, deep forebrain nuclei and diencephalic nuclei also have an integral role in behaviour and cognition. Some cases of dementia have been attributed to deficiency of cholinergic neurotransmission, possibly due to degeneration of the basal nucleus of Meynert. Lesions limited to the basal ganglia, caudate nucleus and thalamus can also cause aphasia, a cognitive function which is therefore not solely controlled by the dominant perisylvian cerebral cortex. The fact that some diseases primarily affecting the subcortical and basal nuclei can cause intellectual decline has led to the term 'subcortical dementia'. Aphasia may therefore indicate a focal cerebral lesion, and its neurological importance must not be disregarded as it may be amenable to surgical treatment. On the other hand the speech disorder may be part of the general impairment of mental faculties due to diffuse diseases such as Alzheimer's, the frontal and temporal lobar atrophy of Pick's disease and subcortical arteriosclerotic encephalopathy (Binswanger's disease). Diagnostic difficulty can arise in these conditions if aphasia preceeds dementia, i.e. before they merge into one another.

Mesulam (1982) described 6 patients with progressive aphasia without generalized dementia, the cause of which was not established. Kirshner *et al.* (1984) described 6 other patients whose illness began with aphasia, with the later development of progressive generalized dementia; again the cause was not found. Yet another form has been described of a familial disorder called hereditary dysphasic dementia; this is transmitted in an autosomal dominant fashion and affects older members in successive generations, the earliest symptoms being reduction in speech output with diminished fluency and a cardinal feature. All the patients became globally aphasic and mute within 5 years and some had parkinsonian features. At autopsy, spongiform degeneration of the external layers of the cerebral cortex and changes in the substantia nigra and locus coaeruleus were found, together with hydrocephalus. Aphasia and dementia may also develop together in Creutzfeldt–Jakob disease, usually progressing rapidly with the other diagnostic features of this condition.

In the subcortical dementias, there is usually slowness of speech and action, difficulty in using previously acquired knowledge, and early and progressive motor abnormalities. Memory is relatively preserved. The Steele–Richardson–Olszewski syndrome (progressive supranuclear palsy) usually starts with parkinsonism, accompanied by slowness and later loss of voluntary eye movements, particularly in vertical directions, and dementia may develop, very rarely as the earliest feature, and pure aphasia would not be expected in this condition.

The distinction of dysphasia from dementia is thus very important. About 10–15% of patients with dementia who come to a neurological unit have treatable causes. These are: normal-pressure hydrocephalus, endogenous depression, brain tumours, hypothyroidism, neurosyphilis and subdural haematomas. About 40% of strokes cause dysphasia, and as a rule a sudden onset with gradual recovery typifies cerebral infarction. Brief recurrent stereotyped disturbances of speech are usually due to transient ischaemic attacks or focal epilepsy. Abrupt onset of dysphasia sometimes following an epileptic attack can occur with an abscess or tumour although the latter usually runs a progressive course. Transient dysphasia can also occur as the aura of migraine attacks.

References

BENSON, D.F. Neurologic correlates of anomia. In H. Whitaker and H.A. Whitaker (eds) *Studies in Neurolinguistics* vol. 4 (1979). New York: Academic Press.

KIRSHNER, H.S. *et al.* Language disturbance: an initial symptom of cortical degenerations and dementia. *Archives of Neurology* (1984), **41**, 491–496.

LECOURS, A.E., BASSO, A., MORASCHINI, S. and NESPOULOUS, J-L. Where is the speech area and who has seen it? In D. Caplan, A.R. Lecours and A. Smith (eds) *Biological Perspectives on Language* (1984). Cambridge (MA.): MIT Press.

MARIN, O.S. and GORDON, B. Neuropsychologic aspects of aphasia. In R. Tyler and D. Dawson (eds) *Current Neurology, Vol. II*, (1979). Boston: Houghton Mifflin.

MESULAM, M-M. Slowly progressive aphasia without generalized dementia. *Annals of Neurology* (1982), **11**, 592–598.

MORRIS, J.C. *et al.* Hereditary dysphasic dementia and the Pick-Alzheimer spectrum. *Annals of Neurology* (1984), **16**, 455–466.

WADE, D.T., HEWER, R.L., DAVID, R.M. and ENDERBY, P.M. Aphasia after stroke: natural history and associated deficits. *Journal of Neurology, Neurosurgery and Psychiatry* (1986), **49**, 11–16.

WEINSTEIN, E.A. Behavioral aspects of jargonaphasia. In J.W. Brown (ed.) *Jargonaphasia* (1981). New York: Academic Press.

11

Subcortical Aphasia

Claus-W. Wallesch and Costanza Papagno

Carl Wernicke (1874) had no doubt that destruction of the left lenticular nucleus resulted in aphasia, which he ascribed to a lesion of fibers converging from the frontal cortex upon the basal ganglia. Classical aphasiologists used the term 'subcortical aphasia' to denote the hypothetical disconnection effect of a subcortical fiber lesion, but the term is now used for those language disturbances resulting from a lesion of the deep nuclei of the cerebral hemispheres, the basal ganglia or the thalamus. Whether a lesion limited to subcortical nuclear structures is really sufficient to produce aphasia is still controversial and unequivocal evidence is scarce. On the other hand, if it was unmistakably proven that the deep nuclei participate in language functions proper — excluding such processes as focussing of attention, memory, consciousness, and drive — this would necessarily have profound implications upon theories concerning the cerebral representation of language.

In the early days of aphasiology, Broadbent (1872) assumed that the corpora striata were the cerebral organs in which words were generated as motor acts. Kussmaul (1877) opposed this view and claimed that the functions of the striate bodies were entirely motor, and — in the case of speech production — purely articulatory.

The first systematic study of the effects of subcortical lesions upon language was undertaken by Pierre Marie's pupil, Moutier, in his monumental doctoral thesis (1908). Following the views of his teacher, Moutier tried to substantiate the theories of the unity of aphasic syndromes and of the 'quadrilateral zone' as its critical focus. Marie's zone extended subcortically and indeed had no limit in the depth of the left hemisphere. Moutier described three patients whose brain lesions were found at autopsy not to extend into the cortex and who were all non-fluently aphasic. Their language symptoms resolved within weeks or months, leaving one patient with a stutter and another with hesitant speech.

The problem whether or not there was a representation of language functions in the deep nuclei was one aspect of cerebral localization and consequently receded into the background when the controversy between holists and localizationists paralysed neuropsychology.

The interest in a possible function of the deep nuclei in language processing started anew when Penfield and Roberts (1959) proposed that thalamic nuclei were engaged in the transmission of information from the posterior to the anterior language areas. By that time neurosurgeons began to stereotactically operate upon the deep nuclei and modern research into their participation in language processes started. Before the results of this research can be presented in detail, some anatomical facts must be considered.

Anatomy and Physiology

The grey nuclei in the depth of the cerebral hemispheres consist of three major ganglia: the lentiform (lentil-shaped) nucleus beneath the insula, the caudate nucleus which stretches along the lateral wall of the lateral ventricle being shaped like a large tadpole, and the thalamus which forms a large part of the wall of the third ventricle (*Figure 1*). The lentiform and caudate nuclei together are part of the basal ganglia and belong to the forebrain, the thalamus to the diencephalon.

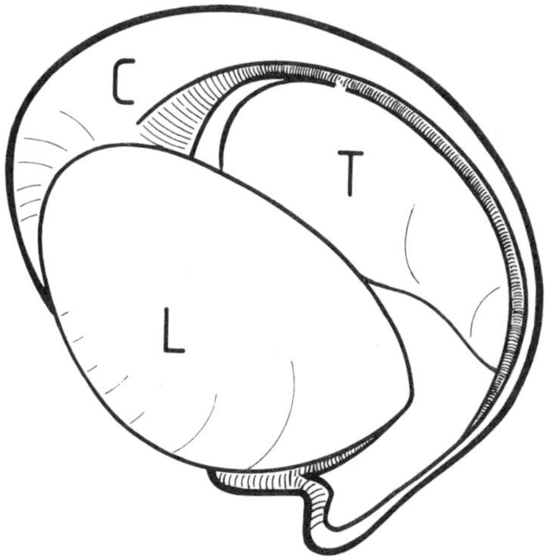

Figure 1 Posterolateral view of the deep nuclei of the left cerebral hemisphere. C: caudate nucleus, L: lenticular nucleus, T: thalamus. Based on a drawing from Nieuwenhuys, R., Voogd, J. and van Huijzen, C. *The Human Central Nervous System* (1978). Berlin: Springer.

The lentiform nucleus is separated both from the thalamus and from the caudate nucleus by the major efferent pathway of the cerebral cortex, the internal capsule, the funnel shape of which matches the nucleus' cone-shaped appearance. The lentiform nucleus is subdivided into two parts: the putamen at the base and the globus pallidus at the tip of the cone.

The caudate nucleus consists of a voluminous head, lateral to the frontal horn, which tapers off to the smaller corpus along the pars centralis of the ventricle and finally to the long tail extending along the temporal horn. Putamen and caudate nucleus together form the neostriatum and are functionally closely connected, their subdivision by the internal capsule and therefore their relative sizes varying among mammalian species (Parent, 1986).

The cerebral cortex of each lobe projects in a topographically organized fashion both upon the caudate nucleus and upon the putamen (Kemp and Powell, 1970). Associative areas of the prefrontal, temporal and parietal cortex are connected mainly with the caudate nucleus (Goldman and Nauta, 1977; Ragsdale and Graybiel, 1981), and the precentral motor cortex mainly with the putamen (Künzle, 1975). These findings indicate that at least in primates the caudate is more closely related to complex and associative behaviour than the putamen (Alexander *et al.*, 1986). Furthermore, for the assumption of nonmotor functions of the basal ganglia, the important fact is that the projections of 'association cortex' increase in phylogenetic ascension (Kemp and Powell, 1970).

Cytoarchitectonically defined cortical areas project upon defined regions within the neostriatum (Kemp and Powell, 1970; Yeterian and van Hoesen, 1978). Such cortical areas which are cortico-cortically connected are linked with overlapping and interdigitated cell groups within the neostriatum (Yeterian and van Hoesen, 1978; van Hoesen *et al.*, 1981; Selemon and Golman-Rakic, 1985). Both Broca's and Wernicke's areas are supposed to project upon the same regions in the head of caudate (Damasio, 1983). The projections from the supplementary motor cortex upon the head of the caudate and from the motor cortex upon the putamen are bilateral (Kemp and Powell, 1970; Künzle, 1975). Apart from cortical afferents, both putamen and caudate receive projections from the substantia nigra and from mainly nonspecific thalamic nuclei (Parent, 1986). The internal structure of the neostriatum is still little understood but there seem to exist two efferent systems which give rise to relatively few excitatory projections and a much larger number of inhibitory collaterals. This output organization indicates an integrative function for the neostriatum (Groves, 1983).

Neostriatal efferents lead to the pallidum and to the substantia nigra in the midbrain. The pallidum receives mainly neostriatal and few thalamic afferents and projects upon the subthalamic nucleus and upon the nuclei of the ventral (VA and VL) and nonspecific thalamus. The pallidal efferents are

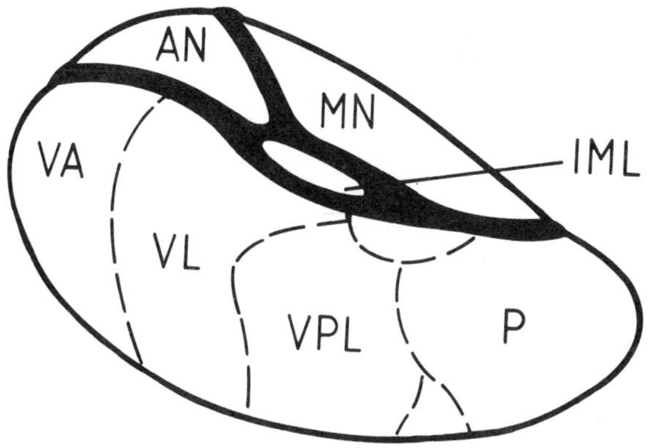

Figure 2 Lateral view of the left thalamus. VA: ventral anterior nucleus, VL: ventral lateral nucleus, VPL: ventral posterolateral nucleus, P: pulvinar, AN: anterior nucleus, MN: medial nuclei, IML: internal medullary laminae and intralaminar nuclei. Based on a drawing from Wallesch, C.W. and Wyke, M.A. Language and the subcortical nuclei. In S. Newman and R. Epstein (eds) *Current perspectives in Dysphasia* (1985). Edinburgh: Churchill-Livingstone.

considered to be inhibitory (Uno *et al.*, 1978; Penney and Young, 1981).

Rosvold and collaborators (e.g. Rosvold and Szwarcbart, 1964) demonstrated behavioral changes in delayed response tasks as occur with frontal lobe pathology following lesions in the head of the caudate; on the basis of their findings, they postulated a frontal lobe system, which included the prefrontal cortex, the head of the caudate, pallidum, substantia nigra and the subthalamic nucleus. In essence, they proposed an interaction of cortical and subcortical structures to occur at least in some cognitive operations.

The thalamus is not a homogeneous structure but consists of more than 30 anatomically and functionally separable nuclei. Y-shaped white matter sheets, the internal medullary laminae, separate the thalamus into five major groups of nuclei, the anterior, medial, ventral, posterior and the 'non-specific' intralaminar and midline nuclei (Walker, 1938; Williams and Warwick, 1975, *Figure 2*). A participation in language processes has been proposed mainly for the ventral anterior (VA) and the ventral lateral nucleus (VL) of the ventral group, and for the pulvinar, which is the largest of the posterior nuclei. In what follows, VA and VL together will sometimes be referred to as ventral thalamus. With respect to their way of cortical projections, the thalamic nuclei have been subdivided into specific (projecting upon circumscribed cortical regions) and nonspecific. As the thalamic nuclei are strongly interconnected with each other, it must be assumed that they do not only act as relays, as was traditionally supposed, but integrate and transform information passing through. Therefore possibly other thalamic nuclei, which are not directly linked with the cortical language areas, may be involved in language processing.

VA and VL are the main thalamic projections of pallidal and cerebellar fibers. Both nuclei also receive afferents from the substantia nigra (Mehler, 1971) and from the limbic, frontal and parietal cortex (Kaitz and Robertson, 1981; Robertson and Cunningham, 1981; Sakai, 1982). They project upon the motor (VL mainly) and premotor (VA mainly) cortex. Wise and Strick (1984) point out, that via VA and VL, the supplementary motor cortex receives a prominent input from the basal ganglia, whereas the premotor cortex receives a major input from the cerebellum. The thalamocortical projections are probably excitatory, but it appears that they act upon inhibitory interneurones (Creutzfeldt, 1983).

According to Mehler (1971) a rigid separation of VA and VL seems rather artificial, as their projectional organization gradually changes between the nuclei. This projectional continuum should be considered when data are discussed which refer to either one of the ventral thalamic nuclei. Evarts *et al.* (1984) have neurophysiologically demonstrated that the function of cortical cells of area 4 are being modulated to a large extent by the thalamic afferent. The VA and VL projection upon areas 4 and 6 of the frontal lobe closes the probably most important loop for subcortical language processing, which runs from almost the whole cerebral cortex to the neostriatum, the pallidum, the ventral thalamus and then to the dorsolateral frontal language area. The function of this loop probably can be modulated by the substantia nigra, the supplementary motor area, other thalamic nuclei, frontal and limbic cortex. Especially for the supplementary motor area an intimate interaction with the loop must be assumed.

The other thalamic nucleus for which a participation in language processing has been specifically claimed is the pulvinar. It is bidirectionally connected with the retrorolandic cortex with the exceptions of the occipital pole and the basal and medial temporal cortex. It is the specific thalamic afferent and efferent projection nucleus for most of the temporoparietal association cortex including the posterior language area. Neurophysiologically, the pulvinar has been demonstrated to contain neurones which are activated with visually guided arm and gaze movements (Acuña *et al.*, 1983).

A role in the pathology of communication has been claimed not only for the specific relay nuclei, which project to defined structures in the cerebral cortex, but also for some of the nonspecific thalamic nuclei, which are supposed to relay arousal from the reticular formation of the brain stem to the cerebral hemispheres (Morrison and Dempsey, 1942), thereby turning on and off cortical processors. The largest of these nonspecific thalamic nuclei, the centrum medianum, was even considered by Penfield and Roberts (1959) to be involved in the transmission of linguistic information from the posterior language area via pulvinar, centrum medianum and the specific prefrontal projections nucleus, the dorsomedian, to the anterior language area.

By far the greatest number of naturally occurring lesions in the deep nuclei are vascular, which necessitates some knowledge of vascular anatomy and pathology for the functional interpretation of subcortical aphasia syndromes.

The putamen with the exception of its anterior pole, the lateral pallidum and the caudate nucleus with the exception of the rostral and basal part of its head, are supplied by lenticulostriate branches of the main stem of the middle cerebral artery (*see* e.g. Lazorthes *et al.*, 1976, for discussion of the vascularization of the deep nuclei). Consequently, the majority of infarctions in these structures and the surrounding white matter result from occlusions of the main stem of the middle cerebral artery (*see* Ringelstein *et al.*, 1985, for aspects of vascular pathogenesis) and effects of ischemia upon the cerebral cortex must be taken into account. The rostral and basal parts of the head of the caudate and the frontal poles of putamen and pallidum receive their blood supply from the anterior cerebral artery by the recurrent artery of Heubner. Most of the pallidum is vascularized by the anterior choroidal artery, which is not a branch of the middle cerebral artery but stems from the internal carotid directly (Krayenbühl and Yasargil, 1965). The area of supply of this artery includes cortex only at the basal surface of the temporal lobe. Therefore the effects of anterior choroidal infarction serve as valid arguments in favour of a participation of the deep nuclei in language functions, as the area of supply of the middle cerebral artery with all its cortical language areas can be considered not ischemic (Wallesch, 1985).

Thalamic vascularization is even more complex and differs inter-individually. According to Percheron (1976) in 60–70% the thalamus receives its principal blood supply from the posterior communicating artery and a lesser amount from the posterior choroidal artery. In the other 30 to 40 per cent the main thalamic blood supply stems from branches of the posterior cerebral artery. Normally, VA and VL are supplied by the tuberothalamic artery from the posterior communicating artery. The pulvinar receives its supply mainly from geniculothalamic branches of the posterior cerebral artery. An inconstant amount of the lateral thalamus is vascularized by the anterior choroidal artery. Since the middle cerebral artery plays no part in supplying the thalamus, symptoms of thalamic infarction cannot be accounted for by middle artery ischemia.

Clinical Evidence

Basal Ganglia

The advent of stereotactic surgery for the relief of parkinsonian symptoms in the late 1950s led to an increasing number of postoperative speech and language alterations, in most instances transient. These disturbances resulted from a lesion of a preoperatively pathological brain. Most operations were performed on the thalamus, but in the early days of stereotaxis (until about 1960) the pallidum was also lesioned. Surgeons used electrical stimulation to determine the optimal site of surgery and, with this procedure, other structures e.g. the head of the caudate (van Buren, 1963) could also be investigated.

Both caudate (van Buren, 1963) and pallidal (Hermann *et al.*, 1966) stimulation resulted in the arrest of ongoing speech. Van Buren (1963) noted that speech arrest under caudate stimulation was not noticed by the patients, who seemed 'unaware that anything out of the ordinary had happened' (p. 156) which differed from patients under cortical stimulation. Impairments of speech following surgery on the pallidum were observed by Cooper (1961), these deficits being mainly dysarthric, although more specific language changes including paraphasia following lesions of the pallidum of the dominant side were also reported (Svennilson *et al.* 1960). On the whole, the evidence derived from stereotactic manipulation of the basal ganglia is scanty and operations upon these structures ceased in the early 60ies following the introduction of L-dopa therapy.

When the CT scan came into general clinical use, an increasing number of language disturbances related to lesions in the basal ganglia and thalamus were reported, including patients who also had cortical damage (e.g. Naeser *et al.*, 1982). In the following, we shall present only those cases where a cortical lesion detectable by CT had been excluded and will then discuss whether cortical dysfunction has to be considered as a possible cause of the deficit. This approach seems imperative, as certain types of deep infarctions are typically caused by middle cerebral artery main stem occlusions, which may also affect cortical language areas (Ringelstein and collaborators, 1985). As there is a wide gap in the metabolic rate necessary for maintenance of structure and the rate needed for proper functioning, brain regions may well be damaged in function following ischemia but appear intact on CT. Microscopic hypoxic damage giving neuronal or synaptic loss may also escape detection by CT and even macroscopic examination at autopsy.

That 'subcortical aphasia' following basal ganglia lesions was the result of cortical hypoperfusion was stressed by Skyhöj Olsen *et al.* (1986), who studied regional cerebral blood flow in aphasic and nonaphasic patients with subcortical lesions of the left hemisphere. They found in 5 aphasic patients with subcortical lesions a focal low-flow area in rCBF, whereas in 5 nonaphasic patients no focal low-flow was noted. The authors interpret their findings as indicating that in 'subcortical aphasia' cortical hypoperfusion is the underlying cause of aphasic symptomatology and, consequently, they 'question the existence of significant aphasic impairment of truly subcortical origin' (p. 408).

These findings certainly constitute important evidence. The lesion size of the patients without aphasia was markedly smaller than that of patients with subcortical lesions with aphasia. With one exception, a caudate haemorrhage, the patients with subcortical lesions without aphasia exhibited damage exclusively in white matter structures. According to Wallesch *et al.* (1983a) the effects of subcortical white matter lesions on language are much less pronounced than that of nuclear lesions. Of those 5 subcortical lesions (Skyhöj Olsen *et al.* 1986) which resulted in aphasia and were investigated with rCBF, 4 showed evidence of middle cerebral artery occlusion on angiography. The fifth, however, had suffered a lentiform nucleus hematoma of 3 cm diameter which, perusal of the CT scans showed, extended into the insula.

A similar investigation was undertaken by Perani *et al.* (in press), who also found cortical hypoperfusion in those patients with left subcortical lesions who were aphasic. These included two patients with thalamic, and two with basal ganglia, lesions. Perani *et al.* consider it unlikely that mass effects or ischemia caused cortical hypoperfusion and suggested a transient depression of function in those cortical structures receiving afferents from the lesioned sites. This mechanism resembles von Monakow's (1914) concept of 'diaschisis'.

Regional cerebral perfusion is closely correlated with regional cerebral metabolism, which has been shown to decrease in the left thalamus in patients suffering from aphasia with superficial CT-lesions (Metter *et al.*, 1981) Conversely, even small thalamic lesions led to cortical hypometabolism in those patients in whom a neuropsychological deficit was present (Baron *et al.*, 1986). In animal experiments, lesions confined to the pallidum resulted in an ipsilateral reduction of cortical metabolism (London *et al.* 1984). Following the argument of Perani *et al.* (in press), the presence of a focal cortical low-flow or hypometabolism area in patients suffering from aphasia with subcortical lesions may give evidence that only a disturbance at any location within a cortical–subcortical language system is present. That the production of language in normal subjects may involve cortical and subcortical structures has been suggested by Wallesch *et al.* (1985) who found, using SPECT, a lateralization of rCBF-increase in left cortical and subcortical sites with language, but not to the same extent with articulatory, tasks. The subcortical flow increase occurred mainly in the left pallidal-anterior thalamic and posterior thalamic regions but the low resolution of the system did not allow a precise location of the region in which blood flow increased.

From Moutier's (1908) pioneering work until the introduction of CT scan in clinical neurology little consideration was given to the possibility of the basal ganglia participating in the cerebral representation of language functions. The first single case reports of aphasia resulting from caudate and putaminal infarctions and haemorrhages, identified using the new diagnostic tool, were published in the late 70s (Hier *et al.*, 1977; Cambier *et al.*, 1979; Kornhuber *et al.*, 1979). The haemorrhages happened to be rather large and compression and edema effects upon the cerebral cortex could not safely be disregarded, and with infarctions the objections mentioned above must be considered. Among the first systematic studies was that of Damasio *et al.* (1982) who described an atypical aphasia syndrome occurring with subcortical infarctions involving the head of the caudate nucleus, the anterior limb of the internal capsule, and the anterior putamen. The most constant feature was the presence of semantic paraphasia. Fluency, presence of phonemic paraphasias, deficits of repetition and comprehension varied among patients. Damasio *et al.* related the language symptomatology to lesions of either the head of the caudate nucleus or to lesions of fibers in the anterior limb of the internal capsule, namely projections from the auditory association cortex to the head of the caudate, or the frontothalamic connections. This syndrome of paraphasic aphasia with lesions in the area of supply of the anterior lenticulostriate branches of the middle cerebral artery had earlier been described by Barat *et al* (1981) and was confirmed by Wallesch (1985), who pointed out that, with this type of lesion, disturbances of cortical functions cannot be excluded, as they usually result from occlusions of the main stem of the middle cerebral artery.

Another syndrome of aphasia was first described by Sterzi and Vallar (1978) and later confirmed by Brunner *et al.* (1982) and Wallesch (1985). Brunner *et al.* found in 8 patients in the acute stage either 'Broca's aphasia with transcortical features or nominal aphasia' (p. 289); in all but two cases they had circumscribed infarctions of the lenticular nucleus as the only subcortical nuclear structure. One of the present authors (C.W.W.), who had investigated all of Brunner's *et al.* patients retrospectively, lay stress upon the transcortical features, namely nonfluent speech and almost intact repetition and diagnosed the respective patients as having transcortical motor aphasia. At reassessment more than 4 months after infarction, 3 patients of Brunner's *et al.* series were diagnosed as having anomic aphasia and altogether 5 patients exhibited some language pathology. Brunner *et al.* interpreted their findings as consistent with a participation in language functions of the loop retrorolandic cortex – neostriatum – pallidum – ventral thalamus – frontal cortex.

The results of Ringelstein *et al.* (1985) suggests that some of the lentiform nucleus infarctions investigated in the Brunner *et al* (1982) study may have resulted from middle cerebral artery embolus and others from cerebral microangiopathy, in which case diffuse vascular encephalopathy may have been present. Unfortunately for the interpretation of the consequences of subcortical strokes, even the angiographic exclusion of middle cerebral artery main stem occlusion indicates only that the vessel was open at the time of angiography but not necessarily so at the time of insult, as occlusions may be transient.

In order to control effects of underlying vascular pathology on cortical tissue, Wallesch *et al.* (1983a) compared chronic ischaemic basal ganglia with white matter lesions for effects upon language functions. This study revealed that there was a lateralization of language deficits to the left with basal ganglia lesions, again in most instances in the lentiform nucleus, but not with white matter lesions. These deficits concerned mainly spontaneous speech, whereas the patients performed almost normally on tasks of repetition, naming and comprehension. However, according to Ringelstein *et al.* (1985), at least for some of the white matter lesions, a different pathogenesis, namely haemodynamic infarction, must be assumed.

Cappa *et al.* (1983) reported 6 patients with basal ganglia lesions and aphasia, and described two syndromes: an atypical nonfluent aphasia sometimes associated with anterior capsular-putaminal lesions and a mild fluent aphasia, sometimes associated with posterior capsular-putaminal lesions. Of these patients, one exhibited a mild fluent aphasia with anomia and semantic paraphasia following a small putaminal haemorrhage and another a mild nonfluent aphasia without dysarthria with a small hematoma in the head of the left caudate; they also presented four negative cases with left subcortical lesions in the CT but no language disorder. As in the study of Skyhöj Olsen *et al.* (1986), these had rather small, mainly white matter, lesions.

Puel *et al.* (1984) presented probably the largest and most thoroughly studied series of 25 patients with left subcortical lesions, which included 15 haemorrhages and 10 infarctions. Of the 25 cases, 21 were aphasic and, of these, 10 exhibited unusual types of aphasia. Some of the hematomas in this series were large and may have caused distance effects upon cortex whilst most of the infarctions probably reflect middle cerebral main stem pathology. However, a number of the patients match even strict criteria: The authors found a fluent atypical aphasia with semantic paraphasia with an anterior putamino-capsular haemorrhage and a non-fluent aphasia with phonemic and semantic paraphasia in a case of haemorrhage in the head of the caudate and parts of the anterior limb of the internal capsule. A small infarction involving pallidum, posterior limb of internal capsule and the body of the caudate also gave rise to semantic paraphasia. Puel *et al.* found non-fluent paraphasic aphasia in three cases of thalamic haemorrhage. The CT lesions in some of these patients were restricted to the white matter. One of these exhibited semantic jargonaphasia with apparently an anterior choroidal infarction involving the knee and the posterior limb of the internal capsule, whilst another with a non-fluent paraphasic aphasia had an anterior limb infarction.

It has already been pointed out that the anterior choroidal artery is not a branch of the middle cerebral artery. It supplies the genu and posterior limb of the internal capsule and parts of the pallidum, but not normally the thalamus proper. Cambier *et al.* (1983) described aphasia with impaired fluency and semantic paraphasia with a left sided infarction; Wallesch (1985) reported two additional cases with lesions of the pallidum and knee of internal capsule, both with non-fluent aphasia. Helgason *et al.* (1986) found only dysarthria in a patient with a lesion confined to the posterior limb of the capsule, and a 'foreign accent syndrome' without aphasia was described by Gurd *et al.* (1987) in a similar patient. Decroix *et al.* (1986) investigated 10 patients with left anterior choroidal infarction and reported 'thalamic aphasia' in 2 cases, a syndrome which seems to have consisted mostly of difficulties in initiating utterances; two further patients experienced transient expressive language deficits. Of 6 patients with left anterior choroidal infarction included in the series of Graff-Radford *et al.* (1985), three exhibited mild language difficulties which were reported not to constitute an aphasic syndrome. Reviewing all these 20 patients with left anterior choroidal infarction who had received language assessment, it seems that aphasia was more pronounced in those cases in which there was a pallidal lesion of some size.

In summary we may conclude from the clinical data presented so far:

1. Anterior choroidal infarction involving the pallidum results in a non-fluent transient aphasia, at least in some cases, whereas those involving only the posterior limb appear rather not to lead to relevant language disturbances. The case of Puel *et al.* (1984) of a Wernicke aphasia with infarction in the genu and posterior limb seems exceptional.
2. Cases of small haemorrhages in the basal ganglia in which direct effects upon cortex can be ruled out with some probability reveal the following picture:
   haemorrhages confined to the head of the left caudate may result in non-fluent aphasia (Cappa *et al.*, 1983; Puel *et al.*, 1984), small putaminal haemorrhages in fluent paraphasic aphasia (Cappa *et al.*, 1983; Puel *et al.*, 1984). In two cases of the latter, the haemorrhage extended in one of the series of Cappa *et al.* to the temporal isthmus, and in one of Puel *et al.* to the anterior limb of the internal capsule.
3. If the anterior limb is involved, semantic paraphasia is a fairly common symptom (Damasio *et al.*, 1982; Puel *et al.*, 1984; Wallesch, 1985). In most of these cases, ischaemia of the cerebral cortex cannot be ruled out, but Wallesch (1985) has pointed out that the aphasia symptomatology with

paraphasias as a central feature does not support cortical dysfunction as the underlying cause of the syndrome.

4. Similarly, transcortical motor aphasia (Sterzi and Vallar, 1978; Brunner *et al.*, 1982 and Wallesch, 1985) occurring with lentiform nucleus lesions is quite distinct from that expected with a lesion of the neighbouring cortex. A relative preservation of repetition in similar cases was also found by Cappa *et al.* (1983). This type of 'subcortical aphasia' most resembles the speech disturbances seen after lesions of the supplementary motor area (*see* Jonas, 1981, for review).
5. Most authors agree that small subcortical lesions of the white matter of the insula (Cappa *et al.*, 1983; Wallesch *et al.*, 1983a), the posterior limb of the internal capsule (Cappa *et al.*, 1983; Helgason *et al.*, 1986) or the centrum semiovale (Fromm *et al.*, 1985; Wallesch *et al.*, 1983a; Ozaki *et al.*, 1986) do not result in language disturbances.

Damasio *et al.* (1982) tried to explain the presence of paraphasia and auditory comprehension deficits in patients with lesions of the anterior limb of the internal capsule by damage to projections which cross it from the auditory cortex to the head of caudate. Wallesch (1985) speculated that the ventral thalamic projection on the frontal language area was involved in gating cortico-cortically transmitted verbal response elements, and its disconnection lead to paraphasia.

From this review of cases of aphasia following lesions of the basal ganglia, it becomes apparent that most of these cases differ from the aphasia syndromes seen with lesions involving the cerebral cortex. Whereas the classical aphasia syndromes affect all levels and modalities of language (Wallesch, in press), the symptomatology of basal ganglia and capsular aphasias is focused upon two deficits, one of lexical processing and one of speech initiation. Of the other aspects of language production, the generation of sentence frames and morphosyntactical operations seem to be left largely unimpaired. Repetition and even naming, both of which are linguistic operations with restricted degrees of freedom, are also frequently not or only mildly disturbed. Those language tasks which involve the highest number of degrees of freedom, namely spontaneous utterances and free choice in the lexicon, are conversely most markedly affected. Some aspects of the disorder resemble transcortical motor aphasia, where the more propositional uses of language are also most affected (Rubens, 1976).

Alexander *et al.* (1986) suggest the existence of nonmotor complex loops from association and prefrontal cortex via caudate, pallidum and ventral thalamus to the prefrontal cortex. These loops are assumed to be important for the spontaneous generation of 'efficient strategies when relying on self-directed task-specific planning' (Taylor *et al.*, 1986). We consider the language deficits occurring with left basal ganglia lesions as consistent with the assumption of a deficit of that faculty.

Thalamus

With the exception of very few clinical observations (e.g. Smyth and Stern, 1938), the thalamus has not been suspected to participate in language functions until the advent of stereotactic neurosurgery. As stereotaxis mainly focused upon two thalamic nuclei, namely the VL for the relief of extrapyramidal motor symptoms, and the pulvinar for pain control, there is an extensive literature regarding these and very little concerning other thalamic structures.

The stereotactic evidence includes electrical stimulation (during operation) and lesion studies. The lesions produced by stereotactic thalamotomy are small (a few millimeters in diameter) and well defined, affecting small areas of the thalamic nuclei only. As the thalamic nuclei are topically organized (Hassler *et al.*, 1979), different targetting approaches may lead to different functional results with respect to language side effects. It has to be kept in mind that most of these investigations have been performed on preoperatively pathologic brains and, further, that the localizing and functional interpretation of electrical stimulation is limited, as there may be current spread and the critical current range for quasi-physiologic stimulation may be small and variable (Ojemann, 1976, 1977).

Ojemann (1975, 1976, 1977, 1983) investigated in great detail naming disturbances with left VL and pulvinar stimulation. These could not be explained on the basis of an interruption of speech as an ongoing motor activity, as had been suggested by Schaltenbrand (1975), as Ojemann's patients were able to read aloud an introductory phrase ('This is a . . .') under stimulation. In addition, Ojemann reported perseverative and repetitive errors. In another series of investigations, Ojemann *et al.* (1971) studied the effects of thalamic stimulation upon verbal short term memory, and found that VL stimulation during the learning period improved, and during the recall phase decreased, performance in a word learning task. The authors concluded that stimulation of the VL nucleus evokes a 'specific alerting response' which turns the patients attention towards external stimuli. Ojemann (1976) described similar effects upon verbal short term memory with pulvinar stimulation. The 'specific alerting response' appeared to be less intense with pulvinar, than with ventrolateral thalamic, stimulation.

Lecours and Lhermitte (1979) and Crosson (1984) provide concise reviews of the thalamic stimulation literature. Lecours and Lhermitte point out that speech disturbances as slurring, tachylalia, arrest and hesitations have been found with thalamic stimulation of either side, but that linguistic phenomena such as palilalia, anomia, perseveration and misnaming were only experienced with dominant VL and pulvinar stimulation.

Following stereotactic lesions, language deficits have been reported in variable percentages, depending probably upon type and (bi-) laterality of the operation performed, age, and preoperative morbidity. In large series of patients with ventral thalamotomy, aphasia was found to occur in 24% (Cooper *et al.*, 1968) to 42% (Selby, 1967) of operations on the left side and in 0% (Bell, 1968) to 25% (Cooper *et al.*, 1968) on the right. The vast majority of authors reports rapid improvement of language deficits. Two studies of the effects of pulvinar thalamotomy (Brown *et al.*, 1971; Vilkki and Laitinen, 1976) failed to find postoperative language impairments.

The following linguistic deficits were described: perseveration with VL-lesions (Allan *et al.*, 1966; Bell, 1968; Ojemann, 1975; Vilkki, 1978), anomia with VL- (Allan *et al.*, 1966, Bell, 1968; Ojemann, 1975), and pulvinar, lesions (Ojemann *et al.*, 1968) and reduced word fluency with VL-thalamotomies (Bell, 1968; Vilkki and Laitinen, 1976; Laitinen and Vilkki, 1977).

A number of studies tried to psychometrically evaluate the outcome of stereotactic thalamotomies (McFie, 1960; Riklan *et al.*, 1960; Shapiro *et al.*, 1973). In the majority, a decrease in verbal subtests with left, mainly VL-, thalamotomies was found. In the investigation of Riklan and Cooper (1975), significant verbal IQ impairments were only present with VL-, but not with pulvinar, lesions. At long term follow-up (Levita *et al.*, 1967), these deficits could no longer be demonstrated.

We conclude that stereotactic stimulation and lesion studies indicate a role of the left VL nucleus in certain language functions, especially naming, and that similar evidence from a smaller number of observations and less consistently has been presented for the left pulvinar.

The consequences upon language of thalamic haemorrhages and infarctions have recently been reviewed by Jonas (1982) and by Crosson (1984). Both authors stress the absence of deficits of language comprehension and repetition in the vast majority of cases. Speech production of patients with left thalamic lesions is characterized by paraphasia or even jargon, perseveration, anomia and, in a smaller number of cases, lack of spontaneity of speech. A predominance of semantic over phonemic paraphasias has been reported (Cappa and Vignolo, 1979; Alexander and LoVerme, 1980). Verbal memory defects have also been noted in a number of cases with left thalamic haemorrhage or infarction (Puel *et al.*, 1986). Syntactic errors are unusual and have been reported without closer specification in only two cases (Bugiani *et al.*, 1969; Fazio *et al.*, 1973). Jonas (1982) drew attention to the disparity between the relative preservation of nonpropositional, and the more severe disruption affecting propositional, speech.

Unfortunately, only few cases with pathology confined to the thalamus have been studied anatomically and neuropsychologically in detail. Graff-Radford *et al.* (1985) in their series of left thalamic infarctions found aphasia in only those three patients who had suffered a stroke in the area of supply of the tuberothalamic artery, which includes the ventral nuclei. Perusal of CT scans given in Graff-Radford *et al.* (1984) reveals that cortical atrophy or lesions were present in the aphasic patients. The authors describe rapid improvement of the language deficits. In three additional patients with ischaemic left ventral thalamic lesions, presumably in the area of supply of the tuberothalamic artery, there appears to be no cortical pathology in the CTs (Gorelick *et al.*, 1984; Bogousslavsky *et al.*, 1986). These patients exhibited reduced speech production, phonemic and semantic paraphasia, anomia and relatively preserved syntax and repetition. A rather similar but fluently aphasic patient with a left ventral thalamic infarction was described by Archer *et al.* (1981). Language pathology in an anatomically verified pulvinar infarction was recently described by Crosson *et al.* (1986), whose patient was fluently aphasic with anomia and mainly semantic paraphasia and relatively preserved repetition and comprehension. Crosson *et al.* stress that anomia and paraphasia were mild when their patient discussed familiar topics, but that speech deteriorated into jargon when unfamiliar topics were raised, and explain these findings on the basis of Crosson's (1985) hypothesis of a thalamic role in semantic monitoring.

A number of negative cases (left thalamic haemorrhage or infarction without language abnormalities) have also been reported. Cappa *et al.* (1986) described 5 patients with posterior thalamic haemorrhages without aphasia. Ventral thalamic vascular lesions in the dominant hemisphere without language symptoms seem to be less frequent but have been described (Mohr, 1983). Wallesch *et al.* (1983 a, b) were unable to find lateralized linguistic or neuropsychological deficits more than 6 months after thalamic stroke but were still able to detect deficits in verbal and nonverbal memory tasks with anterior thalamic lesions of either side (Wallesch *et al.*, 1983b). Wallesch *et al.* (1983a) argue that the cortico – striato – pallido – thalamo – cortical loop they consider involved in expressive language functions may include a number of parallel pathways on the level of the thalamus.

An alternative explanation is given by McFarling *et al.* (1982), who suggest the disruption of a 'specific alerting function' of the VL-nucleus to be the cause of a transient disturbance of the more complex language functions of the cortical regions of projection of the ventral thalamus, an interpretation that obviously relies on Ojemann's (*see* above) results and theory. Luria (1977) had previously tried to explain the 'quasiaphasic' symptoms he encountered in a patient with a large thalamic lesion on the basis of Ojemann's views. Mohr *et al.* (1975) had first described an unusually fluctuating state of pathology with the thalamic haemorrhages: 'When rendered fully alert, the patient appeared virtually intact in language function,... but quickly lapsed into a state of unwonted logorrheic paraphasia resembling delirium' (p. 3). This fluctuating state seems to be characteristic of large left thalamic haemorrhages, and Luria (1977) hypothesized a partial disturbance of cortical tone of vigilance, which he supposed to be of a material-specific nature. Thus, 'the specificity of the speech process was lost, the blocking of already evoked or extraneous associations became impossible, and the selectivity of speech had broken down' (p. 458). Gorelick *et al.* (1984) suggested deficits in lexical access (anomia, semantic paraphasia) separate from deficits in vigilance (leading to neologisms, intrusions, fluctuating performance, jargon, perseverations) in patients with thalamic lesions. The data of Graff-Radford *et al.* (1985) indicate that truly aphasic symptoms occur more with lateral thalamic lesions involving the VA and VL nuclei, whereas disorders of consciousness and vigilance ('Waxing and waning of attention') result more from infarction in the territory of the interpeduncular profundus artery, which supplies mainly nonspecific thalamic nuclei.

In summary, there is solid evidence stemming mainly from clinical studies of small thalamic infarctions that lesions of the ventral thalamic nuclei lead to a distinctive syndrome of aphasia, at least in a considerable number of cases. The salient aspects of language pathology are semantic paraphasia, anomia, relative preservation of repetition and a favourable prognosis. For other thalamic nuclei, the evidence is more equivocal with a number of negative cases reported e.g. by Graff-Radford (1985) and Cappa *et al.* (1986). On the other hand, language disturbances with posterior thalamic lesions have been presented convincingly by Reynolds *et al.* (1979), Alexander and LoVerme (1980) and Crosson *et al.* (1986). Their case reports resemble those of patients with lateral thalamic lesions with the exception that speech production is more fluent in the posterior cases. In general, the clinical evidence of left posterior thalamic lesions is consistent with the observations made with stereotactic manipulation of the pulvinar.

Theoretical Considerations

Any theory of the role of the deep nuclei in language function must deal with the following considerations and questions:

1. Are there linguistic functions specific to the deep nuclei? Is there a supplementary, redundant subcortical representation of language functions? Do the nuclei subserve cortical linguistic function in a specific, but non-linguistic, way or are there only nonspecific effects upon cortical functions, e.g. arousal or alerting?
2. If there was a specific — linguistic or non-linguistic — property of the function of the deep nuclei in the use of language, this should be reflected in the symptomatology of subcortical aphasia. Therefore, subcortical aphasias should differ in quality from language impairments resulting from lesions of the cerebral cortex in the vicinity of the nuclei. Shared features of cortical and basal ganglia pathology would have to be assumed to result from cortical dysfunction, as a null hypothesis would have to be

accepted because damage to the cortex can never be safely ruled out.

3. Lesions of the deep nuclei seem mostly to affect lexical functions, resulting in anomia and mainly semantic paraphasia. The production of neologisms and jargon as described in some cases could also be explained on the basis of disturbed processes of lexicalization, namely by a deficit in access to word forms (Butterworth, 1985). In contrast, the generation of syntactical frames and morphosyntactical operations seem to be largely undisturbed.
4. Language comprehension disturbances appear not to be a prominent feature of subcortical aphasias, but Damasio *et al.* (1982) drew attention to (a) comprehension deficits occurring with lesions involving the head of the caudate and the anterior limb of the internal capsule and (b) projections of the auditory association cortex upon the head of the caudate.
5. Lesions of the deep nuclei appear to affect the more propositional aspects of language most, leaving reactive speech relatively intact. In this, they resemble the effects upon language of lesions of the supplementary motor area (for a review, *see* Jonas, 1981). Repetition was noted to be intact or only mildly disturbed in most cases, and confrontation naming was frequently rapidly restored. In those cases investigated by the present authors, anomia was more severe in conversation than in confrontation naming. Patients suffering from subcortical aphasia thus exhibited a reverse picture of anomia than is usually encountered with anomic aphasics (Wallesch, in press). The word finding deficit thus seems to depend upon the number of degrees of freedom which are potentially available to the patient in any given situation.

The clinical evidence therefore is against the assumption that the 'subcortical aphasias' are caused by cortical damage not visible in the CT. They do not resemble Broca's, Wernicke's, global, conduction, or anomic aphasia. Those which are paraphasic share some features with Wernicke's aphasia, but differ from this syndrome in that they are rather non-fluent and comprehension is largely preserved. Some of them give the clinical impression of transcortical motor aphasia which, however, usually occurs with lesions of cortical structures far from the deep nuclei, e.g. of the supplementary motor area.

As there are only negligible backprojections from the basal ganglia to the cerebral cortex, the thalamus must be regarded as the crucial, and therefore critical, structure of any theory concerning language functions of the deep nuclei. The basal ganglia mainly project to the nuclei VL and VA of the ventral thalamus and the assumption of their involvement in language processes therefore depends upon the assumption of participation of the ventral thalamus.

Theories concerning the possible role of the dominant thalamus in language processes have recently been reviewed by Crosson (1984) who divided the theories described in the literature into five groups:

1. '*Descriptive theories*': According to Crosson (1984) the main exponent of this type of theory is Jonas (1982), who noted similarities between transcortical aphasias and thalamic aphasia. Crosson points out that traditionally the 'transcortical aphasias were thought to be caused by a severing of language cortex from other cortical areas while still maintaining connections between the anterior areas for language formulation and the posterior areas for language decoding' (p. 509) and assumes that transcortical aphasia may also occur with a disconnection of pathways between cortical language areas and subcortical structures. In the view of the present authors, this classical theory of transcortical motor aphasia can account neither for the aphasia syndromes resulting from lesions of the deep nuclei nor of the supplementary motor area. The significance of, and an explanation for, the occurrence of transcortical (mostly motor) aphasia with lesions of these sites will be considered below.
2. '*Non-specific theories*': These propose a thalamic participation in language generation and comprehension, but do not assign a specific function to the thalamus. Crosson quotes as an exponent Brown (1975), who hypothesized that language expressions were first generated in an embryonic form in deep and phylogenetically old brain structures, such as the thalamus, and were then further processed and specified in the forebrain.
3. '*Activation theories*': These rely on the assumption of thalamic alerting mechanisms upon cortical structures. Riklan and Cooper (1975) hypothesized that the more complex language functions required a larger amount of diffuse cortical arousal. Elghozi *et al.* (1978) consider disruption of the activating system to be the main cause of the language disorder in left thalamic lesions, leading to an inactivation of language dynamics (slow speech, pauses, perseverations) and impaired focusing of attention upon language processing, the latter affecting predominantly the propositional use of language (e.g. spontaneous speech, word definitions). They explain the occurrence of semantic paraphasia by the assumption of right hemisphere intrusions resulting from an imbalance between activation of both hemispheres. A related view is Luria's (1977) hypothesis that language specific alerting or vigilance mechanisms had been disrupted in his case of thalamic 'quasi-aphasia'.
4. '*Integration theories*': Penfield and Roberts (1959) first proposed a role for the dominant thalamus in the integration of language. Botez and Barbeau (1971) assumed as one function of cortico-thalamo-cortical loops their involvement in the analysis of language content, including access to the concepts of words which contains recall of memory traces. Cappa and

Vignolo (1979) proposed a contribution of the dominant thalamus to the semantic level of verbal behaviour, namely to the use of words as meaningful units, and compared its participation to that of the 'marginal' language areas. Schuell *et al.* (1965) suggested that thalamic mechanisms participated in feedback processes which were involved in the monitoring of language formulation.

Crosson considered his own theory as integrative and suggested the thalamus was involved in 'a preverbal semantic feedback mechanism that monitors potential language output via the word selection process. This is accomplished through a feedback loop between the anterior areas for language formulation and the posterior centers for semantic decoding. In other words, the dominant thalamus provides the mechanism by which the posterior centers for language decoding monitor verbal output...' (Crosson, 1984, p. 511).

5. '*Multiple function theories*': These theories assign both arousal and integrative functions to the thalamus. A neuroanatomical basis for this view could be the different functions and ways of projection of different, e.g. specific and nonspecific, thalamic nuclei. Crosson (1984) quotes Cooper *et al.* (1968) and Samra *et al.* (1969) as exponents of such theories. As these multiple function theories simply combine other views of thalamic function in language mechanisms they need not be discussed separately.

In summary, mainly three mechanisms have been proposed by which the dominant thalamus may be involved in language processes: (1) by specific or nonspecific activation of cortical structures, (2) by mediation of verbal memory contents, and (3) by participation in semantic selection processes.

Crosson (1984) rightly points out that language and verbal memory impairment can be widely dissociated in cases of thalamic lesions (Squire and Moore, 1979; Michel *et al.*, 1982). Probably the strongest evidence for a connection of lexical and verbal memory processes at the level of the lateral thalamus are Ojemann's (Ojemann *et al.*, 1971) observations that VL, and to a lesser extent pulvinar, stimulation may lead to impaired naming and to systematic changes in a verbal memory task. Ojemann explains these effects on the basis of a common underlying mechanism, namely a highly specific focal alerting and directing of attention, which subserves both language and memory processes. There can be no doubt that thalamic nuclei are part of the cerebral representation of memory functions and it is anatomically plausible that thalamic nuclei interact with each other, but those thalamic nuclei which are part of the memory system (the anterior group of nuclei) are other than those for which a participation in language functions is considered, and their functional separation is reflected in the quoted cases of dissociation. Recently, Crosson (1985) proposed a model of thalamic participation in language functions that was intended to cover most of the available data. He assumed that the dominant thalamus performed a function in semantic monitoring which would explain the predominance of semantic paraphasia in cases of thalamic aphasia, and rightly pointed out that a theory of subcortical language function relies on a complementary theory of cortical language function. He suggested two cortical language areas, a posterior 'language decoder' and an anterior 'language formulator' located in close proximity to a cortical 'motor programmer'. The disturbance of language production in Wernicke's aphasia was though to result from disrupted monitoring processes.

We regard this model of the cortical representation of language functions as not entirely convincing, not only because of its localizationist aspects but, more importantly, because the crucial linguistic operation, the assembly of the sentence, is supposed to be a process situated entirely in the left frontal lobe. The main argument for this assumption is the finding of agrammatism in Broca's aphasia, but agrammatic utterances are not asyntactic but are rule-governed linguistic structures. The present authors very much doubt whether the assembly of sentences or propositions can be localized into a brain structure. Crosson's hypothesis on the cortical distribution of functions leads him to assume that 'in order for preverbal semantic monitoring of language formulation to take place, semantic information must be conveyed from anterior language areas where language is formulated to temporoparietal areas where language is decoded and monitored. The most likely pathway for this transmission is from the anterior language zones to the thalamus via the connections with the ventral anterior thalamus, from ventral anterior thalamus to the pulvinar (probably via the internal medullary lamina) and from the thalamus to the temporoparietal cortex through connections with the pulvinar' (Crosson, 1985, p. 274). This assumption seems implausible for two reasons: whilst similar to Penfield and Robert's hypothesis (with the exception that it works in the opposite direction) it proposes a connection via non-specific thalamus, in which non-specific nuclei would have to perform very specific functions. Furthermore, it cannot account for the fact that lesions to the ventral thalamus disrupt language more severely than does pulvinar damage. Crosson assumes a second function of the VA nucleus: 'In order for anterior cortical mechanisms to produce language, it is also necessary that an optimal arousal level of these mechanisms be maintained. Since it receives afferents from the reticular formation . . , and since it sends efferents to the frontal cortex, the ventral anterior nucleus of the dominant thalamus is the likely site to provide such excitatory influences. The function of the ventral anterior nucleus would be to selectively distribute excitatory influences from the reticular formation to frontal mechanisms for language production . . .' (Crosson, 1985, p. 275). This assumes, however, that the VA nucleus not only serves two very different functions, namely transmission of information from the frontal language cortex and transmission of activation to this cortex, but also acts in two opposite directions. Crosson in fact suggests a 'multiple function theory' for one single thalamic nucleus.

Stretching the functional capabilities of VA nucleus even further, Crosson (1985) assumes it to transmit the outflow of basal ganglia processing to the cortex, suggesting that 'the basal ganglia influence tone in the anterior cortical language areas by regulating the flow of excitatory impulses from the ventral anterior thalamus. If cortical excitation is maintained at too high a level, extraneous material will enter into the encoding (language formulation) and motor-programming processes. If tone is too low, language formulation will be inefficient or not occur spontaneously at all' (p. 277). Crosson suggests a second mechanism of basal ganglia involvement in language, namely a motor release mechanism which allows language segments to be released at the proper time, after semantic monitoring has taken place. 'The purpose of the response release mechanism is to allow a temporary increase in excitation from the ventral anterior thalamus to the anterior language cortex which is timed to allow the motor programming of semantically verified language for speech. This response release function is performed by the head of the caudate nucleus through its input from the anterior and posterior language cortex and its output to the globus pallidus. The reponse release mechanism works as follows. Activity in the caudate head exerts an inhibitory influence over the inhibitory mechanisms of the globus pallidus. Thus, when required, activity from the caudate head will temporarily inhibit pallidal inhibitory mechanisms, thereby releasing the ventral anterior nucleus from pallidal inhibition, which in turn increases excitation to anterior cortical mechanisms allowing the release of semantically verified language for motor programming' (Crosson, 1985, p. 278). Loops involving the basal ganglia and the ventral thalamus seem to be triply involved in Crosson's model, namely by regulating cortical tone, by the response release mechanism and by an involvement in motor programming. In this model, the ventral thalamus serves four separable functions.

Ojemann (1983), on the basis of his stimulation data, proposes a phylo- and onto-genetically oriented model which assumes in the perisylvian cortex a motor-sequencing-phoneme-decoding system surrounded by a short term verbal memory system in the frontal, parietal, and temporal lobes. In this model, the representation of specialized language functions has developed at the interfaces between these systems. Ojemann assumes that frontal sites may be involved in the retrieval of words and syntactic structures during language generation, while sites in the temporoparietal cortex would contain the stores of neural representations of words and syntactical structures.

Ojemann supposes that thalamic alerting processses selectively activate the specific discrete cortical areas appropriate to the particular language processing, and assumes that the thalamocortical specific alerting response is probably the process that must occur simultaneously at anterior and posterior cortical language areas at the onset of naming. Thalamic projections mediating this alerting for language processing would stem from the ventral thalamus for the anterior, and from the pulvinar for the posterior, language areas. Ojemann stresses the potential, but yet little understood, importance of the pallidal afferents for the function of the VL nucleus, considering it likely that the specific alerting response in VL originally developed as part of motor learning, being later utilized for language and verbal memory processes in the dominant hemisphere.

Wallesch's (1984, 1985) model resembles Crosson's in a number of aspects, but also includes important differences, and contains elements of Ojemann's theory. The chief difference from Crosson's views concern cortical functional organization. Wallesch does not assume that language functions are discretely represented on the cerebral cortex in one single location each. Neurophysiological data indicate that the basic functional unit of the cerebral cortex is a barrel-shaped 'module'. These modules were first described for the primary sensory areas (Mountcastle, 1957; Hubel and Wiesel, 1969), but seem to represent a general principle of cortical functional organization (Phillips *et al.*, 1984; Goldman-Rakic, 1984). Szentagothai (1975) defines a module and its boundaries by the thalamic afferents. Phillips and Porter (1977) propose that the VL-afferents transmit 'features of a central command' on the frontal motor cortex. According to Phillips *et al.* (1984), the parallel organization of models is a basic feature of cortical organization, and serves the detection of contingencies on the afferent side of the system (Phillips *et al.*, 1984). Eccles (1977) assumes that on the efferent side a competitive inhibition of neighbouring and functionally parallel modules governs behaviour by a survival (further processing) of the fittest. Goldman-Rakic (1984) supposes that in the prefrontal association cortex the modular machinery could permit combinations and recombinations among inputs that would constitute a highly adaptive and plastic mechanism for information processing. If, now, efferent modules work in parallel and in competition, and if the thalamic afferents transmit features of a central command, then a thalamic gating of the cortical efferents seems plausible. Wallesch (1984) points out that parallel processing within a modular structure in the transmission from posterior to anterior cortex would be profitable for the individual because it would save time and increase the flexibility of responses. The function of the deep nuclei in language acts would then be (1) integrative, in that they have to monitor cortical processing and integrate situational constraints; and (2) goal directed, in that will and intention of the individual have to be integrated into his behaviour (*see* e.g. Groves, 1983, and Alexander *et al.*, 1986, for discussion of the underlying neural circuits).

Evidence in favour of thalamic gating in language production is the almost regular presence of paraphasia with lesions of the thalamus and anterior limb of the internal capsule and the disturbance of lexical processes with lateral thalamic stimulation (Ojemann, 1976).

We assume that the pallidum controls and modulates by inhibition the gating activity of the ventral thalamus which, via inhibitory interneurones, controls (premotor) frontal cortical processing. Pallidal lesions seem quite consistently to result in non-fluent, transcortical motor aphasia. We suppose that a deficit of pallidal inhibition of the ventral thalamus results in a disinhibited gating of language production. This is clinically reflected in the impairment of initiating speech of patients with such lesions, their efforts eventually leading to the release and consequent production of a semantically and syntactically adequate utterance. In the same patients, repetition and in many instances even naming remain largely undisturbed. In these situations of reactive language production, subcortical gating of competing responses is supposed not to be effective, as all parallel organized cortical modules come up with the same response and do not compete. This functional hypothesis can thus explain why the ability to respond of patients with basal ganglia aphasia depends upon the degrees of freedom present in any given situation. The degrees of freedom for the lexical content of a sentence are much greater than with morphosyntactical operations, the latter being restricted by a closely knit set of rules. Thus, there seems to be a functional explanation for the relative preservation of syntax in cases of subcortical aphasia.

Little is known about the intrinsic functional organization of the basal ganglia, which appear to contain a highly complex integrative circuitry with internal and efferent excitatory and inhibitory mechanisms (e.g. Pasik *et al.*, 1979; Rolls *et al.*, 1979; Groves, 1983; Parent, 1986). Consequently, it cannot with the state of the art of lesion analysis be predicted whether the presence of a given neostriatal vascular damage may eventually result in inhibitory or disinhibitory effects upon the ventral thalamus. The clinical diversity of basal ganglia aphasias seems to indicate that both possibilities occur. The clinical aspect of basal ganglia aphasias is consistent with the proposed model that mainly lexical processes are affected and repetition and syntax are preserved.

Our view is quite congruent with that of Rosvold and Szwarcbart (1964) and Taylor *et al.* (1986) in that the head of the caudate, the pallidum and the ventral thalamus are being integrated into a 'frontal lobe system'. In our model, contrary to that of Crosson (1985), the function of the VA and VL nuclei, as far as they concern language, are unitary. These nuclei, together with parts of the basal ganglia, are involved in choosing by gating among a number of possible lexical alternatives. Their function is supposed to be one of integration with the goal of response selection. We assume that, under the control of the frontal cortex, the integrative and focusing organization of the neostriatum (Groves, 1983) is involved in handling multiple degrees of freedom in a given situation and carrying out decisions upon the actual response. We consider situational constraints being transmitted by the converging projections of the retrorolandic cortex upon the neostriatum, and volitional, goal-directed demands by the strong and partly bilateral projection of the prefrontal and supplementary motor cortex (Carman *et al.*, 1965; Kemp and Powell, 1970). With respect to language production, we assume the nuclei to participate in the choice of words as meaningful, conceptually adequate, units (Botez and Barbeau, 1971; Cappa and Vignolo, 1979).

A strong functional link between prefrontal and supplementary motor cortex and basal ganglia is not only anatomically plausible but also made obvious by the similarity of aphasia syndromes encountered with their lesions. Left basal ganglia, prefrontal as well as supplementary motor area, lesions in the dominant hemisphere, all result in transcortical motor aphasia. As Rubens (1976, p. 301f.) summarizes, 'transcortical motor aphasia is one of the labels which have been applied to a symptom complex characterized by a disproportionate disturbance of spontaneous speech, compared to speech evoked through external stimulation. The defect is generally considered to result from loss of frontal lobe volitional influence on the speech apparatus, most often resulting from damage to the dominant frontal lobe, to connections between frontal lobe and the speech area, or to mild damage to the speech area itself. According to Goldstein (*1948, reference given by the present authors*) the transcortical aphasias represent damage of the relations between speech and nonspeech mental processes'.

This statement of Rubens leads to the crucial question concerning the status of subcortical aphasia: Is it really aphasia? A number of authors (e.g. Lichtheim, 1885; Luria, 1970) agree that in transcortical motor aphasia the linguistic apparatus and the instrumental use of language are intact, but that the transmission of 'concepts' (Lichtheim) or 'initial thoughts' (Luria) into language is defective. The classical aphasia syndromes, on the other hand, are characterized by their impairment of the instrumental use of language, of its phonology, lexicon, and syntax. Transcortical motor aphasia constitutes a deficit in the propositional use of language, and we have argued above that the semantic paraphasia in patients with subcortical lesions occurs on the basis of propositionally (situationally and/or intentionally) inappropriate choices.

Two questions remain to be discussed: Why are language disturbances following subcortical lesions unstable and tend to recover rapidly? Why do chronic diseases of the basal ganglia not result in language deficits?

We suggest that the gating (and, conversely, response release) function of the loop via basal ganglia and ventral thalamus upon the frontal language cortex is not exclusive. The nuclei are part of a functional system (e.g. a 'frontal lobe system', Rosvold and Szwarcbart, 1964). There are projections upon the frontal language area from other elements of this system (e.g. frontofrontal connections), and there are bypasses, e.g. the bidirectional frontothalamic connections. The cortical aspects of the frontal lobe system are characterized by their plasticity in functional reorganization (Butters *et al.*, 1974; Wallesch *et al.*, 1983 c), and we assume a similar plasticity to apply to the subcortical aspects of the system.

The assumption of functional plasticity of the system would also explain the relative absence of language disturbances in chronic subcortical disease, but peculiar speech phenomena which indicate disturbed programming of articulatory output, such as palilalia and compulsory speech, have been noted for a long time to occur with extrapyramidal disease. Recently, perhaps encouraged by the theory of 'complex loops' via the basal ganglia (for review, *see* Alexander *et al.*, 1986), a number of investigations have focused on higher mental functions in parkinsonian patients. They produced evidence of a 'frontal lobe dysfunction' (Lees and Smith, 1983; Taylor *et al.*, 1986) and were able to demonstrate in selected patients deficits of lexical retrieval (Matison *et al.* 1982). Both types of observations are consistent with the presented view of the contribution of the deep nuclei to the use of language.

Acknowledgements

During the preparation of the manuscript Dr Wallesch was supported by DFG Heisenberg Grant Wa 509/3, and Dr Papagno by the DAAD.

References

ACUNA, C., GONZALEZ, F. and DOMINGUEZ, R. Sensorimotor unit activity related to intention in the pulvinar of behaving Cebus Apella monkeys. *Experimental Brain Research* (1983), **52**, 411–422.

ALEXANDER, M.L., DELONG, M. and STRICK, P. Parallel organization of functionally segregated circuits linking basal ganglia and cortex. In *Annual Review of Neuroscience 1986* (1986). Palo Alto: The Annual Review Inc.

ALEXANDER, M.P. and LOVERME, S.R. Aphasia after left hemispheric intracerebral haemorrhage. *Neurology* (1980), **30**, 1193–1202.

ALLAN, C.M., TURNER, J.W. and GADEA CIRIA, M. Investigation into speech disturbances following stereotaxic surgery for Parkinsonism. *British Journal of Communication Disorders* (1966), **1**, 55–69.

ARCHER, C.R., ILINSKY, I.A., GOLDFADER, P.R. and SMITH, K.R. Aphasia in thalamic stroke: CT stereotactic localization. *Journal of Computer Assisted Tomography* (1981), **5**, 427–432.

BARAT, M., MAZAUX, J.M. BIAULAC, B., GIROIRE, J.M., VITAL, C.L. and ARNE, L. Troubles du langage de type aphasique et lesions putamino-caudees. *Revue Neurologique* (1981), **137**, 343–356.

BARON, J.C., D'ANTONA, R., PANTANO, P., SERDARU, M., SAMSON, Y. and BOUSSER, M.G. Effects of thalamic stroke on energy metabolism of the cerebral cortex: a positron tomography study in man. *Brain* (1986), **109**, 1243–1259.

BELL, D.S. Speech functions of the thalamus as inferred from the effects of thalamotomy. *Brain* (1968), **91**, 619–638.

BOGOUSSLAVSKY, J., REGLI, F. and ASSAL, G. The syndrome of unilateral tuberothalamic artery territory infarction. *Stroke* (1986), **17**, 434–441.

BOTEZ, M.I. and BARBEAU, A. Role of subcortical structures, and particularly of the thalamus, in the mechanisms of speech and language. *International Journal of Neurology* (1971), **8**, 300–320.

BROADBENT, G. *On the Cerebral Mechanisms of Speech and Thought* (1872). Med. Chir. Trans. London Quoted after Kussmaul (1877).

BROWN, J.W. On the neural organization of language: thalamic and cortical relationships. *Brain and Language* (1975), **2**, 18–30.

BROWN, J.W., RIKLAN, M., WALTZ, J., JACKSON, S. and COOPER, I.S. Preliminary studies of language and cognition following surgical lesions of the pulvinar in man (cryopulvinectomy). *International Journal of Neurology* (1971), **8**, 276–299.

BRUNNER, R.J., KORNHUBER, H.H., SEEMÜLLER, E., SUGER, G. and WALLESCH, C.W. Basal ganglia participation in language pathology. *Brain and Language* (1982), **16**, 281–299.

BUGIANI, O., CONFORTO, C. and SACCO, G. Aphasia in thalamic haemorrhage. *Lancet* (1969), **i**, 1052.

VAN BUREN, J. Confusion and disturbance of speech from stimulation in vicinity of the head of the caudate nucleus. *Journal of Neurosurgery*, **20**, 148–157.

BUTTERS, N., ROSEN, J. and STEIN, D. Recovery of behavioral functions after sequential ablation of the frontal lobe in monkeys. In D.G. Stein, J. Rosen and N. Butters (eds) *Plasticity and Recovery in the Nervous System* (1974). New York: Academic Press.

BUTTERWORTH, B. Jargon aphasia: processes and strategies. In S. Newman and R. Epstein (eds) *Current Perspectives in Dysphasia* (1985). Edinburgh: Churchill Livingstone.

CAMBIER, J., ELGHOZI, D. and STRUBE, E. Hemorrhagie de la tete du noyau caude gauche. Desorganisation du discours et de l'expression graphique, perturbations des series gesturelles. *Revue Neurologique* (1979), **135**, 763–774.

CAMBIER, J., GRAVELLAU, P., DECROIX, J.P., ELGHOZI, D. and MASSON, M. Le syndrome de l'artere choroidienne anterieure. Etude neuropsychologique de 4 cas. *Revue Neurologique* (1983), **139**, 553–559.

CAPPA, S.F., CAVALLOTTI, G.. GUIDOTTI, M., PAPAGNO, C. and VIGNOLO, L.A. Subcortical aphasia: two clinical-CT scan correlation studies. *Cortex*, (1983), **19**, 227–241.

CAPPA, S.F., PAPAGNO, C., VALLAR, G. and VIGNOLO, L.A. Aphasia does not always follow left thalamic haemorrhage: A study of five negative cases. *Cortex* (1986), **22**, 639-647.

CAPPA, S.F. and VIGNOLO, L.A. 'Transcortical' features of aphasia following left thalamic haemorrhage. *Cortex* (1979), **15**, 121–130.

CARMAN, J.B., COWAN, W.M. and POWELL, T.P.S. A bilateral cortico-striate projection. *Journal of Neurology, Neurosurgery and Psychiatry* (1965), **28**, 71–77.

COOPER, I.S. *Parkinsonism: its medical and surgical therapy* (1961). Springfield: Thomas.

COOPER, I.S., RIKLAN, M., STELLAR, S., WALTZ, J.M., LEVITA, E., RIBERA, V.A. and ZIMMERMAN, J. A multidisciplinary investigation of neurosurgical rehabilitation in bilateral Parkinsonism. *Journal of The American Geriatrics Society* (1968), **16**, 1177–1306.

CREUTZFELDT, O.D. Cortex cerebri (1983). Berlin, Heidelberg, New York: Springer.

CROSSON, B. Role of the dominant thalamus in language: a review. *Psychological Bulletin* (1984), **96**, 491–517.

CROSSON, B. Subcortical functions in language: a working model. *Brain and Language* (1985), **25**, 257–292.

CROSSON, B., PARKER, J.C. KIM, A.K. WARREN, R.L., KEPES, J.J. and TULLEY, R. A case of thalamic aphasia with postmortem verification. *Brain and Language* (1986), **29**, 301–314.

DAMASIO, A.R., DAMASIO, H., RIZZO, M., VARNEY, N. and GERSH, F. Aphasia with nonhaemorrhagic lesions in the basal ganglia and internal capsule. *Archives of Neurology*, (1982), **39**, 15–20.

DAMASIO, H. Anatomy of basal ganglia and basal forebrain. Paper read at 28th International Neuropsychological Symposium, Rethymnon, Greece (1983).

DECROIX, J.P., GRAVELEAU, PH., MASSON, M. and CAMBIER, J. Infarction in the territory of the anterior choroidal artery: a clinical and computerized tomographic study. *Brain* (1986), **109**, 1071–1086.

ECCLES, J.C. In K.R. Popper and J.C. Eccles (eds) *The Self and Its Brain* (1977). Berlin: Heidelberg, New York: Springer.

ELGHOZI, D., STRUBE, E., SIGNORET, J.L., CAMBIER, J. and LHERMITTE, F. Quasi-aphasie lors de lesions du thalamus. Relation du trouble du langage et de l'activation elective de l'hemisphere gauche dans 4 observations de lesions thalamiques gauches et droites. *Revue Neurologie* (1978), **134**, 557–574.

EVARTS, E.V., SHINODA, Y. and WISE, S.P. *Neurophysiological Approaches to Higher Brain Functions* (1984). New York: Wiley.

FAZIO, C., SACCO, G. and BUGIANI, O. The thalamic haemorrhage: an anatomo-clinical study. *European Neurology* (1973), **9**, 30–43.

FROMM, D., HOLLAND, A.S., SWINDELL, C.S. and REINMUTH, O.M. Various consequences of subcortical stroke. *Archives of Neurology* (1985), **42**, 943–950.

GOLDMAN, P.S. and NAUTA, W.J.H. An intricately patterned prefronto-caudate projection in the rhesus monkey. *Journal of Comparative Neurology* (1977), **205**, 398–413.

GOLDMAN-RAKIC, P.S. Modular organization of the prefrontal cortex. *TINS* (1984), **7**, 419–424.

GOLDSTEIN, K. *Language and language disturbances* (1948). New York: Grune & Stratton.

GORELICK, P.B., HIER, D.B., BENEVENTO, L., LEVITT, S and TAN, W. Aphasia after left thalamic infarction. *Archives of Neurology* (1984), **41** 1296–1298.

GRAFF-RADFORD, N.R., ESLINGER, P.J., DAMASIO, A.R. and YAMADA, T. Nonhaemorrhagic infarction of the thalamus: behavioral, anatomic, and physiologic correlates. *Neurology* (1984), **34**, 14–23.

GRAFF-RADFORD, N.R., DAMASIO, H., YAMADA, T., ESLINGER, P.J. and DAMASIO, A.R. Nonhaemorrhagic thalamic infarction. Clinical, neuropsychological and electrophysiological findings in four anatomical groups defined by computerized tomography. *Brain* (1985), **108**, 485–516.

GROVES, P.M. A theory of the functional organization of the neostriatum and the neostriatal control of voluntary movement. *Brain Research Review* (1983), **5**, 109–132.

GURD, J., BESSELL, N., BLADON, A. and BAMFORD, J. A case of foreign accent syndrome, with follow-up clinical, neuropsychological and phonetic descriptions. *Poster, 5th European workshop on cognitive neuropsychology* (1987). Bressanone, Italy.

HASSLER, R., MUNDINGER, F. and RIECHERT, T. *Stereotaxis in Parkinson Syndrome* (1979). Berlin: Heidelberg, New York: Springer.

HELGASON, C., CAPLAN, L.R., GOODWIN, J. and HEDGES, T. Anterior choroidal artery infarction. *Archives of Neurology* (1986), **43**, 681–686.

HERMANN, K., TURNER,J.W., GILLINGHAM, F.J. and GAZE, R.M. The effects of destructive lesions and stimulation of the basal ganglia on speech mechanisms. *Confinia Neurologica* (1966), **27**, 197–207.

HIER, D.B., DAVIS, K.R., RICHARDSON, E.P. and MOHR, J.P. Hypertensive putaminal haemorrhage. *Annals of Neurology* (1977), **1**, 152–159.

VAN HOESEN, G.W., YETERIAN, E.M. and LAVIZZO-MOUREY, R. Widespread cortico-striate projections from temporal cortex of rhesus monkey. *Journal of Comparative Neurology* (1981), **199**, 205–219.

HUBEL, D.H. and WIESEL, T.N. Anatomical demonstration of columns in the monkey striate cortex. *Nature (Lond.)* (1969), **221**, 747–750.

JONAS, S. The supplementary motor region and speech emission. *Journal of Communication Disorders* (1981), **14**, 349–373.

JONAS, S. The thalamus and aphasia, including transcortical aphasia: a review. *Journal of Communication Disorders* (1982), **15**, 31–41.

KAITZ, S.S. and ROBERTSON, R.T. Thalamic connections with limbic cortex, II. Corticothalamic projections. *Journal of Comparative Neurology* (1981), **195**, 527–545.

KEMP, J.M. and POWELL, T.P.S. The cortico-striate projection in the monkey. *Brain* (1970), **93**, 525–546.

KORNHUBER, H.H., BRUNNER, R.J. and WALLESCH, C.W. Basal ganglia participation in aphasia. In O.D. Creutzfeldt, H. Scheich and C. Schreiner (eds) *Hearing Mechanisms and Speech* (1979). Berlin, Heidelberg, New York: Springer.

KRAYENBÜHL, H. and YASARGIL, M.G. *Die zerebrale Angiographie* (1965). Stuttgart: Thieme.

KÜNZLE, H. Bilateral projections from precentral motor cortex to the putamen and other parts of the basal ganglia. An autoradiographic study in *Macaca fascicularis. Brain Research* (1975), **88**, 195–209.

KUSSMAUL, A. *Die Störungen der Sprache* (1877). Leipzig: Vogel.

LAITINEN, L.V. and VILKKI, J. Observations on physiological and psychological functions of the ventral oral internal nucleus of the human thalamus. *Acta Neurologica Scandinavica* (1977), **55** 190–212.

LAZORTHES, G., GOUAZE, A. and SALOMON, C. *Vascularization et Circulation de l'encephale* (1976). Paris: Masson.

LECOURS, A.R. and LHERMITTE, F. *L'aphasie* (1979). Paris: Fleammearion.

LEES, A.J. and SMITH, E. Cognitive deficits in the early stages of Parkinson's disease. *Brain* (1983), **106**. 257–270.

LEVITA, E., RIKLAN, M. and COOPER, I.S. A psychological comparison of unilateral and bilateral thalamic surgery. *Journal of Abnormal Psychology* (1967), **72**, 251–254.

LICHTHEIM, L. On aphasia. *Brain*, (1885), **7**, 433–484.

LONDON, E.D., MCKINNEY, M., DAM, M., ELLIS, A. and COYLE, J.T. Decreased cortical glucose utilization after ibotenate lesion of the rat ventromedial globus pallidus. *Journal of Cerebral Blood Flow and Metabolism* (1984), **4**, 381–390.

LURIA, A.R. *Traumatic Aphasia* (1970). Den Haag: Mouton.

LURIA, A.R. On quasi-aphasic speech disturbances in lesions of the deep structures of the brain. *Brain and Language* (1977), **4**, 432–459.

MCFARLING, D., ROTHI, L.J. and HEILMAN, K.M. Transcortical aphasia from ischaemic infarcts of the thalamus: a report of two cases. *Journal of Neurology, Neurosurgery and Psychiatry*, (1982), **45**, 107–112.

MCFIE, J. Psychological effects of stereotaxic operations for the relief of Parkinsonian symptoms. *Journal of Mental Science* (1960), **106**, 1512–1517.

MATISON, R., MAYEUX, R., ROSEN, J. and FAHN, S. 'Tip-of-the-tongue' phenomenon in Parkinson disease. *Neurology* (1982), **32**, 567–570.

MEHLER, W.R. Idea of a new anatomy of the thalamus. *Journal of Psychiatric Research* (1971), **8** 203–217.

METTER, E.J., WASTERLAIN, C.G., KUHL, D.E., HANSON, W.R. and PHELPS, M.E. 18FDG Positron emission computed tomography in a study of aphasia. *Annals of Neurology* (1981), **10**, 173–183.

MICHEL, D., LAURENT, B., FOYATIER, N., BLANC, A. and PORTAFAIX, M. Infarctus thalamique paramedian gauche. *Revue Neurologique* (1982), **138**, 533–550.

MOHR, J.P. Thalamic lesions and syndromes. In A. Kertesz (ed.) *Localization of Lesion in Neuropsychology* (1983). New York: Academic Press.

MOHR, J.P., WATTERS, W.C. and DUNCAN, G.W. Thalamic haemorrhage and aphasia. *Brain and Language* (1975), **2**, 3–17.

VON MONAKOW, C. *Die Lokalisation im Grosshirn* (1914). Wiesbaden: Bergmann.

MORRISON, R.S. and DEMPSEY, E.W. Mechanisms of thalamocortical augmentation and repetition. *American Journal of Physiology* (1942), **135**, 281–292.

MOUNTCASTLE, V.B. Modality and topographic properties of single neurones of cats somatic sensory cortex. *Journal of Neurophysiology* (1957), **20**, 615–622.

MOUTIER, F. *L'Aphasie de Broca* (1908). Doctoral thesis, Paris.

NAESER, M.A., ALEXANDER, M.P., HELM-ESTABROOKS, N., LEVINE, H.L., LAUGHLIN, S.A. and GESCHWIND, N. Aphasia with predominantly subcortical lesion sites *Archives of Neurology* (1982), **39**, 2–14.

OJEMANN, G.A. Language and the thalamus: Object naming and recall during and after thalamic stimulation. *Brain and Language* (1975), **2**, 101–120.

OJEMANN, G.A. Subcortical language mechanisms. In H. Whitaker and H.A Whitaker (eds) *Studies in Neurolinguistics* vol. 1 (1976). New York: Academic Press.

OJEMANN, G.A. Asymmetric function of the thalamus in man. *Annals of The New York Academy of Science* (1977), **299**, 380–396.

OJEMANN, G.A. Brain organization for language from the perspective of electrical stimulation mapping. *The Behavioural and Brain Sciences* (1983), **2**, 189–230.

OJEMANN, G.A., FEDIO, P. and VAN BUREN, G. Anomia from pulvinar and subcortical parietal stimulation. *Brain* (1968), **91**, 99–116.

OJEMANN, G.A., BLICK, K. and WARD, A. Improvement and disturbance of short term verbal memory with human ventrolateral thalamic stimulation. *Brain* (1971), **94**, 225–240.

OZAKI, I., BABA, M., NARITA, S., MATSUNAGA, M. and TAKEBE, K. Pure dysarthria due to anterior internal capsule and/or corona radiata infarction: a report of five cases. *Journal of Neurology, Neurosurgery and Psychiatry* (1986), **49**, 1435–1437.

PARENT, A. *Comparative Neurobiology of the Basal Ganglia* (1986). New York: Wiley.

PASIK, P., PASIK, T. and DIFIGLIA, M. The internal organization of the neostriatum in mammals. In I. Divac and R.G.E. Öberg (eds) *The Neostriatum* (1979). Oxford: Pergamon.

PENFIELD, W. and ROBERTS, L. *Speech and Brain Mechanisms* (1959). Princeton: Princeton University Press.

PENNEY, J.B. and YOUNG, A.B. GABA as the pallidothalamic neurotransmitter: implications for basal ganglia function. *Brain Research* (1981), **207**, 195–199.

PERANI, D., VALLAR, G., CAPPA, S., MESSA, C. and FAZIO, F. Aphasia and neglect after subcortical stroke. *Brain* (1987, in press).

PERCHERON, G. Les arteres du thalamus humain. Arteres et territoires thalamiques paramedians de l'artere basilaire communicante. *Revue Neurologique* (1976), **132**, 309–324.

PHILLIPS, C.G. and PORTER, R. *Corticospinal Neurones* (1977). London: Academic Press.

PHILLIPS, C.G., ZEKI, S. and BARLOW, H.B. Localization of function in the cerebral cortex. *Brain* (1984), **107**, 327–362.

PUEL, M., DEMONET, J.F., CARDEBAT, D., BONAFE, A., GAZOUNAUD, Y., GUIRAUD-CHAUMEIL, B. and RASCOL, A. Aphasies sous-corticales. *Revue Neurologique* (1984), **140**, 695–710.

PUEL, M., CARDEBAT, D., DEMONET, J.F., ELGHOZI, D., CAMBIER, J., GUIRAUD-CHAUMEIL, B. and RASCOL, A. Le role du thalamus dans les aphasies sous-corticales. *Revue Neurologique* (1986), **142**, 431–440.

RAGSDALE, C.W. and GRAYBIEL, A.M. The fronto-striatal projections in the cat and monkey and its relationship to inhomogeneities established by acetylcholinesterase histochemistry. *Brain Research* (1981), **208**, 259–266.

REYNOLDS, A.F., TURNER, P.T., HARRIS, A.B., OJEMANN, G.A. and DAVIS, L.E. Left thalamic haemorrhage with dysphasia: a report of five cases. *Brain and Language* (1979), **7**, 62–73.

RIKLAN, M. and COOPER, I.S. Psychometric studies of verbal functions following thalamic lesions in humans. *Brain and Language* (1975), **2**, 62–73.

RIKLAN, M., DILLER, L. WEINER, H. and COOPER, I.S. Psychological studies on effects of chemosurgery of the basal ganglia in Parkinsonism. *Archives of General Psychiatry* (1960), **2**, 22–31.

RINGELSTEIN, E.B., ZEUMER, H. and SCHNEIDER, R. Der Beitrag der zerebralen Computertomographie zur Differentialtypologie und Differentialtherapie des ischämischen Grosshirninfarktes. *Fortschritte Neurologie und Psychiatrie* (1985), **53**, 315–336.

ROBERTSON, R.T. and CUNNINGHAM, T.J. Organization of corticothalamic projections from parietal cortex in cat. *Journal of Comparative Neurology* (1981), **199**, 569–585.

ROLLS, E.T., THORPE, S.J., MADDISON, S., ROPER-HALL, A., PUERTO, A. and PERRETT, D. Activity of neurones in the neostriatum and related structures in the alert animal. In I. Divac and R.G.E. Öberg (eds) *The Neostriatum* (1979). Oxford: Pergamon.

ROSVOLD, H.E. and SZWARCBART, M. Neural structures involved in delayed-response performance. In J.M. Warren and K. Akert (eds) *The Frontal Granular Cortex and Behaviour* (1964). New York: McGraw Hill.

RUBENS, A.B. Transcortical motor aphasia. In H. Whitaker and H.A. Whitaker (eds) *Studies in Neurolinguistics* vol. 1 (1976). New York: Academic Press.

SAKAI, S.T. The thalamic connectivity of the primary motor cortex (MI) in the raccoon. *Journal of Comparative Neurology* (1982), **204**, 238–252.

SAMRA, K., RIKLAN, M., LEVITA, E. ZIMMERMAN, J., WALTZ, J.M., BERGMANN, L. and COOPER, I.S. Language and speech correlates of anatomically verified lesions in thalamic surgery for Parkinsonism. *Journal of Speech and Hearing Research* (1969), **12**, 510–540.

SCHALTENBRAND, G. The effects on speech and language of stereotactical stimulation in the thalamus and corpus callosum. *Brain and Language* (1975), **2**, 70–77.

SCHUELL, H., JENKINS, J.J. and JIMINEZ-PABON, E. *Aphasia in Adults* (1965). New York: Harper & Row.

SELBY, G. Stereotactic surgery for the relief of Parkinson's disease. Part 2. An analysis of the results in a series of 303 patients (413 operations). *Journal of Neurological Science* (1967), **5**, 343–375.

SELEMON, L.D. and GOLDMAN-RAKIC, P.S. Longitudinal topographic organization and interdigitation of cortocostriatal projections in the rhesus monkey. *Journal of Neuroscience* (1985), **5**, 776–794.

SHAPIRO, D.Y., SADOWSKY, D.A., HENDERSON, W.G., and VAN BUREN, J.M. An assessment of cognitive functions in postthalamotomy Parkinson patients. *Confinia Neurologica* (1973), **35**, 144–166.

SKYHÖJ, OLSEN, T., BRUHN, P., and ÖBERG, R.G.E. Cortical hypoperfusion as a possible cause of 'subcortical aphasia'. *Brain* (1986), **109**, 393–410.

SMYTH, G.E. and STERN, K. Tumours of the thalamus. A clinico-pathological study. *Brain*, (1938), **61**, 339–373.

SQUIRE, L.R. and MOORE, R.Y. Dorsal thalamic lesion in a case of human memory dysfunction. *Annals of Neurology* (1979), **6**, 503–506.

STERZI, R. and VALLAR, G. Frontal lobe syndrome as a disconnection syndrome: report of a case. *Acta Neurologica* (1978), **33**, 419–425.

SVENNILSON, E., TORVIK, A., LOWE, R. and LEKSELL, L. Treatment of Parkinsonism by stereotactic thermolesions in the pallidal region. *Acta Psychiatrica et Neurologica Scandinavica* (1960), **35**, 358–377.

SZENTAGOTHAI, J. The 'module-concept' in cerebral cortex architecture. *Brain Research*, (1975), **95**, 475–496.

TAYLOR, A.E., SAINT-CYR, J.A. and LANG, A.E. Frontal lobe dysfunction in Parkinson's disease: the cortical focus of neostriatal outflow. *Brain*, (1986), **109**, 845–883.

UNO, M., OZAWA, N. and YOSHIDA, M. The mode of participation of pallido-thalamic transmission investigated with intracellular recording from cat thalamus. *Experimental Brain Research*, (1978), **33**, 493–507.

VILKKI, J. Effects of thalamic lesions on complex perception and memory. *Neuropsychologia* (1978), **16**, 427–437.

VILKKI, J. and LAITINEN, L.V. Effects of pulvinotomy and ventrolateral thalamotomy on some cognitive functions. *Neuropsychologia*, (1976), **14**, 67–78.

WALKER, E. *The Primate Thalamus* (1938). Chicago: Chicago University Press.

WALLESCH, C.W. Zur Repräsentation höherer Hirnleistungen in den tiefen Kernen des Grosshirns. *Habilitationsschrift*, (1984). Freiburg University.

WALLESCH, C.W. Two syndromes of aphasia occurring with ischaemic lesions involving the left basal ganglia. *Brain and Language*, (1985), **25**, 357–361.

WALLESCH, C.W. Aphasia. In M. Swash and J. Oxbury (eds) *Clinical Neurology* vol. 2, (in press). Edinburgh: Churchill-Livingstone.

WALLESCH, C.W., KORNHUBER, H.H., BRUNNER, R.J., KUNZ, T., HOLLERBACH, B. and SUGER, G. Lesions of the basal ganglia, thalamus and deep white matter: differential effects on language functions. *Brain and Language* (1983a), **20**, 286–304.

WALLESCH, C.W., KORNHUBER, H.H., KUNZ, T. and BRUNNER, R.J. Neuropsychological deficits associated with small unilateral thalamic lesions. *Brain*, (1983b), **106**, 141–152.

WALLESCH, C.W., KORNHUBER, H.H., KÖLLNER, C., HAAS, J.C. and HUFNAGL, J.M. Language and cognitive deficits resulting from medial and dorsolateral frontal lobe lesions. *Archiv Psychiatrie Nervenkrankheiten* (1983c), **233**, 279–296.

WALLESCH, C.W., HENRIKSEN, L., KORNHUBER, H.H. and PAULSON, O.B. Observations on regional cerebral blood flow in cortical and subcortical structures during language production in normal man. *Brain and Language* (1985), **25**, 224–233.

WERNICKE, C. *Der aphasische Symptomencomplex* (1874). Breslau: Cohn & Weigert.

WILLIAMS, P.L. and WARWICK, R. *Functional Neuroanatomy of Man* (1975). Edinburgh: Churchill-Livingstone.

WISE, S.P. and STRICK, P.L. Anatomical and physiological organization of the non-primary motor cortex. *TINS* (1984), **7**, 442–446.

YETERIAN, E.M. and VAN HOESEN, G.W. Cortico-striate projections in the rhesus monkey: the organization of certain cortico-caudate connections. *Brain Research* (1978), **139**, 43–63.

12

The Relationship Between Aphasia and Motor Apraxia

Klaus Poeck

Introduction

Before attempting a discussion of the relationship between aphasia and motor apraxia, the latter term should be made explicit. This necessitates comment on symptoms or syndromes which will be excluded from discussion, even though they are traditionally subsumed under the heading of 'the apraxias'.

There are two types of motor apraxia, the ideomotor and the ideational variant (summarized in Poeck, 1982). For reasons discussed below, it cannot even be certain that these two, which make up the core of the apraxias, belong to the same class of neuropsychological syndromes. Constructional apraxia should be treated apart, because it is basically a spatial and not a motor disturbance; it is, so to speak, the efferent aspect of visuo-spatial disorientation which, again, might not be a unitary symptom but rather the result of visual, proprioceptive, or vestibular dysfunction due to parietal lobe damage. Similarly, two other syndromes, which have been given the epitheton of apraxia will not be considered here because their relationship to the motor apraxias is not evident. On the contrary, they can be easily explained on a different basis. 'Dressing apraxia' (Brain, 1956), although highly esteemed in Anglo-American teaching in neurology, is definitely but one of the many consequences of spatial disorientation and in most cases also of left-sided neglect. The so-called 'apraxia of gait' (Meyer *et al.*, 1960) fails to fulfill the basic requirement for the diagnosis of motor apraxia, which is that the patient not only abstains from certain movements or actions, or carries them out in a clumsy way, but even more so performs 'parapractic' movements. This crucial term, coined by Hugo Liepman (1905), can be defined on the basis of modern studies on the quality of apraxic movements (Poeck and Kerschensteiner, 1975; Lehmkuhl, Poeck and Willmes, 1983) as movements whose elements have been incorrectly selected and are being produced in incorrect sequences. Both aspects: selection of elements of a movement and their sequential ordering are equally important, hence it does not do justice to the phenomena of apraxia when they are viewed exclusively as disorders in sequencing.

Kimura (1977) lays great emphasis on the sequential impairment of movements after left hemisphere brain damage. She describes this sequential deficit as 'problems in making the transition from one position to another'. Admittedly, apraxic patients do have these problems, but any study of apraxia in terms of the quality of the faulty elements distorting the required movements will demonstrate that there is more in apraxia than just a deficit in sequencing (*see* our studies cited above). Considering selection and sequencing, we have a first analogy between language and movement which will be discussed in detail later in this chapter. Another important reason for the exclusion of dressing and gait disturbance is more theoretical in nature: A subgroup or variant of apraxia must make sense in neurophysiological terms. Apraxia — that is, ideomotor apraxia — is observed for movements of *certain parts of the body* having a distinct representation in the motor system. Hence there is oral and limb apraxia, the latter affecting the upper and/or lower limb(s) usually to a similar degree (Lehmkuhl, Poeck and Willmes, 1983; Poeck, 1985), although the legs are rarely tested. There is, however, no cerebral representation for *certain actions* like dressing, so that a patient cannot be apraxic for certain types of performances any more than he can be aphasic for verbs or adjectives. Apraxia, like aphasia, must be viewed as a multi-modal disturbance.

Localized Relationship Between Aphasia and Motor Apraxia and its Possible Significance

The relationship between aphasia and apraxia has been discussed in the literature almost exclusively under two aspects: Both syndromes affect only *human* expression and communication. Animals do not develop apraxia as a consequence of a brain lesion, no matter where the lesion is located (Ettlinger, 1969). Both syndromes are related to lesions in the hemisphere dominant for language, and this is true for ideomotor as well as ideational apraxia. Recently De Renzi *et al.* (1980) have maintained that motor apraxia is also found to a considerable extent in patients with right-sided brain lesions. They found 20% of unselected right brain damaged patients showing signs of apraxia, which is in contrast to the experience of many researchers and also to our systematic study (Lehmkuhl, Poeck and Willmes, 1983). This controversial finding is most likely an artifact of the cut-off score which they established on purely empirical grounds, without cross validation or use of a discriminant analysis procedure.

It is well known that patients with right-sided language dominance develop, as a rule, ideomotor apraxia after right-sided brain damage (Poeck and Kerschensteiner, 1971). Only in very rare instances has a dissociation of hemispheric dominance for praxis and language been discussed (Heilman *et al.*, 1973; Heilman *et al.*, 1974). For ideational apraxia, there is only one case on record where it was due to right-sided brain damage, and the patient had right-sided or at least bilateral language representation (Poeck and Lehmkuhl, 1980).

These two lines of evidence might suggest that motor apraxia is in some way language dependent. 'Language dependent' can mean that a symptom or a syndrome is brought about by a disconnexion of a certain cortical area from the language area (Geschwind, 1965). The disconnexion hypothesis implies that verbal concepts govern motor actions of the 'higher' order that we term praxis. Geschwind has some very good arguments to support his point, e.g. the occurrence of sympathetic dyspraxia of the left hand after a supracapsular lesion of the left hemisphere or anterior callosal lesion, and the fact that lesions of the left hemisphere, which could not possibly disconnect either the language area or the adjacent fields from the motor areas, do not produce motor apraxia. The fact that ideational apraxia cannot be explained in a disconnexion model would not speak against Geschwind's views because of the important structural differences between the two variants of apraxia (Poeck and Lehmkuhl, 1980; Poeck, 1982, *see* also below).

The experience that ideomotor apraxia manifests itself not only on verbal command but also on imitation would not necessarily preclude verbal mediation. The important objection against a verbal-motor disconnexion model stems from the generally accepted experience that apraxic patients are also unable to perform meaningless, non-symbolic movements. So the role of verbal mediation, although certainly present in the execution of meaningful movements, as in any other verbalization activity, does not seem to be the crucial factor for praxis.

'Language dependent' could, in a more restricted sense, imply that a symptom or a syndrome is the direct consequence of aphasic language disorder. This problem has been discussed for a variety of left-hemisphere symptoms by Poeck and Orgass (1971). However, aphasia and both types of apraxia vary independently. While it is true that all patients with oral apraxia and bilateral ideomotor limb apraxia as well as all patients with ideational apraxia are aphasic in the initial stage of the disease, there can be recovery of language functions in the presence of persisting apraxia and vice versa.

So this does not appear to be a fruitful line of reasoning either, although the common advent of language and praxis in the phylogenetic development of the brain should be given some meaningful interpretation. A tentative and highly speculative consideration is that both activities, language and praxis, require the formation of concepts. Certainly, one important step in the phylogenetic development of the human brain as well as in child development was the liberation from instinctive and reflexive behaviour in favour of conceptual behaviour. It has repeatedly been maintained that conceptual behaviour is linked to left hemisphere activity (Basso *et al.*, 1971; Cohen *et al.*, 1980; Basso *et al.*, 1981). The fact that aphasia and apraxia are both left hemisphere syndromes (the term left hemisphere being used here somewhat loosely, yet correctly for the very great majority of patients) would neither indicate a dependence of one syndrome upon the other nor suggest a mere coincidence devoid of any meaning. Rather, both syndromes would be (loosely) linked to a common denominator. This would still leave room for the view that conceptual thinking was made possible by the development of language functions.

The problem with this reasoning is that certainly there is no evidence for the assumption that either ideomotor apraxia or aphasia can be traced back to a conceptual disturbance. Moreover, as will be shown below, there is no well defined structural relationship between aphasic and apractic errors.

Symptomatic Relationship Between Aphasia and Motor Apraxia

One important technical problem is that, in contrast to the considerable agreement on how language should be tested in aphasic patients, there is more diversity with regard to what motor tasks should be given to patients with left hemispheric damage. Most clinical studies to which common teaching on apraxia refers are based on a limited repertoire of oral or limb movements which are partly meaningful and partly meaninglesss, and which lend themselves to easy bedside use. Pertinent tasks are listed e.g. in De Renzi, Pieczuro and Vignolo (1966) or, more recently, in Poeck (1986), the latter paper including also lists of bimanual movements and movements of the legs. A systematic study on axial movements was published by Poeck, Lehmkuhl and Willmes (1982).

Motor functions after left hemisphere damage have, however, also been tested with regard to more basic skills, like a tapping test (Heilman, 1975), performance on the pursuit rotor (Heilman *et al.*, 1975) and speed of arm movements towards a target (Wyke, 1967). In non-brain damaged subjects, Lomas and Kimura (1976) have found that sequential hand and arm movements were particularly impaired on the right by concomitant speaking. Freund (1985) and Freund and Hummelsheim (1985) have studied motor performance in patients with CT evidence of a lesion restricted to frontal lobe structures sparing the precentral gyrus. They gave their patients a battery of standardized dexterity tests calling for steadiness, tracking, aiming with one hand, aiming with both hands, tapping, manipulation rate, and they also measured speech of finger movements and the ability to perform synchronous or alternating windmill movements of the arms. The majority of the patients showed degradation and decomposition of movements when coordination of both arms was required. These studies are certainly of great importance for the conceptualization of those motor functions which are in the realm of the left hemisphere, and they might eventually help to enrich the concept of ideomotor apraxia. At present, however, they cannot be discussed in the context of this chapter, because performance on the above mentioned motor tasks was not systematically related to performance on 'clinical' apraxia tasks. Furthermore, the aphasiological data are at best confined to the statement that aphasia was present or absent, which does not permit considerations of the structural relationship between the motor and language deficit.

The same is true of studies on *motor learning* after left hemisphere damage (Kimura, 1977). A comparison of the acquisition of motor versus language skills in left brain damaged patients would be most desirable, but this study still has to be done. It would certainly meet some theoretical problems, because the aim of the aphasic patient in speech therapy is the reacquisition of a system of communication whose highly complex rules he mastered before and has only lost in part. In contrast, the acquisition of tapping or aiming or correctly carrying out the movements with the manual sequence box (Kimura, 1977) requires highly artificial performances of no communicative value. Also, it should not be overlooked that aphasic errors are observed in spontaneous behaviour, while (ideomotor) apraxic patients are not impaired in movements within their natural context.

Mateer and Kimura (1977) have done a study on non-verbal oral movements in aphasic patients, and they have compared their motor performance to some aspects of their linguistic performance. The most interesting feature of these experiments is that, in addition to the usually applied single movements of the 'stick out tongue' type, the authors introduced serial oral movements which are not included in the tasks of other researchers. They found patients with non-fluent aphasia, but not those with fluent aphasia, impaired in imitating simple discrete movements of the oral musculature. In contrast, fluent aphasics demonstrated a highly significant impairment in multiple oral movements. Scores for single phoneme production were lowest in the non-fluent group, production of multiple phonemes of the 'ba-da-ga' type was strikingly impaired in the fluent aphasic group.

Although the design of this study is impressive, several objections can be raised which suggest some caution vis-à-vis the authors' conclusion that 'deficits in co-ordinating oral movements are fundamental to most aphasic impairments'. First, the groups are small (4 non-fluent versus 8 fluent aphasics). Second, and more important, the supercategories fluent and non-fluent are ill-suited for a refined qualitative analysis of both linguistic and motor performance. In the non-fluent group, the patients may have Broca's, global or transcortical motor aphasia, and the fluent group might include Wernicke's aphasia with or without semantic or phonemic jargon, amnesic or conduction aphasia. These subgroups differ so profoundly with respect to linguistic performance, localization and extent of brain lesion that one should not build a very strong hypothesis on the results of this interesting experiment. Certainly, when Kimura (1976) goes so far as to suggest that speech should be considered primarily as another, albeit special, complex motor function, she neglects the non-motor aspects of oral communication which are generally made explicit in the distinction between speech and language. That language cannot be considered a sequential activity has been strongly argued by Poeck and Huber (1977). A critical approach to the poorly defined concept that the left hemisphere harbours 'symbolic functions' is certainly in place, but the view that 'the fundamental left hemispheric function is the execution of certain motor functions which lend themselves readily to communication' (Kimura, 1973) is not warranted considering the wealth of other researchers' findings both in the field of aphasia and apraxia.

Given that most aphasic patients — not only those with Broca's aphasia (*see* Kerschensteiner and Poeck, 1974; Poeck und Kerschensteiner, 1975) — have oral apraxia, and given further that a global analysis shows a high positive correlation between the *quantitative* occurrence of phonemic paraphasias and the degree of oral apraxia (de Renzi *et al.*, 1965, Kerschensteiner and Poeck, 1974), the question must be discussed to what extent the deficit in oral movements might influence language performance. Obviously, this could occur in two ways:

1. First, the patient could be so severely apractic that he is unable to utter a sound. He could, when addressed, either produce no oral movement at all or produce random oral movements which do not result in voiced and articulated speech. This condition is termed anarthria. The view that anarthria is the most severe form of oral apraxia is hard to defend. Patients with ideomotor apraxia of the limbs, even in its most striking degree, are not *unable* to move the limbs but rather produce sequences of inadequate, mostly perseverative movements, and they do so only in the testing situation, as will be repeatedly stressed in this chapter.
2. A second and more interesting question is whether the deficit in the selection and sequential ordering of phonemes which leads to phonemic paraphasias is linguistic or motor in nature. This problem has been studied initially by Burns and Canter (1977), and these authors have convincingly demonstrated that in Wernicke's aphasia the quality of

phonemic paraphasias bears no relationship to the presence of oral apraxia. The thorny problem of apraxia of speech will not be discussed here (*see* Martin and Rigrodsky, 1974). Also, the intrinsic types of phonemic errors, i.e. substitution, anticipation, elision and augmentation are not all seen in oral apraxia, anticipation being virtually absent. Our analysis of error type in both linguistic and motor performance did not yield a common pattern. Dysarthria has not, to the present author's knowledge, been studied with respect to presence or absence of oral apraxia, let alone in terms of quality of errors.

The language disturbance does not offer any explanation for the syndrome of either ideomotor or ideational apraxia. In spite of their aphasia, the patients frequently make adequate comments on the movements they are unable to carry out or on the nature of the objects they are unable to use to achieve a certain goal.

For the occurrence of aphasic symptoms, the Jacksonian distinction between propositional and automatic language is valid. Without going deeper into the problem of left or right hemisphere contributions to language performance, it can be safely stated that propositional language is always considerably more affected in aphasia.

The aphasias can be reasonably divided into various subgroups of standard and non-standard aphasia, which can be distinguished by certain combinations of symptoms. Yet, they have certain essential features in common, e.g. in principle they affect all linguistic components: phonology, lexicon, syntax/semantics, although to a different degree. Furthermore, they affect all modalities of language performance: speaking and understanding, writing and reading. Finally, the expressive and receptive aspect is always compromised, again to a different degree, which contributes to the distinction of clinical syndromes. The standard aphasic syndromes have a coordinate and not a super- and sub-ordinate relationship.

Can motor apraxia reasonably be viewed in similar categories? Ideomotor apraxia manifests itself only if it is tested for, in other words, out of context, if analytical praxic competence is required. The patients have no problems performing spontaneously the very movements impaired on verbal commands or on imitation.

It does not appear appropriate to refer to this dichotomy in terms of the propositional-automatic dissociation known in the aphasias, because this is not a 'more or less' but rather an 'all or none' phenomenon. Furthermore, one should not treat the propositional-automatic situation in the aphasias at the relatively basic left–right hemisphere level of conceptualization, where automatic is equated with emotional and this with right hemisphere language. Any neurolinguistic analysis, for instance of the naming performance of aphasic patients, clearly demonstrates that the patients are superior when naming is required in a referential, and inferior when in a classificatory, situation. Since this has nothing to do with the emotional aspect of language, it has to be explained at a linguistic level (Poeck *et al.*, 1974) and there is no parallel to this — and similar — language behaviour in ideomotor apraxia.

Geschwind (1965) points out that the difference between spontaneous movements and movements on verbal command or on imitation is an anatomical one, the input to the motor system stemming from the 'motivational cortex' as motor physiologists tend to call it today in one case, and from the posterior language area or the visual association cortex in the other. In terms of the disconnexion model this view is well founded. Again, very few aphasic symptoms can be explained profitably as disconnexion phenomena.

We have looked into the problem of subtypes of ideomotor apraxia, both for apraxia as such and for apraxia in relation to aphasia. An extensive qualitative analysis not only with respect to parts of the body but also with respect to error types (*see* below) has yielded essentially negative results. For error types in oral apraxia, we found that the profiles for the four major subtypes of aphasia ran virtually parallel to each other and to the profile for the whole group of 101 patients (Poeck and Kerschensteiner, 1975). When we extended this type of study on the basis of 88 patients with aphasia and ideomotor apraxia to cover oral, upper limb, lower limb and bimanual movements, meaningful as well as meaningless ones, tested in the verbal and in the imitative mode of examination, we again did not find subtypes of apraxia, be they characterized by affection of certain parts of the body or by certain configurations of errors. Also, there was no structural similarity with the subtypes of aphasia. Theoretically, one could have expected, for example, predominance of fragmentary movements in patients with Broca's aphasia or of augmentation of movements in Wernicke's aphasia and of perseveration of movements in global aphasia. In addition, the degree of severity of apraxia could have corresponded to the degree of aphasia. None of these expectations was confirmed: error types were not differentially distributed across the subtypes of aphasia, and there was no correspondence in degree of severity between aphasia and apraxia (Lehmkuhl, Poeck and Willmes, 1983). These negative findings are in contrast to the statement by Kertesz (1979) that there is a strong correspondence between performance in language comprehension tasks and degree of apraxia. Furthermore, it has not been demonstrated that ideomotor apraxia also has a receptive aspect. Weniger and Müller (1978) have shown that apraxic patients are able to identify the meaning of photographed gestures in a multiple choice set of four situations where only one was appropriate.

For ideational apraxia, the situation is different, but this is a motor disorder at another level (Poeck and Lehmkuhl, 1980 a,b; Poeck, 1982). We have recently carried out a study (Lehmkuhl and Poeck, 1981) in which we demonstrated that patients with ideational apraxia have a disturbance in the conceptual organization of actions. A test was designed that has sufficient similarity to the clinical examination for ideational apraxia but does not include the actual use of objects. Series of photographs representing well defined steps in everyday actions were presented to patients in random order, and the task was to put them in correct sequence. Patients *without* ideational apraxia, even though they were brain damaged, performed the task with no problem in deciding the order of the pictures. In contrast, the patients *with* ideational apraxia were hesitant and quite often could not decide which pictures fit together. Severity of aphasia was not greater in the subgroup with than without ideational apraxia. The results of this study strongly suggest that ideational apraxia, in contrast to ideomotor apraxia, is not characterized by defective motor programming but rather by defective conceptualization of actions.

Preliminary observations indicate that patients with ideational apraxia also have problems when they are to judge correct and incorrect sequences of pictures, but these observations await confirmation which, hopefully, will be produced by a systematic study we have recently started. The problem of coordinate or superordinate relation between subtypes of apraxia does not pose itself, given that we did not find subtypes of apraxia. Even the relation between ideomotor and ideational apraxia cannot be considered as one of superordination, because the presence of ideomotor apraxia is no prerequisite for the occurrence of ideational apraxia. In other words: the latter is not the more severe expression of the former.

Structural Relationship Between Aphasia and Apraxia

In spite of the great functional importance of speaking and moving for human interaction and in spite of the common organization of praxis and language in the same hemisphere, it is only aphasia that has been studied closely with regard to the structure of the disorder. While the introduction of linguistic methods to aphasia research has yielded both a closer insight into the phenomena of aphasia and a strong impetus for research, studies into apraxia were limited to the assessment of the patients passing or failing a given task. The distorted segments of apraxic movements are in general not described in detail, let alone analyzed with the purpose of detecting regular features.

The discrepancy between the refined methods applied to the analysis of aphasic speech and the crude way of assessing apraxic movements is primarily due to the lack of an adequate method for the segmentation and analysis of movements. It is true that David Efron has applied very sophisticated methods of recording and description of expressive movements in his pioneer study on gestural behaviour (1941). Interestingly enough, he used the term linguistic to denote the referential aspect of symbolic movements. He confined his analysis, however, to movements as a whole and did not break them down into single components, probably because this was not required by the scope of his study.

The first author to systematically apply the methods of structural linguistics to the study of normal movements was Birdwhistel (1970). He recognized that body posture, movements and facial expression are patterned behaviour, and he tried to describe a hierarchy of elements in analogy to the description of speech units at different hierarchical levels. He developed an '-emic' system in which kinemes and kinemorphs as units of movement correspond to phonemes and morphemes in the description of language. He also used a system of notation permitting the precise description of the single elements within a motor sequence. The science of kinesics, as he saw it, is concerned with the grouping of only those movements which are of significance for the communication process. More recently, Ulatowska, Kumin and Kaplan, (1974), considering the common communicative aspects of language and motor behaviour, studied the symbolic gestural behaviour (so-called emblems) of aphasics and normals with regard to the production and understanding of an emblem as a whole. These authors have also categorized several modes of failure observed in their patients.

Some years ago we hypothesized that, similar to aphasia, there might exist regularities in the distortion of motor elements in apraxia. We hoped that the systematic analysis of these elements would permit insight into the structure of apraxic movements and into the relationship between aphasia and apraxia. Consequently, we empirically developed a method permitting the quantitative and qualitative assessment of the single components constituting apraxic movements (Kerschensteiner and Poeck, 1974, Poeck und Kerschensteiner, 1975). To describe the movements in this study on oral apraxia, we elaborated a code permitting the transcription of the characteristics of the single components of a motor sequence. We differentiated between four categories: substitution, augmentation, deficient performance and other types of error.

The common feature of substitutions was that the required oral movement was replaced by a finite motor, verbal or acoustic reaction. In this respect, we tentatively spoke of semanticlly different movements. In augmentations, the patient produced additional movements or noises. In deficient performance there was either no reaction or fragmentary execution. Furthermore, we discovered a behaviour similar to the *conduite d'approche* in the language behaviour of aphasic patients, when they correct a phonemic or semantic paraphasia through several stages of approach. Quite similarly, patients approached the correct execution of a movement through several stages of failure. The code we developed permitted the transcription of movements which could then be subjected to mathematical analysis. (For details the reader is referred to the original publications.) In the context of this chapter it is stressed that perseveration emerged as the most characteristic behaviour in apraxia. It has been known since Liepmann's (1905) studies that perseveration is an important feature of apraxia. We have, in our two studies on oral and other types of ideomotor apraxia, evaluated the role of perseveration under conditions of a detailed error analysis, and found an extremely high proportion of perseveration errors. For instance, in the oral apraxia study 75 errors out of a total of 1985 were perseverations. It was surprising how many steps were bridged by perseveration. If we gave our patients 14 tasks for oral apraxia, we could detect even in task no. 13 elements of the movement the patient had carried out in task no. 1. The recognition of these perseveratory elements was, of course, only possible because we did not limit ourselves to a simple pass or fail judgement on the movement as a whole but considered the elements of the movements separately. The strength of the perseveratory tendency can also be judged by the rate of perseveratory errors made on imitation after the execution of the task on verbal command. Here, the patient repeated the error he had made in the version on verbal command against the visual evidence of the correct execution of the movement by the examiner. The role of perseveration has also been stressed by Kimura (1977) and Mateer and Kimura (1977). It should be pointed out that perseveration is not indicative of apraxia after frontal lesions as was suggested by Luria (1966), as it is found with any localization of lesion.

In our study we have strongly stressed analogies between structural linguistics and our approach to analysis and interpretation of apraxic symptoms, but this analogy remained limited to the phonological/kinemic and semantic/conceptual components. Our data did not permit the interpretation of the apraxic motor sequences on a level corresponding to the syntactic component in linguistics. This was not surprising in the light of Birdwhistel's (1970) statement that he was unable to discover a grammar in normal communicative movements.

The impact of our qualitative studies on a theory of ideomotor apraxia is that apraxia can no longer be viewed as a mere deficit in sequential activity. Rather, the selective activity must be given equally careful consideration. This calls strongly for a more refined analysis of the functional elements which both performances, speaking and moving, have in common and those which are differentially germane to each of them.

Conclusions

The relationship between aphasia and motor apraxia has been discussed at various levels. At the neurological level, all reliable data speak strongly for a localization of the lesion underlying both syndromes in the hemisphere dominant for language. At the semiotic and structural level there are certain similarities: language and praxis are structured activities whose elements must be adequately selected and then organized in an appropriate order. By virtue of these structural similarities there must necessarily be similarities in the configuration of errors which may be morphological, semantic and sequential in nature. At this point, however, the correspondence ends. There is no parallel variation in degree of severity, there is no relation between subtype of aphasia and error pattern in apraxia. In fact, there are no subtypes of apraxia, except for the neurologically determined predilection for parts of the body. Comparative studies of aphasia and apraxia did not suggest that disturbances of gesture and pantomime are the outflow of a higher order central communication disorder (*see also* Goodglass and Kaplan, 1963). On the other hand, both activities cannot simply be viewed as but two aspects of a higher order motor disturbance related to left brain damage. If there is a common psychological factor, this can only be seen in the conceptual activity of the left hemisphere, but it should be admitted that this is a vast superstructure which cannot at present be discussed in sufficiently precise terms.

Acknowledgements

For stimulating discussions and critical comments the author is indebted to Ria de Bleser, W. Hartje, W. Huber, M. Kerschensteiner, F.-J. Stachowiak and W. Sturm.

References

BASSO, A., DE RENZI, E., FAGLIONI, P. and SPINNLER, H. Neuropsychological evidence for the existence of cerebral areas critical to the performance of intelligence tasks. *Brain* (1973), **96**, 715–728.

BASSO, A., CAPITANI, E., LUZZATI, C. and SPINNLER, H. Intelligence and left hemisphere disease: the role of aphasia, apraxia and size of lesion. *Brain* (1981), **104**, 721–734.

BIRDWHISTEL, R.L. *Kinesics and Context* (1970). Philadelphia: University of Pennsylvania Press.

BRAIN, W.R. *Speech Disorders: Aphasia, Apraxia, and Agnosia* (1965). Washington: Butterworths.

BURNS, M.S. and CANTER, G.J. Phonemic behavior of aphasic patients with posterior cerebral lesions. *Brain and Language* (1977), **4**, 492–507.

COHEN, R., KELTER, S., ENGEL, D., LIST, G. and STROHNER, H. Zur Validität des Token Tests. *Nervenarzt* (1976), **47**, 357–361.

CRITCHLEY, M. The language of gesture (1971). New York: Haskell House Publishers.

DE RENZI, E., PIECZURO, A. and VIGNOLO, L.A. Oral apraxia and aphasia. *Cortex* (1966), **2**, 50–73.

DE RENZI, E., MOTTI, F. and NICHELLI, P. Imitating gestures. A quantitative approach to ideomotor apraxia. *Archives of Neurology* (1980), **37**, 6–10.

EFRON, D. *Gesture and Environment* (1941). New York: King's Crown.

ETTLINGER, G. Apraxia considered as a disorder of movements that are language-dependent: Evidence from cases of brain bisection. *Cortex* (1969), **5**, 285–289.

FREUND, H.-J. Motor disturbances after frontal lobe lesions in man. *Experimental Brain Research* **58**, Al–A17. In Cerebral events in voluntary movement: the supplementary motor and premotor areas.

FREUND, H.-J. and HUMMELSHEIM, H. Lesions of premotor cortex in man. *Brain* (1985), **108**, 697–733.

GESCHWIND, N. Disconnexion syndromes in animals and men, Part II. *Brain* (1965), **88** 585–644.

GOODGLASS, H. and KAPLAN, E. Disturbance of gesture and pantomime in aphasia. *Brain* (1963), **86**, 703–720.

HEILMAN, K.M., COYLE, J.M., GONYEA, E.F. and GESCHWIND, N. Apraxia and agraphia in a left-hander. *Brain* (1973), **96**, 21–28.

HEILMAN, K.M., GONYEA, E.F. and GESCHWIND, N. Apraxia and agraphia in a right-hander. *Cortex* (1974), **10**, 284–288.

HEILMAN, K.M. A tapping test in apraxia. *Cortex* (1975), **11**, 259–263.

HEILMAN, K.M., SCHWARTZ, H.D. and GESCHWIND, N. Defective motor learning in ideomotor apraxia. *Neurology (Minneap.)* (1975), **25**, 1018–1020.

KERSCHENSTEINER, M. and POECK, K. Bewegungsanalyse bei buccofacialer. Apraxie. *Nervenarzt* (1974), **45**, 9–15.

KERTESZ, A. *Aphasia and Associated Disorders* (1979). New York: Grune and Stratton.

KIMURA, D. The neural basis of language qua gesture. In H. Whitaker and H.A. Whitaker (eds) *Studies in Neurolinguistics* vol. 2 (1976). New York: Academic Press.

KIMURA, D. Acquisition of motor skill after left hemisphere damage. *Brain* (1977), **100**, 527–542.

LEHMKUHL, G. and POECK, K. A disturbance in the conceptual organization of actions in patients with ideational apraxia. *Cortex* (1981), **17**, 153–158.

LEHMKUHL, G., POECK, K. and WILLMES, K. Ideomotor apraxia and aphasia: An examination of types and manifestations of apraxic symptoms (1983). **21 (3)**, 199–212.

LIEPMANN, H. Die linke Hemisphäre und das Handeln. *Münch. med Wschr.* (1905), **52**, 2322–2326, 2375–2378.

LIEPMANN, H. Der weitere Krankheitsverlauf bei dem einseitig Apraktischen und der Gehirnbefund auf Grund von Serienschnitten. *Monatsschrift fin Psychiatrie und Neurologie* (1905), **16**, 289–311.

LIEPMANN, H. Über die Funktionen des Balkens beim Handeln und die Beziehungen von Aphasie und Apraxie zur Intelligenz. In *Drei Aufsätze aus dem Apraxiegebiet* (1908). Berlin: Karger.

LOMAS, J. and KIMURA, D. Intrahemispheric interaction between speaking and sequential manual activity. *Neuropsychologia* (1976), **14**, 23–33.

MARTIN, A.D. and RIGRODSKY, S. An investigation of phonological impairment in aphasia, part I. *Cortex* (1974), **10**, 317–328.

MATEER, C. and KIMURA, D. Impairment of nonverbal oral movements in aphasia. *Brain and Language* (1977), **4**, 262–276.

MEYER, J.S. and BARRON, D.W. Apraxia of gait: A clinico-physiological study. *Brain* (1960), **83**, 261–284.

POECK, K. and ORGASS, B. The concept of the body schema: A critical review and some experimental results. *Cortex* (1971), **7**, 254–277.

POECK, K. and KERSCHENSTEINER, M. Ideomotor apraxia following right-sided cerebral lesion in a left-handed subject. *Neuropsychologia* (1971), **9**, 359–361.

POECK, K., KERSCHENSTEINER, M. STACHOWIAK, F.-J. and HUBER, W. Die amnestische Aphasie. *Journal of Neurology* (1974), **207**, 1–17.

POECK, K. and KERSCHENSTEINER, M. Analysis of the sequential motor events in oral apraxia. In K.J. Zülch, O Creutzfeldt and G.C. Galbraith (eds) *Cerebral Localization* (1975). Berlin: Springer.

POECK, K. and HUBER, W. To what extent is language a sequential activity? *Neuropsychologia* (1977), **15**, 359–363.

POECK, K. and LEHMKUHL, G. Ideatory apraxia in a left handed patient with right-sided brain lesion. *Cortex,* (1980), **16**, 273–284.

POECK, K. und LEHMKUHL, G. Das Syndrom der ideatorischen Apraxie und seine Lokalisation. *Vervenarzt* (1980), **51**, 217–225.

POECK, K. The two types of motor apraxia. *Archives of Italian Biology* (1982), **120**, 361–369.

POECK, K. Clues to the nature of disruptions to limb praxis. In E.A. Roy (ed.) *Advances in Psychology 23, Neuropsychological Studies of Apraxia and Related Disorders* (1984), pp. 99–109. Amsterdam: North Holland.

POECK, K. The clinical examination for motor apraxia. *Neuropsychologia* (1986), **24 (1)**, 129–134.

ULATOWSKA, H., KUMIN, L and KAPLAN, E. Symbolic gestural behavior of aphasics and normals under three task conditions. Unpublished observations.

WENIGER, D. and MÜLLER, R. Recognition and imitation of gestures in brain damaged patients. Paper presented at *the International Neurosychological Symposium* in Oxford, England, June 19-23, 1978.

WYKE, M. Effect of brain lesions on the rapidity of arm movement. *Neurology (Minneap.)* (1967), **17**, 1113–1120.

13

Speech Fluency in Aphasia

Uri Hadar and F. Clifford Rose

Introduction

The use of terms reflecting the concept of speech fluency in the clinical description of various forms of aphasia occurred very early in the study of language disturbances following brain damage. Wernicke (1908) noted that patients with 'sensory' aphasia tend to 'speak rapidly and use a comparatively rich vocabulary' (p. 271) and Pick (1931) described speech in motor aphasia as 'slow, hesitant and with choppy intonation' (p. 14) adding that 'the flow of speech in such patients . . . is generally abnormal' (p. 16). These statements reflected a line of thought that ascribed theoretical importance to the concept of speech fluency, as in Wernicke's (1908) recognition of 'two opposite types of arrested or still fluent speech' (p. 322), but it was not until the 1960s that the term 'fluency' acquired a primary role in the classification of aphasic syndromes, a development triggered by quantitative analyses of spontaneous speech, especially rate (Howes, 1964) and phrase length (Goodglass *et al.*, 1964). Aphasic patients, it was found, tended to speak either in very short phrases (under 3 words per phrase) and at a distinctly low speech rate (under 100 words per minute) or in long phrases (over 5 words per phrase) and high speech rate (over 175 words per minute) (Goodglass *et al.*, 1964; Howes, 1964). While these characteristics were compatible with the increasing evidence for a demarcation between two major classes of aphasic syndromes, they proved resistant to explanatory labelling (e.g., sensory versus motor, receptive versus expressive or anterior versus posterior), and a purely descriptive distinction, with reference to speech ouput only, looked attractive (Geschwind, 1966). The distinction between fluent and nonfluent patients was strengthened by enlarging the battery of fluency parameters with measures of hesitancy, pausing, prosodic structure, etc., and was supported by anatomical findings localizing the lesion in the two groups of patients, with a tendency for fluent patients to have posterior, and nonfluent anterior, lesions (Benson, 1967).

Yet problems soon arose. Firstly, while some fluency parameters discriminated successfully between groups of patients, others did not, e.g., patients tended to have either high or low, but not intermediate, scores on measures such as phrase length, frequency of pause and prosodic line but, on measures such as paraphasia or perseveration, many scores fell inside the intermediate range of values (Kerschensteiner *et al.*, 1972; *Table 1*). This

Table 1 **Rank order of variables according to discriminating power between two classes of aphasic patients (after Kerschensteiner *et al.*, 1972, with permission).**

Class	*1* *−1*	*2* *0*	*3* *1*	x^2	*Variable*
●	18	1	0	36	Phrase length
○	0	0	17		
●	19	0	0	36	Pauses
○	0	7	10		
●	19	0	0	36	Prosody
○	0	1	16		
●	18	1	0	32.99	Rate of speaking
○	0	3	14		
●	13	55	1	32.21	Effort
○	0	0	17		
●	13	4	2	28.82	Articulation
○	0	0	17		
●	18	1	0	18.75	Word choice
○	1	3	13		
●	15	4	0	13.12	Verbal paraphasias
○	4	7	6		
●	8	9	2	11.68	Literal paraphasias
○	2	4	11		
●	12	3	4	10.13	Perseveration
○	2	5	10		

raised the questions of whether or not fluency constituted a unitary group of speech features and, if so, which features characterized this group. Of particular importance was the distinction between articulatory/phonetic and linguistic aspects of speech fluency, without which the unitary nature of the groups could not be preserved. Studies often mixed articulatory measures of fluency, such as speech rate, with linguistic measures such as vocabulary, whilst the nature of other measures (e.g., hesitancy, prosody, etc.) proved highly controversial.

Secondly, even where patients were unambiguously divided between high and low fluency groups, aetiologies differed substantially (Kerschensteiner *et al.*, 1972), findings supported in a comprehensive CT scan study (Knopman *et al.*, 1983) which revealed the inaccuracy of the claim that fluent patients had posterior, and nonfluent anterior, lesions (Benson, 1967). Nonfluency, defined as composite measures of spontaneous speech, could arise from lesions in almost any area of the cortex and, although damage to the foot of the Rolandic fissure correlated most strongly, lesions were found *both* anteriorly and posteriorly (*Table 2*).

These difficulties arose from failure to consider the nature of the various fluency measures with consequent descriptive and conceptual ambiguities. This chapter attempts to clarify some of these issues by a systematic presentation of the available data.

Definition of Fluency and its Constituents

Certain measures have been more or less generally accepted as constituting speech fluency, notably speech rate (words or syllables, per unit time), phrase length (words or syllables per utterance) and prosody (the adequacy of pitch transitions and stress assignment). 'Pronunciation' or 'articulation', a measure of intelligibility of words or syllables was also widely accepted. 'Effort' referred to initiation difficulties, either as syllabic repetitions (stutter or groping) or as the inability to start speech with an unstressed item. 'Pauses' were stoppages in the flow of speech that were either inadequately long (relative to phonation) or placed at non-grammatical junctures, i.e. inside the boundaries of words or clauses (Benson, 1967; Kerschensteiner *et al.*, 1972; Wagenaar *et al.*, 1975; Knopman, 1983).

Besides these accepted measures, less conventional ones were occasionally employed, for example, Benson (1967) regarded 'press of speech', the inability to stop speaking, as a fluency feature. Perseveration was also regarded as fluency related, albeit not without reservations (*ibid*: Kerschensteiner *et al.*, 1972), but these were problematic categories because they could be uttered either fluently or not, for example. Bleser and Poeck (1983) reported both fluent and nonfluent production in highly perseverative

Table 2 Regional involvement in fluent versus nonfluent patients at 6 months postonset: incidence of region sparing in non-fluent patients and region involvement in fluent patients (after Knopman *et al.*, 1983, with permission).

Region		No. of nonfluent patients (N=17)* *without lesion*	No. of fluent patients (N=32)† *with lesion*	x^2	p
Superior premotor		9	3	7.02	0.008
Inferior frontal anterior		7	6	6.39	0.012
Inferior frontal posterior		6	9	4.73	0.030
Middle frontal anterior		10	1	9.15	0.003
Middle frontal posterior		10	2	6.85	0.009
Lower anterior rolandic		1	8	18.55	<0.0001
Lower posterior rolandic		2	6	19.14	<0.0001
Upper anterior rolandic		3	3	22.98	<0.0001
Upper posterior rolandic		4	4	17.32	<0.0001
Suprasylvian supramarginal		6	13	1.70	0.192
Anterior insula		2	11	10.82	0.001
Posterior insula		1	17	6.72	0.004
Posterior superior temporal		8	14	0.10	0.754
Hemispheral white matter	A	4	4	17.33	<0.0001
	B	4	9	8.63	0.003
	C	0	7	24.08	<0.0001
	D	1	9	16.80	<0.0001
	E	3	13	6.22	0.013
Putamen globus pallidus		3	11	8.40	0.004
Internal capsule posterior		6	4	11.89	0.0006
Internal capsule anterior		9	4	7.02	0.008

* Group I
† Groups IIb and III

patients, whose speech comprised a single consonant–vowel (CV) syllable. In this chapter we shall not consider as measures of fluency speech press and perseveration, nor measures of quality of spontaneous speech such as vocabulary range and the grammatical classes that constitute it, paraphasias, etc. This methodological approach may be economically expressed by defining fluency as *the quality that emerges from the regulation of quantity*, where 'quantity' is defined as the temporal aspect of speech production (Lehiste, 1976). This definition will be helpful in considering the basic sources of fluency disturbance.

A variety of definition problems occurred even with the most widely accepted, and ostensibly simple, measures. For instance, Howes (1964) considered normal rates as ranging from 100 to 175 words per minute (wpm), aphasic patients being either nonfluent (less than 100 wpm) or 'hyper' fluent (over 175 wpm), but for Benson (1967) the cut-off values were respectively 50 and 150, while Kerschensteiner *et al.* (1972) failed to observe in aphasic patients speech rates greater than 150 wpm, possibly because their subjects spoke German, not English. Accordingly, *their* cut-off values were respectively 50 and 90.

Another typical problem was the inclusion of non-language sounds in the computation of output volume, especially where rate or length were computed as syllables (rather than words) per unit, as grunts or approximation (groping) syllables could be either included in or excluded from the computed value (Kerschensteiner *et al.*, 1972).

Some measures of fluency were formulated in so vague a fashion that findings could depend on subjective interpretation as, for example, Benson's (1967) definition of 'prosody' disturbance: 'speech is halting and uneven with pauses breaking the phrases or even the words into unusual groupings. Inflection may be entirely absent or almost constant producing a monotonous output, or may be supplied to normally unstressed syllables producing a colourfully abnormal pattern' (p. 375). This, as well as other similar definitions, already included many fluency measures (rate, phrase length, intonation, application of stress, etc.), but without qualification. Examiners could diagnose a prosody disturbance as an overall impression, rather than a specific evaluation of a fluency problem, and it is not surprising that 'prosody' has repeatedly proved a most powerful, if over-generalized, discriminative measure (Benson, 1967; Kerschensteiner *et al.*, 1972). This ambiguity could be overcome by using acoustic measures to define terms such as 'halting', 'uneven' or 'monotonous', and a number of recent studies have employed such measures (e.g., Danly and Shapiro, 1982; Ryalls, 1981, 1982; Kent and Rosenbek, 1982).

More theoretical difficulties with past fluency studies concern the manner in which they proceeded, beyond determining the discriminative power of each measure, to explain the role of a certain fluency feature in shaping other speech deficits. The construal of fluency deficits in an explanatory framework must refer to models of speech production and the fashion in which they relate one speech feature to another. Current models usually discuss this with reference to levels of description, that is, speech segment (phoneme and syllable), word, and phrase levels (e.g., Garrett, 1984). Each fluency measure may have level-specific manifestations which are qualitatively different from each other, for example, the segment level manifestation of decreased speech rate is increased syllable duration and syllable segregation (Kent and Rosenbek, 1983), while its word level manifestation is non-grammatical pauses (indicating problems in lexical access) (Butterworth, 1980). There are essential differences between these two types of fluency problems, the former presenting a primarily articulatory impairment, as in speech apraxia (Kent and Rosenbeck, 1983), while the latter reflects the primarily linguistic impairment of naming or lexical access (*see* Bay, 1962). Moreover, both are essentially different from the decrease in speech rate originating in an inability to initiate or maintain the continuity of speech with items that do not receive phrase level stress, as in agrammatic Broca's aphasia (Goodglass, 1976). With this concept of level-specific manifestations, the functional diversity of fluency impairments (Knopman *et al.*, 1983) is not surprising, emphasizing the heterogeneous nature of fluency problems.

In the following sections we review recent findings obtained with advanced acoustic methods, taking into account the principle of level-specific description and elaborating on some theoretical implications.

Segmental Fluency Deficits I: Speech Errors

Although some of the best known studies of fluency in aphasia have included phonemic and lexical substitutions, the adequacy of this inclusion is controversial. In fluent aphasia, where substitutions often establish the primary production disorder, the hypothesis of a fluency deficit contributes little to our understanding of the origin and nature of substitutions since, despite occasional counter-arguments (Johns and Darley, 1970), no phonetic or articulatory consistencies can be traced in the available corpus of substitutions (Lecours and Rouillon, 1976; Buckingham, 1981; Nespoulous *et al.*, 1985). Even where substitutions were recognized as reflecting articulatory or phonetic deficits, as in phonetic disintegration or speech apraxia, there are considerable difficulties in establishing the existence of a phonetic fluency disorder through detailed analysis.

One source of speech errors lies in the serial ordering of sounds (or articulatory-gestures) in a given utterance, as when a perfectly articulated phoneme is transposed backwards in anticipation or forward in reiteration. This kind of deficit may reflect the impaired ability to organize speech gestures in a prescribed sequence (LaPointe and Johns, 1975), but could also reflect difficulties in selecting phonemes from the phonological lexicon (Klich *et al.*, 1979). Monoi *et al.* (1983) interpreted their findings, whereby conduction aphasics tended to make transposition errors while Broca's asphasics made other substitution errors, as indicative of phonological and phonetic deficits respectively. The thesis of a pnonetic deficit in segmental errors of nonfluent patients could be supported by showing that substitutions involve the *simplification* of speech gestures, for example, the high resistance of vowels to substitution suggests that slower articulatory gestures are affected less than rapid ones, such as in stop consonants (/b/, /p/, /t/, etc.).

In testing this hypothesis, Shankweiler and Harris (1966) found that the stop consonants were affected significantly more than the much 'slower' fricatives and affricatives (/s/,/f/ʃ/, etc.). Monoi *et al.* (1983) confirmed the preservation of vowels in motor aphasia, and argued that a motor theory of substitutions could still apply through concepts of gestural complexity rather than gestural velocity, but this thesis has not been subsequently developed to offer testable predictions. Comparable difficulties occurred with the interpretation of feature similarity between the target phoneme and the actual production. Both Klich *et al.* (1979) and Monoi *et al.* (1983) found that fewer features differentiated actual from target productions in nonfluent patients while more features did so in fluent patients; the latter interpreted this as implying phonetic, and the former as phonological, simplification. Klich *et al.* (1979) did not, of course, suggest that the pattern of errors in fluent patients reflected non-phonological deficits, thus leaving the differential patterns of error in the two groups unaccounted for (*see* also Nespoulous *et al.*, 1985).

The area where evidence for simplification in speech errors has proved least controversial concerns the devoicing of voiced consonants (e.g., /b/→/p/, /d/→/t/, etc.). The perception of sounds as voiceless originates either in the absence of glottal pulsing (in fricatives such as /s/), or in the late onset of pulsing after the release of supraglottal occlusion, i.e., the long latency of voice onset time (VOT). Long VOTs, especially on initial stops, occurred primarily in nonfluent patients, often in the absence of obvious word- or phrase-level language disturbances (Blumstein *et al.*, 1977, 1980; Freeman *et al.*, 1978, Hoit-Dalgaard *et al.*, 1983). Specifically, while in normals and fluent aphasics VOT for voiced stops was usually less than 25 ms, in apraxic and Broca's aphasics as a group VOT exceeded 50 ms. Comparable delays were found in syllables starting with voiced, but not with voiceless, consonants (Kent and Rosenbek, 1983). Moreover, voice control in apraxic patients seems highly variable both in accuracy, reflected in variability of the formants (Ryalls, 1981), and in timing, where abnormally early onset of voicing, especially towards voiced fricatives, has also been observed (Kent and Rosenbek, 1983). Tuller (1984) found that Broca's aphasics, despite displaying increased VOTs for initial stops, continued to show the pattern of bipolar distribution of VOT values between voiced and voiceless targets. This could mean that they preserve the ability to distinguish between the two categories on a phonemic level (and fail on phonetic implementation), but could also mean that they possess the ability to differentiate phonetically between the classes (*ibid*). Tuller (1983) also found that VOTs were poor predictors of vowel duration prior to final stops, an important property of voicing in final syllabic positions. She argues that this disproves the simplistic concept of a global phonetic disturbance in Broca's aphasia, as speech sounds are not universally affected. Rather, phonetic position, and with it the continuity of articulation, must be taken into account.

Another group of speech errors is created by reiterations and approximations of target speech units. Like speech errors, reiteration phenomena could be divided into those where the phonetic integrity of the target phoneme remains intact, and those where it is disturbed. The former, referred to as 'stutter' (Darley *et al.*, 1975), represents a large set of disturbances, both phonetic, reflected in the impaired transition between differential articulatory targets, and phonemic, reflecting the perseveration of phonemic units (Buckingham, 1979). The latter, referred to as 'groping' (Wertz *et al.*, 1983) is characterized by phonetic disintegration in the narrow sense, i.e. by voicing problems. The only study to address groping as a distinct phenomenon merely attempted to determine the degree to which successive approximations actually converged upon the target phonation through configurational similarity of the formants (Kent and Rosenbek, 1983); this, together with the frequency of groping phenomena, could offer a measure of the degree of phonetic disturbance.

As for stutter, one of its most impressive features is the degree of functional diversity with which it is associated. In patients with left hemisphere damage, stutter may accompany Broca's aphasia and speech apraxia, but a case was also made for a specific syndrome of cortical stutter, where no other speech disturbances were shown (Helm *et al.*, 1978; Rosenbek *et al.*, 1978). This disturbance, it was argued, resembles developmental stutter in occurring with similar frequency (20–40% of syllables), primarily at initial positions and in showing improvement with repeated trials (Quinn and Andrews, 1977). Stutter is also a frequent accompaniment of parkinsonian speech disturbances, which usually also involve disturbances of rate, rhythm, volume and intonation (Rosenbek *et al.*, 1978; Koller, 1983). Unlike in developmental and post-stroke cases, parkinsonian stutter appears unpredictable, resistent to positive adjustment, persistent in singing and progressive (Koller, 1983). Cases have been reported of stutter in more diffuse neurological conditions such as presenile (Quinn and Andrews, 1977) and dialysis dementia (Rosenbek *et al.*, 1978). Recently some cases of stutter following right hemisphere damage were reported (Rosenbek *et al.*, 1978; Horner and Massey, 1983; Fleet *et al.*, 1985), where the stutter was often extended to word and phrase levels.

To phonetically explain substitution and voicing deficits in non-fluent aphasics, Darley *et al.*, (1975) and then Kent (1983) and Kent and Rosenbek (1983) differentiated between disorders of positioning, sequencing and timing. 'Positioning' refers to the accuracy with which the articulators obtain the required positions for specific speech segments. The prime indicator of positioning problems is acoustic variability, i.e. the wide variation of acoustic features in repeated productions of the same segment in the same phonetic context (Ryalls, 1981; Kent and Rosenbek, 1983). Perceptually, this may result in substitution or distortion of the target segment and therefore act to create those errors that do not involve transpositions or VOT problems.

To account for errors that originate in positioning problems, McNeilage (1982) adapted his concept of a co-ordinate space (MacNeilage, 1970), where speech segments were represented in the form of the related postural values of each articulator. Crudely, each segment /x/ is represented in the co-ordinate space as a vector (Tx, Lx, Jx, Gx . . .) where Tx, Lx, etc. specify the positions of the tongue, lips, etc. (More accurately, each vector represents an equivalence class such that variation in the position of one articulator is compensated by 'conjugate' variations in the others, resulting in an equivalent final position.) In these terms, positioning disorders may arise either from a failure to implement an intact articulatory 'vector', as in dysarthria, or from partial damage to the co-ordinate space itself with the consequent mis-representation of segments ('programming disorder'), as in speech apraxia (Darley *et al.*, 1975; Kent, 1983). In the absence of phonetic disintegration, the demarcation of central positioning problems from disorders of phonemic selection may be extremely difficult as both may show substitutions (DeRenzi *et al.*, 1966; Klich *et al.*, 1979). This difficulty resulted in a split between those researchers for whom all simplification is phonemic (e.g., Buckingham, 1979) and those for whom it is articulatory (e.g., Johns and Darley, 1970).

'Sequencing' disorders, manifested in transpositions, involve the impaired sequential ordering of separable speech gestures, irrespective of the phonetic integrity of the individual gestures. Conceptualized as the central mapping (or projection) of a sub-space of the articulatory co-ordinate space into a one dimensional ('linear') space, sequencing does not concern the regulation of the time-dependent suprasegmental features (quantity, pitch and volume. *See* Lehiste, 1976). Accordingly, transpositions can, and often do, occur with intact phonemic selections, no segmental distortions and, indeed, no fluency problems.

'Timing' refers to the synchronicity, succession or separation of points that are critical for the execution of articulatory gestures ('phase points') such as onset, termination and peak acceleration (or peak intensity change), either *among the articulators* or *between phonatory and articulatory gestures.* In problems of inter-articulatory timing, like in those of positioning, phonetic distortions occur but, unlike in positioning deficits, the articulators actually obtain their target position, albeit out of phase with each other. Distortions are therefore likely to have distinctive-features characteristics other than voicing or markedness (*see* Nespoulous *et al.*, 1985). These may originate either in the mapping from multidimensional to linear representations, or in a separate executive function that regulates quantity, but not in co-ordinate space representations. In the next section we shall argue that autonomous timing problems may generate the other deficits associated with speech apraxia.

Problems of timing between the phonatory and articulatory systems are reflected in voicing deficits, that is, either in longer VOT or in its increased variability. These may be, and are often seen as, the result of impaired co-ordination between phonatory and articulatory gestures that are autonomously represented. But, we shall argue, they may also reflect the peripheral outcome of a timing deficit superimposed upon intact co-ordination (*see* next section).

The hypothesis of three separate types of segmental motor disturbance is useful in categorizing speech errors and differentiating dysarthria from apraxia (Darley *et al.*, 1975), but it presents a number of difficulties. Firstly, in speech apraxia all three types of disturbance tend to occur together in one way or another, which raises the possibility that a unitary deficit is involved. Secondly, the concept of representation and symbol manipulation is inherently deterministic and does not explain the wide variability in performance of identical tasks by the same individuals (Scott Kelso and Tuller, 1981). Thirdly, none of the three accounts for articulatory slowness as an independent deficit. These difficulties are discussed in the next section.

Segmental Disorders II: Duration

The most consistent disturbances of fluency at the segmental level are the prolongation and segregation of syllables, the former referring to the length of the spectrographic nuclei that acoustically represent speech segments, and the latter to the insertion of pauses between them, with perceptual loss of the continuity of sound inside word boundaries (Kent and Rosenbek, 1983). Accounts of syllable prolongations in the so-called 'motor' aphasics have been available for quite some time (DeRenzi *et al.*, 1966; Johns and Darley, 1970) but rigorous acoustic studies have been only recently conducted.

In a detailed analysis of speech spectrograms of normals and speech apraxia patients, Kent and Rosenbek (1983) found that the duration of syllables of the latter were usually more than two standard deviations longer than those of the former. While this proved a general feature across the whole range of speech segments, it was especially marked for vowels, where patients displayed syllable durations of up to ten times longer than the normal average (*Figure 1*). Less marked were the prolongations of liquids and fricatives (e.g., /s/. /l/, etc.) while consonant durations in monosyllabic utterances were often similar to those of normals (*Figure 1*).

Kent and Rosenbek (1983) also found that syllable prolongation was greater in longer words. Interestingly, in another careful spectrographic study, where the relationships between vowel and word duration were systematically investigated, apraxic patients again displayed vowel prolongations but, like normals, *reduced* vowel durations with the increase in word length ('vowel reduction') (Collins *et al.*, 1983). Thus, while vowel duration in /please/ averaged around 270 ms, the respective value in /pleasing/ was around 230 ms and in /pleasingly/ around 210 ms (*ibid*). Although it is possible that vowel reduction applies only to syllabic extensions (as in Collins *et al.*, 1983; DiSimoni and Darley, 1977), others have failed to confirm this; despite the assertion that vowel reduction is a robust feature of speech with remarkable resistance to change (Collins *et al.*, 1983), further data are required to disentangle this issue. No overall effect of word position on syllable duration was observed although some prolongations occurred consistently in one position in a certain context, and not in other positions or contexts (Kent and Rosenbek, 1983).

Syllable segregation is the second constituent of the segmental fluency disturbances related to speech rate. To assess its variation in apraxic patients independently of prolongation, Kent and Rosenbek (1982) computed the ratio between the sum of the durations of syllabic nuclei and the total utterance duration. They found that while for normals this ratio ranged from 0.54 to 0.62, for apraxic patients it ranged from 0.20 to 0.47. Another aspect of syllable segregation refers to fundamental frequency (f_0). In normals and mildly affected patients the continuation of phonation after intersyllable pauses is marked by maintenance of f_0 level, perceived as a degree of prosodic continuity. With the more severely affected patients this feature is sometimes lost, resulting in increased perceptual 'choppiness' of phonation (Kent and Rosenbek, 1982). In another related acoustic measure Kent and Rosenbek (1983) found that the intensity envelope (the range of maximum and minimum intensity values) was more limited in apraxic patients than in normals. This can not be considered formally as a segmental deficit, but it is not inconceivable that both segmental prolongation and the failure to create the normal level of pulmonary air pressure (Ryalls, 1981) originate in the same deficit (*see* below).

Unlike the descriptive clarity of the available data with regard to prolongation and segregation of syllables, their motor origin is not so obvious, particularly when considered in relation to substitutions and reiterations. The mechanisms of positioning, sequencing and timing, previously employed to explain speech errors, do not explain articulatory slowness as such, but there is direct evidence to that effect in speech apraxia (Itoh *et al.*, 1980). If slowness presents as an independent deficit, how is it related to speech errors and is it possible that an elementary mechanism may give rise to both slowness and co-ordination problems? Action-theoretical or

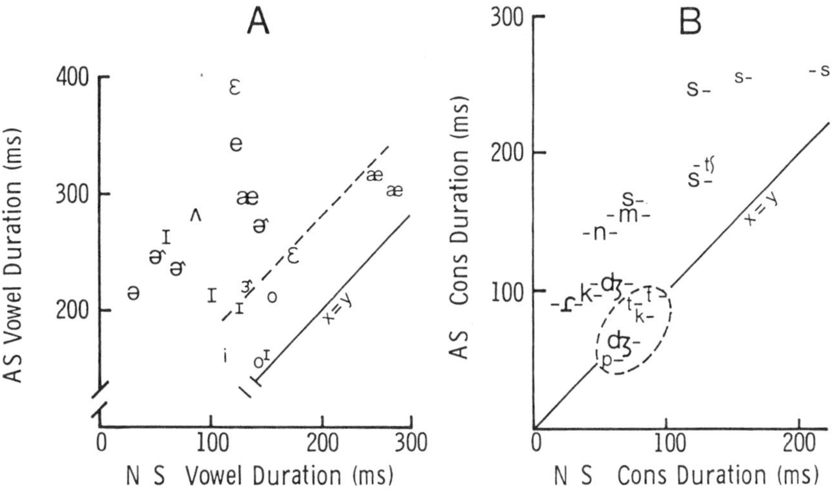

Figure 1 Segment durations for apraxic speakers (AS) plotted against those of normal speakers (NS). Small phonetic symbols represent segments in monosyllablic words, and large in longer words.
(A) Vowel duration. The dashed region nearly separates data for monosyllabic versus longer words, indicating longer durations in longer words.
(B) Consonant duration. Position of consonants in a word is shown by position of dashes, eg, s- is word initial, -s- is medial and -s is final. The dashed line encloses symbols showing no group differences (after Kent & Rosenbek, 1983, with permission).

dynamic views on apraxic disorders suggest that central mechanisms can not, and should not, be called upon to explain every discernible feature of the deficit. Some features may emerge as peripheral consequences of a generalized central disorder (Scott Kelso and Tuller, 1981). In the case of speech apraxia all deficits may principally result in a failure to time the increase in muscle tone following the initial burst of the lower motor neurone. Let us examine this idea further.

Viewed as a mass-spring system, muscle function is fully specified by two parameters: length and tension (Bizzi *et al.*, 1982). Crudely, the length of the muscles subserving an integral system (body segment or body part) determines their postural *position*, whilst tension determines their postural *power*. Similarly, final length determines final position of a certain gesture, while tension determines its speed or velocity. The timing of the increase in muscle tension, based on the timing of motor-neurone (MN) recruitment, determines the acceleration of a given gesture (Desmedt, 1983). We suggest that most apraxic speech deficits may be explained as a generalized disturbance in the timing of MN recruitment, with consequent delays in the increase of muscle tension in *both* the phonatory and the articulatory systems.

Delay in MN recruitment may directly explain syllable prolongation and segregation. Firstly, it results in slow gestural acceleration and delayed peak velocity, segregating syllabic nuclei (assuming that peak velocity coincides with syllabic nuclei). Secondly, the anatomic restriction of articulatory amplitudes links delayed acceleration with reduced velocities (slowness), which explains syllabic prolongation. As for *positioning problems*, it is well known that in rapid movements such as articulatory gestures velocity and accuracy correlate (Schmidt *et al.*, 1985), and so reduced velocity is sufficient to explain inaccurate positioning. Inter-articulatory *timing problems* may result from an equalizing effect in the timing of tension rise. If articulators A1 and A2 normally reach final positions simultaneously by virtue of differential MN recruitment latencies (TL1 and TL2, respectively determined by passive properties of A1 and A2), and if the deficit imposes a minimum latency MTL which is greater than both TL1 and TL2, then, except when in initial positions, the timing of A1 and A2 will also be disturbed (this mechanism should offer predictions about the precise nature of inter-articulatory timing problems in a specific task). Finally, assuming that MN recruitment is also disturbed in the phonatory system this may explain *voicing problems*. The normal VOT for voiced stops may be a peripheral consequence of co-activation of voicing with supraglottal release, 15–25 ms being the time it takes the intrinsic laryngeal muscles to reach the level of tension required for voicing. The increased latencies of MN recruitment in the phonatory system may result in the laryngeal muscles reaching their voicing level of tension after 55 ms or more, with the consequence of un-voicing.

The hypothesis of increased recruitment latencies does not account, of course, for sequencing problems (transpositions), which may be viewed, in line with other approaches, as non-apraxic in nature. The occurrence of transpositions in speech apraxia does not necessarily imply a sequencing motor problem as this could result from extra-load on an intact system, comparable to effects of tiredness or anxiety.

Word-level Fluency Problems in Aphasia

Unlike segmental fluency problems, those at word level do not concern articulation or motor control, but instead involve difficulties in accessing or retrieving words, which are probably the most distinctly linguistic of all aphasic disturbances (Bay, 1962). Word-finding problems concern the issue of fluency as they often result in pauses, filled or unfilled. Especially significant in this respect are those pauses that occur at non-grammatical junctures, that is, not between clause or sentence boundaries (Butterworth, 1980). These affect non-fluent more than fluent patients (Knopman *et al.*,

Table 3 Mean duration of pauses prior to paraphasic and neologistic productions in a patient with jargonaphasia (after Butterworth, 1979, with permission).

	Error category					
	Verbal paraphasias	A	B	C	D	E
N	35	12	8	21	55	68
Mean delay (sec)	.135	.233	.250	.348	.494	.301
			.295			

t-tests verbal paraphasias versus A + B + C
$t(74) = 1.66$, $p < .05$ (one-tailed)
A + B + C versus D
$t(94) = 1.85$, $p < .05$ (one-tailed)
A: Neologisms phonologically related to a prior word
B: Neologisms phonologically related to a following word
C: Neologisms phonologically related to a target word
D: Neologisms not related to a real word
E: Other neologisms

1984), but tend to occur in their pure form in fluent patients, creating the syndrome of anomia or nominal aphasia (Benson, 1979). In some fluent patients word finding problems appear to concern rate-related, 'on line' linguistic operations, in which case they may be seen also as presenting with a 'fluency' problem, albeit not in the usual sense of the term. Seeing this requires a closer look at the pattern of pauses in fluent aphasia.

The speech of fluent aphasics usually involves the substitution, transposition, omission, etc. of words and phonemes, creating paraphasias and neologisms. In one case, pause lengths of a jargonaphasic patient were correlated with his speech-error types (Butterworth, 1979), where it was found that errors unrelated to a target item were preceded by pauses of significantly longer durations than other productions in identical grammatic categories (*Table 3*). This indicated that searches for target lexical items which ended up empty handed took longer to complete than those ending with partial or complete success (*ibid*). The reduction of jargon in spontaneous speech is often marked by increased pauses and silences, as though the ability to reduce speech rate makes output processing more compatible with retrieval and accessing. This co-ordination of rate dependent processes between articulatory output and lexical search is an aspect of fluency that has so far been given little attention but may prove of much importance for the management of speech disorders of the so-called fluent aphasics.

Word-level functions during spontaneous speech minimally involve the search for items in two discernible lexicons: semantic and phonological. Crudely, the representation of word meanings is said to be organized in a semantic lexicon, whilst word sounds are represented in the phonological lexicon. Difficulties in accessing the semantic lexicon implicate posterior–superior regions of the left temporal lobe, whilst problems in accessing the phonological lexicon also implicate the insula and putamen (Knopman *et al.*, 1984). This region links the phonological–semantic distinction with fluency, being implicated in nonfluent aphasia (Knopman *et al.*, 1983): patients with a predominantly phonological disturbance, reflected in 'phonemic jargon' (Lecours and Rouillon, 1976) could be expected to show greater dysfluency than other jargonaphasics on account of the lack of feature similarity between jargon and target items. (Recall that pause length was found to increase in the absence of similarity between jargon and target items, presumably due to the failure in lexical search (Butterworth, 1979)).

Finally, one aspect of word-level fluency has acquired a special status due to its simple application for assessment purposes, namely, 'verbal fluency', defined as the production-rate of words of a given class (Bolter *et al.*, 1983), specified by semantic or phonological constraints such as, respectively, animal names or words starting with a selected letter. This measure of fluency is generally outside the scope of the present chapter, but it is interesting that, like word-level fluency problems generally, impairment of verbal fluency does not localize in any simple fashion and may be displayed by both anterior and posterior aphasics, as well as non-aphasic right hemisphere patients (Joannette *et al.*, 1984).

Phrase-level Fluency in Aphasia

Aphasic distortions of speech features at higher than segment or word level were first systematically reported in a seminal paper by Monrad-Krohn (1947). He observed a patient with left hemisphere brain damage whose melodic line had changed and whose speech acquired a foreign accent. Such disturbances of prosody usually occur in patients with right hemisphere lesions (Ross, 1981) but none had been associated with speech fluency.

The first observations on phrase level features directly concerning speech fluency in aphasia were made by Goodglass *et al.* (1967) who reported that agrammatic Broca's aphasics have great difficulty in initiating speech with any but a stressed item. Moreover, unstressed items other than in initial sentence positions were also likely to be omitted by these patients. On the strength of these findings, later replicated by Gleason *et al.* (1975), Goodglass (1976) suggested that Broca's aphasics suffer from a central motor disorder that renders 'mobilizing' the articulatory system effortful and raises its movement thresholds. As a result the speech of Broca's patients is dysfluent, slow and choppy, but not necessarily phonemically distorted.

Kean (1977) suggested a theory of agrammatism in Broca's aphasia, where the impaired production of unstressed items was construed as a phonological, linguistic deficit rather than an articulatory phonetic one. In her theory the stressed/unstressed distinction separates content (nouns, verbs) from function (articles, prepositions) words, and underlies the agrammatic tendency to omit the latter. In both Goodglass's and Kean's formulations nonfluency in Broca's aphasia was conceived of as a phrase level deficit, but conceptualized in articulatory terms in the former and in linguistic terms in the latter.

More recent studies of Broca's aphasia, using advanced acoustic methods, also report phrase-level deviations from normal patterns (Danly and Shapiro, 1982; Ryalls, 19892; Cooper *et al.*, 1984), and give a rather consistent, if incomplete, description of the nature of the fluency disturbance of Broca's patients in terms of prosodic deficits, that is, in terms of the abnormal regulation of pitch, volume and quantity. Ryalls (1982) found longer articulatory durations and reduced speech rate, which he ascribed to segmental prolongation rather than articulatory segregation or pauses. However, this in itself does not imply a disturbance in segmental control: while Broca's patients tend to lengthen segments in initial sentence positions they tend to shorten them at final positions (Danly and Shapiro, 1982). Indeed, word-length in final positions was *not* significantly different between Broca's aphasics and normals (*ibid.*; Cooper *et al.*, 1984), suggesting that in Broca's aphasia reduction in rate and increase in segmental duration closely interact with phrase level factors such as position. This pattern of final segmental shortening was in marked contrast with the normal pattern of final lengthening (*ibid.*; also Lehiste, 1976).

Another acoustic parameter that appears relevant to the fluency problems of Broca's aphasics is that of fundamental frequency (f_0), which is the acoustic correlate of pitch and intonation. Ryalls (1982) found that, in middle positions, the f_0 range (its top to bottom variation) of Broca's patients was more limited than that of normals by an average of approximately 20%. Danly and Shapiro (1982) had similar findings, but they observed that Broca's aphasics were still able to produce the pattern of f_0 declination, i.e. the lowering of f_0 level from initial to final positions. f_0 levels were found generally higher in Broca's aphasia by 40% to 50% (Danly and Shapiro, 1982; Cooper *et al.*, 1984), especially in initial positions (f_0 resetting). Danly and Shapiro (1982), but not Cooper *et al.* (1984), found that the specific levels of f_0 resetting depended upon phrase length. In cases where f_0 values were

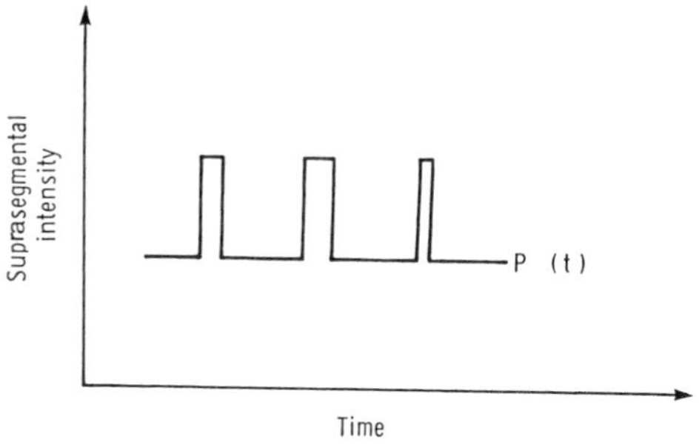

Figure 2 Schematic illustration of a hypothetical function (P) representing the mode of suprasegmental transition in patients with Broca's aphasia. Sharp initial and final transitions are connected with 'flat' transitions.

especially high in initial positions, amplitude also tended to be of higher values than normal (Danly and Shapiro, 1982).

The general pattern of speech prosody in Broca's aphasia may be construed by reference to a function of P of f_o, amplitude (A) and syllable duration (D) such that $P(t) = F(f_o(t), A(t), D(t))$, where t represents time and F is a function of f_o, A and D that is monotonous in the sense that it rises and falls with them. The above findings on Broca's aphasia may now be presented as the alternation of P between sharp and flat transition, the former applying to initial and final, and the latter to middle positions (*Figure 2*). This pattern is consistent with Goodglass's (1976) concept of difficulty in 'mobilizing' the articulatory system and the consequent rise in speech onset thresholds, as P values derived from acoustic studies were remarkably high in initial positions. But the present ideas offer more than a graphic illustration of initiation difficulties.

Hadar (1985) suggests that the function P could be used to characterize an ideal prosodic structure., based upon considerations of economy of action

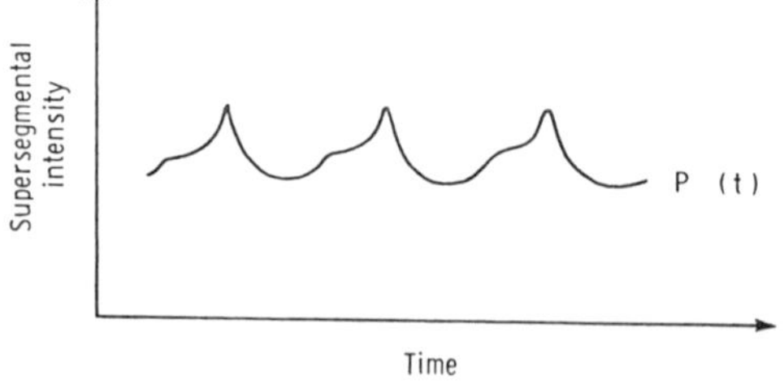

Figure 3 Schematic illustration of a hypothetic function (P) representing the mode of suprasegmental transition in 'normal' speech, making use of economy principles. Suprasegmental peaks, representing stressed syllables, are smoothly connected.

(Lindblom, 1983). Specifically, for efficient use of energy resources, the motor system needs to be able to build upon the elastic oscillations of a moving body part, and increase or decrease the amplitude of movement in phase with peripheral oscillations. This requires the tuning of the central system to peripheral specifications, graphically represented as the smooth transition of P between peak values (*Figure 3*). The comparison of this ideal pattern with that of Broca's aphasics reveals a failure to smoothly connect between prosodic peaks, and this, in turn, reflects a failure to increase or decrease P values in phase with peripheral oscillations. Broca's aphasia, it appears, is 'bound up with disturbance of motor timing and the rhythmic structure of the utterance', and involves 'an oscillator which controls speech rhythm or intonational pattern' (Brown, 1982, pp. 453; 454). These formulations suggest that prosodic control should offer a prime route for the treatment of Broca's aphasia, which is supported by the fact that, more than any other group, Broca's patients improved their fluency with exercises designed to improve prosodic control (Hadar *et al.*, 1987).

The psychomotor treatment of phrase-level fluency problems in aphasic patients both reflects and emphasises the role of non-articulatory movements (of the hands, head or feet) in regulating the prosodic speech features. This role has long been recognized, especially in respect of the regulation of rhythm (Condon and Ogston, 1967), volume and stress (Dittman, 1972) and speech onset (Hadar *et al.*, 1984). Indeed, aphasic disturbances appear to be accompanied by a compensatory increase in the ratio of gesture to verbalization: while the ratio for normals was 0.16, for aphasics it was 0.40 (Feyereisen, 1982). This increase could be ascribed in part to symbolic functions of gesture, but the fact that non-fluent have a higher ratio than fluent patients (0.42 and 0.38 respectively) suggests the predominance of phonetic factors. Note that the regulation of rhythm through gesture also inspired the development of a technique ('gestural reorganization') for the treatment of segmental problems such as in speech apraxia (Wertz *et al.*, 1983).

Conclusion

The idea that fluency as a concept has explanatory value in aphasia has a long history. Its use as a diagnostic tool can be traced back to Wernicke's formulations and followed in modern times through Geschwind's and Benson's work. However, the usefulness of the concept of fluency can not be sustained without adapting its operational measures to recent findings and research techniques, especially acoustic analysis. This chapter offers such an update, directly motivated by some of the difficulties encountered in past research, especially addressing the ambiguity of past fluency measures, the inability to distinguish between articulatory and linguistic effects on fluency and the belief that it represents a homogeneous entity. Instead, we suggest, the concept of fluency offers a framework for the investigation of time-dependent speech processes, both linguistic and articulatory/phonetic (the regulation of quantity).

While time-dependent processes involved in aphasic articulation have attracted considerable research, especially on segmental level, their role in lexical and linguistic processing has not, and only a few attempts have been made to address this issue, notably by Butterworth and co-workers. Although there is little new to offer in this respect, a concerted effort in this direction is long overdue.

A more espoused territory, if still grossly under-investigated, is the study of time-dependent processes on phrase level. Investigating the role of articulatory processes in creating some of the agrammatic deficits in Broca's aphasia should prove of considerable potential, not least for its possible applications to therapy. Whilst current conceptual paradigms do not encourage research along these lines, the increased availability of advanced techniques for acoustic analysis may change this state of affairs. Such an investigation, we feel, should compare inferences from syntactic structure with those from rhythmic/prosodic features. To illustrate, the hypothesis that agrammatism involves the reduced availability of closed class items (determiners, conjunctives, etc.) implies that the utterance of phrases such as (1) 'John is back' (in reading aloud, repetition, etc.) should produce more errors than that of phrases such as (2) 'John came back', because the former and not the latter contain a closed class item. The opposite prediction arises from the hypothesis of a primary deficit in regulating smooth prosodic transitions, because (1) involves the prosodic pattern illustrated in *Figure 2*, i.e., sharp initial and final transitions connected with a flat transition, whilst phrase (2) involves three successive items that receive stress and requires the regulation of a rhythmic oscillator over three cycles. In our formulations this task should prove especially vulnerable in Broca's aphasia.

The study of time-dependent factors on the segmental level has acquired during the past two decades a degree of specificity that probably ensures continuing interest in the subject, not least because of a high degree of involvement of experimental phoneticians. In explaining the available data we have sympathy with the style of analysis offered by action theorists, especially where the continuity in control strategies is assumed between speech and other motor performances, which motivated some speculation on the nature of motor disorder in apraxia of speech. Global theoretical convictions notwithstanding, the competition between action-theoretical and programming/representational models is valuable, both in encouraging research and in complementing each other on some issues (e.g., serial ordering).

References

BAY, E. Aphasia and nonverbal disorders of language. *Brain* (1962), **85**, 411–426.

BENSON, D.F. Fluency in aphasia: Correlation with radioactive scan localization. *Cortex* (1967), **3**, 373–394.

BENSON, D.F. Neurological correlates of anomia. In H. Whitaker and H.A. Whitaker (eds) *Studies in Neurolinguistics, Vol. 4* (1979). New York: Academic Press.

BIZZI, E., CHAPPLE, W. and HOGAN, N. Mechanical properties of muscles: implications for motor control. *Trends in the Neurosciences* (1982), 395–398.

BLESER, R. DE and POECK, K. Analysis of prosody in the spontaneous speech of patients with CV-recurring utterances. *Cortex* (1985), **21**, 405–416.

BLUMSTEIN, S.E., COOPER, W.E., ZURIF, E.B. and CARAMAZZA, A. The perception and production of voice onset time in aphasia. *Neuropsychologia* (1977), **15**, 371–383.

BLUMSTEIN, S.E., COOPER, W.E. GOODGLASS, H., STALENDER, S. and GOTTLIEB, J. Production deficits in aphasia: A voice onset time analysis. *Brain and Language* (1980), **9**, 153–170.

BOLTER, J.F., LONG, C.J. and WAGNER, M. The utility of the Thurstone word fluency test in identifying cortical damage. *Clinical Neuropsychology* (1983), **5**, 77–82.

BROWN, J.W. Hierarchy and evolution in neurolinguistics. In M.A. Arbib, D. Caplan and J.C. Marshall (eds) *Neural Models of Language Processes* (1982). New York: Academic Press.

BUCKINGHAM, H.W. Explanations in apraxia with consequences for the concept of apraxia of speech. *Brain and Language*, (1979), **18**, 202–226.

BUCKINGHAM, H.W. Where do neologisms come from? In J.W. Brown (ed.) *Jargonaphasia* (1981). New York: Academic Press.

BUTTERWORTH, B. Hesitation and the production of verbal paraphasias and neologisms in jargonaphasia. *Brain and Language* (1979), **8**, 133–161.

BUTTERWORTH, B. Evidence from pauses. In B. Butterworth (ed.) *Language Production, Vol. I* (1980). London: Academic Press.

COLLINS, M., ROSENBEK, J.C. and WERTZ, R.T. Spectrographic analysis of vowel and word duration in apraxia of speech. *Journal of Speech and Hearing Research* (1983), **26**, 224–230.

CONDON, W.S. and OGSTON, W.D. A segmentation of behavior. *Journal of Psychiatric Research* (1967), **5**, 221–235.

COOPER, W.E., SOARES, C., NICOL, J., MICHELOW, D. and GOLOSKIE, S. Clausal intonation after unilateral brain damage. *Language and Speech* (1984), **27**, 17–24.

DANLY, M. and SHAPIRO, B. Speech prosody in Broca's aphasia. *Brain and Language* (1982), **16**, 171–190.

DARLEY, F.L., ARONSON, A.E. and BROWN, J.R. *Motor Speech Disorders* (1975). Philadelphia: Saunders.

DERENZI, E., PIECZURO, A. and VIGNOLO, L.A. Oral apraxia and aphasia. *Cortex*, (1966), **2**, 50–73.

DESMEDT, J.E. Size principle of motorneuron recruitment and the calibration of muscle force and speed in man. In J.E. Desmedt (ed.) *Motor Control Mechanisms in Health and Disease* (1983). New York: Raven Press.

DiSimoni, F.G. and Darley, F.L. Effect on phoneme duration control of three utterance length conditions in an apractic patient. *Joural of Speech and Hearing Disorders* (1977), **42**, 257–264.

Dittman, A.T. The body movement — speech rhythm relationship as a cue for speech encoding. In A.W. Siegman and B. Pope (eds) *Studies in Dyadic Communication* (1972). New York: Academic Press.

Feyereisen, P. Temporal distribution of coverbal hand movements. *Ethology and Sociobiology* (1982), **3**, 1–9.

Fleet, S.W. and Heilman, K.M. Acquired stuttering from a right hemisphere lesion of a right-hander. *Neurology* (1985), **35**, 1343–1346.

Freeman, F.J., Sands, E.S. and Harris, K.S. Temporal coordination of phonation and articulation in a case of verbal apraxia: A voice onset time study. *Brain and Language*, (1978), **6**, 106–111.

Garrett, M.F. The organization of processing structure for language production: Applications to aphasic speech. In D. Caplan, A.R. Lecours and A. Smith (eds) *Biological Perspectives on Language* (1984). Cambridge (MA): MIT Press.

Geschwind, N. Discussion of a paper by Wepman and Jones. In E.C. Carterette (ed.) *Brain Function, Vol. III* (1966). Los Angeles: University of California Press.

Gleason, J.B., Goodglass, H., Green, E., Ackerman, N. and Hyde, M.R. The retrieval of syntax in Broca's aphasia. *Brain and Language* (1975), **2**, 451–471.

Goodglass, H. Agrammatism. In H. Whitaker and H.A. Whitaker (eds) *Studies in Neurolinguistics I* (1976). New York: Academic Press.

Goodglass, H., Quadfasel, F.A. and Timberlake, W.H. Phrase length and the type and severity of aphasia. *Cortex* (1964), **1**, 133–153.

Goodglass, H., Fodor, I.G. and Schulhoff, C. Prosodic factors in grammar: Evidence from aphasia. *Journal of Speech and Hearing Research* (1967), **10**, 5–20.

Hadar, U. *The Relevance of Articulatory Processes in Broca's Aphasia to Agrammatism* (1985). Unpublished manuscript, Charing Cross and Westminster Medical School, London.

Hadar, U., Steiner, T.J. and Clifford Rose, F. The involvement of head movement in speech production and its implications for language pathology. In F.C. Rose (ed.) *Progress in Aphasiology* (1984). New York: Raven Press.

Hadar, U., Twiston Davies, R., Steiner, T.J. and Clifford Rose, F. Psychomotor Therapy: A general framework and preliminary results. *Aphasiology* (1987, in press).

Helm, N.A., Butler, R.B. and Benson, D.F. Acquired stuttering. *Neurology* (1978), **28**, 1159–1165.

Hoit-Dalgaard, J., Murray, T. and Kopp, H.G. Voice-onset-time production and perception in apraxic subjects. *Brain and Language* (1983), **20**, 329–339.

Horner, J. and Massey, E.W. Progressive dysfluency associated with right hemisphere disease. *Brain and Language* (1983), **18**, 71–85.

Howes, D. Application of the word-frequency concept to aphasia. In A.V.S. de Reuck and M. O'Connor (eds) *Disorders of Language* (1964). London: Churchill.

Itoh, M., Sasanuma, S., Hirose, H., Yoshioka, H. and Ushijima, T. Abnormal articulatory dynamics in a patient with apraxia of speech: X-ray microbeam observation. *Brain and Language*, (1980), **11**, 66–75.

JOANETTE, Y. and GOULET, P. Is verbal fluency really reduced among right brain-damaged right-handers. Poster presented at *the Aphasia Academy Meeting*, Los Angeles (1984).

JOHNS, D. and DARLEY, F.L. Phonemic variability in apraxia of speech. *Journal of Speech and Hearing Research* (1970), **13**, 556–583.

KEAN, M-L. The linguistic interpretation of aphasic syndromes: Agrammatism in Broca's aphasia. *Cognition* (1977), **5**, 9–46.

KENT, R.D. The segmental organization of speech. In P.F. MacNeilage (ed.) *The Production of Speech* (1983). New York: Springer Verlag.

KENT, R.D. and ROSENBEK, J.C. Prosodic disturbance and neurologic lesion. *Brain and Language* (1982), **15**, 259–261.

KENT, R.D. and ROSENBEK, J.C. Acoustic patterns of apraxia of speech. *Journal of Speech and Hearing Research* (1983), **26**, 231–249.

KERSCHENSTEINER, M., POECK, K. and BRUNER, E. The fluency-nonfluency dimension in the classification of aphasic speech. *Cortex* (1972), **8**, 233–247.

KLICH, R.J., IRELAND, J.V. and WEIDENER, W.E. Articulatory and phonological aspects of consonant substitutions in apraxia of speech. *Cortex* (1979), **15**, 451–470.

KNOPMAN, D.S., SELNES, O.A., NICCUM, N., RUBENS, A.B., YOCK, D. and LARSON, D. A longitudinal study of speech fluency in aphasia: CT correlates of recovery and persistent nonfluency. *Neurology* (1983), **33**, 1170–1178.

KNOPMAN, D.S., SELNES, O.S., NICCUM, N. and RUBENS, A.B. Recovery of naming in aphasia: relationship to fluency, comprehension and CT findings. *Neurology* (1984), **34**, 1461–1470.

KOLLER, W.C. Dysfluency (stuttering) in extrapyramidal disease. *Archives of Neurology* (1983), **40**, 175–177.

LAPOINTE, L.L. and JOHNS, D.F. Some phonemic characteristics of apraxia of speech. *Journal of Communication Disorders* (1975), **8**, 259–269.

LECOURS, A.R. and ROUILLON, F. Neurolinguistic analysis of jargonaphasia and jargon agraphia. In H. Whitaker and H.A. Whitaker (eds) *Studies in Neurolinguistics, Vol. 2* (1976). New York: Academic Press.

LEHISTE, I. Suprasegmental features of speech. In N.J. Lass (ed.) *Contemporary Issues in Experimental Phonetics* (1976). New York: Academic Press.

LINDBLOM, B. Economy of speech gestures. In P.F. MacNeilage (ed.) *The Production of Speech* (1983). New York: Springer-Verlag.

MCNEILAGE, P.F. Motor control of serial ordering of speech. *Psychological Review* (1970), **77**, 182–196.

MCNEILAGE, P.F. Speech production mechanisms in aphasia. In S. Grillner, B. Lindblom, J. Lubker and E. Persson (eds) *Speech Motor Control* (1982). New York: Pergamon Press.

MONOI, H., FUKUSAKO, Y., ITOH, M. and SASANUMA, S. Speech sound errors in patients with conduction and Broca's aphasia. *Brain and Language* (1983), **20**, 175–194.

MONRAD-KROHN, G.H. Dysprosody or the altered 'melody of language'. *Brain* (1947), **70**, 405–415.

NESPOULOUS, J-L., DORDAN, M., SKA, B., CAPLAN, D. and LECOURS, A.R. Production deficits in Broca's and conduction aphasia. In E. Keller and M. Copnik (eds)

Motor Sensory Processes of Language (1985).

PICK, A. *Aphasia* (trans. by J.W. Brown) (1931). Springfield: Charles C. Thomas.

QUINN, P.T. and ANDREWS, G. Neurological stuttering — a clinical entity? *Journal of Neurology, Neurosurgery and Psychiatry* (1977), **40**, 699–701.

ROSENBEK, J.C., MESSERT, B., COLLINS, M. and WERTZ, R.T. Stuttering following brain damage. *Brain and Language* (1978), **6**, 82–96.

ROSS, E.D. The aprosodias: functional-anatomic organization of the affective components of language in the right hemisphere. *Archives of Neurology* (1981), **38**, 561–569.

RYALLS, J.H. Motor aphasia: acoustic correlates of phonetic disintegration in vowels. *Neuropsychologia* (1981) **19**, 365–374.

RYALLS, J.H. Intonation in Broca's aphasia. *Neuropsychologia* (1982), **20**, 355–360.

SCHMIDT, R.A., SHERWOOD, D.E., ZELAZNIK, H.N. and LEIKIND, B. Speed-accuracy trade-offs in motor behavior: Theories of impulse variability. In H. Heuer, U. Kleinbek and K-H. Schmidt (eds) *Motor Behavior: Programming, Control and Acquisition* (1985). Berlin: Springer.

SCOTT KELSO, J.A. and TULLER, B. Towards a theory of apractic syndromes. *Brain and Language* (1981), **12**, 224–245.

SHANKWEILER, D. and HARRIS, K.S. An experimental approach to the problem of articulation in aphasia. *Cortex* (1966), **2**, 277–292.

TULLER, B. On categorizing aphasic speech errors. *Neuropsychologia* (1984), **22**, 547–557.

WAGENAAR, E., SNOW, C and PRINS, R. Spontaneous speech of aphasic patients: A psycholinguistic analysis. *Brain and Language* (1975), **2**, 281–303.

WERNICKE, C. The symptom-complex of aphasia. In A. Church (ed.) *Diseases of the Nervous System* (1908). New York: D. Appleton.

WERTZ, R.T., LAPOINTE, L.L. and ROSENBEK, J.C. *Apraxia of Speech in Adults: The Disorder and its Management* (1984). New York: Grune and Stratton.

IV

Assessment

14

The Assessment of Non-verbal Abilities in Aphasic Subjects

Maria A. Wyke

The assessment of non-linguistic aspects of cognitive function is an essential part of the examination of the aphasic patient. This information is of fundamental importance for interpreting the case and for planning adequate rehabilitation. But before describing the available methods of evaluation it is necessary to touch upon the more theoretical aspects of the problem, i.e. to discuss whether the presence of a language disorder fundamentally affects the patient's intellectual capacity and to comment on the non-verbal cognitive deficits which are known to coexist with the breakdown of language function. The problem of the relationship between thought and language remains largely unsolved. The various attempts to understand and define the nature of the relationship have been largely philosophical, although the neurologist and the psychologist have both attempted to elucidate several aspects of this difficult problem. In all fields of enquiry the hypotheses advanced largely represent diametrically opposed views. One is that no distinction between language and thought can be established (monistic theories); the other that language and thought are totally independent (dualistic theories). The subject has been reviewed in detail by Zangwill (1964, 1969), Critchley (1970), and Lebrun and Hoops (1974).

Most early neurologists favoured some type of monistic theory. For instance, Hughling Jackson (1878) thought aphasia to be a disturbance of symbolic thinking and expression; Pierre Marie (1926) viewed aphasia, especially Wernicke's aphasia, as an intellectual disorder and Head (1926) argued that intellectual insufficiency in aphasia could be ascribed wholly to the defective use of language. Head added, however, that when the lesion was extensive the intellectual changes resulted from coincidental disease of the brain. Goldstein's (1948) position, which later gave rise to a great deal of psychological inquiry, was somewhat similar. He considered that an intellectual deficit consisting of an impairment of abstract thought was found in a high proportion of aphasic patients, especially those with amnesic aphasia. More recently Bay (1962), on the basis of a study designed to analyse drawings and models of aphasic patients, concluded that these showed evidence of a breakdown or restriction of intellectual capacities.

Intelligence Tests in Aphasia

With the advent of psychometric tests the question asked by neurologist and psychologist alike changed drastically. The emphasis was no longer on the relationship between thought and language but rather on that between language and intelligence, or more specifically between aphasia and measurements of intellectual ability. It was at this point that the dualistic theories, i.e. those which postulate independence of thought and language, began to flourish.

The first research workers to use intelligence tests with a group of aphasic subjects were Weisenburg, Roe and McBride (1936). Their study showed that while aphasics performed poorly in intelligence tests of a verbal nature, their performance in non-verbal tests was adequate. At present there is substantial evidence to show that aphasic patients are impaired in tests of verbal intelligence (Meyers, 1948; Andersen, 1950, 1951; Reitan, 1954, Archibald, Wepman and Jones, 1967). What remains controversial is whether, and if so, the extent to which, non-verbal abilities are also affected by the breakdown of language function. Research in this field has followed two lines of enquiry. Attempts have been made firstly to establish whether *general* intelligence — as measured by non-verbal tests — remains intact, and secondly to delineate specific aspects of non-verbal cognitive function which might suffer as a direct consequence of the presence of an aphasic disorder. The principal contribution to understanding the relationship of aphasic disorders and non-verbal intelligence has come from the use of Raven's Progressive Matrices (1956, 1965). The test is considered a good tool for assessment of the intellectual ability of aphasics for two reasons: it correlates highly with other tests of intelligence (Hall, 1957) and it has a zero correlation with verbal comprehension (Basso *et al.*, 1973). The results of other studies indicate that aphasics do not show significant impairment in the test. For instance, Zangwill (1964) found that the performance of patients with motor, jargon and amnesic aphasia was adequate, except in cases where the speech disorder was associated with constructional apraxia. Similarly other studies (Arrigioni and De Renzi, 1964; De Renzi and Faglioni, 1965) have found no difference between aphasics and non-aphasics in the performance of the test. Basso *et al.* (1973) found impairment in some aphasics but interpreted their results as showing that the failure was not due to language disorder but was instead related to the fact that language areas overlap with other areas involved in the performance of several, verbal and non-verbal, intellectual tasks. It is worth noting, however, that impairment on the Raven's matrices has been found even when the severity of the aphasia has been taken into consideration. Thus Archibald, Wepman and Jones (1967) found that global aphasics in particular showed significant impairment on the test. Also, positive correlations have been found (Kertesz and McCabe, 1975; Edwards, Ellmans and Thompson, 1976) between the scores on the Raven's matrices and the severity of aphasia — severity being assessed on the basis of scores obtained on various aphasia batteries.

Many questions remain unanswered despite the extensive research carried out on the Raven's matrices performance of aphasics. Furthermore, several findings are contradictory — which makes it difficult to judge the validity of the test. For instance, Arrigioni and De Renzi (1964) used Raven's matrices in a study designed to investigate the relationship between constructional apraxia and hemisphere locus of lesion. They found that while patients with left-sided lesions did worse than those with right-sided cerebral damage, there was no significant difference between the patients with and without aphasia. On the other hand, Colonna and Faglioni (1966), in a study of the performance on spatial intelligence tests of patients with unilateral brain damage, found that, while there were no significant differences between the performance of patients with left or right hemisphere lesions, the aphasics performed worse on the Raven's matrices than non-aphasics. Contradictory results have also been found with the use of the two versions of the test (Raven, 1956, 1965). Bailey, Powell and Clarke (1981) demonstrated a negative correlation between severity of aphasia and the scores obtained in the coloured matrices while there was no significant correlation between the severity of language disorder and the scores on the standard black and white version of the test. Reasons such as these should discourage assessments of non-verbal intelligence in aphasic patients based solely on the use of the Raven's matrices.

Specific Cognitive Disabilities and Aphasia

The search for one test of the non-verbal intelligence of aphasics has been disappointing. The reasons for this have been discussed by Piercy (1964) who suggests that instead of seeking a single suitable test of non-verbal intelligence it would be more profitable to examine the non-verbal deficits which are most rather than least associated with aphasia.

At present, there is a substantial number of experimental studies designed to examine non-verbal deficits that coexist with aphasia; and in the following pages an attempt will be made to draw together information on those aspects of defective cognition thought to result from the breakdown of language function. The various clinical and experimental studies are reviewed here under four main headings: disorders of auditory function; disorders of visual function; disorders of conceptual thought; and disorders of non-verbal memory. Special emphasis is given to those studies considered relevant to the assessment of non-verbal abilities in aphasic patients.

Disorders of Auditory Function

Auditory discrimination

Interest in disorders of auditory function in aphasics has centred round the topic of defects of sequential perception. This originates from Lashley's (1951) views on the problem of serial order in behaviour. He considered that both language comprehension (auditory perception) and language expression (organization of movements) require an orderly sequential integration of the elements of speech. Following this a great deal of research using tasks which required temporal ordering was carried out on aphasics.

Defects in the sequential perception of aphasics were first reported by Efron (1963). He tested brain-damaged subjects with two temporal discrimination tasks using visual and auditory stimuli. Efron presented two coloured light flashes — red and green — separated by intervals which varied from 0 to 600 milliseconds. The subject was required to indicate whether the red or the green appeared first. The second test involved the delivery of two tones both of 10-millisecond duration, but of different pitch, and again the subject had to report which came first. His subjects were 12 patients, 11 of whom were reported as having 'some degree of aphasia', and five controls. He showed that a defect in sequence discrimination of sound was found only where there was some aphasia present and he postulated that the area of the brain concerned with input sequence analysis of auditory stimuli was located in the left temporal region where language function is organized. On the other hand the area of the brain concerned with the sequencing of visual stimuli was located somewhat more posteriorly. Efron's findings on aphasics have been corroborated by other studies, although a few contradictory observations have been recorded mostly explained by differances in test procedures and in the selection and classification of aphasic patients (Edward and Auger, 1965; Holmes, 1965; Swisher and Hirsh, 1972; Brookshire, 1972; Tallal and Newcombe, 1978; Chedru, Bastard and Efron, 1978).

So there is convincing evidence that aphasics are impaired in their perception of the temporal order of verbal and non-verbal stimuli. On the other hand, the relationship of such impairment to the breakdown of language remains largely unexplained. Efron (1963) was aware that his study could not show other than a coincidental relationship between aphasia and the defect in sequence discrimination. Swisher and Hirsh (1972) likewise concluded that the deficits in the ordering of auditory stimuli shown by aphasic subjects could not be claimed to be the cause of their poor comprehension of language but were rather only a part of their pattern of deficits. By contrast Tallal and Newcombe (1978), on the basis of a significant correlation found between poor performance in their task (ability to respond to rapidly changing verbal and non-verbal stimuli) and the number of errors made on the Token Test (Boller and Dennis, 1979), have claimed that the auditory impairment is directly related to the comprehension of language. Such a claim, however, cannot be fully accepted until the role of three variables — the impairment in temporal discrimination, the degree of comprehension impairment, and the site of the lesion responsible for the aphasia — have been taken into consideration. It is valuable to note that a practical application of these findings has been made by Poeck and Pietron (1981) who tested the comprehension of a group of aphasic subjects using two types of presentation: one at a normal speed and another in which the commands were 'stretched' without altering their frequency. They found that stretching of the commands led to a significant improvement in understanding in the aphasic group.

Finally it is important to comment on an observation which has direct relevance to the problem of assessment of aphasics. It comes from Holmes (1965), who carried out a study similar to that of Efron and found that the responses of aphasics were more impaired when there was no spatial separation between the stimuli presented (visual or acoustic). Furthermore, the aphasics' performance improved dramatically when the acoustic stimuli which they had to discriminate were presented to different ears (e.g. low pitch in left and high pitch in the right); such improvement does not happen in normal subjects tested in similar conditions (Hirsh and Sherrick, 1961). It seems, therefore, that the time available for auditory processing is not the only variable that can affect the aphasics' performance. The spatial separation of the stimuli appears also to be important for the analysis of acoustic stimuli.

Disorders of recognition of meaningful sounds

The failure of some aphasics to recognize meaningful sounds has been frequently reported as a feature of the language disorder. But it was not until 1966 that the first systematic study was carried out. Spinnler and Vignolo (1966) studied a group of brain-damaged patients with and without aphasia to analyse the nature of the impairment, its incidence in different clinical forms of aphasia, and its relationship with disorders of auditory verbal comprehension. Their test consisted of the presentation — on a tape recorder — of 10 easily recognizable meaningful sounds (e.g. the neighing of a horse, the song of a canary, gunshots). The subjects were asked to listen to the sound and to indicate which one of four given pictures was the natural source. The alternatives given to the subject were: a picture of the correct source of the sound; a picture of an item which had an 'acoustic' relationship to the sound, a picture depicting an object with a 'semantic' connection, and finally one of an item which had no relationship with the presented sound. An example is: the presented sound = a song of a canary; the correct response = a picture of a singing canary; the 'acoustic' response = a card depicting a man whistling; the semantic response = a card showing a crowing cock; the unrelated ('odd') response = the picture of a train in motion.

The results of this test showed that only the aphasic patients, and especially those who had comprehension deficits, demonstrated evidence of defective sound recognition. Analysis of the type of errors made by the aphasics disclosed a greater number of 'semantic' than 'acoustic' errors. On the basis of this observation Spinnler and Vignolo suggested that the aphasics' failure to recognize meaningful sounds was not due to an impairment of their acoustic perception but rather to an inability to associate the perceived sound with its correct meaning. Moreover, they considered that such a deficit of association — defined as the inability to put together different aspects of the same concept (Vignolo, 1982) — was not exclusive to the auditory modality but represented an intermodal defect. Finally they postulated that the semantic associative disorder was the common factor underlying defects both in sound recognition and in auditory language comprehension. This observation was confirmed by a study of Doehring *et al.* (1967) who replicated the investigation using the same material. The authors agreed fully with the interpretation proposed by Spinnler and Vignolo. A further study extending the analysis to recognition of meaningful and meaningless sounds (Faglioni *et al.*, 1969) found that aphasics performed as well as controls in the discrimination of meaningless sounds whilst failing to identify the meaningful ones.

In a more recent investigation the interpretation of the aphasics' failure to recognize meaningful sounds has been challenged (Strohner *et al.*, 1979). In all previous studies the 'semantic' association choice was a picture of a meaningful related object producing a sound (e.g. a crowing cock, for the sound of the song of a canary). In the test of Strohner *et al.* the semantic choice was a meaningfully related, but silent, object (e.g. for the sound of a frog the semantically related item was a lizard). The result of their investigation confirmed previous findings — except that aphasics did not produce a larger number of semantic than acoustic errors. For this reason the authors claimed that the difficulties encountered by the aphasics in the sound–picture matching task were not a simple failure of association, as had been claimed before, but reflected a wider deficit: an inability to analyse and extract features from a stimulus or from the concept represented by the stimulus. Although the nature of the deficit remains a matter for debate, the results of the different studies have provided convincing evidence that the failure of aphasics to recognize meaningful sounds is not primarily a deficit of acoustic discrimination.

Disorders of Visual Function

Figure-ground discrimination

The first systematic study to show a specific deficit of visual perception in aphasics was that of Teuber and Weinstein (1956). They tested a group of brain-injured subjects and a normal control group with the Gottschaldt (1929) Hidden Figures Test. This test requires the subject to find, by tracing with a pencil, a given figure embedded within a larger display. The brain-injured subjects were grouped by locus of lesion, presence or absence of visual field defect, somatosensory deficits, aphasia or post-traumatic epilepsy. The results showed that the control subjects performed significantly better than any of the brain-injured groups, and that aphasics performed worst of all. The deficits culd not be attributed to their language disorder nor to a general decline of intelligence and it was concluded that aphasia was associated with a perceptual defect which transcended language, but which was not identical to intellectual deterioration. Teuber and Weinstein interpret the deficit as one of defective 'intellectual organization' a disturbance which manifests itself only partly in the difficulties which aphasic patients experience in linguistic reception and expression. This observation has been substantiated by a later study (Russo and Vignolo, 1967) using the same test. The patients were however grouped according to the laterality of their brain lesion — this was not done by Teuber and Weinstein. Russo and Vignolo found, like Teuber and Weinstein, that aphasics performed poorly in the Hidden Figure Test, and that the more severe the aphasia, the worse the performance was. But they further found that patients with right-hemisphere lesions also performed poorly; to explain this result they suggested that an individual's performance in tests which require the ability to make figure–ground discriminations is in fact dependent upon two abilities: a language ability (or a reasoning ability closely related to language) and a visuo-spatial ability, the latter being subserved by the right cerebral hemisphere.

Despite these studies, the association of deficits of figure–ground discrimination with the break-down of language remains to some extent puzzling as the performance of other complex tasks of visual recognition, such as the perception of incomplete figures or of overlapping shapes, has been shown to be unaffected by the presence of aphasia (De Renzi and Spinnler, 1966).

Colour perception

Considerable attention has been paid to the association of abnormalities of colour perception with brain lesions, and to colour naming difficulties in aphasic patients (see Critchley, 1965; Oxbury *et al.*, 1969; Scotti and Spinnler,

1970; Wyke and Holgate, 1973). By contrast, little work has been done on the performance of aphasic patients in colour tasks which do not have explicit verbal requirements.

The original report on this subject was provided by De Renzi and Spinnler (1967) in a study concerned with the performance on colour tasks by patients with unilateral hemisphere damage. The study included a test which required the subjects to colour 25 outline drawings of objects with specific colour characteristics (e.g. strawberry, banana, postbox). The aphasics performed significantly worse on this test than any other brain damaged group. De Renzi and Spinnler established that the deficits could not be accounted for either by the language disorder or by the presence of primary perceptual defects. They considered that there was a more general involvement of mental abilities and argued that the nature of the deficit was one of inadequate conceptualization. These findings have been corroborated and extended in several studies (De Renzi *et al.*, 1972; Cohen and Kelter, 1979) which attempted to show more systematically that the poor performance of aphasics is not due to primary perceptual deficits or inadequate verbal comprehension. At present the consensus is that the colour deficit is a disorder of conceptual thought. The implication of this finding to the non-verbal assessment of the aphasic patient will be discussed next.

Disorders of Conceptual Thought

The above studies, especially those concerned with the performance of aphasics in tests involving the recognition of meaningful sounds and the matching of colour-to-object, strongly suggest that a defect of conceptualization is present and that this defect transcends the breakdown of language. For some time there has been a growing reluctance to interpret such a defect in Goldsteinian terms (Teuber, 1966). At this point, therefore it may be helpful to restate Goldstein's views and examine the extent to which the analysis of other research workers differs from his.

The analysis of 'categorical (or abstract) attitude' in clinical psychology stems from the work of Goldstein (1924). The terms 'abstract and concrete behaviour' had been used previously (*see* Pikas, 1966 for historical review), but it was Goldstein and his associates who introduced them as an explanation for the disorders of cognitive function occurring in patients with brain lesions. The clinical description emerged from the observations of brain-damaged patients in sorting tasks. Gelb and Goldstein (1925) considered that when sorting skeins of wool of different colours for instance, the concrete colour was not perceived as an independent singular entity but was considered more as a representative of the concept of red, yellow, blue etc. Several years later a battery of five sorting tasks to evaluate abstract attitude was developed by Goldstein and Scheerer (1941). The basic idea was that normal adults show an ability not only to sort objects into conceptual categories but also to sort them out afterwards into other categories, while patients with brain damage do not have this ability. An early experimental report on the use of the Goldstein Scheerer battery with aphasic patients comes from Brown (1955), who also tested a control group of normal subjects. The inclusion of a control group was important, as the work of Goldstein had been criticized because no attempt had been made to carry out a normative study. Brown's investigation found no significant differences in abstract ability between the two groups on four of the five tests. On one task (the Stick-test), however, the performance of the aphasics was significantly poorer than that of the matched controls.

In recent years there has been a renewed interest in this topic and several reports of the failure of aphasic patients on conceptual tasks have appeared in the literature. De Renzi *et al.* (1966) used a modified version of the Weigl's Sorting Test (Weigl, 1927). They assessed a group of aphasic and non-aphasic patients and also a normal control group and a brain damaged group with lesions restricted to the right hemisphere. The data obtained showed that the poorest performance was seen when the lesions were associated with aphasia. From this evidence they concluded that aphasic subjects had a specific defect of 'abstract thinking', and claimed that those areas of the brain which subserved language behaviour also specialized in tasks of a symbolic nature. Similar observations have come from other sources, for instance the investigations of Kelter *et al.* (1976) and Cohen *et al.* (1980). Both groups used a picture-to-picture matching task. The subject was shown three pictures arranged so as to form an inverted triangle. The two pictures at the top represented 2 objects; one of these was linked conceptually to the third picture below. For example in the upper corners were the pictures of a frog and a snail and the picture underneath (the clue picture) was a kangaroo. The patients were asked to point out the picture which was more closely linked with the clue picture. The test had 3 parts based on the nature of the conceptual links. One set relied on attributes shared by the objects, the second on common actions, and the third on common situations. On those parts of the test involving common attributes and actions the performance of the aphasics was significantly worse than that of the controls. The authors conjectured that in the case of patients with Wernicke's aphasia the nature of the failure illustrated a lack of 'analytical competence'.

The co-existence of a conceptual deficit and aphasia has not been universally accepted. Criticism has derived especially from studies dealing with 'pantomime' interpretation (*see* Peterson and Kirshner, 1981 for a review). Some authors (Duffy *et al.*, 1975; Gainotti and Lemmo, 1976; Varney, 1978) have found a close relationship between the severity of aphasia and the ability to carry out tasks requiring the interpretation of pantomime gestures. The findings have been variously described as disorders of representative ability or failures of symbolic thought. Other studies, however, (Seron *et al.*, 1979; Feyereisen *et al.*, 1981) have failed to establish a close association between the severity of aphasia and impairment in the interpretation of pantomime gestures and have alleged that failure in this task is not necessarily, attributable to a linguistic deficit. These differences of opinion arise, to a certain extent, from differences in the terms used to describe the abilities tested by the various tasks. Thus, the terms, 'analytic behaviour', 'analytic competence', 'abstract and conceptual thinking' and 'symbolic function' seem to imply slightly different mechanisms of concept formation. But none of these expressions has emerged as a new explanation of abstract behaviour. There seems to be, therefore, no justification for discarding the terms used by Goldstein and his associates.

Until there is more uniformity in the delineation of the underlying process, and a better description of what each task attempts to test, it is likely that discrepancies of interpretation will continue to arise. Meanwhile, the claim that some form of conceptual disorder is associated with some types of aphasia should be taken as a significant observation for the assessment of the non-verbal abilities of these patients.

Disorders of Memory for Non-verbal Material

The discussion here is restricted to studies which have examined disorders of non-verbal memory associated with aphasia. Two main questions are addressed. The first is whether the nature of the pictorial material used in memory tests is an important factor in the assessment of non-verbal memory deficits in these patients; that is to say, whether there are differences in the memorization when the stimulus presented is meaningful and easily verbalized, or non-meaningful and therefore difficult to verbalize. The second is whether disorders of memory function in aphasic subjects relate solely to deficits of immediate recall or to those of delayed recall as well.

The types of material and the methods of testing used by different research workers have varied considerably but the findings have been surprisingly consistent. De Renzi and Spinnler (1966) used coloured drawings of animals; Boller and De Renzi (1967) presented pictures of both realistic objects and nonsense shapes, whilst Kelter *et al.* (1977) used drawings of objects and photos of snow-flakes — these were considered extremely difficult to code verbally, although easy to discriminate visually. The methods of testing also varied among the authors. They were: simple recognition; paired associations (i.e. presenting pairs of cards and later showing one card to the subject and asking him to select its associate from a set of cards); and 'forced choice' (i.e. showing stimulus card and after intervals of time asking the subject to select the original picture from a set of cards). All studies found significant impairment in patients with aphasia. De

Renzi and Spinnler (1966) and Boller and De Renzi (1967) showed that the scores of aphasics were worse than those of any other brain damaged group. Moreover, aphasics scored poorly whether the material was meaningful or meaningless. They considered, however, that it was impossible to establish a close relationship between the aphasic deficit and the disorders of memory for two reasons: firstly, the scores of aphasics in memory tests have no relationship to the severity of the aphasia and secondly, the possibility of verbal encoding of the nonsense shapes could not be discounted. Kelter *et al.* (1977) divided the aphasics into two groups: fluent and non-fluent. Analysis of their results demonstrated that while both groups scored lower than the normal subjects, but equally poorly, when the interval between presentation and recall was left free (i.e. the subjects had no other task to carry out and could therefore use the interval as a time for 'rehearsal'), there was a difference between fluent and non-fluent aphasics if the interval was filled with another task — sorting playing cards according to suit — most likely preventing 'rehearsal' of the presented stimulus. In the 'non-rehearsal' conditions fluent aphasics showed impairment in their ability to recognize drawings of objects and snow-flakes whilst non-fluent aphasics were impaired only in the latter. Kelter *et al.* interpreted their findings in terms of the verbal-loop hypothesis of Glanzer and Clark (1962) which postulates that subjects encode experience into language and store the linguistic encoding for later use thus permitting the subject to return to the world of experience by forming a 'verbal loop'. The time taken to perform the encoding will depend both on the complexity of the stimulus presented and on the linguistic ability of the person encoding the experience (*see* also Brewer, 1969). Kelter *et al.* (1977) proposed that, as the perceptual processing includes a covert verbalization, non-fluent aphasics who have special difficulty in verbalizing are likely to be impaired only in tasks (such as the snow-flakes) which require complex verbal labelling, whilst fluent aphasics will show impairment in tasks involving both familiar and unfamiliar objects because of the presence of word finding difficulties and paraphasic errors.

The observation that aphasic subjects might have difficulty with verbal encoding has been made previously, in a study carried out by Goodglass *et al.* (1974). This study intended to explore the problem of covert mediation in aphasic subjects directly by using a simple test of matching from visual memory developed by Conrad (1964), who had found that lists of letters comprising acoustically similar items were less well remembered than lists containing items which were acoustically distinctive. Some years later Conrad (1971) made a similar observation using pictures rather than letters. The subjects were asked to recall immediately after presentation two sets of pictures. One had homophonic names (bat, cat, rat, mat) whilst the other was composed of pictures with non-homophonic names (girl, fish, spoon, horse). Although the procedure did not require verbalization of the stimuli the subjects' performance was significantly worse when the stimuli were identified by homophonic names. The poor performance was interpreted as an interference effect which provided strong evidence of the acoustic encoding of visually presented material.

Goodglass *et al.* used this technique to test a group of aphasic subjects and a group of brain-damaged patients without aphasia. They included in addition to the Conrad tests a test requiring the recognition of nonsense figures. Their results provided proof of the absence of covert verbal mediation in aphasic subjects. The evidence was twofold; first, the phenomenon of interference shown in normal subjects with the homophonic set of pictures was absent in the aphasic group but present in non-aphasic patients with brain-damage; furthermore, there was no significant improvement in the performance of aphasic patients in the visual memory test when the pictures represented familiar objects rather than nonsense figures. By contrast, subjects without aphasia produced considerably better scores with the meaningful pictures than with the nonsense shapes.

There is one further point that requires comment. This relates to a discrepancy between the findings of De Renzi and Spinnler (1966) and those of Kelter *et al.* (1977) in respect of the performance of aphasic subjects in delayed memory tasks. De Renzi and Spinnler tested recall after an interval of 60 seconds, which was filled with a distracting activity (an inquiry into the patient's illness). They found that the lowest scores in the delay task were related not to aphasia but to other variables such as the presence of visual field defects and slow reaction times. On the other hand, Kelter *et al.* who used a 10 second delay period found a greater impairment in aphasic patients and particularly in fluent aphasics where the interval between presentation and recall was *not* filled with another distracting activity. The discrepancy in these results, most likely stems from the different intervals used, and from the different tasks carried out in the intervening period. Furthermore, Dr Renzi and Spinnler did not segregate the various categories of aphasia.

Although much more research is required before many aspects of the impairment of non-verbal memory in aphasic patients are clarified, evidence so far collected suggests that the following considerations should be borne in mind when testing aphasic subjects:

1. These patients show convincing evidence of impairment in short and delayed memory for pictorial material.
2. The impairment is present both for meaningful (pictures of familiar objects, animals etc.), and meaningless material (e.g. nonsense shapes), and for meaningful material which is easily discriminable but not easily verbalized (e.g. pictures of snow-flakes).
3. The use of covert verbal mediation by the aphasic group is restricted.
4. In delayed memory tasks the interval between presentation and recall and

the activities carried out during this period are both factors that must be taken into consideration.

Assessment

In the preceding pages an attempt has been made to outline the principal non-verbal defects which constitute part of the breakdown of language. From this account it is clear that any evaluation of the various components of language function should not be divorced from an inquiry into non-verbal defects. A dual evaluation would provide a firmer base for constructing a rehabilitation programme: for example, a therapist often conducts an assessment of an aphasic patient using material which either requires high level colour discrimination or offers compensatory strategies involving pattern recognition or the ability to memorize pictorial material, without realizing that deficits in these abilities may coexist with aphasia.

It is essential, however, to distinguish between two areas of non-verbal dysfunction. The first comprises those cognitive deficits which occur in *association* with aphasia due to an overlap of the brain regions which can produce a language breakdown with those which subserve high level perceptual-motor functions, such as praxis, personal and extrapersonal orientation and visual recognition. The presence of these associated deficits has been reviewed by Weinstein (1965) and more recently by Kertesz (1979); and tests to evaluate these functions frequently form part of the aphasic assessment. One notable example is that offered by Goodglass and Kaplan (1972) whose test battery contains various tasks designed to evaluate parietal lobe dysfunction. Their manual provides a description of test procedures for administration and scoring and statistical values for the aphasic subject's performance — with reference to constructional apraxia, finger agnosia, acalculia and right–left disorientation.

The second area of assessment comprises the deficits that *coexist* with the break-down of language, and for these there is no available test battery providing normative values. Test procedures and statistical values for the performance of aphasic and non-aphasic subjects have to be derived from the scattered studies published in different journals. A list of the tests described in this chapter together with suitable alternatives is presented in *Table 1*. The list does not represent a test 'battery' but merely a guideline for the selection of tests which might prove useful in demarcating areas of impairment.

The final choice should be determined by the aims of the assessment. When testing is carried out for a clinical purpose, that is to determine the nature and extent of the deficits of a particular individual, test selection and interpretation should be guided by such factors as the age, sex and cultural

Table 1 **Tests for the assessment of disorders of non-verbal cognitive function**

I Disorders of auditory function
- (i) Temporal sequencing
  - Efron (1963)
  - Tallal and Newcombe (1978)
  - Test of Rhythm (Seashore *et al.*, 1960)
- (ii) Recognition of meaningful sounds
  - Vignolo (1982)
  - Doehring (1967)
  - Faglioni *et al.* (1969)
  - Strohner *et al.* (1979)

II Disorders of visual function
- (i) Figure–ground discrimination
  - Gottschaldt's Hidden Figure Test (Thurstone, 1944)
  - Overlapping Drawing Test Poppelreuter (1917)
- (ii) Colour perception
  - Colour form Matching
  - De Renzi and Spinnler (1967)
  - Wyke and Holgate (1973)
  - Cohen and Kelter (1979)
- (iii) Disorders of conceptual thought
  - Goldstein and Scheerer (1941)
  - Kelter *et al.* (1976)
  - Cohen *et al.* (1980)
  - Payne and Hewlett (1960)
  - Weigl's Test — Modified (De Renzi *et al.*, 1966)
- (iv) Disorders of memory
  - De Renzi and Spinnler (1966)
  - Boller and De Renzi (1967)
  - Kelter *et al.* (1977)
  - Goodglass *et al.*, (1974)

level of the subject, in addition to the patient's clinical history and clinical examination. It is essential in a clinical assessment to make a close observation of the patient's performance, and not to record the outcome of the test as only a simple pass or fail. To do this would preclude the examiner from understanding the reasons for failure. For instance, a low score in the Picture Arrangement subtest of the WAIS may be due to a perceptual disorder, an inability to understand a temporal sequence of events, or a deficit in interpretation. When the assessment is made for a research purpose, however, selection of the tests has to be determined by a conceptual framework. That is to say the test selection should satisfy the requirements of a theoretical model.

Concluding Remarks

The work which has been carried out so far on non-verbal deficits in aphasic patients has been limited. Most research workers have considered individual cognitive skills and have not attempted therefore, to perform a systematic analysis of a constellation of non-verbal deficits in the same group of patients. Furthermore, most of the studies have considered aphasic subjects as a unitary group. Those few that have tried to examine differential performances according to the type of aphasia have not employed a consistent method of classification. Some studies have thus grouped their subjects on the basis of an anatomical–functional division (such as Broca, or Wernicke aphasia) while others have employed a more linguistic criterion (such as fluent and non-fluent aphasia). A great deal of research is required to unravel the nature and extent of the non-verbal deficits that coexist with aphasia. Attempts to develop a suitable test battery for this purpose will encounter, however, all the pitfalls which occur when developing one to assess the breakdown of language. The difficulty which arises when faced with such a task has been discussed by Benton (1967). He points out that the problems are quite formidable, starting with the building of a conceptual framework which will determine what tests to employ to assess non-verbal deficits and ending with time consuming practical tasks: for instance the determination of reliability, validity and level of difficulty, the collection of normative data which must take into consideration factors of age, sex and cultural status; the correcting of scores to compensate for the influence of age and educational level where this is necessary and the transformation of scores into standard scores or ranks in order to obtain a valid picture of an individual patient's strengths and weaknesses. The use of such a battery for the purpose of a clinical assessment will still carry the danger of providing information only on those disturbances which fit a preconceived theoretical model and, as pointed out by Osgood (1963), among others, a battery developed on these terms is likely to be only as adequate as the theory on which it rests.

References

ANDERSEN, A.L. The effect of laterality localization of brain damage on Wechsler–Bellevue indices of deterioration. *Journal of Clinical Psychology* (1950), **6**, 191–194.

ANDERSEN, A.L. The effects of laterality localization of focal brain lesions on the Wechsler–Bellevue subtests. *Journal of Clinical Psychology* (1951), **7**, 149–153.

ARCHIBALD, Y.M., WEPMAN, J.M. and JONES, L.V. Non-verbal cognitive performance in aphasic and nonaphasic brain damaged patients. *Cortex* (1967), **3**, 276–294.

ARRIGIONI, G. and DE RENZI, E. Constructional apraxia and hemispheric locus of lesion. *Cortex*, (1964), **1**, 170–197.

BAILEY, S., POWELL, G. and CLARKE, E. A note on intelligence and recovery from aphasia: the relationship between Raven's Matrices Scores and change on the Schonell Aphasia Test. *British Journal of Disorders of Communication* (1981), **16**, 193–203.

BASSO, A., DE RENZI, E., FAGLIONI, P., SCOTTI, G. and SPINNLER, H. Neuropsychological evidence for the existence of cerebral areas critical to the performance of intelligence tasks. *Brain* (1973), **96**, 715–228.

BAY, E. Aphasia and Non-verbal Disorders of Language. *Brain* (1962), **85**, 411–426.

BENSON, A.L. Problems of test construction in the field of aphasia. *Cortex* (1967), **3**, 32–58.

BOLLER, F. and DENNIS, M. (eds) *Auditory Comprehensioh Clinical and Experimental Studies with the Token Test* (1979). New York: Academic Press.

BOLLER, F. and DE RENZI, E. Relationships between visual and memory defects and hemispheric locus of lesion. *Neurology* (1967), **17**, 1052–1082.

BREWER, W.F. Visual memory, verbal encoding and hemispheric localization. *Cortex* (1969), **5**, 145–151.

BROOKSHIRE, R.H. Visual and auditory sequencing by aphasic subjects. *Journal Communication Disorders* (1972), **5**, 259–269.

BROWN, I. Abstract and concrete behaviour of dysphasic patients and normal subjects. *Journal of Speech and Hearing Disorders* (1955), **20**, 37–42.

CHEDRU, F., BASTARD, V. and EFRON, R. Auditory micropattern discrimination in brain damaged subjects. *Neuropsychologia* (1978), **16**, 141–149.

COHEN R. and KELTER, S. Cognitive impairment of aphasics in a colour-to-picture matching task. *Cortex* (1979), **15** 235–245.

COHEN, R., KELTER, S. and GERHILD, W. Analytical competence and language impairment in aphasia *Brain and Language* (1980), **10**, 331–347.

COLONNA, A. and FAGLIONI, P. The performance of hemisphere damage patients on spatial intelligence tests. Cortex (1966), **2**, 293–307.

CONRAD, R. Acoustic confusions in immediate memory. *British Journal of Psychology* (1964), **55**, 75–84.

CONRAD, R. The chronology of the development of covert speech in children. *Developmental Psychology* (1971), **5**, 398–405.

CRITCHLEY, M. Acquired anomolies of colour perception of central origin. *Brain* (1965), **88**, 711–724.

CRITCHLEY, M. Thinking and speaking: verbal symbols in thought. *Aphasiology and other Aspects of Language* (1970), pp. 159–173. London: Edward Arnold Ltd.

DE RENZI, E. and FAGLIONI, P. The comparative efficiency of intelligence and vigilance tests in detecting hemispheric cerebral damage. *Cortex* (1965). **1**, 410–433.

DE RENZI, E., FAGLIONI, P., SAVOIARDO, M. and VIGNOLO, L.A. The influence of the hemispheric side of the cerebral lesion on abstract thinking. *Cortex* (1966), **2**, 399–420.

DE RENZI, E., FAGLIONI, P., SCOTTI, G. and SPINNLER, H. Impairment in associating colour to form concomitant with aphasia. *Brain* (1972), **95**, 293–304.

De Renzi, E. and Spinnler, H. Visual recognition in patients with unilateral cerebral disease. *Journal of Nervous and Mental Disease* (1966), **142**, 515–525.

De Renzi, E. and Spinnler, H. The influence of verbal and non-verbal defects on visual memory tasks. *Cortex* (1966), **2**, 322–336.

De Renzi, E. and Spinnler, H. Impaired performance on colour tasks in patients with hemispheric damage. *Cortex* (1967), **3**, 194–216.

Doehring, D.G., Dudley, J.G. and Coderre, L. Programmed instruction in picture-sound association for the aphasic. *Folia Phoniatrica* (1967), **19**, 414–426.

Duffy, R.L., Duffy, J.R. and Pearson, K.L. Pantomime recognition in aphasics. *Journal of Speech and Hearing Research* (1975), **18**, 115–132.

Edwards, A.E. and Auger, R. The effect of aphasia on the perception of precedence. In *Proceedings 73rd American Psychological Association Convention* (1965), pp. 207–208.

Edwards, S., Ellmans, J. and Thompson, J. Language and intelligence in dysphasia: are they related? *British Journal Disorders of Communication* (1976), **11**, 83–94.

Efron, R. Temporal perception, aphasia, and déjà-vu. *Brain* (1963), **86**, 403–424.

Faglioni, P., Spinnler, H. and Vignolo, L.A. Contrasting behaviour of right and left hemisphere damage patients on a discriminitive and semantic task of auditory recognition. *Cortex* (1969), **5**, 366–389.

Feyereisen, P., Seron, X. and De Macar, M. Interpretation de differentes categories de gestes chez deq sujets aphasiques. *Neuropsychologia* (1981), **19**, 515–521.

Gainotti, G. and Lemmo, M.A. Comprehension of symbolic gestures in aphasia. *Brain and Language* (1976), **3**, 451–460.

Gelb, A. and Goldstein, K. Psychologische Analysen hirnpathologischer Falle X uber Farbennamen-amnesie. *Psychologische Forschung* (1925), **6**, 127–199.

Glanzer, M. and Clark, W.H. Accuracy of perceptual recall: An analysis of organization. *Journal of Verbal Learning and Verbal Behaviour* (1962), **1**, 289–299.

Goldstein, K. Uber die gleichartige funktionelle Bedingtheit der Symptome bei organischen und psychischen Krankheiten im besonderem uber den funktionallen Mechanisms der Zwangsvorgange. *Monatsschirft zur Psychiatrie und Neurologie* (1924), **57**, 191–209.

Goldstein, K. *Language and Language Disturbances* (1948). New York: Grune and Stratton.

Goldstein, K. and Scheerer, M. *Abstract and Concrete Behaviour An Experimental Study with Special Tests* (1941). Psychological Monographs American Psychological Association.

Goodglas', H., Denes, G. and Calderon, M. The absence of covert verbal mediation in aphasia. *Cortex* (1974), **10**, 264–269.

Goodglass, H. and Kaplan, E. *The Assessment of Aphasia and Related Disorders* (1972). Philadelphia: Lea and Fehiger.

Gottschaldt, K. Uber den Einfluss der Erfahrung auf die Wahrnehmung von Figuren. *Psychologische Forschung* (1929), **8** 261–317, **12**, 1–87.

Hall, J.C. Correlation of modified form of Raven's Progressive Matrices (1938) with the Wechler Adult Intelligence Scale. *Journal of Consultant Psychology* (1957), **21**, 23–26.

HEAD, H. *Aphasia and Kindred Disorders of Speech* (1926). Cambridge University Press.

HIRSH, I.J. and SHERRICK, C.E. Perceived order in different sense modalities. *Journal of Experimental Psychology* (1961), **62**, 423–432.

HOLMES, H. *Disordered Perception of Auditory Sequential Patterns in Aphasia* (1965). PhD Thesis Harvard University.

JACKSON, J.H. On affections of speech from disease of the brain. *Brain* (1878), **1**, 304–330.

KELTER, S., COHEN, R., ENGEL, D., LIST, G. and STROHNER, H. Aphasic disorders in matching tasks involving conceptual analysis and covert naming. *Cortex* (1976), **12**, 383–394.

KELTER, S., COHEN, R., ENGEL, D., LIST, G. and STROHNER, H. Verbal coding and memory in aphasics. *Neuropsychologia* (1977), **15**, 51–60.

KERTESZ, A. and MCCABE, P. Intelligence and Aphasia: Performance of Aphasics on Raven's coloured progressive matrices (R.C.M.P.). *Brain and Language* (1975), **2**, 387–395.

KERTESZ, A. *Aphasia and Associated Disorders: Taxonomy Localization and Recovery* (1979). New York: Grune and Stratton, Inc.

LASHLEY, K.S. The problem of serial order in behaviour. In A. Jeffress (ed.) *Cerebral Mechanisms in Behaviour* (1951), pp. 112–136. New York: Wiley.

LEBRUN, Y. and HOOPS, R. (eds) *Intelligence and Aphasia* (1974). Neurolinguistics 2. Amsterdam: Sweets and Zeitlinger B.V.

MARIE, P. *Travaux et memoires 1* (1926). Paris: Masson.

MEYERS, R. Relation of 'thinking and language': An experimental approach using dysphasic patients. *Archives of Neurology and Psychiatry* (1948), **60**, 119–139.

OSGOOD, C.E. and MIRON, M.S. (eds) *Approaches to the Study of Aphasia* (1963). University of Illinois Press.

OXBURY, J.M., OXBURY, S.M. and HUMPHREY, N.K. Variety of colour anomia. *Brain* (1969), **92** 847–860.

PAYNE, R.W. and HEWLETT, J.H.G. Thought disorders in psychotic patients. In H.J. Eysenck (ed.) *Experiments in Personality 2*, Psychodiagnostics and Psychodynamics) (1960). New York: Humanities Press.

PETERSON, L.N. and KIRSHNER, H.S. Gestural Impairment and gestural ability in aphasia: A review. *Brain and Language* (1981), **14**, 333–348.

PIERCY, M. The effects of cerebral lesions on intellectual functions: A review of current research trends. *British Journal of Psychiatry* (1964), **110**, 310–352.

PIKAS, A. *Abstraction and Concept Formation an Interpretative Investigation into a Group of Psychological Frames of Reference* (1966). Cambridge, Massachusetts: Harvard University Press.

POECK, K. and PIETRON, H.P. The influence of stretched speech presentation on token test performance of aphasic and right brain damage patients. *Neuropsychologia* (1981), **19**, 133–136.

POPPELREUTER, W. *Die psychischen schadigimgen durch Köpfschuss im Kriege* 1914–1916 (1917). Leipzig: Voss.

RAVEN, J.C. *Standard Progressive Matrices* (1956). London: H.K. Lewis.

RAVEN, J.C. *Guide to Using Coloured Progressive Matrices* (1965). London: H.K. Lewis.

REITAN, R.M. Intelligence and Language functions in dysphasic patients. *Diseases of the Nervous System* (1954), **14**, 2–8.

RUSSO, M. and VIGNOLO, L.A. Visual figure–ground discrimination in patients with unilateral cerebral disease. *Cortex* (1967), **3**, 113–127.

SCOTTI, G. and SPINNLER, H. Colour perception in unilateral hemisphere damage patients. *Journal of Neurology, Neurosurgery and Psychiatry* (1970), **33**, 22–28.

SEASHORE, C.E., LEWIS, D. and SAETVEIT, J. *Seashore Measures of Musical Talents Manual* (revised), (1960). New York: Psychological Corporation.

SERON, X., VAN DER KAA,, M.A., REMITZ, A. and VANDERLINDEN, M. Pantomime interpretation and Aphasia. *Neuropsychologia* (1979), **17**, 661–667.

SPINNLER, H. and VIGNOLO, L.A. Impaired recognition of meaningful sounds in aphasia. *Cortex* (1966), **2**, 337–348.

STROHNER, H., COHEN, R., KELTER, S. and WOLL, G. 'Semantic' and 'acoustic' errors in aphasic and schizophrenic patients in a sound–picture matching task. *Cortex* (1979), **14**, 391–403.

SWISHER, L. and HIRSH, I.J. Brain damage and the ordering of two temporally successive stimuli. *Neuropsychologia* (1972), **10**, 137–152.

TALLAL, P. and NEWCOMBE, F. Impairment of auditory perception and language comprehension in dysphasia. *Brain and Language*, **5** 13–24.

TEUBER, H.L. and WEINSTEIN, S. Ability to discover hidden figures after cerebral lesions. *American Medical Association Archives of Neurology and Psychiatry* (1956), **76**, 369–379.

TEUBER, H.L. Kurt Goldstein's role in the development of neuropsychology. *Neuropsychologia* (1966), **4**, 299–310.

THURSTONE, L.L. *A Factorial Study of Perception* (1944). Chicago: University of Chicago Press.

VARNEY, N.R. Linguistic correlates in pantomime recognition in aphasic patients. *Journal of Neurology, Neurosurgery and Psychiatry* (1978), **41**, 564–568.

VIGNOLO, L.A. Auditory agnosia In the Neuropsychology of Cognitive Function. Proceedings of Royal Society Discussion Meeting held on 18th and 19th November 1981 (1982). D.E. Broadbent and Weiskrantz (eds). London: The Royal Society.

WEIGL, E. Zur Psychologie Sogenannter Abstrations prozesse. *Zeitschrift fur Psychologie* (1927), **103**, 2–45.

WEINSTEIN, S. Deficits concomitant with aphasia or lesions of either cerebral hemisphere. *Cortex* (1965), **1**, 154–169.

WEISENBURG, T., ROE, A. and MCBRIDE, K. *Adult Intelligence: A Psychological Study of Test Performance* (1935). New York.

WYKE, M. and HOLGATE, D. Colour-naming defects in dysphasic patients — a qualitative study. *Neuropsychologia* (1973), **11**, 451–461.

ZANGWILL, O.L. Intelligence in aphasia in A.V.S. De Reuck and M. O'Connor (eds) *Disorders of Language* (1964), pp. 261–274. London: Churchill.

ZANGWILL, O.L. Intellectual status in aphasia. P. Vinken and G. Brujn *Handbook of Clinical Neurology* (1969), **4**, pp. 105–111. Amsterdam: Elsevier.

15

The Assessment of Verbal Comprehension

Ruth Lesser

Basic to a consideration of assessment of verbal comprehension is a definition of how the term 'verbal comprehension' is being used. As frequently happens in the study of aphasia, it has various interpretations for different students in the field. For some it is synonymous with the reception of verbal material by the hearer. Such an interpretation distinguishes auditory and visual aspects of reception, and the assessment of reading comprehension is unequivocally separated from the assessment of auditory verbal comprehension. This is the approach used in most test batteries.

To other students of aphasia, verbal comprehension more interestingly draws on central processes in language rather than peripheral. The closest equivalent of verbal comprehension for them is 'linguistic knowledge', as first used by transformational grammarians in distinguishing competence from performance in language use. Whether linguistic knowledge be accessed through reading or listening is immaterial within such a framework. The one exception is the phonological level of language organization, which relates primarily to speech perception through the auditory modality (if we leave aside such issues as phonological recoding during reading, the use of lip-reading information or the perception of finger-spelling by the profoundly deaf). Prominent amongst the interests of students of this school has been the investigation of the comprehension of grammar as a central process, with questions of restriction of comprehension due to limitation of auditory memory relegated to secondary importance as concerning performance rather than competence. That the issues are not as clear as this will emerge later in this chapter.

To yet another school, verbal comprehension comes close to 'understanding', with its implications of appreciation of concepts and the use of language in the mental manipulation of ideas. For those who hold this view, semantic and pragmatic aspects of language and the effect of aphasia on intellectual ability are the main focus of attention. The assessment of verbal comprehension as part of testing in an intelligence scale exemplifies this approach.

A fourth approach to the analysis of verbal comprehension in aphasia emphasises processing stages in the transmission of information from the ear to some form of response — repetition or writing to dictation. It is concerned with the dissociation of components in these processes and the possible separate malfunctioning of alternative routes, and uses models for auditory comprehension which have been initially adapted from investigations of difficulties in reading.

The association of these four interpretations of verbal comprehension with the separate disciplines concerned with aphasia may already be evident from the summary given above. The first approach is traditionally that of the clinic oriented speech pathologist or neurologist; the second is that of the linguist; the third is that of the clinical psychologist in the role of psychometrician; the fourth is that of neuropsychologist. The approach taken in this chapter will attempt a synthesis of these interpretations, but give most emphasis to the last, drawing on the eclectic use that has been made of linguistic theory in information-processing models of aphasia.

Having delimited our usage of verbal comprehension, we are still left with some practical problems in its investigation for assessment. Firstly, verbal comprehension, however defined, cannot be directly measured but only inferred. In attempting to assess comprehension we can control the stimuli we give, but what we actually score is the overt response the individual makes, the verbal or gestural output rather than direct comprehension of the input. It is therefore uncertain to what extent a patient's response reflects comprehension, however defined, or other aspects influencing the organization and execution of a response. Secondly, the variables which influence comprehension as such are not easy to control. Presenting a picture first, or providing an introductory sentence, can significantly improve the scores of patients with severe comprehension difficulties (Pierce and Beekman, 1985). There are many such situational clues in a natural setting to which a patient may be sensitive, leading to the appearance of good comprehension. Conversely, people who are not brain-damaged or aphasic, but who are unaccustomed to formal clinical testing may, in their anxiety, produce results which might be scored as indicative of some impairment of comprehension. Both a natural setting and a formal controlled setting have their disadvantages, therefore, when aphasic people are examined. These are sociolinguistic aspects of assessment and the mores and expectations of the particular speech community have consequences for scores on formal tests which may need to be taken into consideration (Noll and Lass, 1980). A third problem is the transitory nature of an act of comprehension. Speech can be tape-recorded and replayed several times for analysis. Writing also endures in a concrete form. The mental processes of verbal comprehension, however, occur in a temporal context which is shaped by a conjunction of many factors and experiences, and is essentially unrepeatable and unavailable for later analysis except in the examiner's coded form as scores. To an even greater degree than the assessment of speech and writing, therefore, the assessment of comprehension is vulnerable to the preconceptions and theory biases of the assessor, who may often assume with dubious justification that what has been manipulated in the stimulus is indeed what is being measured in the score.

These problems present dilemmas to the investigator. They account in part for the simplification of assumptions which are generally made in designing clinical tests of comprehension in aphasia batteries, and for the relatively recent development of more theoretically motivated procedures in research studies. (For reviews of the historical development of ideas about auditory comprehension in aphasia, *see* Boller, Kim and Mack, 1977; Boller, 1978; Brookshire, 1978a; Riedel, 1981; and for general reviews of the principles of assessment in aphasia from clinical perspectives *see* Linebaugh, 1979; Sarno and Höök, 1980; Spreen and Risser, 1981; Davis, 1983 and Chapey, 1986).

One moral to be drawn from the complexity of problems in examining comprehension, and the relative immaturity of techniques of assessment, is that a number of different approaches need to be used, in assessing individuals, as a cross check on the validity of the inferences which can be made. In particular, we need to use several media of response to establish the common factor which is consistent throughout them. The types of responses which have been employed frequently include pointing to identify an object, picture or word; selecting a symbol to show discrimination of whether two items are the same or different; sorting and arranging of printed words; oral repetition; manipulation of objects or tokens; writing; representational gesture. All these methods have been used as single tasks and claimed as assessing verbal comprehension. Yet the method affects the results. The limitations are evident of using a spoken response to measure comprehension in those people who by definition produce abnormal speech. It has also been shown, however, that methods of response which do not require speech give variable results. For example, in examining aphasic patients' perception of the phonemes of speech, Blumstein, Baker and Goodglass (1977) obtained disparate results depending on whether patients were asked to point to cards indicating that pairs of syllables were the same or different, or whether they were asked to point to a written symbol for the word. Evidently the tasks were either drawing on different mental processes (as psycholinguistic models would predict, since the second task requires reading) or prompting different strategies. The requirement to manipulate objects to show comprehension of sentences gives different results from the requirement to select a ready-made display (Mack, 1981). Input variables which may seem relatively trivial to the naive examiner can be crucial, such as the order of presentation and number of choices (Lenneberg *et al.*, 1978) and the use of live or tape recorded voice (Green and Boller, 1974). The amount of time given for auditory presentation and the delay before a response is required also influence the results (Baker and Goodglass, 1979; Blumstein *et al.*, 1985).

So is the amount of practice and training in responding given to the patient; by use of a careful induction procedure with a globally aphasic patient Deloche *et al.* (1981) were able to demonstrate a retained ability to categorize words which would not otherwise have been suspected. Clearly what the examiner is scoring in any procedure aimed at measuring comprehension is the end product of a number of complex interactions in the processing of information and the organization of responses.

In examining verbal comprehension there are therefore at least four dimensions to be taken into consideration. Firstly, there is the linguistic dimension, i.e. the store of knowledge about the rules and meanings of language which the individual brings to an act of comprehension. Secondly there is the dimension of the modalities of language behaviour. The existence of patients who have more conspicuous deficits in one modality than in others (reading or writing or speaking or listening), or who may present with a modality-specific disorder, has encouraged the analysis of deficits in the processing of information through one particular channel. There has been, in particular, a large number of studies of acquired disorders of verbal comprehension through the modality of reading (*see* Coltheart, 1985, for a review), many of them concerned with patients who also have supramodal disorders of language. For deep dyslexia, for example, the essential criterion is the making of semantic errors in reading aloud (e.g. reading 'projector' as 'camera'), a characteristic also of a central language disorder in aphasia. Peripheral damage clearly can affect only one modality (for example, in dysarthria or in deafness) but the question of the extent to which higher cortical damage can also be specific to one modality-related system is open to some dispute (*see* Beauvois's 1982, discussion of optic aphasia). Thirdly there is the dimension of automaticity and emotional relevance. This is as yet a skimpily charted area in the examination of comprehension in aphasia despite the attention drawn to it by Jackson and Goldstein several decades ago, but there are some signs that it may be particularly relevant to global and Wernicke's aphasic patients, whose comprehension on formal tests appears to be minimal but who nevertheless function much better in everyday life than these test results would imply. Boller *et al.* (1979), for example, have shown that emotionally relevant phrases are understood better (or at least responded to more appropriately) than are neutral phrases, and Landis, Graves and Goodglass (1982) have reported that emotionally loaded words can be read aloud more easily than neutral words. Personally relevant questions are better understood by severely aphasic people than impersonal ones (Wallace and Canter, 1985), although this may be a function of greater familiarity. The fourth dimension which needs to be employed in assessing comprehension is that of the dynamics of processing language, both in the temporal aspects of language performance (such as attention, intermittency of perception, the use of working memory, the discrimination of temporal sequence), and in higher level processing limitations, which may consistently or sporadically mar the operations of language, such as the effect of reduced processing capacity on syntactic abilities.

In view of all these factors, the theoretical bias to which one is justified in resorting in assessing comprehension in aphasia depends on the purpose for which the assessment is undertaken. When there are so many potentially interacting and complex factors, and at this relatively early stage of development of knowledge of brain-language behaviour relationships, a stochastic approach is easily defended. I shall therefore use the motivation for assessment as the framework for this chapter in discussing the methods which have been used for assessing verbal comprehension.

Broadly speaking there are three motivations. Firstly, there may be a need to establish whether an individual person is aphasic or not. For the medical practitioner this may be the prime motivation. Secondly, the assessor's aim may be to obtain information about the behaviour in the clinic or in daily living of someone already diagnosed as aphasic and to use this information as a basis for selecting amongst the present range of techniques of intervention and management. This may be the speech therapist's main concern. Thirdly, all the disciplines associated with aphasia share a need to understand its nature and the cognitive bases of its behavioural phenomena as part of the development of psycholinguistic and neurolinguistic models. The pursuit of this aim advances on two fronts, the analysis of systems and the examination of control and access dynamics in the utilization of these systems. Built into this third motivation is also the desire to use such information-processing models as an improved rationale for therapy.

Aphasic or not Aphasic?

We shall not be concerned here with discussion of differential diagnosis between aphasia and disorders not clearly associated with focal brain damage which can sometimes resemble some varieties of fluent aphasias, i.e. dementia, schizophrenia and confused language. For such differential diagnosis other measures, medical, psychiatric, or analysis of spoken language, are more useful than measures of verbal comprehension, although preserved ability to perform a test of verbal comprehension can play a role (for reviews *see* Halpern, Darley and Brown, 1973; Chedru and Geschwind, 1972).

The decision as to whether a patient is aphasic or not depends upon the definition of aphasia as well as on the motivation for wishing to index an individual with a label. Most (but not all) definitions of aphasia necessarily include in it some impairment of verbal comprehension; the labelling of a patient as aphasic therefore implies not only impaired speech but also impaired comprehension.

Impaired verbal comprehension with retained oral speech, however, may also be classed as an aphasia. One such condition, 'word-deafness', will be discussed later. The second condition in which oral speech is unimpaired but verbal comprehension is affected, albeit more subtly than in word-deafness, is a result of non-dominant hemisphere damage and is described as 'non-aphasic'. The existence of this condition deserves some mention here because of its implications for the preparation of materials for assessing verbal comprehension after brain damage.

Non-aphasic right-brain-damaged patients show a number of subtle deficits in the apprehension of linguistic materials. These have been characterized as involving pragmatic, lexical-semantic, affective, prosodic and visuo-spatial abilities. For example, such patients have difficulty in integrating the elements of a story into a coherent narrative, and making appropriate inferences, although they retain the ability to remember isolated details and wordings (Wapner, Hamby and Gardner, 1981). They also show some impairment in rejecting antonyms which are not obvious opposites (e.g. accepting 'tie' as an antonym of 'win' rather than 'lose') (Gardner *et al.*, 1978). Lesser (1974) and Gainotti (1981) have described a selective semantic-lexical impairment of language comprehension in right hemisphere damaged patients. Impaired recognition of affect and emotional expression has also been reported (Gainotti, 1972; Tucker *et al.*, 1977; Tompkins and Flowers, 1985). Weintraub *et al.* (1981) and Ross (1981) have also identified in such patients disturbances in the recognition of prosody which relate to denotative meaning rather than to the emotional or connotative aspects of word meaning or sentence intonation. Disturbed visuo-spatial processing after right brain damage has also been invoked to account for deficits in comprehending some kinds of comparative sentences (Caramazza *et al.*, 1976). A test for verbal comprehension disorders which is to result in a diagnosis of aphasia, when this is not immediately evident in conversational speech, therefore needs to be as little contaminated as possible with variation in affective, visuo-spatial or prosodic elements and is more likely to be successful if it draws on syntactic rather than subtle lexical-semantic distinctions.

There are, of course, a number of general prescriptions (e.g. concerning standardization, reliability, validity) for the design of formal tests (Nunally,

1970) and some which particularly apply to the design of formal tests of aphasia (summarized by Porch, 1967; Benton, 1967; Spreen and Risser, 1981). But there are also requirements which are not so much those of a test battery as such but which are specifically relevant to the diagnosis of the presence of aphasia through a measure of verbal comprehension.

De Renzi and Vignolo (1962) list five features which a test should have if it is to be clinically useful in revealing minimal receptive disorders: it should be linguistically difficult and intellectually easy, be short so as not to exceed memory capacity at any (adult) age, and also not require special apparatus. The particular nature of material which is at one and the same time intellectually simple but linguistically difficult they define as 'lack of redundancy'. There should be no extra-linguistic cues for comprehension from the situation or from the nature of the objects used, nor should there be duplication of linguistic cues within the sentence, but each word should be indispensable.

Carroll (1972) comments that tests of verbal comprehension, as used in educational measurement, tend to be significantly correlated with intelligence tests, even those of a non-verbal nature such as a figure analogies test. He questions whether it is possible 'to distinguish "pure" comprehension of language tests from processes of inference, deduction and problem solving that often accompany the reception of language tests' (page 3). He cites evidence from Davis, however, that factors of a truly linguistic comprehension (i.e. lexical knowledge, grammatical knowledge and the ability to locate facts in paragraphs) can be experimentally distinguished from an inferential factor requiring the examiner to go beyond the data given. In the disordered adult, comprehension abilities are to be compared not with a standard obtained from developmental norms but with the adult's own pretraumatic abilities which are (except in some surgical cases) unknown. What one patient may have always found beyond his scope may represent a significant decrement for another person.

There are a number of factors which could have shaped the pretraumatic linguistic skills of the aphasic adult, and which may therefore be inextricably involved with his present abilities. Froeschels (1970) suggests that an important influence is 'ideational type', i.e. whether the patient was more developed in optic or acoustic or motor-kinaesthetic skills. The motor-kinaesthetic type, for example, would rely on slight lip movements when doing mental arithmetic, and would be more severely affected by an aphasia in which articulation difficulties were prominent. Educational level is another factor related to reading and also to facility with oral and aural language. But even at the same educational level, Day (1970) has suggested that some people operate more in terms of language than others: some are 'stimulus-bound', some 'language-bound'. Hunt, Lenneberg and Lewis (1975) have also shown that 'high-verbal' and 'low-verbal' students, all intelligent and presumed to be without brain-damage, are nevertheless consistently distinguishable by a range of cognitive tasks; for example, the high-verbal are more sensitive than the low-verbal to sequential order. Yet a deficit in serial processing has often been linked to aphasia, without control for pre-traumatic linguistic skills.

Cultural factors and local speech-community habits can also be reflected in scores on formal standard verbal comprehension tests and this sociolinguistic aspect of test use is often unwisely ignored. Identification of what is pathological and what is cultural in an individual patient is by no means obvious. For example, use of 'is' as a plural auxiliary may be a normal feature of the speech and comprehension of one community, but may also be a sign of a pathological reduction in a well-educated aphasic adult from that community.

A clinical test for the presence of an aphasic disorder of verbal comprehension must therefore be sensitive to all these caveats and accommodate the range of sociolinguistic communities and individual abilities in the language. Three of the tests which have attempted this are described below.

The oldest of these is Marie's 'Three paper test'. Marie's original 1906 version (Cole and Cole, 1971) went as follows:

> 'Of the three unequal pieces of paper placed on this table, you will give me the largest one, you will crumple the middle-sized one and throw it down, and, as to the smallest, you will put it in your pocket.'

Each version used by other clinics is slightly different (for example, in Paris the patient now has to 'give me the little one, put the middle-sized one on your knees, throw away the big one'). This short test clearly makes no claims to be standardized, and the presentation varies as much as the content. Its load on short-term auditory memory must vary according to the speed of the examiner's delivery and the opportunity the patient has to rehearse (or perform) the gestures required at the same time as he listens.

The 'hand-eye-ear tests' are the best known of a set of tests devised by Head (1926) to detect aphasia. Originally, they included a modality comparison: the patient was first asked to imitate gestures in which the left or right hand touched the left or right ear or eye, then to execute these actions by copying them from drawings, then to execute them from oral commands and from written commands and finally to write down the actions performed by the examiner. The ability to perform ipsilateral actions could be compared with that to perform crossed actions and with that to recognize left–right relationships on someone else's body. Rather than testing comprehension the tests may therefore measure spatial abilities and body awareness (Boller, 1979). Modifications of another of Head's tests, the 'coin-bowl' test in which patients were asked to follow oral and written instructions to place coins, have been used in examining comprehension in aphasia. Such tests, however, are more useful in exploring the type of aphasia than in detecting its presence.

A popular means of detecting aphasia and quantifying the severity of the disorder of auditory verbal comprehension is now the Token Test in its variety of versions. It was devised in Milan (De Renzi and Vignolo, 1962) with the express purpose of detecting receptive disorders in patients in whom comprehension appeared to be unimpaired on standard clinical testing, even when the investigation had been 'far more thorough than a routine clinical examination of aphasia'. It has been extremely successful in this respect; through this test, it has become clear that many patients with expressive disorders but without apparent disorders in comprehension do in fact have difficulty in understanding language, and it has stimulated research into the nature of these difficulties.

The aims of its designers were that it should not tax memory or intellect, but should contain considerable difficulties on a linguistic level. The linguistic difficulties should be attributable not to complexity of structure, nor to low-frequency words, but to lack of redundancy. It provides no extra-linguistic cues for comprehension from the situation or from the nature of the objects used. Comprehension of each word is required for success on the task.

The test's authors used a set of twenty tokens 'like those used in card games'. They were of two shapes (circles and rectangles) of five colours (red, green, blue, yellow, white) and two sizes. The examiner speaks a sentence and the patient indicates comprehension by picking up or moving one or two tokens (or sometimes by touching several) according to the instruction. The essential content of the first set of sentences is a colour and a shape word, and of the second a colour, a shape and a size word, in each case identifying a single token. The third and fourth parts double these contents, and in each case two tokens have, therefore, to be identified. For the fifth and final part the patient needs to decode syntactic structure and grammatical particles. Locative propositions, conditionals, relative conjunctions and adverbs are included, and the verb also varies significantly from 'pick up' or 'take' to 'put' or 'touch'. Sipos and Tägert (1972) recommended the use of only this last part of the test as being sufficient to reveal receptive disorders.

Research studies of versions of the Token Test are copious. They have confirmed that it satisfactorily distinguishes aphasic from non-aphasic with an accuracy of from 84% to 91% (Boller and Vignolo, 1966; Orgass and Poeck, 1966; Spellacy and Spreen, 1969; Swisher and Sarno, 1969; Van Dongen and Van Harskamp, 1972; Hartje, Kerschensteiner, Poeck and Orgass, 1973).

Some studies endorse the designers' claim that test performance is independent of intellectual ability (Orgass and Poeck, 1966; Boller and Vignolo, 1966), while others have found a significant correlation with intelligence scores in aphasic or control subjects (Van Dongen and Van

Harskamp, 1972). In adults the correlation with age is not significant (Orgass and Poeck, 1966; Swisher and Sarno, 1969) but the test discriminates different levels of ability with age in children (Orgass and Poeck, 1966; Whitaker and Noll, 1972; Noll and Lass, 1979). Token Test ratings have correlated with clinical ratings of overall severity (Orgass and Poeck, 1966; Swisher and Sarno, 1969) but not with functional ratings (Needham and Swisher, 1972).

Modifications which have been made are a change in terminology from 'rectangles' to 'squares' and from 'pick-up' to 'touch', and a random instead of ordered presentation of tokens. The test has been shortened to its sixteen most discriminating items (Spellacy and Spreen, 1969), to a selection of items from each part (Spreen and Benton, 1969) and to the final section only (Sipos and Tägert, 1972) which correlates at over .9 with the complete test. Less abstract versions have been tested (Kreindler, Gheorghita and Voinescu, 1971; Martino, Pizzamiglio and Razzano, 1976; Lohmann and Prescott, 1978; Lesser, 1979); these studies suggest that it is not the use of tokens as such which gives the test its sensitivity. Another substantial revision is that made by McNeil and Prescott's Revised Token Test (1978). This uses standardized materials and presentation, a balanced number of occurrences of each type of word (substituting the monosyllabic 'black' for 'yellow'), extensions of the last section and a 15-point qualitative scoring scale similar to that used in the Porch Index of Communicative Ability (Porch, 1967). The relative merits of pass–fail and of weighted scoring (one point per item correctly interpreted within a sentence) have also been investigated (Spellacy and Spreen, 1969).

In an attempt to redirect attention back to a commonly acceptable version of the test, its originator published normative data for a shortened 36-item 15 minute version, which diagnosed 93% of 200 aphasic subjects and 95% of 215 normal subjects correctly (De Renzi and Faglioni, 1978). The version uses black tokens instead of blue ones, to reduce colour discrimination difficulties. Pass–fail scoring for each sentence is used with a .5 score if a repetition is needed. Although this study found that the effect of age on test scores was negligible, there was a highly significant correlation with educational level and De Renzi suggests an adjustment of scores for years of schooling. The mid-score of this shortened test, 17, may be taken as the division line for the differentiation of non-fluent aphasic patients into the two categories of Broca's aphasia (with a score of 17 or more) and global aphasia (under 17).

Apart from severity, the type of aphasia, according to conventional classifications, seems to make little difference to scores. Non-fluent aphasics are no less impaired in comprehension as assessed by this test than are the fluent (Orgass and Poeck, 1966; Poeck, Kerschensteiner and Hartje, 1972; De Renzi and Faglioni, 1978), and they show a similar rank order of difficulty of items in the last section (Poeck, Orgass, Kerschensteiner and Hartje, 1974). The divorce of Token Test results from the particularities of a speech disorder is supported by evidence that people who are not overtly aphasic despite left brain damage make a significant number of errors on the test (Boller, 1968).

Slight impairment has been reported after right brain damage, but attributed to difficulties in visual scanning (Swisher and Sarno, 1969). Zaidel (1977, 1979) has used a technique for prolonging presentation of an image to one visual field to examine the different capacities on the Token Test of the right and the left hemispheres in split-brain and hemispherectomized patients. He concludes that the right hemisphere makes no specific contribution to normal Token Test performance.

Besides being incorporated into test batteries (e.g. the Neurosensory Center Comprehensive Examination for Aphasia, the Multilingual Aphasia Examination, and the Aachen Aphasia Test), the Token Test has been used in therapy as a training procedure to assist recovery of comprehension (Holland and Sonderman, 1974; West, 1973).

Just what qualities make this test difficult for aphasics has been the subject of discussion. Leischner (1974), criticizing its adoption in clinics as the prime means of assessing auditory comprehension, describes it as 'too polyvalent and artificial, influenced by attention, concentration, fatigue, difficulty in differentiation amongst similar tasks, optic gnostic disturbances' Nevertheless, at least four studies have attempted a qualitative analysis of errors on its last section based on the linguistic characteristics of the sentences (Whitaker and Noll, 1972; Poeck *et al.*, 1974; Noll and Randolph, 1978; Whitaker and Whitaker, 1979). Whitaker and Noll's analysis (of children's errors) relates the difficulty of items in the last section to the implicit cases associated with the different verbs used. For example, 'touch' is particularly difficult because the implicit instrument case ('with your hand') is negated in a sentence such as 'touch the red square with the green circle'. The difficulty of eight sentences can be attributed, they suggest, to this shift from an implicit to an overt instrumental case. Lesser (1976) has suggested that one problem in such qualitative interpretations of Token Test results is the loading this test has on short-term verbal and non-verbal memory.

This wealth of research attention has led to the use of the Token Test for purposes which extend beyond its original aim of detecting minimal receptive difficulties. One of its more extreme modifications is Peuser and Schriefers' (1980) Three-Figure-Test, which has a specific aim of differentiating the type of errors made into lexical and syntactic. The test, given in both an auditory and a reading version, uses 20 sets of four representations of a red circle paired with a blue square or a green triangle. The construction of the sentences is declarative rather than imperative, and varies between affirmative and negative, and active and passive, e.g. *Das grune Dreieck wird von dem roten Kreis nicht bedeckt* (The green triangle is not covered by the red circle). The patient's task is to select one of the four representations, the three incorrect ones showing omission of the negative, wrong shape or inversion of active–passive. This test presents some problems of ambiguity in an English translation, which makes a qualitative analysis of error type less reliable. For an examination of the quality of the disorder of verbal comprehension in aphasia (as distinct from its presence and its degree of severity), most examiners have therefore preferred to use a more flexible paradigm than that provided by the Token Test format.

Assessment for Diagnosis of Type of Aphasia and for Remediation

Observation of Behaviour

By its very nature the detection of receptive disabilities in people with apparently good verbal comprehension requires some structuring of the situation through a formal test format such as the Token Test provides. Clinical observation is not sufficient. When the purpose of the assessment, however, is diagnosis of the type or quality of aphasia, with management and remediation in mind, observation of the patient's communicative abilities in an informal situation forms a valuable part of the assessment procedure. We will return later to the question of quantifying functional communication, including comprehension, in daily living and outside a clinical setting. For the time being we will consider those aspects of the patient's behaviour from which the clinician may derive a preliminary estimate of his comprehension at a first meeting at the bedside or in a consulting room.

The clinician will observe facial and eye responses to greetings, gestures requesting repetition, or self-correctional or delaying strategies which indicate that the patient is aware of inaccuracies in his speech. McNeil and Kozminsky (1980) list five strategies used by patients to help their auditory comprehension, i.e. vocal or subvocal rehearsal of the stimulus, delay before replying, abnormally hurried response, request for a repetition and request for a cue. They report that of these the self-employed delay is the least useful tactic and that even the other strategies frequently fail. The patient's response to cuing (Goodglass and Stuss, 1979) can also be indicative of the level of disturbance of linguistic abilities, and consequently of comprehension. Lubinski, Duchan and Weitzner-Lin (1980) have offered a useful taxonomy for analysing communicative breakdowns in videotaped conversations between aphasic patient and a partner. Sparks (1979) suggests examination guidelines for the continuing assessment of a patient, both on first meeting and during therapy sessions; these are based on twenty aspects of behaviour which the clinician can observe or formally test. The guidelines which specifically concern comprehension relate to peripheral hearing, comprehension during conversation (including comprehension of gestural communication), variability of auditory comprehension which is not related to known degrees of difficulty, the effect of different methods of presenting auditory stimuli (e.g. the patient's dependency on lip-read support, or on slowness of presentation), the benefit derived from thematic organization of stimuli, the improvement in comprehension when attention to a stimulus is demanded and press of fluent speech is reduced, and evidence of self-criticism.

More structured methods of recording and quantifying communication, including auditory comprehension, will be described shortly in the section on Functional Comprehension.

In a different tradition are the sub-tests of auditory comprehension which are incorporated into many standard aphasia tests.

Sub-tests of Comprehension in Aphasia Batteries

Almost every battery of aphasia tests aimed at a comprehensive survey of the patient's language abilities includes sections examining auditory verbal comprehension and the understanding of written language. The motivations for these batteries are varied. Several aim at a brief assessment of abilities over a sample of behavioral tasks and describe themselves as screening tests. When they succeed in their aim for brevity they lend themselves to convenient test–retest comparisons in the assessment of the evolution of the aphasia and the evaluation of intervention. In as much as they try to answer relatively simple questions about the patient's behaviour (e.g. can he point to pictures by name? can he write short words to dictation?) they serve as an indication of the level of residual abilities rather than providing any direct inferences for therapy based on a specified model of language or of language dysfunction. In the absence of such a model it is difficult to examine their construct validity. Most, moreover, do not claim to be standardized, allowing the examiner some freedom with its inherent disadvantages as well as clinical attractions and are therefore untested for reliability.

Examples of such screening tests in English are: Halstead and Wepman's Screening for Aphasia (1949), Eisenson's Examining for Aphasia (1954), the Orzeck Aphasia Evaluation (1966), Russell, Neuringer and Goldstein's Aphasia Screening Test (1970), Emerick's Appraisal of Language Disturbance (1971), Sklar's Aphasia Scale (1973), Whurr's Aphasia Screening Test (1974), Keenan and Brassell's Aphasia Language Performance Scales (1975), shortened versions of Schuell's test by Thompson and Enderby (1979) and Powell, Bailey and Clark (1980), and Reitan's (1984) Aphasia Screening Test.

Besides these relatively brief screening tests, there is a number of more comprehensive clinical batteries which have gained currency in the English-speaking world, and whose theoretical bases have been more explicitly discussed. They may be broadly characterized into three types. Firstly, there are those which have developed within the tradition of making comparisons of performances in different combinations of input and output channels. These include the Language Modalities Test for Aphasia (Wepman and Jones, 1961), the Neurosensory Center Comprehensive Examination for Aphasia (Spreen and Benton, 1969), the Queensland University Aphasia and Language Test (Jordan and Tyrer, 1973) and the Multilingual Aphasia Examination (Benton and Hamsher, 1978).

Secondly, some batteries have been developed within the theory of aphasia as essentially homogeneous and distinguishable only by degrees of severity, although presenting as superficially disparate syndromes because of overlaid dysfunctions of visual, visuo-motor or sensorimotor processing. Batteries developed within this tradition aim at differential diagnosis according to the presence or absence of these additional dysfunctions; these batteries offer more direct implications for the appropriate therapeutic approach, generally recommending a stimulation technique for the aphasia component of the patient's disorder together with procedures aimed specifically at remedying the accompanying deficits. They are also direct in their concern for establishing the prognosis for recovery, and in particular in detecting those patients with an irreversible syndrome who will not recover functional language and for whom other forms of management than direct therapy are indicated. The two principal batteries within this category are the Minnesota Test for the Differential Diagnosis of Aphasia (MTDDA) (Schuell, 1965) and the Porch Index of Communicative Abilities (PICA) (Porch, 1967). Scores on the MTDDA are used to categorize the patient into one of five major or two minor categories, each of which is associated with a general prognosis and recommended treatment. The PICA has a more individualized approach. The percentile difference between the mean of the nine lowest subtest scores and the mean of the nine highest subtest scores is described as the 'High–Low Gap', a large gap indicating potential scope for improvement and a low gap the reverse.

The PICA is one of the few tests of aphasia which has attempted both adequate standardization and within-subtest homogeneity. It was innovatory in its incorporation of qualitative dimensions (efficiency, promptness, completeness, spontaneity of responsiveness, as well as the usual dimension of correctness) into a quantitative scoring scheme, statistical manipulations of which must consequently be used with discretion. It was also exceptional in not attempting to measure auditory or reading comprehension directly: it scores only through responses which are classified as verbal (i.e. oral), graphic or gestural, and makes inferences about comprehension through the pattern of scores. These may reflect a number of requests for a repetition of the instruction, or, within subtests, a slowness at grasping the nature of the task ('slow rise time') or rapid loss of attention with fatigue. Linebaugh (1979)

Table 1 **Sub-tests related to auditory verbal comprehension in some comprehensive batteries**

Auditory input	*LMTA*	*MTDDA*	*NCCEA*	*BDAE*	*MAE*	*WAB*	*LNNB*
Speech sounds		(in minimal pair words PP)					O IB W S-D
Letter names		PW	O (words)	PW	O (words)	PW W	
Number names	O W	O	O	PW	O	PW O W	W
Spelled words	O			O		O	O
Non-words			O				
Colour names			PO	PO	PO	PO	
Shape names			PO	PP	PO	PP	
Body part names				IB		IB	IB
Action names	W O	W	O (sentences) O	PP	O (spell) W		
Object and other names	W PP O PW	PP W PW O	O (sentences) PO O	PP O	O (spell) W PO	PO PP O W	PP O W
Modifiers (including left–right)			O	IB	O (spell) W	IB	IB
Series of object names		PP		PO		PO	IB W
Phrases		O		O	PP	O O	PP W
Declaratives	O PP PW	O W	O W		O	O	O
Imperatives		MO O W	O PO MO	MO IB	O PO MO	MO W	PP MO
Interrogatives		Y-N W		Y-N O	O	Y-N	O
Texts		Y-N O		Y-N			O

Non-verbal responses:

S-D	Signal same-different discrimination
MO	Move objects (or tokens or letters)
Y-N	Signal agreement or disagreement
PO	Point to objects or tokens
PP	Point to pictures
IB	Indicate or move body parts (other than as incidental to pointing)
PW	Point to written material

Table 1 (continued)

Verbal responses:

O	Oral response required
W	Written response required

LMTA:	WEPMAN, J.M. and JONES, L.V. *Language Modalities Test for Aphasia* (1961). Chicago: Education Industry Service
MTTDA:	SCHUELL, H. *Minnesota Test for the Differential Diagnosis of Aphasia* (1965). Minneapolis: University of Minnesota Press.
NCCEA:	SPREEN, O. and BENTON, A.L. *Neurosensory Center Comprehensive Examination for Aphasia* (1969). Victoria, Canada: University of Victoria.
BDAE:	GOODGLASS, H. and KAPLAN, E. Boston Diagnostic Aphasia Examination. In *The Assessment of Aphasia and Related Disorders* (1972, 1983). Philadelphia: Lea and Febiger.
MAE:	BENTON, A.L. and HAMSHER, K. *Multilingual Aphasia Examination* (1978). Iowa: University Hospitals.
WAB:	KERTESZ, A. *Western Aphasia Battery* (1980). London, Canada: University of Western Ontario.
LNNB:	GOLDEN, C.J., HEMMEKE, T.A. and PURISCH, A.D. *The Luria–Nebraska Neuropsychological Battery* (1980). Los Angeles: Western Psychological Services

comments also that the PICA is unique in ordering subtests according to decreasing task difficulty so as to minimize learning effects, whereas other tests begin with the easy tasks.

Based on the premise that aphasia represents a reduction in the processing efficiency of the brain, Porch (1986) has made suggestions as to how PICA scores can be interpreted as guidelines for therapy.

The third category of batteries is those which have as a prime aim the classification of patient into a syndrome which has a neuro-anatomical correlate. English-language batteries which comprise this third category are the Boston Diagnostic Aphasia Examination (BDAE) (Goodglass and Kaplan, 1972, 1983), the Western Aphasia Battery (WAB) (Kertesz, 1980), Luria's Neuropsychological Investigation (Christensen, 1974) and its standardized form the Luria-Nebraska Neuropsychological Battery (Golden, Hemmeke and Purisch, 1980). The three last batteries include measures of non-verbal abilities, and therefore provide a wider assessment of the sequelae of brain-damage other than aphasia. As a consequence, they also lend themselves to diagnosis of the presence of aphasia in individuals where this may be questioned, as well as to differential diagnosis within aphasia. Luria's batteries are unique in their systematic exploration derived from linguistic theory (i.e. amongst phonemic, lexical semantic, grammatical and pragmatic aspects of comprehension), although, as we shall describe in a later section, these dimensions have been used selectively by a number of later researchers as a basis for research measures into the nature of aphasia.

A summary of how these batteries examine auditory verbal comprehension is given in *Table 1*. It should be noted, however, that these batteries do not use the quality of disturbances of auditory comprehension to define aphasic syndromes, but only the degree of the disturbance (Poeck, 1983). For general reviews of the batteries see Sarno and Höök (1980), Spreen and Risser (1981), and Muller, Munro and Code (1981).

Functional Comprehension

The test batteries so far described examine verbal comprehension in a clinical rather than a more natural every-day setting. Yet studies of functional communication corroborate the frequent observations of therapists and relatives that there are significant differences between this and the results of formal clinical tests (Ulatowska, Macaluso-Haynes, Mendel-Richardson, 1976; Needham and Swisher, 1972). Assessment of functional comprehension therefore forms an important part of the investigation of the aphasic individual. Four measures have been published which attempt to cope with the difficulties of quantifying communicative competence in aphasia. The Functional Communication Profile (Taylor, 1965) uses ratings of 15 behaviours to describe the patient's 'understanding' and to describe his functional reading levels. The 15 comprehension behaviours range from awareness of gross environmental sounds, through understanding verbal directions to understanding rapid complex conversation. The 5-point scale ratings are based on the assessor's observation of the patient and from relatives' accounts. Although they are avowedly subjective, reasonably good inter-assessor reliability is reported.

A more recent assessment is Holland's (1980) measure of Communicative Abilities in Daily Living (CADL). Holland asks, amongst other questions, under what circumstances normal people are called upon to demonstrate that they comprehend communicative acts in the course of a day and attempts to reproduce these circumstances, through role playing. In one section, for example, the patient is asked to pretend he is in a doctor's office and is handed an appointment card and the building directory. He is then asked what floor he has to go to for the doctor's office, and how much time he will have to wait before the appointment is due. The scoring system on this assessment does not, of course, distinguish comprehension from other aspects of communication, but in the questionnaires to relatives and other observers of the patient which are used in association with CADL some questions are asked which bear directly on comprehension. The observer is asked, for example, if the patient requested a repetition of the message or that the speaker should slow down or that the message be written instead of spoken. The Edinburgh Functional Communication Profile (Skinner, Wirz and Thompson, 1984) attempts a more linguistically oriented quantification of communicative exchanges, and uses the speech-act categories of greeting, acknowledging, responding and requesting, together with propositional and problem-solving speech. It does not directly quantify auditory comprehension, although since the rating scales used are concerned with adequacy and appropriateness, this can be inferred.

'Appropriateness of the exchange' is the substance of Penn's (1985) Profile of Communicative Appropriateness (PCA). This assessment of pragmatic behaviour, designed for clinical description and prediction, includes sociolinguistic sensitivity (such as use of polite forms, self-correction, reference to the interlocutor) and responses which involve 'knowledge of the rules of discourse and an understanding of the speaker's intention with regard to a particular utterance' (p. 19).

Other investigators have also used case-history forms or questionnaires to relatives to obtain information as to functional comprehension (*see* Chapey, 1986). A possible weakness in such questionnaires, however, is the relative's interpretation of comprehension as including intellect and mental integrity with consequent denial of disturbance.

Apart from Luria's investigation, none of these test batteries or functional profiles has focussed on the attempt to distinguish different types of disorders within comprehension as distinct from comparing comprehension with production in order to classify the patient. Since the preparatory work was begun for even the most recent of the batteries, however, an increasing number of psycholinguistic research studies of aphasia has pointed towards the existence of components in comprehension which may be differently impaired in different types of aphasia. Consistent with the notion of aphasia as a central disturbance of language, it has been suggested that the forms of breakdown which can be distinguished in speech can also be distinguished in comprehension (i.e. as phonological, syntactic or lexical-semantic). *Table 1* offers a framework for such dissociations which will be elaborated in the next section. This is in sharp contrast to the differentiation of syndromes of aphasia according to contrasts of speech and comprehension, which has been the major alternative to the unitary concept of aphasia for the last century.

Psycholinguistic Assessment

Since the test batteries have not been derived from information-processing models, the assessment of individual patients against such criteria requires the use of specialized measures drawn from research studies or other tests. The present application of such measures is in testing hypotheses about an individual's level of breakdown in processing language and in using such case studies to support or modify the models. At the time of writing, various researchers are compiling and standardising batteries of assessment

Table 2. Components of language/processes in auditory comprehension which may be differentially impaired by brain damage.

Linguistic Level	*Some Psycholinguistic components distinguished and examined*
Sounds	Discrimination of seriation/ Rhythm/Pitch
	Phonemic categorical perception
	Phonemic categorial perception
Lexicon	Phonemic/Syllabic analysis
	Non-analytic mapping of sound to sense
	Semantic-associative relations
	Hierarchical relations
Grammar	Derivation
	Function words/Inflections
	Linear relations in surface structure
	Sentence parsing/Thematic roles
Prosody and Paralinguistics	Lexical stress
	Intonation and sentence stress
	Speaker identification/Voice quality
Discourse and language use	Illocutionary force/Use of humour and metaphor/Social appropriateness/Turn-taking etc.

materials based on psycholinguistic models, eg. Kay, Lesser and Coltheart (forthcoming).

In respect of the studies of normal subjects on which psycholinguistic models are based there are a number of current controversies concerning the structures, processes and dynamics of speech perception and auditory verbal comprehension. One is the question of how far comprehension proceeds in a top-down direction (with the hearer drawing on a store of linguistic knowledge to interpret messages in an approximate way in large meaningful chunks, which can be revised if they prove inappropriate), and how far it proceeds in a bottom-up direction, with small units decoded in order to build up larger ones (i.e. phonemes decoded before a word is understood, words decoded before a sentence is understood). Warren's (1970) demonstration that phonemes can be 'perceived' which have been deleted from a stimulus is evidence that at least some top-down processing takes place. Two other, not unrelated, questions are how far speech perception and comprehension are achieved in temporally ordered stages or operate in parallel, and to what extent such processes are interactive or independent.

For want of better guidance from psycholinguistic processing models, a number of assumptions have therefore to be made about the underlying linguistic and cognitive structures and processes when assessing aphasic patients. In turn data from such assessments can be illuminating in confirming or contradicting such models (despite the caveats required in using the behavioral output of a damaged and reorganized brain to make inferences about undamaged brains).

The assumption made in the psycholinguistic assessment of comprehension in aphasia is that some of the levels of description and elements used in linguistics have psychological validity as mental structures (see Table 2). Specifically distinctions are made between single lexical items, phrase-level relationships and sentence-level constructions. Several further distinctions are also made within each of these levels. Selective impairment of these mental processes by brain damage supports the claim in cognitive neuropsychology that the human brain has a modular organization.

In respect of lexical items semantic units (or 'lexemes' which are independent of any particular configuration as a word) may be conceptualized as being distinct from 'words' which have a configuration which can be realized as a phonological form. The phonological aspects of words can be further examined independently of word meaning e.g. in the same–different discrimination of phonemes, or in respect of the interface between sound and meaning, e.g. in the linking of a heard word with its referent. Yet a further distinction can be drawn between the phonemic aspects of phonology (the distinctive feature characterization of phonemes as a sound system and the rules for their combination) which are necessarily segmental, and the suprasegmental aspects of phonology. The placement of stress accent in polysyllabic words can distinguish, for example, *'conduct* as a noun and *con'duct* as a verb.

At the phrase and sentence level the distinctions which have been applied to the study of aphasia are less well psychologically motivated. It has seemed useful to preserve the distinction between phrase and sentence level, since there is some possibility that these may be differentially impaired (Saffran, Schwartz and Marin, 1980). Within phrase level relations in English most attention has been paid to the distinction between content words (nouns, verbs etc.) and function words, the latter group including ones in noun phrases (e.g. articles, pronouns), in verb phrases (e.g. auxiliary verbs including modals) and in adverbial phrases (e.g. locative prepositions). In some languages some of these phrase relationships are realized by inflections on content words rather than by separate function words, so it is assumed that grammatical inflections and function words serve the same psycholinguistic operation. The principal indices which have been used to show that constructions are operating at a sentence level, rather than at a phrase level, employ subject–object reversals, embedded clauses, passive transformations and wh-interrogatives.

The interface between syntax and lexical semantics in aphasia has also been studied through comprehension tasks, particularly in respect of how thematic rules can be extracted from verbs.

At the suprasentential level attempts have also been made to examine aphasic abilities in comprehending narrative and discourse. Speech act theory has been applied both to the grammatical use of prosody to distinguish interrogatives from affirmatives and to the context-dependent use of utterances as indirect requests. The influence of emotional relevance to the immediate context on comprehension has also been considered.

There is yet another aspect of the assessment of verbal comprehension in aphasia which it will be necessary to include in our survey of psycholinguistic methods. All the parameters of examination listed so far have been hypothetical structures and processes in the abstract rather than of their use 'on-line' i.e. their dynamic, temporal employment during acts of comprehension. To draw on a medical analogy, they have been concerned with the linguistic anatomy of the mental substrate of language rather than its linguistic physiology. The on-line dynamics of auditory verbal comprehension form a relatively uncharted area, but one of major importance to aphasia. It holds the key to the interpretation of a patient's errors of comprehension as due to impairment of structures and processing systems as such, or as due to problems in the on-line use of such systems. Our review of the assessment of comprehension will conclude with some comments about its dynamics and the evidence that can be obtained about this from the patient's capacity for learning.

Measures Using Single Items

Segmental phonological

It has been suggested that most patients with poor levels of auditory verbal comprehension on clinical batteries (Wernicke's aphasics, global aphasics, and the word-deaf) have some impairment of phonemic discrimination. The possible exceptions are those who suffer from transcortical sensory aphasia, a distinguishing characteristic of which is the ability to echo utterances. The degree to which poor phonemic discrimination, when it exists, may contribute to the comprehension deficit, and its importance to each syndrome, is disputed (Blumstein, 1981; Riedel, 1981). By analogy with the models proposed for reading processes, once the preliminary sensory analysis of the signal has been achieved, direct lexical access to words drawing on contextual information without their detailed serial phonological analysis may be the preferred route (Neisser, 1967). This claim has some support from computer systems which employ natural speech perception. HERESAY (Rumelhart, 1977), for example, showed how minimal an analysis of the acoustic waveform was necessary. It distinguished amongst only three types of signal: those with periods of constant frequency which it classified as vowels; those with high frequency noise which it classified as fricatives; and those with periods of silence which it classified as stop consonants. Using this minimal acoustic information it drew on the pragmatic likelihood of the instructions to be expected in a chess game.

There is also evidence from studes of dichotic listening (Wood, 1973) and the isolated right hemisphere in split-brain patients (Zaidel, 1978) that some capacity to understand words is available in the right hemisphere, which is presumed to process auditorily but not phonemically. In Wernicke's aphasia, following unilateral damage, errors of comprehension of high frequency words may therefore not be solely or even predominantly attributable to a disorder of phonological decoding. They may be the result of a slippage of a semantic-phonological interface (a mapping of the phonological lexicon on to the semantic lexicon) or of a more radical lexical-semantic impairment itself. Baker, Blumstein and Goodglass (1981) report that Wernicke's aphasics are disproportionately disadvantaged, in comparison with Broca's aphasics, on a task of phonological discrimination when the semantic load is increased. Confirmation, however, that phonological discrimination does indeed also play a role in such a task of matching words to pictures was obtained from the observation that both types of patients made more errors on discriminations involving only one distinctive feature than those involving two.

In the rare syndrome known as word-deafness, patients have a complete inability to make phonological discriminations and a profound disorder of auditory comprehension while retaining reading comprehension and well-articulated, meaningful speech. Such patients generally have bilateral brain damage and a history of sudden onset of deafness following cortical damage (Goldstein, 1974). Michel, Peronnet and Schott (1980) examined one such patient, found an absence of scalp recorded auditory evoked potentials, and suggested that for the words the patient was able to recognise auditorily after priming with reading he was using a Gestalt recognition of the amplitude shape of the speech sounds. Von Stockert (1982) describes a young man with word-deafness after brain damage through a gun-shot wound in an attempted suicide; his inability to comprehend single spoken words increased with the length of the word, but he benefited from lip-read information. Miceli (1982) found that the phonological disorder in a woman with gross impairment of comprehension of spoken language and meaningful sounds, but intact comprehension of written language, was limited to a disorder in the analysis of stop consonants. Specifically her problem appeared to be in processing the feature of place of articulation. It has been suggested that there are sub-types of Wernicke's aphasia (Hécaen, Dubois and Marcie, 1968; Goldblum and Albert, 1972; Riedel, 1981), some of them with a greater component of the phonological disorder, as in word-deafness, and some with a greater semantic or 'cognitive-associative' disturbance. Two studies (Varney and Benton, 1979, and Blumstein, Cooper, Zurif and Caramazza, 1977) have shown that a defect in the ability to discriminate phonemes may be relatively independent of the ability to link them with a lexical label.

For these reasons it is desirable for assessment of auditory verbal abilities, at the single item level, to include measures of phonological abilities which are independent of word meaning, as well as those which require meaning to be processed.

Under the first heading, and assuming that tapes of synthesized speech objectively controlled for voice onset time, etc. are not yet readily available in most clinics, the assessor may wish to use an auditory discrimination task of word pairs such as Wepman's (1958) or a test in which contrasts of distinctive features are more systematically balanced such as those devised by Naeser (1974), Blumstein, Baker and Goodglass (1977) and Shewan (1980a). Other measures which test phonological abilities independently of meaning (and which use knowledge of vowels as well as consonants) are to ask the patient to select from the alphabet those letters which rhyme with 'tea', and to ask him to pronounce (read aloud and/or repeat after the examiner) non-words.

To establish the relative severity of phonological or semantic disorder, results from such meaning-independent measures can be compared with those from tests in which the meaning of words must be used, e.g. tests in which heard words have to be matched with pictures. Typically the patient has to select from four choices the appropriate picture (Pizzamiglio and Massa, 1968; Goldman, Fristoe and Woodcock, 1970; Lesser, 1974; Naeser,

1974; Baker *et al.*, 1981). A useful format is that of Gainotti, Caltagirone and Ibba's (1975) Verbal Sound and Meaning test, which provides in its three incorrect choices one phonemically related, one semantically related and one unrelated. This allows the examiner to compare phonemically motivated and semantically motivated errors directly.

The ability of patients to evoke phonological sound images without speech may also be examined using a method devised by Peters and Zaidel (Zaidel, 1978). This test requires patients to match pictures that 'sound alike but mean different things'; for example, the four pictures shown might be drawings of a nail (metal), nail (finger), hammer and mail, i.e. the two extra pictures are semantic and phonological distractors. With one of the homophone illustrations omitted, the patient may also be asked to find pictures of words that rhyme.

The clinical assessment of comprehension abilities at the segmental phonological level might therefore include (1) a measure of same–different discrimination using pairs of words, distinguished by one or two distinctive features; (2) the selection of rhyming alphabet letters; (3) reading and repetition of non-words; (4) a picture-choice test with semantic and phonologically contrastive distractors; (5) a homophone test.

Suprasegmental phonological

An assessment can also be made of comprehension of the suprasegmental phonological feature of lexical stress. Blumstein and Goodglass (1972) devised a picture-choice test which contrasted 20 sets of words like 'greenhouse' and 'green house' or ''convict' and 'con'vict' where the placement of stress is a dominant factor in distinguishing meaning. This test has also been used by Weintraub, Mesulam and Kramer (1981) with non-aphasic right brain damaged subjects. The conclusion is that, though this and other aspects of the comprehension of prosody may be impaired by right brain damage, they are relatively spared by aphasia. Two other studies in different languages corroborate this, those of Mihailescu, Botez and Kreindler (1970) with Rumanian patients and Sasanuma, Tatsumi and Fujisaki's study of discrimination of word accent types in Japanese aphasic patients (quoted by Blumstein, 1981). Other aspects of prosody are more readily examined through the use of longer utterances than single words, and will be referred to later. Assessment of retention of the ability to use stress and intonational information in comprehension is particularly relevant to the management of the severely aphasic.

Lexical semantics

The simplest measure of the integrity of semantic fields in the patient's lexicon is to use a picture choice test, with target word and two or three distractors selected from word association norms (Pizzamiglio and Appicciafuoco, 1967; Lesser, 1974; Gainotti, Caltagirone, Miceli and Masullo, 1981; Bishop and Byng, 1984). Such a test may be given aurally and then presented for reading as a control for the centrality of the disorder. A measure of lexical–semantic integrity which does not require the use of pictures is to ask patients to sort printed words into those which are closely associated with a target word, those which are loosely associated and those which are unrelated. Dérouesné and Lecours (1972), Lesser (1978) and Fulton (1980) have used such a measure, using a forced choice with 12 words for each target word. It is notable that the above measures have also been used with right-brain-damaged subjects, who show a significant decrement below normal controls in such tasks although not in other verbal and non-verbal comprehension tests. The tasks may therefore be useful in detecting subclinical semantic–conceptual disorders in the right brain damaged.

Some other assessments of lexical–semantic discrimination are those devised by Zurif, Caramazza, Meyerson and Galvin (1974) and Grober, Perecman, Kellar and Brown (1980). Zurif and his colleagues asked patients to indicate which two out of three words were more closely associated, using all the possible triads out of a set of 12 printed words. These were selected for the contrast of human (mother, wife, cook, partner, knight, husband) versus non-human (shark, trout, dog, tiger, turtle, crocodile), of ferocious (shark, tiger, crocodile) versus neutral (dog, trout, turtle) and of distinction by presuppositional feature (male or female) or of distinction by residual features (married, activity performed).

The task devised by Grober and her colleagues was to present the patient with a target word labelling a category such as 'vehicle', 'furniture', 'tool', and to provide a series of 16 pictures or printed names for typical and atypical members of that category, similar members of a related category and unrelated words. Both Broca-type and Wernicke-type patients were able to reject unassociated words and to accept typical category members with a fair degree of success. Wernicke-type patients were, however, significantly worse on the words at the fuzzy boundary of the category, i.e. the atypical members and the members of related categories. Grober suggests that posterior aphasics do not distinguish between defining features and residual features in deciding on category membership. When a word has only the defining features (an atypical member) or only the residual features (a member of a related category), they are uncertain as to its classification. When it has both features (typical member) or neither (unrelated), classification is easier.

For patients who fail to comprehend some spoken or written names of objects Warrington (1981) describes methods of probing for partial knowledge of the words' meaning. For example, a mixed list of 20 object names and 20 animal names is presented, with the patient asked to decide whether each name is an animal or not; he is then asked, for each animal, whether it is a bird or not, following which the animal list is presented again for him to decide whether it is foreign or not, and then bigger than a cat or not. By this means it can be ascertained whether superordinate information is available to the patient, even though specific information is not. Warrington also draws attention to the possibility that comprehension of different semantic categories of words may be selectively impaired or preserved. She describes patients with selective impairment of concrete as opposed to abstract words (the reverse of the expected order of deficit) and with selective impairment of object names as opposed to names of living things, or of living things as opposed to object names. The patients were tested by being asked to define the words, if they were fluent speakers, or by being given a task of matching the spoken word with a picture, in the case of a severely aphasic woman. Warrington suggests that there are distinct neural substrates for different categories of words, reflecting for example whether they are organized in terms of physical properties and functions for the user (object names) or a hierarchical tree structure (living things) or on a continuum of meaning (abstract words).

Funnell (1982) has reported findings which suggest that a critical influence on verbal semantics in aphasics is the degree of independence a word has in its sensory representation. Independence reflects the degree to which a word evokes an image directly rather than through the mediation of another word (e.g. 'fur' would be rated low in independence since it is evoked in terms of 'cats', 'coats' etc. rather than directly). The tasks that Funnell used with four patients were reading aloud a word list, writing words to dictation and selecting words from a list to match a spoken word. For a semantic system operating with lowered efficiency words of high independence may be easier to retrieve than those which require the mediation of other semantic elements.

Other factors besides category membership and number of associates are known to influence word-retrieval and recognition, i.e. concreteness, imageability, word-length, operativity, emotional relevance, age of acquisition, part of speech and frequency (for a review of studies of these *see* Lesser, 1978). That aspect of lexical semantics which may be best described as 'Knowledge of the World' can be examined by means of a test such as the Pyramids and Palm Trees Test (Howard and Patterson, 1980). The patient is asked, for example, to choose between a palm tree and a pine tree when shown a picture of a pyramid. The examination of the relevance of part of speech will be discussed in the next section. Probably the most easily examined variable from the above list is word frequency, through a standard picture vocabulary test, such as the Peabody Picture Vocabulary Test (Dunn, 1965), the English Picture Vocabulary Test 3 (Brimer and Dunn, 1968), the Listening for Meaning Test (Brimer, 1981) or the British Picture Vocabulary Scales (Dunn, Dunn, Whetton and Pintillie, 1982). In the devising of verbal materials for assessment of aphasic patients a large number of variables need to be taken into consideration, such as frequency, the abstract-concrete dimension (or dimensions), category size and regularity of spelling. Lists of sources of such materials may be found in Brown (1976) and Lesser and Trewhitt (1982).

Measures Using Phrase Constructions

In this section we shall discuss abilities related to sensitivity to function words and grammatical inflections (which have also been termed grammatical or closed class items). These include determiners, articles, prepositions, verb particles, pronouns, auxiliary verbs and intensifiers, and constitute what it is difficult to think of as other than a psychologically heterogeneous group. The distinction between content and function words, however, is relevant in studying aphasia, since the speech of patients can be contrasted by their facility in the use of these respective classes.

It has been claimed (Bradley, Garrett and Zurif, 1980; Zurif, 1980; Berndt and Caramazza, 1981) that function words play a crucial role in the comprehension of sentences by permitting the assignment of class relationships to the content words and in this way providing the framework for recognition of the syntactic constituents of the sentence, such as noun phrase and adverbial phrase. Indeed our ability to assign sentence structure to 'jabberwocky' such as 'the slithy toves did gyre and gimble in the wabe' is evidence of this role. Zurif (1980) has proposed that there are therefore separate mental processes for retrieving function words and content words, and that Broca's aphasics have a disruption of the specialized mechanism for retrieving the former. His evidence is that, on a test of recognizing whether printed letter strings are real words, Broca's aphasics, unlike normal control subjects and other kinds of aphasics, are not slower in rejecting nonsense words which incorporate a content word than those which incorporate a function word (Bradley, Garrett and Zurif, 1980). That the Broca's aphasics recognize the inbuilt words of both types can be assumed from the fact that they are sensitive to the effect of their word frequency; they do not, however, appear to be less delayed by function words than by content words. The syntactic role of function words therefore appears to be impaired in them; such words are treated as if they were content words. It should be noted, however, that the soundness of this implication tests on the reliability of the evidence that normal subjects are affected by the frequency ratings of content words and not by the frequency ratings of function words in a lexical decision task; this evidence has been called into question by Gordon and Caramazza (1982) and by Kolk and Blomert (1985).

The extent of the role, however, which function words play in the surface structure parsing of sentences needs to be considered. It is more likely to be in the assignment of surface phrase structure as a preliminary to the assignment of subject-predicate constituents rather than as directly cuing these major constituents. Although a sentence such as 'The horse that was raced past the barn fell' is more quickly understood than 'The horse raced past the barn fell' (Bever, 1970) we can still assign its constituents to the latter without the function words which mark the embedded clause. Syntactic constituents can also be assigned to sentences which contain no function words, such as 'Deer ignore sheep', which can be unambiguously distinguished from 'Sheep ignore deer'. Moreover, although function words provide clues to phrase structure in 'The ball was kicked to the goalkeeper', 'The ball was kicked by the goalkeeper' and 'The ball was kicked by the goalpost', the surface phrase structure does not provide all the information needed for the assignment of sentence-level constituents.

Impairment of the recognition of function words does not necessarily compromise the ability to recognize syntactic constituents, therefore, and Saffran, Schwartz and Marin (1980) and Berndt (1987) have claimed that two distinctive deficits may occur in agrammatism. These concern respectively grammatical markers and sentence structure. It has also been suggested that comprehension of sentence structure may itself be differentially impaired, in respect of firstly, extraction of thematic roles at a functional level of representation and secondly, extraction of information derived from surface structure order at the positional level of representation (Lesser, 1987).

Noun phrases

Some of the research measures used to examine patients' sensitivity to function words do not lend themselves easily to a clinical assessment because they use reaction times (Swinney, Zurif and Cutler, 1980; Goodenough, Zurif and Weintraub, 1977). In respect to the use of articles in noun phrases, however, Goodenough's technique can be adapted to provide qualitative data. Sets of three figures are shown to the patient, such as a white circle, a black circle and a black square, and the patient's response is noted to the inappropriate instructions 'Touch the round one' and 'Touch a square one' or 'Touch the square one'. Agrammatic patients are predicted to respond to 'the' and 'a' phrases as if their meaning is the same.

Sensitivity to the indefinite article may also be examined by means of a picture-choice test in which the presence or absence of the article distinguishes a count or mass noun ('He's buying a lamb' versus 'He's buying lamb', or 'He needs a change' versus 'He needs change') (Lesser, unpublished observations).

If the patient is indeed insensitive to the role of function words, this will show in reading tasks as well as auditory. Again the method of triads may be used, this time in asking a patient to pair together two out of three words drawn from a sentence. Differential sensitivity to articles and to possessive pronouns in noun phrases has been shown by this method (Zurif, Green, Caramazza and Goodenough, 1976). Kolk (1978), however, has shown that some patients not only fail to recognize the links between article or pronoun and noun but also between adjective and noun; he compared triads drawn from sentences like 'This girl fed my kitten' with those from sentences like

'Rich people pay high taxes'. Use of such a method may therefore reveal in a patient a more radical disruption of the ability to interpret sentence structure which cannot be attributed to insensitivity to function words. A disadvantage in using the method of triads in clinical assessment is the number of presentations which are required for words from each sentence, i.e. ten presentations for a five word sentence. The patient's ability to understand the general meaning of the sentence and of the content items also needs to be confirmed, as well as understanding of the task. Kolk's paper describes in detail the technique to be used.

Three other techniques which have been used to examine patients' ability to understand pronouns are those of Whitaker (1971), Grober and Kellar (1981) and Blumstein, Goodglass, Statlender and Biber (1983). Whitaker presented a written passage describing an episode concerning a man and woman identified throughout by proper nouns. The patient was asked to substitute pronouns in the appropriate places. Grober and Kellar studied the influence of semantic factors on pronoun assignment in aphasia. They tested the influence of implied causality in the main verb of conjoined sentences, such as 'Bob scolded Tom because he was annoyed/Bob scolded Tom because he was annoying' (in which the assignment of 'he' to Bob or Tom is influenced by the meaning of 'scold'). The degree to which aphasics are sensitive to such influences can be assessed by giving them a picture choice of referents for the pronoun when they hear the sentence. This can also be used to detect the extent to which 'he' and 'she' can be distinguished.

Comprehension of reflexive pronouns was the object of Blumstein *et al.*'s (1983) study. Aphasic patients made more errors in assignment of the reflexive pronoun when there was a longer anaphoric gap, as in 'The boy watching the chef bandaged himself' compared with 'The boy watched the chef bandage himself'. This examines the anaphoric use of pronouns (their use in referring to an antecedent, often in an earlier sentence), and therefore is also relevant to the examination of patients' use of narrative and discourse, which we shall discuss later.

Discrimination of the dimensions of gender and plurality in pronouns is one of the elements examined in the picture choice test of syntactic comprehension devised by Parisi and Pizzamiglio (1970). Patients make very few errors on the discrimination of gender, and discrimination of plurality is also relatively well preserved (Lesser, 1974). Shewan (1976) using a four choice picture test of syntactic comprehension also noted that pronoun discriminations were relatively easy. Inclusion of such items in a test of comprehenaion may therefore be useful as an index of the patient's residual abilities and attention to the task. A test designed for children, which is being used increasingly to assess the ability of aphasics to understand syntactic elements, is Bishop's Test for the Reception of Grammar (TROG) (1982).

The possessive construction in noun phrases has also been used in the assessment of syntactic comprehension by asking patients to judge the referent for phrases like 'mother's brother' and 'father's sister'. Luria (1966) considers failure in such a task to be diagnostic of semantic aphasia. Such relational terms however, involve, in English, the ordering of the words and raise the question of how patients cope with serial organization, which we shall come back to later.

Prepositional phrases

Another discrimination which has been incorporated into these picture tests is between pairs of locative prepositions such as in 'The cat is jumping onto the wall', 'The cat is jumping from the wall'. Smith (1974) used a test of the comprehension of locative prepositions in which the patient was asked to arrange objects in specified positions to conform with instructions such as 'Put the coin in the bowl', or prepositions of time such as in 'Touch the cup after the ribbon'. The propositions which Smith used were *on, under, in, beside, with, and, or, by, from, before, after, over, in front of, behind, off, about, upside down* and *next to*, together with the qualifier *only*. She found that this test differentiated between patients who made errors on the choice of objects and those who failed to produce the correct relationships between the objects. A test presented in this way is difficult for many aphasic patients, and it is instructive to compare it with a somewhat different presentation used by Goodglass, Gleason and Hyde (1970) from which patients make fewer mistakes. With this the patients were shown sets of three pictures, illustrating, for example, a girl in front of a car, or behind a car or next to a car, and were asked to point to 'the girl behind the car'. As Smith points out, with such a task there is a movable figure with a fixed referent, and the patients could achieve the correct result by attending only to the position of the movable figure in the picture. Mack (1981) also noted that aphasic patients made fewer errors on a modified Token Test when asked to touch prearranged tokens than when asked to arrange them.

Seron and Deloche's (1981) experiment was a compromise between the two conditions. Here patients had to move one object with reference to a stationary one, and the prepositions tested were only the three, *in, on* and *under*. Seron and Deloche first used three pairs of toy objects so selected that each pair had a conceptual bias towards one of the prepositions, i.e. coin *in* a money box, soap *on* a hand basin, shoes *under* a bed. In a second experiment they replaced the movable objects with a small grey cube and the referents with small green wooden constructions designed to encourage *in, on* and *under* positions. The type of construction used was 'put the x in/on/under the y'. Broca's aphasics were more successful with the context biassed relationships than with the others, but the authors concluded that Wernicke's aphasics were not influenced by this factor.

Seron and Deloche's data suggest that, of these three prepositions, there were fewest errors with *in*. Picture-choice tests using a wider range of prepositions also suggest that prepositions are not equal in the comprehension problems they pose for some aphasics. Lesser (1974) found that three pairs of prepositions out of the eight tested accounted for the highest number of mistakes (*from/to*; *behind/beside*; *between/beside*), with others being considerably easier (*behind/in front of*; *in/outside*; *up/down*; *in/under*; *near/away from*). There are differences of length and of phonological distinctiveness in these types of prepositions as well as in transitivity and number of implied relationships (*between* necessarily implies three entities).

Understanding of these relational words is therefore clearly not an all-or-none affair in most patients. Differences of results with different presentations suggest that a critical factor may be the patient's ability to attend to more than one operation at a time. Despite failures with some kind of presentation, the patient may retain awareness of the concept of 'in-ness'. Indeed, failures of syntactic comprehension of other kinds in sentence decoding may also be due to limitations in the patient's on-line processing capacity rather than of his understanding of single elements (Friederici, 1982). Since a large number of items have to be used in binary choice tests, because of the 50% chance of random success, in assessing a patient's knowledge of prepositional relationships it may be preferable to begin with a task requiring movement of objects such as Seron and Deloche's, minimizing processing demands by keeping one element in the relationship fixed. Using instructions such as 'Draw a cross under the circle' or 'Put the key under the box' may of course involve the decoding of sentence structure as well as phrase structure if the topic of the sentence is not already given or presupposed from the context.

Verb phrases

Picture-choice tests have also been used to examine the patient's recognition of differences of meaning in auxiliary verbs, and in verb inflections, notably the plurality distinctions of *is/are* and the verb inflection *-s*. The modal *will* has also been examined as an indicator of future tense, together with inflectional endings signifying present and past tenses (Doktor and Taylor, 1969; Parisi and Pizzamiglio, 1970; Lesser, 1974). Pierce (1979) describes a sentence comprehension test using a choice of three vertically arranged photographs for 16 sentences each of the following types: negation, locative phrase using 'to', reversible passive, irregular past tense, regular past tense and future tense. Sensitivity to the extensive range of tense meanings which can be conveyed in the English language ('He will have been working there now for 20 years') has not yet been reported as being examined in aphasia.

Detection of syntactic deviances in utterances produced by the examiner is another technique which has been used in attempting to assess the patient's syntactic knowledge. Gardner, Denes and Zurif (1975) reported that the most difficult syntactic judgement for posterior patients was that concerning incorrect verb forms (*He giving the cat milk*). Grossman and Haberman (1982) asked both fluent and non-fluent aphasics to make judgements of the grammaticality of 152 sentences, 60% of which contained violations of agreement between pronoun and verb, e.g. 'I is reading a newspaper'. They used both simple sentence frames and those with passive or interrogative structures and report that the Broca's aphasics were influenced by the sentence structure and the fluent aphasics by type of pronoun–verb agreement (number and person agreement). Bliss, Tikofsky and Guilford's (1976) test of sensitivity to syntactic violations required patients to repeat agrammatic and grammatical sentences aloud; they had considerable difficulty in repeating sentences which included syntactic violations such as *Mary has changes them* or *Mary is hits me.*

Martin, Wasserman, Gilden, Gerstman and West (1975) have also used repetition to compare aphasic patients' difficulties with inflected words (e.g. *crossed*) with uninflected words ending in the same phonemic cluster (e.g. *breast*) or in a cluster which never occurs as an inflectional ending (e.g. *trump*). Since words with inflectional endings result in the most errors, Martin concludes that the aphasic's processing of the perceptual stimulus involves segmentation into the units of stem + inflection, which overloads the limited capacity processor more than the single stem items do. In a second experiment, Martin, Kornberg, Hoffnung and Gerstman (1978) varied the inflections used between the allomorphs of *-s* as the plural *-s* on nouns, and the verb inflection -s and *-d* indicating the present and past tense. They presented the words for repetition both in isolation and cued with a phrase context which disambiguated the inflection (*Three slaps, he slaps, he had slapped*). A control condition was also used in which the same words were converted into non-words by a change of vowel. The patients' sensitivity to the inflections was confirmed by the greater proportion of omissions of phonemes with the real inflected words in comparison with the non-words for which there was a higher incidence of substitution errors. For the words given a context the number of omission errors decreased, and there was an increase in the substitution of one inflection for another. Martin suggests that, assuming that omission errors are due to decay in short-term memory, and that the word is divided into its two units of stem and inflection, the presence of heightened expectancy from the context condition assists in the maintenance of the vulnerable second unit, the inflection. Martin's experiments can be used to justify the employment of repetition as a test of comprehension, since they support the belief that higher linguistic processess generally enter even into this limited task. A repetition task comparing contextualized and context-free words can therefore be a legitimate test of a patient's ability to process verb phrases, provided that his articulatory abilities permit this.

Measures Using Sentence Constructions

In understanding sentences one aspect of the process which is separable from the use of function words in parsing is word order. Although it has been claimed that aphasics are not deficient in this aspect of grammar (Goodglass, 1968), evidence has recently been accumulating to cause this to be questioned. The principal instruments used have been sentences in which the positioning of the indefinite article determines structure and sentences which remain plausible when subject and object are reversed.

Heilman and Scholes (1976) used a picture-pointing task in attempting to show that agrammatic aphasics fail to use the positioning of the definite article to disambiguate sentences. They read out to the patients a series of 20 sentences, the meaning of which it was claimed depended on detecting the positioning of *the* to distinguish indirect object and direct object, e.g. 'He showed his friend's lion the tracks' and 'He showed his friends the lion tracks'. For each sentence sets of four pictures were used, two illustrating the object contrasts and two, used as checks on the patient's ability to understand the content words, illustrating a different pair of sentences from the series, such as 'The man showed her boys the hats', 'The man showed her the boys' hats'. The verb 'showed' was used throughout, and the agent was always a man. Wernicke's aphasics performed at chance on this task. Broca's and conduction aphasics were able to reject the pictures using the incorrect content items but were impaired in selecting between the syntactic contrasts. The sentences were not presented from tape, and the researchers do not comment on the intonation, stress and juncture patterns which differentiate the two types of sentences, but the patients would not seem to have been able to benefit from such prosodic information to disambiguate the pairs of sentences. Two factors may have contributed to the confusion of the aphasics: the difference in plausibility between the two situations illustrated, in some cases, and the length of the seven-word sentences which may have exceeded the patient's verbal memory span. How much the disorder of syntactic comprehension which some agrammatic aphasics show is dependent on their reduced verbal memory span and how much on the limits of their syntactic processing will be discussed later.

A further means of examining the use of the position of the indefinite article to interpret sentence structure is illustrated by Caplan, Matthei and Gigley's (1981) experiment with gerundive constructions. For this they asked patients to manipulate toy figures to show the meaning of sentences of the following types: 'Can you show Bill walking the dog' (where *Bill* forms part of the direct object) 'Can you show Bill the walking dog' (where *the walking dog* is the direct object) and 'Can you show Bill the walking of the *dog*' (where the gerundive *walking* is the direct object and may be interpreted as an intransitive act in which the dog walks, or as a transitive act in which a third agent walks the dog). Although this experiment was conducted only with patients diagnosed as Broca's aphasics, it was found that they fell into two subgroups, four who utilized grammatical structures to differentiate amongst the sentences, and six who appeared to overgeneralize on the basis of the first type 'Bill walking the dog' — possibly applying a kernel Subject-Verb-Object strategy. It was noted that this latter group were all older than the other group.

An examination of how far patients rely on word order as indicative of subject–object relations and how far they attend to inflectional markers of these syntactic roles is possible in German, where the definite article accompanying subject and object can be distinguished as in the nominative or accusative case; word order can therefore be reversed without changing meaning (Von Stockert and Bader, 1976; Heeschen, 1980). Heeschen's picture choice test showed that Broca's aphasics tend to choose a more plausible situation in preference to a less plausible situation signalled by the inflectional cues (such as a recruit shouting at an officer).

A method of examining the integrity of syntactic knowledge, which avoids problems of auditory memory in examining word order, is to use a written Sentence Order Test. The principle suggested by Von Stockert (1972) is to compare the patient's ability to reconstitute short sentences which are segmented at phrase constituent boundaries with those which are segmented within the phrase and keep the boundaries intact. The segmented sentences can be written (in block capitals to avoid cuing the first word) on cards for the patient to arrange. Von Stockert suggests presenting the cards out of sequence and angled at 90 degrees. An example of the first type is THE/ GIRL FROM/LONDON IS/CLEVER, compared with a presentation THE GIRL/FROM LONDON/IS CLEVER. Von Stockert used simple declaratives (e.g. The young lady opened the door), sentences with embedded phrases (as in the example above), wh- questions (When did your father go?) and imperatives (Sing a song for your mother!). Kremin and Goldblum (1975) adapted this test, adding adverbial phrases, passives and negatives. These investigators also report a dissociation in some patients between the ability to order telegrammatic messages such as MOUSE EAT CHEESE and the sentences with function words. They interpret this as showing retention of semantic and syntactic abilities respectively.

The preference of Broca's aphasics for semantic information over syntactic information conveyed by word order has been shown in picture choice studies by Caramazza and Zurif (1976) and Deloche and Seron (1981). Caramazza and Zurif use centre-embedded sentences with strong semantic constraints (*The wagon that the horse is pulling is green*) or ones which were plausibly reversible (*The cat that the dog is biting is black*) or ones which were semantically implausible (*The dog that the man is biting is black*). Broca's aphasics performed at chance on the latter two types of sentences; they were as likely to choose a picture showing the reversed situation as the picture represented by the sentence. Deloche and Seron's picture choice test concentrated on simple declarative reversible sentences, but presented the sentences in written form. In this version also Broca's aphasics were found to prefer the pictures showing plausible situations, and to make significantly fewer correct choices when the sentences were equally plausible in either order. These authors also found that Wernicke's aphasics were helped when the left–right position of the figures in the picture corresponded to the left–right position of subject and object in the printed sentence; Broca's aphasics did not appear to use such a mapping strategy. The spatial position of the figures is of no assistance to aphasics when sentences are given auditorily (Lesser, unpublished data). Nevertheless, it would seem to be wise, in preparing assessment material, to control for this factor, so as to allow for comparisons of reading and auditory presentations in examining the strategies patients use.

Lesser (1974) noted in her version of Parisi and Pizzamiglio's (1970) picture test of syntactic comprehension that constructions which depended on the decoding of word order were the most difficult for aphasic patients. This finding was corroborated in a more detailed study in which the comprehension of sentences requiring the decoding of word order was compared with those in which order was not critical (Lesser, 1984), using both reading and listening as inputs and picture-choice, manipulation of objects, sentence arrangement and writing as responses. The auditory interpretation of 'word order' sentences resulted in proportionately more errors in the aphasic group in comparison with three control groups (non-brain damaged, right brain damaged, and 7–11 year old children) than did that of sentences in which the underlying subject–object relationships or 'thematic roles' are assigned by lexical information (as in *The doctor wonders what to take/advises what to take. The shop is keen to buy/cheap to buy. The lion is eager to kill/easy to kill*).

Schwartz, Saffran and Marin (1980) have also studied the problem of whether Broca's aphasics have a specific difficulty in understanding reversible sentences. They used both noun-phrase/verb/noun-phrase sentences (*The dancer applauds the clown. The square shoots the circle*) and ones including adverbial complements (*The square is above the circle*). The task was to make a choice from two pictures on listening to the sentence spoken twice. Two of their five subjects responded correctly to active sentences, but not to passives, which all subjects found difficult. Schwartz and her colleagues include the list of sentences they used in their paper; unfortunately it did not include any comparable assessment of the patients' ability to perform a picture-pointing task successfully when listening to sentences which do not depend on the correct decoding of word order.

A task which is frequently given to aphasic people is to ask them to respond to sentences in which an adverbial clause marks the temporal order of events, e.g. 'Before you touch the book, give me the pen'. Ansell and Flowers (1982a), using a Token Test type of array, have shown that the errors made by patients, who can understand the words 'before' and 'after' presented singly, do not indicate that they use a strategy of assuming that the order of mention coincides with the order of events. Since the majority of their errors are order errors it may be that such instructions overtax their working syntactic memory even though they can respond to the lexical information in the sentence, or to the syntactic information in the adverbials when presented in isolation. In a further study of these patients who had relatively preserved auditory comprehension, Ansell and Flowers (1982b), noted good comprehension of reversible sentences in which the order of mention coincided with the underlying actor-action-object relations (e.g. 'It was the woman that shot the man') in contrast to ones where the order of mention does not (e.g. 'It was the farmer that the painter kicked'). Such results suggest that word order can be processed in working memory if the syntactic relations are simple and that difficulties only arise when a more complex syntactic operation is required due to the clefting of the sentence moving the object to initial position.

Shewan's test of sentence comprehension (Shewan and Canter, 1971) is now commercially available (Shewan, 1980b), and this includes measures of the effect of syntactic complexity, sentence length and word frequency on comprehension. It does not include plausibly reversible sentences, and therefore cannot be used as a test of the patient's use of word order, but it provides a choice of four pictures for each sentence, and therefore can be relatively short (21 test items). The syntactic constructions which the test examines are active, passive, affirmative and negative sentences. Two of the sentences include contrasts of adjectives and three include contrasts of pronouns; the remaining error possibilities are in selection of pictures showing incorrect nouns or verbs or, in five cases, omitting a negative. The range of the test is therefore limited. A more comprehensive test, using a similar range of sentences as Parisi and Pizzamiglio's (1970) test, but with the advantage of a four picture choice, is under preparation by Naeser (personal communication).

It will be evident from the above that there is not only a paucity of available published material for the assessment of sentence-level comprehension, but that there are many areas yet to be explored in research studies against an uncertain theoretical background of the role played by syntactic decoding in comprehension. Investigation has been even more rudimentary of patients' comprehension of suprasentential structures in narrative and the use of anaphora.

Measures Using Narrative and Conversational Discourse

Ulatowska, Macaluso-Haynes and North (1981) have suggested that there is a dissociation between sentence-level and discourse-level competence in aphasia. The production of narrative discourse lends itself more easily to a structural analysis than does its comprehension and the examination of the comprehension of narrative has been predominantly of retention of its content rather than of the effect of its structure. It is therefore more relevant to an examination of verbal memory than linguistic competence, but what evidence there is so far supports Ulatowska's suggestion.

Waller and Darley (1978) have tested the effect of giving patients picture or verbal prompts to assist their recall of tape-recorded narratives, as evaluated through their answers to yes/no questions. The researchers comment on the surprising ability of the patients to comprehend the narratives even when less cohesive texts were used, with and without the prompts, and suggest that this shows the retention of basic inferential abilities in aphasia.

Kerschensteiner, Poeck, Huber and Stachowiak (1975) recommend using, for the narrative part of the assessment of auditory comprehension, short paragraphs consisting of six sentences about everyday situations. After the patient has heard the text he is asked a question, the answer to which can be given by pointing to one of five pictures showing different versions of the situation. An example of such a text (modified for English) is:

> 'Mr Butler works in an office. He has volunteered to do his colleagues' work during their holidays. But, after being ill himself for a week, Mr Butler cannot cope with the piles of files on his desk. He's got himself into a pretty kettle of fish. That's what comes of his ambition. Which picture shows the situation he is in?'

One of the incorrect pictures illustrates the literal interpretation of the idiomatic expression in the narrative, the other three showing an incorrect lexical item for agent, action or situation described in the key sentences of the narrative.

The research reported on this and similar measures of comprehension of narrative after brain-damage (reviewed by Foldi, Cicone and Gardner, 1983) suggests that it is right-brain-damaged patients rather than the left-brain-damaged aphasic who show an intrinsic impairment: 'Aphasic patients show a surprising ability to detect the sense of the passage, or the underlying message or effect that is intended' (p. 81). Such tests may therefore form a useful addition to a battery of comprehension measures, in helping to establish the relative integrity of 'right-hemisphere functions', influential on prognosis for recovery. They are as yet, however, at an early stage of development. Brookshire and Nicholas (1984), for example, have shown that it is fluent and mixed aphasic patients, rather than those with right brain damage, who are impaired on comprehending narrative paragraphs when this is tested by asking them questions about the main ideas or details of the stories.

Narrative is, of course, only one aspect of discourse. Another, perhaps more important, aspect for aphasia is conversation. The structure and processes of conversation, as relevant to children's acquisition and aphasic disorders respectively have been discussed by McTear (1985) and by Davis and Wilcox (1985) and Lesser and Milroy (1987). Penn's PCA for aphasic adults has already been referred to. Examining comprehension needs to be undertaken, not in isolation, but as part of conversational analysis in all its aspects including turn-taking, exchanges, content, coherence, repairs of communication failures and clarifications. Some selected aspects of conversational comprehension, however, will be discussed in the next section.

Measurement of Aspects of Language Use

Intonation and voice quality

The changes which have been occurring in linguistics over the last few years have sharpened an interest in the functional use of language, in contrast to its abstract structure and its propositional content (Lyons, 1981). The notion of illocutionary force is an extension of observations made by Austin (1962) concerning the performative nature of some utterances which are not so much declarative statements but are themselves acts, e.g. 'I promise to pay you £5', 'I now declare you man and wife'. This notion of the illocutionary force of utterances (as an addition to their locutionary force which was what had previously occupied linguistic theory) has in turn brought an emphasis on the context of utterances, leading to a theory of Speech Acts (Searle, 1969) in which the contextual interpretation of an utterance is more important than its logical content. For example, in saying 'That radiator is hot', the speaker may be making a complaint, giving a friend advice to sit elsewhere, asking a question etc. Most speech acts are culture-specific in that their interpretation is dictated by the social rules and conventions of politeness in the speaker's society, although it is assumed that speech acts in all cultures can be distinguished by their functions of making statements, asking questions and issuing commands. These are often distinct from their structural form of declarative, interrogative and imperative; 'Would you pass the salt', 'Can you open the door for me' are, typically, requests. Intonation, and tone of voice, as well as contextual expectancy, give information as to the illocutionary force of such utterances.

Most of the investigations of aphasic individuals outlined in the last few sections have been within an information-processing framework of language as a mental activity. This represents one advance from the examination of aphasia within the modality-focused approach which dominates the formal batteries. However, equally important is the development of the sociolinguistic examination of aphasia and its concern for the functional use of language as an important aspect of communication in social interaction. Indeed a consideration of some of the material used in the psycholinguistic studies (where for example 'The farmer kills the robber' is considered a reversible and *plausible* utterance) shows the need for maintaining contact with the natural use of language. Sentences such as 'The ball was kicked by John', 'This girl fed my kitten' may describe common situations, and be propositionally accurate, but are in fact highly unlikely to be uttered.

Some evidence points to the preservation of aphasic awareness of the illocutionary force of utterances, even in severely impaired aphasic patients (Boller and Green, 1972; Green and Boller, 1974); they respond differently to commands, yes/no questions and wh- questions ('Stand up'. 'Are you wearing a necktie?'. 'Where were you born?').

Lonie and Lesser (1983) examined this aspect of comprehension in global aphasics by testing whether they could distinguish between pairs of sentences spoken with intonation appropriate to a statement or a question ('He's coming tomorrow.' 'He's coming tomorrow?') or a question or a command ('Will you stop now?' 'Will you stop now!').

Severely aphasic patients perform worse when listening to tape recorded voices than to live voices (Green and Boller, 1974). The unfamiliarity of the task may have been one reason why aphasic patients had difficulty in judging whether the different intonation contours of a computer synthesized phrase 'See you soon' were declarative or interrogative in intent in Fink's (1969) study. Severely aphasic patients also seem to have some degree of impairment in relating the emotional tone of utterances to pictures showing angry, happy and sad facial expressions, but mildly impaired aphasics fare better than the right brain damaged nonaphasic (Schlanger, Schlanger and Gerstman, 1976). Feyereisen (cited by Riedel, 1981) reports that ability in such tasks correlates with the severity of the comprehension deficit in aphasia.

Assal, Buttet and Zanger (1978) found that left brain damaged patients (whether aphasic or not) were on the whole better than right brain damaged patients on a test of deciding whether two short sentences were uttered by the same speaker. The pairs of speakers were either men, women and children from the same geographical area or women from different countries, or women from the same geographical area. Assessment of an aphasic patient's ability to recognize voices is clearly of potential use in indicating the severity of the comprehension disorder.

Context

Voice quality and the illocutionary force of intonation contours are aspects of speech acts which draw on sufficient general paralinguistic knowledge to be examined out of specific contexts. The contextual use of speech acts, however, has been examined by Wilcox, Davis and Leonard (1978; Davis and Wilcox, 1985). They used utterances with the illocutionary force of requests, but with the syntactic forms 'Can you . . .', 'Will you . . .', 'Can't you . . .', Won't you . . .', e.g. 'Will you close the door?', 'Can't you answer the phone?'. Two people were videotaped in four settings, an office, a kitchen, a hallway and a living room during brief interactions where one of these utterances was used. The videotaped listener's response was either an appropriate action as requested, or the inappropriate production of 'yes', or some other activity. Only the severely impaired aphasics failed to recognize which was the appropriate response. Wilcox and her colleagues also examined in a similar way the patients' abilities to understand speech acts which imply negative requests, as in 'Must you tap the pencil?', 'Should you erase the board?'. When patients' scores on standard clinical tests of auditory comprehension were compared with their understanding of speech acts in context, no systematic relationship was found; success rate was much higher on the latter task. Now that videotape equipment is more readily available in clinics, Wilcox's method has become practical as part of an asessment procedure.

An aspect of auditory comprehension which may be significant is the emotional relevance of what is said. Boller, Cole, Vrtunski, Patterson and Kim (1979) compared patients' comprehension of sentences which had emotional content for the patient ('Are you an alcoholic?' 'What would you do if you won a million dollars?') with neutral ones ('Are you an American?', 'What would you do if you had a red notebook?'). The emotionally loaded sentences were subdivided into high and low emotional groups. The patients, who were all severely impaired, showed significantly better comprehension of the high emotional sentences than the neutral. Comprehension was assessed not only by whether the patient spoke a correct or appropriate answer, but also by whether he used relevant gestures or changed behaviour.

Observations concerning emotional relevance may offer some explanation for the dissociation between assessment on clinical examinations and on functional profiles which has been reported.

The Dynamics of Auditory Verbal Comprehension

Limitations of working memory, of discrimination and recall of sequence, of attention, of speed of processing, of ability to change set, and intermittency of perception and fatiguability, are some of the factors which have been invoked to account for problems of auditory verbal comprehension in aphasia. Obtaining an estimate of the extent to which the patient's abilities are influenced by such dynamics of processing is of relevance to theories of aphasia, since they may be evidence of effects of operational deficits rather than a loss of linguistic knowledge as such. (It is a moot point as to whether linguistic knowledge can be distinguished from linguistic processing, since this implies that mental structures can exist independently of their operation; but let us leave this question aside for the present purposes). An awareness of these limitations in the patient, and of the circumstances under which he performs most favourably is necessary for the planning of therapy. It is also of relevance to examine how far the limitations referred to above are specific to verbal material rather than visuo-performative material, and how far, within verbal material, the different modalities of reading and listening are impaired.

The comparison of memory for concatenated items of the same grammatical class with memory for syntactically organized strings of the same length provides an indication of how far the comprehension problems of a patient may be due to syntactic processing and how much to overloading of working memory. Lesser (1976) found that the majority of aphasics in her sample could point to more named items than they could successfully process items of information combined into the syntactic structure of a noun phrase. Albert (1976) and Lesser (1976) have described pointing span tests using common objects which can easily be employed in a clinic.

Another technique for examining the relationship between auditory working memory and syntactic comprehension has been used by Caramazza, Zurif and Gardner (1978). This probes for memory of words; patients listened to a sentence, were given a word from it and asked to recall (or recognize) the word that followed it. The seven-word sentences were varied for syntactic complexity (*Bob hit a ball to the boy. John holds the bike that is broken. The bike that John holds is broken.*) Errors when a function word had to be recalled to a content word prompt were significantly greater than in the reverse condition. In the experiment of Caramazza *et al.* there was no effect of syntactic complexity amongst the sentence types, and it would seem that seven word sentences may generally exceed the memory span of aphasic patients.

Using the objects from the Porch Index of Communicative Ability, Berry (1978) has proposed an exploration of auditory comprehension, the Advanced Auditory Battery, which includes pointing span as well as the carrying out of instructions which require the comprehension of sentence structure. Tompkins, Rau, Marshall, Lambrecht, Golper and Phillips (1980) studied Berry's battery and report that the aphasics' behaviour on the 3-item pointing span subtest was significantly impaired, though not on the two-item span. In the comprehension of sentences by normal subjects, span limit is not critical if information is recoded at a higher level. The degree to which some aphasic patients can make use of such higher level syntactic recoding may be examined by a comparison of their performance on these two types of tests.

In the light of the possibility already referred to that aphasic patients may have specific difficulties with the decoding of sequence, of words as well as of other units, pointing span needs to be investigated both with a free recall of items and with ordered recall. Berry's Advanced Auditory Battery promises therefore to be a useful tool in assessing comprehension.

A further measure of the limits of syntactic processing in Broca-type aphasics may be obtained by using a comparison suggested by Goodglass, Blumstein, Gleason, Hyde, Green and Statlender (1979). This is between the ability to comprehend an embedded sentence such as 'The man greeted by his wife was smoking a pipe' with its equivalent expressed as two concatenated clauses 'The man was greeted by his wife and he was smoking a pipe'. The test method used was a four-picture choice. The propositional content of each condition is the same, so that a memory deficit as such cannot account for improved performance of concatenated over embedded sentences, particularly as the former are longer.

Performance on tests of syntactic comprehension varies as a function of the amount of processing time allowed as well as the syntactic complexity (Lasky, Weidner and Johnson, 1976; Weidner and Lasky, 1976). In their three-picture choice test these investigators found that subjects showed greater comprehension of short active–affirmative, active–negative and passive–affirmative sentences when the sentences were spoken at slower than normal rate and when 1-second pauses were given at phrase boundaries (e.g. *The woman . . . is helped . . . by the man*). It has also been demonstrated that performance on Token Test instructions improves with increase of pause time between the sentences (Liles and Brookshire, 1975) and within the sentences (Fehst and Brookshire, 1980). It has been claimed that slower presentation can also assist the patient when the requirement is only to point to a single object by name and syntactic comprehension cannot be invoked (Salvatore and Davis, 1979). Baker and Goodglass (1979), however, found that it is only Wernicke's aphasics who require long decoding times for single words (c 650 ms compared with the 200 ms of Broca's aphasics) and Blumstein, Katz, Goodglass, Shrier and Dworetsky (1985) report that slowed speech helps only the decoding of syntax. In their 7-picture choice test of lexical matching, Gardner, Albert and Weintraub (1975) noted a dramatic facilitation in global aphasia when the word was inserted in a sentence which was spoken slowly at a rate of one word per second, even when this sentence provided no contextual information specific to the word (e.g. *cat* in 'You see a cat that is nice'). Katz (cited by Blumstein, 1981) reports that comprehension is not necessarily facilitated by increasing the duration of the words or the pauses between them, but by increasing the silent intervals of major syntactic breaks. Porch (1986) emphasises the need to consider processing dynamics in aphasia, and notes that PICA scores may be interpreted as showing 'Tuning-in' problems or 'tuning-out' problems which suggest that the patient 'lacks the ability to keep his system locked into the task or to handle cumulative noise that might build up during the task' (p. 296).

Reaction time measures need to be used with caution in examining aphasic comprehension, since responses are often so delayed that automatic mental processing becomes overlaid with deliberate strategies. Studies which have used such measures include those of Baker and Goodglass (1979) on recognition of object names, Milberg and Blumstein (1981) on semantic priming in a lexical decision task, and Tyler (1985, 1987) on real-time comprehension as examined by probes as agrammatic and other patients listened to sentences.

Measures of the ability to focus attention in aphasia have been described by, amongst others, Kreindler and Fradis (1978), Diggs and Basili (1978) and De Renzi and his colleagues. Kreindler and Fradis' nonverbal measure is to ask the patient to respond each time he hears a certain sound out of a series of sounds recorded on a tape. For example, he might be asked to listen for the sound of a barking dog or a bell repeated at different intervals in a series of other sounds. Aphasics are reported as making 14 times as many errors on such a test lasting 20 minutes, and omitting 6 times as many occurrences of the sounds. Using instructions from the Token Test, De Renzi, Faglioni and Previdi (1978) and Diggs and Basili (1978) showed that even mildly aphasic patients performed worse when the instructions had been recorded against a background of speech babble. Unlike normal control subjects their performance deteriorated more with such competing babble than with competing white noise, thus implicating a specific overloading of speech processing mechanisms rather than auditory threshold. Since, in everyday life, some auditory verbal comprehension often has to take place against competing babble, using similar measures of comprehension against distractors may help in quantifying functional communicatory abilities and in the counselling of relatives.

Ability to Learn

For the planning of intervention and management one of the most important aspects of the assessment of comprehension in aphasia is the investigation of the patient's ability to learn. This is important whether a didactic approach is used in therapy, or whether therapy is based on encouraging compensatory strategies or on the belief that verbal stimulation will release otherwise unavailable resources in the patient's language system. Whatever the theoretical basis for therapy the decision to use direct intervention rather than other forms of management and counselling implies a faith that the patient will show some ability to learn. Yet, as Spreen and Risser have pointed out (1981, p. 117) 'None of the existing assessment procedures provide a fully adequate opportunity to judge this capacity' for relearning language. These authors recommend the use of a brief series of items which can be presented to the patient to a specified criterion on one session, and the repetition of this procedure the following day so that learning can be measured by comparison of the number of trials to criterion then required. La Pointe's Base 10 system (1976) provides a useful format for such a procedure. The use of careful training procedures in responding can reveal unsuspected retention of comprehension in a severely handicapped patient (Deloche, Andreewsky and Desi, 1981). The patient described in this study was unable, before training, to point to pictures, objects or body parts upon oral requests, or to carry out simple commands such as 'close your eyes'. He was trained first to point to a calendar when he heard the name of a month. Then he learned to associate each finger on the experimenter's hand with a word from a five-word list, following which he had 75% success in showing recognition, by this method, of the odd word out in a list of five spoken words in which four were closely related (e.g. bonnet, helmet, cap, beret, bread).

A systematic procedure for assessing learning potential in severely affected aphasics, based on procedures used with educationally subnormal children, has been outlined by Horner and La Pointe (1979). The performance variables they suggest need to be included are: rate of learning (trials to criterion); stimulability (reactions to cues and prompts); response pattern (stability over time and across conditions); carry-over from clinic to home; and generalization to untrained items. Horner and La Pointe used five symbols selected from the Bliss symbolic system, whose referents the patient had to learn to say. The procedure was repeated over 14 days to assess learning potential. These researchers suggest (p. 109) that 'routine and periodic evaluation of learning potential through measurement of specified performance variables might have predictive value for an aphasic individual's responses to treatment and for eventual recovery. Description of "learning potential" of the aphasic person, particularly at the time of the initial evaluation, may eventually strengthen our prognostic statements and enhance treatment planning.'

Summary

The complexity of verbal comprehension has been emphasised in the earlier part of this chapter, together with the problems involved in its assessment. It is clear that tests of comprehension in formal batteries, though providing guidelines for further investigations, are not sufficient in themselves. It is also evident that the psycholinguistic investigations of comprehension which have been undertaken extensively over the last few years need to be continued into new areas, and that from them a resource of new assessment materials can be developed with practical clinical applications.

For example, in respect of the most studied aspect of verbal comprehension, the comprehension of single content words, psycholinguistic models now offer us an analysis for an individual patient's disorder in terms of selective disruptions amongst acoustic-phonemic analysis, the phonological lexicon and the semantic lexicon, the last being itself potentially distinguishable in respect of high and low-imagery words. The implications of an assessment using such a model with a Wernicke's aphasic who proves to have a modality specific impairment in comprehending low-imageability words may be that priming the semantic lexicon by the reading route can facilitate auditory comprehension (S. Franklin, personal communication).

The use of psycholinguistic measures is likely to continue to be eclectic and individualized, selecting from the standardised batteries which are being developed. Although there are many areas of psycholinguistic processing which have been barely explored, such studies will always need to be complemented by assessment of comprehension in language use. Developments in linguistic and sociolinguistic theory have applications in the investigation of comprehension, and are likely also to prove useful in examining aspects of paralinguistic and social use of language which may be preserved in aphasia. They have a value in the assessment of functional communication in both aphasic and non-aphasic patients. Finally an assessment of neurodynamics is pertinent to aphasia, not least for its potential for distinguishing verbal-specific processing difficulties from the more general consequences of brain damage; amongst these dynamics an important aspect is the individual's potential for learning so as to benefit from therapy procedures. Such factors underline the importance of regarding the assessment of verbal comprehension in aphasia not as an isolated task but as a part of a comprehensive neuropsychological and neurolinguistic examination in which behaviour can be related to the mental processes serving language, the functional and contextual use of language, the intactness of the patient's other cognitive and affective abilities and the compensatory and adaptive strategies which can be employed.

References

ALBERT, M.L. Short term memory and aphasia. *Brain and Language* (1976), **3**, 28–33.

ANSELL, B.J. and FLOWERS, C.R. Aphasic adults' understanding of complex adverbial sentences. *Brain and Language* (1982a), **15**, 82–91.

ANSELL, B.J. and FLOWERS, C.R. Aphasic adults' use of heuristic and structural linguistic cues for sentence analysis. *Brain and Language* (1982b), **16**, 61–72.

ASSAL, G., BUTTET, J. and ZANGER, E. Prosodic aspects in the reception of language. In Y. Lebrun and R. Hoops (eds.) *Problems of Aphasia* (1979). Lisse: Swets and Zeitlinger.

AUSTIN, J.L. *How to do Things with Words* (1962). Oxford: Clarendon.

BAKER, E., BLUMSTEIN, S.E. and GOODGLASS, H. Interaction between phonological and semantic factors in auditory comprehension. *Neuropsychologia* (1981), **19**, 1–16.

BAKER, E. and GOODGLASS, H. Time for auditory processing of object names by aphasics. *Brain and Language*, (1979), **8**, 355–366.

BENTON, A.L. Problems of test construction in the field of aphasia. *Cortex* (1967), **3**, 32–53.

BENTON, A.L. and HAMSHER, K. *Multilingual Aphasia Examination* (1978). Iowa City: Benton Laboratory of Neuropsychology.

BERNDT, R.S. Symptom co-occurrence and dissociation in the interpretation of aggramatism. In M. Coltheart, G. Sartori and J. Rob (eds.) *The Cognitive Neuropsychology of Language* (1987). London: Lawrence Erlbaum.

BERNDT, R.S. and CARAMAZZI, A. Syntactic aspects of aphasia. In M.T. Sarno (ed.) *Adult Aphasia* (1981). New York: Academic Press.

BERRY, W.R. Testing auditory comprehension in aphasia: a clinical alternative to the Token Test. In R. Brookshire (ed.) *Clinical Aphasiology* (1976). Minneapolis: BRK.

BEVER, T.G. The cognitive basis for linguistic structures. In J.R. Hayes (ed.) *Cognition and the Development of Language* (1970). New York: Wiley.

BISHOP, D.V.M. *Test for the Reception of Grammar* (1982). Department of Psychology, Manchester University.

BISHOP, D.V.M. and BYNG, S. Assessing semantic comprehension: methodological considerations and a new clinical test. *Cognitive Neuropsychology*. (1984), **1**, 233–244.

BLISS, L.S., TIKOFSKY, R.S. and GUILFORD, A.M. Aphasics' sentence repetition behaviour as a function of grammaticality. *Cortex* (1976), **12**, 113–121.

BLUMSTEIN, S.E. Phonological aspects of aphasia. In M.T. Sarno (ed.) *Adult Aphasia* (1981). New York: Academic Press.

BLUMSTEIN, S., BAKER, E. and GOODGLASS, H. Phonological factors in auditory comprehension in aphasia. *Neuropsychologia* (1977), **15**, 19–30.

BLUMSTEIN, S., COOPER, W., ZURIF, E. and CARAMAZZA, A. The perception and production of voice onset time in aphasia. *Neuropsychologia*, (1977), **15**, 371–383.

BLUMSTEIN, S. and GOODGLASS, H. The perception of stress as a semantic cue in aphasia. *Journal of Speech and Hearing Research* (1972), **15**, 800–806.

BLUMSTEIN, S., GOODGLASS, H. STATLENDER, S. and BIBER, C. Comprehension strategies determining reference in aphasia: a study of reflexivization. *Brain and Language* (1983), **18**, 115–127.

BLUMSTEIN, S., KATZ, B., GOODGLASS, H. SHRIER, R and DWORETSKY, B. The effects of slowed speech on auditory comprehension in aphasia. *Brain and Language* (1985), **24**, 246–265.

BOLLER, F. Comprehension disorders in aphasia: a historical review. *Brain and Language* (1978), **5**, 149–165.

BOLLER, F. Introduction: Testing for Comprehension: a short history of Comprehension Tests up to the Token Test. In F. Boller and M. Dennis (eds.) *Auditory Comprehension* (1979). New York: Academic Press

BOLLER, F., COLE, M., VRTUNSKI, B., PATTERSON, M. and KIM, Y. Paralinguistic aspects of auditory comprehension in aphasia. *Brain and Language* (1979), **7**, 164–174.

BOLLER, F. and GREEN, E. Comprehension in severe aphasics. *Cortex*, (1972), **8**, 382–394.

BOLLER, F., KIM, Y. and MACK, J.L. Auditory comprehension in aphasia. In H. Whitaker and H.A. Whitaker (eds.) *Studies in Neurolinguistics* Vol. 3 (1977). New York: Academic Press.

BOLLER, F. and VIGNOLO, L.A. Latent sensory aphasia in hemisphere damaged patients: an experimental study with the Token Test. *Brain* (1966), **89**, 815–830.

BRADLEY, D.C., GARRETT, M. and ZURIF, E.B. Syntactic deficits in Broca's aphasia. In B. Caplan (ed.) *Biological Studies of Mental Processes* (1980). Cambridge Mass.: MIT.

BRIMER, M.A. *The Listening for Meaning Test* (1981). Newnham, Glos: Education Evaluation Enterprises.

BRIMER, M.A. and DUNN, L.M. *English Picture Vocabulary Test* (1968) Bristol: Educational Evaluation Enterprises.

BROOKSHIRE, R.H. and NICHOLAS, L.E. Comprehension of directly and indirectly stated main ideas and details in discourse by brain-damaged and non-brain-damaged listeners. *Brain and Language* (1984), **21**, 21–36.

BROOKSHIRE, R.H. Auditory comprehension and aphasia. In D.F. Johns (ed.) *Clinical Management of Neurogenic Communication Disorders* (1978a). Boston: Little Brown.

BROOKSHIRE, R.H. A Token Test battery for testing auditory comprehension in brain-injured adults. *Brain and Language* (1978b), **6**, 149–157.

BROWN, A.S. Catalog of scaled verbal material. *Memory and Cognition* (1976), **4**, 1S–45S.

CAPLAN, D., MATTHEI, E. and GIGLEY, H. Comprehension of gerundive constructions by Broca's aphasics. *Brain and Language*, (1981), **13**, 145–160.

CARAMAZZA, A., GORDON, J., ZURIF, E.B. and DE LUCA, D. Right hemisphere damage and verbal problem solving behaviour. *Brain and Language* (1976), **3**, 41–46.

CARAMAZZA, A. and ZURIF, E.B. Dissociation of algorithmic and heuristic processes in language comprehension. *Brain and Language* (1976), **3**, 572–582.

CARAMAZZA, A., ZURIF, E.B. and GARDNER, H. Sentence memory in aphasia. *Neuropsychologia* (1978), **16**, 661–669.

CARROLL, J.B. Defining language comprehension: some speculations. In J.B. Carroll and R. Freedle (eds) *Language Comprehension and the Acquisition of Knowledge* (1972). Washington: Winston.

CHAPEY, R. The assessment of language disorders in adults. In R. Chapey (ed.) *Language Intervention Strategies in Adult aphasia* (2nd edn) (1986). Baltimore: Williams and Wilkins.

CHÉDRU, F. and GESCHWIND, N. Disorders of higher cortical functions in acute confusional states. *Cortex* (1972), **8**, 396–411.

CHRISTENSEN, A.L. *Luria's Neuropsychological Investigation* (1974). Copenhagen: Munksgaard.

COLE, M.F. and COLE, M. *Pierre Marie's Papers on Speech Disorders* (1971). New York: Hafner.

COLTHEART, M. Cognitive neuropsychology and the study of reading. In M. Posner and O, Marin (eds.) *Attention and Performance* XI (1985). Hillsdale: Lawrence Erlbaum.

DAVIS, G.A. *A Survey of Adult Aphasia* (1983). Englewood Cliffs, N.J.: Prentice-Hall.

DAVIS, G.A. and WILCOX, M.J. *Adult Aphasia Rehabilitation: Applied Pragmatics* (1985). Windsor: NFER-Nelson.

DAY, R. *Temporal order judgements in speech: are individuals language-bound or stimulus-bound?* (1970). Status Report in Speech Research, Haskins Lab.

DELOCHE, G., ANDREEWSKY, E. and DÉSI, M. Note: lexical meaning: a case report, some striking phenomena, theoretical implications. *Cortex* (1981), **17**, 147–152.

DELOCHE, G. and SERON, X. Sentence understanding and knowledge of the world: evidences from a sentence-picture matching task performed by aphasic patients. *Brain and Language* (1981), **14**, 57–69.

DE RENZI, E. and FAGLIONI, P. Normative data and screening power of a shortened version of the Token Test. *Cortex* (1978), **14**, 41–49.

DE RENZI, E., FAGLIONI, P. and PREVIDI, P. Increased susceptibility of aphasics to a distractor task in the recall of verbal commands. *Brain and Language* (1978), **6**, 14–21.

DE RENZI, E. and VIGNOLO, L.A. The Token Test: a sensitive test to detect receptive disturbances in aphasia. *Brain* (1962), **85**, 665–678.

DÉROUESNÉ, J. and LECOURS, A.R. Two tests for the study of semantic deficits in aphasia. *International Journal of Mental Health* (1972), **1**, 14–24.

DOKTOR, M. and TAYLOR, O.L. *A generative transformational analysis of syntactic comprehension in adult aphasics* (1969). Paper presented to ASHA Convention.

DUNN, L.M., DUNN, L.M., WHETTON, C. and PINTILLIE, D. *British Picture Vocabulary Scales* (1982). Windsor: NFER-Nelson.

EISENSON, J. *Examining for Aphasia* (1954). New York: Psychological Corporation.

EMERICK, L.L. *The Appraisal of Language Disturbance* (1971). Marquette: Northern Michigan University.

FEHST, C. and BROOKSHIRE, R. Aphasic subjects' use of within-sentence pause time in a sentence comprehension task. In R. Brookshire (ed.) *Clinical Aphasiology* (1980). Minneapolis: BRK.

FINK, R. *Experiments in the perception of intonation by aphasic and normal speakers of English*. PhD Thesis, University of Rochester.

FOLDI, N.S., CICONE, M. and GARDNER, H. Pragmatic aspects of communication in brain-damaged patients. In B.J. Segalowitz (ed.) *Language Functions and Brain Organization* (1983). New York: Academic Press.

FRIEDERICI, A.C. Syntactic and semantic processes in aphasic deficits: the availability of prepositions. *Brain and Language* (1982), **15** 249–258.

FROESCHELS, E. Observations on aphasia and ideational type. *Journal of Communication Disorders* (1970), **3**, 65–67.

FULTON, L. *A study of the semantic systems of aphasics* (1980). Undergraduate Dissertation, Department of Speech, University of Newcastle upon Tyne.

FUNNELL, E. *Sensory Semantics: one key to language processes and a basis for therapy*. Paper presented at Colloquium on Psycholinguistics and Language Pathology, University of Newcastle upon Tyne, November 1982.

GAINOTTI, G. Studies on the functional organization of the minor hemisphere. *International Journal of Mental Health* (1972), **3**, 78–82.

GAINOTTI, G., CALTAGIRONE, C. and IBBA, A. Semantic and phonemic aspects of auditory language comprehension in aphasia. *Linguistics* (1975), **154/5**, 15–29.

GAINOTTI, G., CALTAGIRONE, C., MICELI, G. and MASULLO, C. Selective semantic-lexical impairment of language comprehension in right-brain-damaged patients. *Brain and Language* (1981), **13**, 201–211.

GARDNER, H., ALBERT, M. and WEINTRAUB, S. Comprehending a word: the influence of speed and redundancy on auditory comprehension in aphasia. *Cortex* (1975), **11**, 155–162.

GARDNER, H., DENES, G. and ZURIF, E. Critical reading at the sentence level in aphasia. *Cortex* (1975), **11**, 60–72.

GARDNER, H., SILVERMAN, J., WAGNER, W. and ZURIF, E. The appreciation of antonymic contrasts in aphasia. *Brain and Language* (1978), **6**, 301–317.

GOLDBLUM, M.C. and ALBERT, M.L. Phonemic discrimination in sensory aphasia. *International Journal of Mental Health* (1972), **1**, 25–29.

GOLDEN, C.J., HEMMEKE, T.A. and PURISCH, A.D. *The Luria-Nebraska Neuropsychological Battery* (1980). Los Angeles: Western Psychological Services.

GOLDMAN, R., FRISTOE, M. and WOODCOCK, R.W. *Test of Auditory Discrimination* (1970). Circle Pines: American Guidance Service

GOLDSTEIN, M.V. Auditory agnosia for speech (pure word deafness): a historical review with current implications. *Brain and Language* (1974), **1**, 195–204.

GOODENOUGH, C., ZURIF, E. and WEINTRAUB, S. Aphasics' attention to grammatical morphemes. *Language and Speech* (1977), **20**, 11–19.

GOODGLASS, H. Studies on the grammar of aphasics. In S. Rosenberg and J.H. Koplin (eds) *Developments in Applied Psycholinguistics Research* (1968). New York: Macmillan.

GOODGLASS, H., BLUMSTEIN, S., GLEASON, J.B., HYDE, M., GREEN, E and STATLENDER, S. The effect of syntactic encoding on sentence comprehension in aphasia. *Brain and Language* (1979), **7**, 201–209.

GOODGLASS, H., GLEASON, J.B. and HYDE, M. Some dimensions of auditory language comprehension in aphasia. *Journal of Speech and Hearing Research* (1970), **13** 595–606.

GOODGLASS, H. and KAPLAN, E. *The Assessment of Aphasia and Related Disorders* (1972, 1983). Philadelphia: Lea and Febiger.

GOODGLASS, H. and STUSS, D.T. Naming to picture versus description in three aphasic subgroups. *Cortex* (1979), **15**, 199–211.

GORDON, B. and CARAMAZZA, A. Lexical decision for open- and closed-class words: failure to replicate differential frequency sensitivity. *Brain and Language* (1982), **15**, 143–160.

GREEN, E. and BOLLER, F. Features of auditory comprehension in severely impaired aphasics. *Cortex* (1976), **10**, 133–145.

GRICE, H.P. Logic and conversation. In P. Cole and J.L. Morgan (eds) *Syntax and Semantics, 3, Speech Acts* (1975). New York: Academic Press.

GROBER, E. and KELLAR, L. Semantic influences on pronoun assignment. *Applied Psycholinguistics* (1981), **2**, 253–268.

GROBER, E., PERECMAN, E., KELLAR, L. and BROWN, J.W. Lexical knowledge in anterior and posterior aphasics. *Brain and Language* (1980), **10**, 318–330.

GROSSMAN, M. and HABERMAN, S. Aphasics' selective deficits in appreciating grammatical agreements. *Brain and Language* (1982), **16**, 109–120.

HALPERN, H., DARLEY, F.L. and BROWN, J. Differential language and neurologic characteristics in cerebral involvement. *Journal of Speech and Hearing Disorders* (1973), **38**, 162–173.

HALSTEAD, W. and WEPMAN, J.M. Aphasia Screening Test. *Journal of Speech and Hearing Disorders* (1949), **14**, 9–15.

HARTJE, W., KERSCHENSTEINER, M., POECK, K. and ORGASS, B. Cross validation study on the Token Test. *Neuropsychologia* (1973), **11**, 119–121.

HEAD, H. *Aphasia and Kindred Disorders of Speech* Vols 1 and 2. (1926). London: Cambridge University Press.

HECAEN, N., DUBOIS, J. and MARCIE, P. La désorganisation de la réception des signes verbaux dans l'aphasie sensorielle. *Revue d'Acoustique* (1968), **3/4**, 287–305.

HEESCHEN, C. Strategies of decoding actor-object-relations by aphasic patients. *Cortex* (1980), **16**, 5–19.

HEILMAN, K.M. and SCHOLES, R.J. The nature of comprehension errors in Broca's, Conduction and Wernicke's aphasics. *Cortex* (1976), **12**, 258–265.

HEILMAN, K.M., SCHOLES, R. and WATSON, R.J. Auditory affective agnosia: disturbed comprehension of affective speech. *Journal of Neurology, Neurosurgery and Psychiatry* (1975), **38**, 69–72.

HOLLAND, A. *Communicative Abilities in Daily Living* (1980). Baltimore: University Park Press.

HOLLAND, A.L. and SONDERMAN, J.C. Effects of a program based on the Token Test for teaching comprehension skills to aphasics. *Journal of Speech and Hearing Research* (1974), **17**, 589–598.

HORNER, J. and LA POINTE, L.L. Evaluation of learning potential of a severe aphasic adult through analysis of five performance variables using novel pictorial stimuli. In R. Brookshire (ed.) *Clinical Aphasiology* (1979). Minneapolis: BRK.

HOWARD, D. and PATTERSON, K. Pyramids and Palm Trees Test (1980). Unpublished observations.

HUNT, E., LENNEBERG, C. and LEWIS, J. What does it mean to be high verbal? *Cognitive Psychology* (1975), **7**, 194–227.

JORDAN, J.M. and TYRER, J.H. Standardisation of the Queensland University Aphasia and Language Test 'QUALT). *British Journal of Communication Disorders* (1973), **8**, 105–115.

KAY, J. LESSER, R. and COLTHEART, M. The Psycholinguistic Assessment of Language in Aphasia (forthcoming). London: Lawrence Erlbaum.

KEENAN, J.S. and BRASSELL, E.G. *Aphasia Language and Performance Scales* (1975). Murfressboro: Pinnacle Press.

KERSCHENSTEINER, M., POECK, K., HUBER, W. and STACHOWIAK, F.J. Die Untersuchung auf Aphasie. *Acta Neurologica* (1975), **2**, 151–157.

KERTESZ, A. *The Western Aphasia Battery* (1980). London, Canada: University of Western Ontario.

KOLK, H.H.J. Judgement of sentence structure in Broca's aphasia. *Neuropsychologia* (1978), **16**, 617–625.

KOLK, H.H.J. and BLOMERT, L. On the Bradley hypothesis concerning agrammatism:

the non-word interference effect. *Brain and Language* (1985), **26**, 94–105.

KREINDLER, A. and FRADIS, A. *Performances in Aphasia* (1971). Paris: Gauthier-Villers.

KREINDLER, A., GHEORGHITA, N. and VOINESCU, I. Analysis of verbal reception of complex order with three elements in aphasics. *Brain* (1971), **92**, 375–386.

KREMIN, H. and GOLDBLUM, M.C. Étude de la compréhension syntaxique chez les aphasiques. *Linguistics* (1975), **154/5**, 31–46.

LANDIS, T., GRAVES, R. and GOODGLASS, H. Aphasic reading and writing: possible evidence for right hemisphere participation. *Cortex* (1982), **18**, 105-112.

LAPOINTE, L.L. Aphasia therapy: some principles and strategies for treatment. In D.F. Johns (ed.) *Clinical Management of Neurogenic Communicative Disorders* (1978). Boston: Little Brown.

LASKY, E.Z., WEIDNER, W.E. and JOHNSON, J.P. Influence of linguistic complexity, rate of presentation and interphrase pause time on auditory verbal comprehension of adult aphasic patients. *Brain and Language* (1976), **3**, 386–395.

LEISCHNER, A. Die neuropsychologisch-hirnpathologische Untersuchung. *Archives Psychiatrica Nervenkranze* (1974), **219**, 53–77.

LENNEBERG, E., POGASH, K., COHLAN, A. and DOOLITTLE, J. Comprehension deficit in acquired aphasia and the question of its relationship to language acquisition. In A. Caramazza and E. Zurif (eds.) *Language Acquisition and Language Breakdown*. Baltimore: Johns Hopkins.

LESSER, R. Verbal comprehension in aphasia: an English version of three Italian Tests. *Cortex*, (1974), **10**, 247–263.

LESSER, R. Verbal and non-verbal memory components in the Token Test. *Neuropsychologia* (1976), **14**, 79–85.

LESSER, R. *Linguistic Investigations of Aphasia* (1978). London: Edward Arnold.

LESSER, R. Turning tokens into things: linguistic and mnestic aspects of the initial sections of the Token Test. In F. Boller and M. Dennis (eds.) *Auditory Comprehension: Clinical and Experimental Studies with the Token Test* (1979). New York: Academic Press.

LESSER, R. Sentence comprehension and production in aphasia: an application of lexical grammar. In F.C. Rose (ed.) *Advances in Neurology, Vol. 42, Progress in Aphasiology* (1984). New York: Raven Press.

LESSER, R. Cognitive neuropsychological influences on Aphasia Therapy. *Aphasiology* (1987). **1**.

LESSER, R. and MILROY, L. Two frontiers in aphasia therapy. Bulletin of the College of Speech Therapists (1987), **420**, 1-4.

LESSER, R. and TREWHITT, P. *An annotated Bibliography of Verbal Materials: for use in psycholinguistic and neurolinguistic experimentation* (1982). Newcastle upon Tyne: Grevatt and Grevatt.

LILES, B.Z. and BROOKSHIRE, R.H. The effects of pause time on auditory comprehension by aphasic subjects. *Journal of Communication Disorders* (1975), **8**, 221–235.

LINEBAUGH, C.W. Assessing the assessments: the adequacy of standardised tests of aphasia. In R. Brookshire (ed.) *Clinical Aphasiology* (1979). Minneapolis: BRK.

LOHMANN, L. and PRESCOTT, T.E. The effects of substituting 'objects' for 'forms' on the Revised Token Test: performance of aphasic adults. In R. Brookshire (ed.) *Clinical Aphasiology* (1978). Minneapolis: BRK.

LONIE, J. and LESSER, R. Intonation as a clue to speech act identification in aphasic and other brain-damaged people. *International Journal of Rehabilitation Research* (1983), **6**, 512–513.

LUBINSKI, R., DUCHAN, J. and WEITZNER-LIN, B. Analysis of breakdowns and repairs in aphasic adult communication. In R. Brookshire (ed.) *Clinical Aphasiology* (1980). Minneapolis: BRK.

LURIA, A.R. *Higher Cortical Functions in Man* (1966). New York: Basic Books.

MCNEIL, M.R. and KOZMINSKY, L. The efficacy of five self-generated strategies for facilitating auditory processing. In R. Brookshire (ed.) *Clinical Aphasiology* (1980). Minneapolis: BRK.

MCNEIL, M.R. and PRESCOTT, T.E. *Revised Token Test* (1978). Baltimore: University Park Press.

MCTEAR, M. *Children's Conversation* (1985). London: Blackwell.

MARTIN, A.D., KORNBERG, S., HOFFNUNG, A. and GERSTMAN, L. The effect of grammatic context on repetition by aphasic adults. In R. Brookshire (ed.) *Clinical Aphasiology* (1978). Minneapolis: BRK.

MARTIN, A.D., WASSERMAN, N., GILDEN, L., GERSTMAN, L. and WEST, J.A. A process model of repetition in aphasia. *Brain and Language* (1975), **2**, 434–450.

MARTINO, A.A., PIZZAMIGLIO, L. and RAZZANO, C. A new version of the Token Test for aphasics: a concrete objects form. *Journal of Communication Disorders* (1976), 91–95.

MICELI, G. The processing of speech sounds in a patient with cortical auditory disorder. *Neuropsychologia* (1982), **20**, 5–20.

MICHEL, F., PERONNET, F. and SCHOTT, B. A case of cortical deafness: clinical and electrophysiological data. *Brain and Language* (1980), **10**, 367–377.

MIHAELESCU, L., BOTEZ, M.I. and KREINDLER, A. Decoding of correct and wrong word stress in aphasic patients. *Revue Roumaine de Neurologie* (1970), **7**, 65–74.

MILBERG, W. and BLUMSTEIN, S.E. Lexical decision and aphasia: evidence for semantic processing. *Brain and Language* (1981), **14**, 371–385.

MULLER, D.J., MUNRO, S.M. and CODE, C. *Language Assessment for Remediation* (1981). London: Croom Helm.

NAESER, M.A. *The relationship between phoneme discrimintion, phoneme picture perception and language comprehension in aphasia* (1974). Paper presented to Academy of Aphasia.

NEEDHAM, E.C. and SWISHER, L.P. A comparison of three tests of auditory comprehension for adult aphasics. *Journal of Speech and Hearing Disorders* (1972), **37**, 123–131.

NEISSER, V. *Cognitive Psychology* (1967). New York: Appleton-Century-Crofts.

NOLL, J.D. and LASS, N.J. Use of the Token Test with children: two contrasting socioeconomic groups. In F. Boller and M. Dennis (eds.) *Auditory Comprehension: Clinical and Experimental Studies with the Token Test* (1979). New York: Academic Press.

NOLL, J.D. and RANDOLPH, S.R. Auditory semantic, syntactic and retention errors made by aphasic subjects on the Token Test. *Journal of Communication Disorders* (1978), **11** 543–553.

NUNALLY, J.C. *Psychometric Theory* (1967). New York: McGraw-Hill.

ORGASS, B. and POECK, K. Clinical validation of a new test for aphasia. *Cortex* (1966), **2** 222–243.

ORZECK, A.Z. *The Orzeck Aphasia Evaluation* (1966). Los Angeles: Western Psychological Services.

PARISI, D. and PIZZAMIGLIO, L. Syntactic comprehension in aphasia. *Cortex* (1970), **2**, 204–215.

PENN, C. Profile of Communicative Appropriateness: a clinical test for the assessment of pragmatics.. *South African Journal of Communication Disorders* (1985), **32**, 18–23.

PEUSER, G. and SCHRIEFERS, H. Sentence comprehension in aphasics: results of administration of the 'Three-Figures Test' (TFT). *British Journal of Disorders of Communication* (1980), **15**, 157–164.

PIERCE, R.S. A study of sentence comprehension of aphasic subjects. In R.H. Brookshire (ed.) *Clinical Aphasiology* (1979). Minneapolis: BRK.

PIERCE, R.S. and BEEKMAN, L.A. Effects of linguistic and extralinguistic context on semantic and syntactic processing in aphasia. *Journal of Speech and Hearing Research* (1985), **28**, 250–254.

PIZZAMIGLIO, L. and APPICCIAFUOCO, A. Semantic comprehension in aphasia. *Journal of Communication Disorders* (1971), **3**, 280–288.

PIZZAMIGLIO, L. and MASSA, A. Versione italiano di un test di intelligibilità multipla. *Rivista di Psicologia* (1968), **62**, 137–147.

POECK, K. What do we mean by 'aphasic syndromes'? A neurologist's view. *Brain and Language* (1983), **20**, 79–89.

POECK, K., KERSCHENSTEINER,M. and HARTJE, W.A quantitative study on language understanding in fluent and non-fluent aphasia. *Cortex* (1972), **8**, 299–304.

POECK, K., ORGASS, B., KERSCHENSTEINER, M. and HARTJE, W. A qualitative study on Token Test performance in aphasic and non-aphasic brain damaged patients. *Neuropsychologia*, (1974), **12**, 49–54.

PORCH, B.E. Therapy subsequent to the Porch Index of Communicative Ability (PICA). In R. Chapey (ed.) *Language Intervention Strategies in Adult Aphasia* (1986). Baltimore: Williams and Wilkins.

POWELL, G.E., BAILEY, S. and CLARK, E. A very short form of the Minnesota Aphasia Test. *British Journal of Social and Clinical Psychology* (1980), **19**, 189–194.

REITAN, R.M. Reitan — Indiana Aphasia Kit for Adults (1984). Tucson, AZ: Neuropsychology Press.

RIEDEL, K. Auditory comprehension in aphasia. In M.T. Sarno (ed.) *Adult Aphasia* (1981). New York: Academic Press.

ROSS, E.D. The aprosodias: functional-anatomic organisation of the affective components of language in the right hemisphere. *Archives of Neurology* (1981), **38**, 561–569.

RUMELHART, D.E. *Introduction to Human Information Processing* (1977). New York: Wiley.

RUSSELL, E.W., NEURINGER, C. and GOLDSTEIN, G. *Assessment of Brain Damage: a Neuropsychological Key Approach* (1970). New York: Wiley.

SAFFRAN, E.M., SCHWARTZ, M.J. and MARIN, O.S.M. Evidence from aphasia: isolating the components of a production model. In B. Butterworth (ed.) *Language Production* (1980). New York: Academic Press.

SALVATORE, A.P. and DAVIS, K.D. Clinical treatment of auditory comprehension deficits in acute and chronic aphasic adults: an experimental analysis of within-message pause duration. In R. Brookshire (ed.) *Clinical Aphasiology* (1979). Minneapolis: BRK.

SARNO, M.T. and HÖÖK, O. *Aphasia: Assessment and Treatment* (1980). Stockholm: Almqvist and Wiksell.

SCHIENBERG, S. and HOLLAND, A. Conversational turntaking in Wernicke's aphasia. In R. Brookshire (ed.) *Clinical Aphasiology* (1980). Minneapolis: BRK.

SCHLANGER, B., SCHLANGER, P. and GERSTMAN, L. The perception of emotionally toned sentences by right hemisphere damaged and aphasic subjects. *Brain and Language* (1976), **3**, 396–463.

SCHUELL, H.R. *The Minnesota Test for the Differential Diagnosis of Aphasia* (1965). Minneapolis: University of Minnesota Press.

SCHWARTZ, M., SAFFRAN, E. and MARIN, O.S. The word order problem in agrammatism: comprehension. *Brain and Language* (1980), **10**, 249–262.

SEARLE, J. *Speech Acts* (1969). London: Cambridge University Press.

SERON, X. and DELOCHE, G. Processing of locatives 'in', 'on' and 'under' by aphasic patients: an analysis of the regression hypothesis. *Brain and Language* (1981), **14**, 70–80.

SHEWAN, C.M. Error patterns in auditory comprehension in adult aphasics. *Cortex* (1976), **12**, 325–336.

SHEWAN, C.M. Phonological processing in Broca's aphasics. *Brain and Language* (1980a), **10**, 71–88.

SHEWAN, C.M. *Auditory Comprehension Test for Sentences* (1980b). Chicago: Biolinguistics Inst.

SHEWAN, C.M. and CANTER, C.J. Effects of vocabulary, syntax and sentence length on auditory comprehension in aphasic patients. *Cortex* (1971), **7**, 209–226.

SIPOS, J. and TÄGERT, J. Kurzverfahren zur Erfassung von aphasischen Störungen. *Nervenarzt* (1972), **43**, 207–211.

SKINNER, C., WIRZ, S. and THOMPSON, I. *The Edinburgh Functional Communication Profile* (1984). Buckingham: Winslow.

SKLAR, M. *Sklar Aphasia Scale* (1973). Los Angeles: Western Psychological Services.

SMITH, M.D. On the understanding of some relational words in aphasia. *Neuropsychologia* (1974), **12**, 377–384.

SPARKS, R.W. Parastandardised examination guidelines for adult aphasia. *British Journal of Disorders of Communication* (1978), **13**, 135–146.

SPELLACY, F. and SPREEN, O. A short form of the Token Test. *Cortex* (1969), **5**, 390–397.

SPREEN, O. and BENTON, A.L. *Neurosensory Center Comprehensive Examination for Aphasia* (1969). Brit. Columbia: University of Victoria.

SPREEN, O and RISSER, A. Assessment of aphasia. In M.T. Sarno (ed.) *Acquired Aphasia* (1981). New York: Academic Press.

STACHOWIAK, F.J., HUBER, W., POECK, K. and KERSCHENSTEINER, M. Text comprehension in aphasia. *Brain and Language* (1977), **4**, 177–195.

SWINNEY, D., ZURIF, E. and CUTLER, A. Effects of sentential stress and word class upon comprehension in Broca's Aphasia. *Brain and Language* (1980), **10**, 132–145.

SWISHER, L.P. and SARNO, M.T. Token Test scores of three matched patient groups. *Cortex* (1969), **3** 264–273.

TAYLOR, M. *Functional Communication Profile* (1953). New York: University Medical Center.

THOMPSON, J. and ENDERBY, P. Is all your Schuell really necessary? *British Journal of Disorders of Communication* (1979), **14**, 195–201.

TOMKINS, C., KAU, M., MARSHALL, R., LAMBRECHT, K., GOLPER, L. and PHILLIPS, D. Analysis of a battery assessing mild auditory comprehension involvement in aphasia. In R. Brookshire (ed.) *Clinical Aphasiology* (1980). Minneapolis: BRK.

TOMPKINS, C.A. and FLOWERS, C.R. Perception of emotional intonation by brain-damaged adults: the influence of task processing levels. *Journal of Speech and Hearing Research* (1985), **28**, 527–538.

TUCKER, D.M., WATSON, R.T. and HEILMAN, K.M. Discrimination and evocation of affectively intoned speech in patients with right parietal disease. *Neurology* (1977), **27**, 947–950.

TYLER, L.K. Real-time comprehension processes in agrammatism: a case study. *Brain and Language* (1985), **26**, 259–275.

TYLER, L.K. Spoken language comprehension in aphasia: a real-time processing perspective. In M. Coltheart, G. Sartori and R. Job (eds.) *The Cognitive Neuropsychology of Language*. London: Lawrence Erlbaum.

ULATOWSKA, H., MACALUSO-HAYNES, S. and MENDEL-RICHARDSON, S. The assessment of communicative competence in aphasia. In R. Brookshire (ed.) *Clinical Aphasiology* (1976). Minneapolis: BRK.

ULATOWSKA, H., MACALUSO-HAYNES, S. and NORTH, A.J. Production of narrative and procedural discourse in aphasia. In R. Brookshire (ed.) *Clinical Aphasiology* (1980). Minneapolis: BRK.

VAN DONGEN, H.R. and VAN HARSKAMP, F. Token Test: a preliminary evaluation of a method to detect aphasia. *Neurochirurgia, Amsterdam* (1972), **75**, 129–134.

VARNEY, N.R. and BENTON, A.L. Phonemic discrimination and auditory comprehension in aphasic patients. *Journal of Clinical Neuropsychology* (1979), **1**, 65–74.

VON STOCKERT, T.R. Recognition of syntactic structure in ataxic patients. *Cortex* (1972), **8**, 323–354.

VON STOCKERT, T.R. On the structure of word deafness and mechanisms underlying the fluctuation of disturbances of higher cortical functions. *Brain and Language* (1982), **16**, 133–146.

VON STOCKERT, T.R. and BADER, L. Some relations of grammar and lexicon in aphasia. *Cortex* (1976), **12**, 49–60.

WALLACE, G.L. and CANTER, G.J. Effects of personally relevant language materials on the performance of severely aphasic individuals. *Journal of Speech and Hearing Disorders* (1985), **50**, 385–390.

WALLER, M.R. and DARLEY, F.L. The influence of context on the auditory comprehension of aphasic subjects. In R. Brookshire (ed.) *Clinical Aphasiology* (1978). Minneapolis: BRK.

WAPNER, W., HAMBY, S. and GARDNER, H. The role of the right hemisphere in the apprehension of complex linguistic materials. *Brain and Language* (1981), **14**, 15–33.

WARREN, R.M. Perceptual restoration of missing speech sounds. *Science* (1970), **167**, 392–393.

WARRINGTON, E.K. Neuropsychological studies of verbal semantic systems. *Phil. Trans. R. Soc. Lond.* (1981), **B295**, 411–423.

WEIDNER, W.E. and LASKY, E.Z. The interaction of rate and complexity of stimulus on the performance of adult aphasic subjects. *Brain and Language* (1976), **3**, 34–70.

WEINTRAUB, S., MESULAM, M.M. and KRAMER, L. Disturbances in prosody: a right hemisphere contribution to language. *Archives of Neurology* (1981), **38**, 742–744.

WEPMAN, J.M. *Auditory Discrimination Test* (1958). Chicago: Language Research Associates.

WEPMAN, J.M. and JONES, L.V. *Language Modalities Test for Aphasia* (1961). Chicago: Education Industry Services.

WEST, J.A. Auditory comprehension in aphasic adults: improvements through training. *Archives of Physical Medicine and Rehabilitation* (1973), **54**, 78–86.

WHITAKER, H.A. *On the Representation of Language in the Human Brain* (1971). Edmonton: Linguistic Research.

WHITAKER, H.A. and NOLL, J.D. Some linguistic parameters of the Token Test. *Neuropsychologia* (1972), **10**, 395–404.

WHITAKER, H.A. and WHITAKER, H. Lexical, syntactic and semantic aspects of the Token Test: a linguistic taxomony. In F. Boller and M. Dennis (eds) *Auditory Comprehension: Clinical and Experimental Studies with the Token Test* (1979). New York: Academic Press.

WHURR, R. *An Aphasia Screening Test* (1974). London: Whurr.

WILCOX, M.J., DAVIS, G.A. and LEONARD, L.B. Aphasics' comprehension of contextually conveyed meaning. *Brain and Language* (1978), **6**, 362–377.

WOOD, C.C. Levels of procxessing in speech perception: neurophysiological and information processing analyses. Status Report on Speech Research 35/36 (1973). Haskins Lab.

ZAIDEL, E. Unilateral auditory language comprehension on the Token Test following cerebral commissurotomy and hemispherectomy. *Neuropsychologia* (1977), **15**, 1–8.

ZAIDEL, E. Lexical organization in the right hemisphere. In P. Buser and A. Rougeul-Buser (eds.) *Cerebral Correlates of Conscious Experience* (1978). Amsterdam: Elsevier.

ZURIF, E.B. Language mechanisms: a neuropsychological perspective. *American Scientist* (1980), **68**, 305–311.

ZURIF, E.B., CARAMAZZA, A., MEYERSON, R. and GALVIN, J. Semantic feature representations for normal and aphasic language. *Brain and Language* (1974), **1**, 167–187.

ZURIF, E., GREEN, E., CARAMAZZA, A. and GOODENOUGH, C. Grammatical intuitions of aphasic patients: sensitivity to functors. *Cortex* (1976), **12**, 183–186.

16

The Assessment of Verbal Expression

A. Damien Martin

Introduction

> The plan throughout has been to interpret the aphasic performances in terms of the normal, placing the former in relation to the latter quantitatively and comparing the two from the point of view of method and quality.... Each aphasic is judged on the basis of the median performance, and of the normal variability characteristic in that performance.
>
> (Weisenburg and McBride, 1935, pp. 3–4)

Assessment in aphasiology has evolved from two separate sources, the structured non-standardized procedures of clinical researchers like Henry Head, and the psychometric model. Although Moutier outlined an extensive battery of procedures derived from intelligence tests (Weisenburg and McBride, 1935) as early as 1908, the application of formal psychometric concepts to the study of aphasia did not become dominant until the landmark Weisenburg and McBride study. Since then, assessment in aphasiology has been practically synonymous with standardized testing and, because of this synonymy, the standardized test for aphasia stands as the major epistemological context for assessment.

The great advantage of Weisenburg and McBride's contribution to assessment in aphasiology was that, through the psychometric model, they gave clear cut answers to two questions basic to the study of aphasia: what is the nature of normal functioning and what is the nature of the disorder? A norm is defined for each test and the disorder becomes any deviation from that norm.

While this clarity of definition gave focus and strength to the research that was to follow, the underlying conceptualization of what was actually tested created problems (Benton, 1967). Standardized tests defined intelligence and aphasia as that which was being tested, an impossible intellectual tautology. This particular difficulty has been discussed extensively elsewhere, especially for the IQ test (Block and Dworkin, 1976). While not addressed directly here, circular definitions must be kept in mind as a pervasive factor in the assessment of verbal expression.

There are five major issues in assessment of any kind: the purpose of assessment; what to assess; how to elicit behaviour to assess; how to organize observations; and finally, how to interpret that which is observed.

Since our discussion focuses on verbal expression, the second issue has been decided arbitrarily. Therefore, this essay is organized around the other four issues. However, a focus on the assessment of verbal expression carries with it the false connotation that one can evaluate verbal expression separate from considerations like comprehension, cognitive functioning, and interpersonal relationships. This is a reductionist view that does damage not only to the rich complexity of language functioning, but to the total process of assessment no matter the focus. Therefore, while maintaining primary attention to verbal expression, other aspects of language functioning will not be ignored.

Purpose of Assessment

Assessment is usually undertaken for reasons of basic research, diagnosis, or therapeutic planning. The role of assessment in basic research is too broad for this essay and therapeutic considerations are outside the scope of our discussion. Diagnosis, however, is the most frequent purpose of assessment and is closely related to both basic research and to therapeutic planning.

Most diagnostic typologies depend heavily on two aspects of verbal expression, fluency and characteristics of speech. Roughly defined as the amount of speech per unit of time, fluency lies on a continuum from no speech to the 'press of speech' seen sometimes with Wernicke's aphasia and bipolar illness. Many characteristics of verbal expression are dependent on the degree of fluency. For example, a characteristic profile of the Broca's aphasic shows no paraphasias in running speech (Goodglass and Kaplan, 1976). Since the Broca's aphasic produces no running speech and therefore cannot have paraphasias in running speech, this is not an unexpected finding. However, paraphasias do occur in Broca's aphasia (Critchley, 1970). Conversely, the Wernicke's aphasic will produce paraphasias in a range from every utterance to at least once per minute of conversation. In other words, the diagnostic characteristic depends on opportunity for error as reflected in fluency. Similarly, melodic line, phrase length, and grammatical form are all dependent on the amount of speech that is produced.

Diagnostic categories, like any form of organization, have severe limitations that must be kept in the forefront of the examiner's attention. A major objection to all classification systems is the loss of information inherent in the system through a concentration on the more obvious symptoms. As Schuell and her colleagues put it:

> When an 'amnesic' patient, asked what you pound with replies, 'You pound with — we know that thing — what it is. We have him back down there — we do down there — the pound bench,' it is obvious he could not readily retrieve the word hammer. Presumably he is trying to tell us he knows what you pound with, and that he has a hammer downstairs on his workbench. Isn't it obvious that he is also having a little trouble discriminating gender of pronouns, and structuring and sequencing a message, as well as, or perhaps because of, trouble finding words?
>
> On the other hand, when a 'syntactical' patient, asked what he did today, responds, 'Eat — doctor — go — I can't say it — you know? — haircut,' it is obvious that he has difficulty generating sentences. It may be less obvious that he can't think of the word *breakfast*, his doctor's name, or a label for *barber shop*, that his retrieval vocabulary is confined to common words of high immediate utility, and that he uses common grammatical combinations on occasion. (pp. 101–102)

Goldstein summarized the problem when he criticized diagnostic classification systems because 'they produce a misconception of the facts because they neglect a finer analysis of the symptoms or analyze them from a theoretical point of view which leads to the overlooking of many of the phenomena' (1948, p. x).

Apraxia of Speech

One diagnostic category, apraxia of speech, deserves special consideration as a supposedly purely expressive disorder separate from dysarthria and aphasia.

Prior to 1900, movement disorders were described within a context of perceptual or symbolic disruption. In 1900, Liepmann attempted to describe and explain one brain damaged individual's difficulty with movements involving his right limbs. Liepman called this problem apraxia, a term derived from the Greek word *praxis* meaning deed, action or act, and the prefix *a* meaning without. To explain the phenomenon, he used the then popular psychological model called Association Theory. Liepman's use of Association Theory focused attention on movement as movement, separate from perception and, to a certain extent, from symbolic function (DeAjuriaguerra and Tissot, 1975).

Association Theory outlined three consecutive stages in the execution of any act: first, memory traces of the *idea* of movement; second, an *association* between the idea and the third stage, memory traces of the *motor image* of the act. That is, the idea of an action like lighting a candle (first stage) is also represented by a memory of the motor movement necessary for the act (the third stage); and the two are connected by an association (second stage).

Apraxias involved the first two stages only. A disruption of the idea is an 'ideational apraxia' and a disruption of association is an ideomotor apraxia.

Paralysis or weakness (dysarthria in speech) affected the third stage. Apraxia of speech is, in essence, a form of ideomotor apraxia, a disruption of the association between the phoneme as idea and the motor image of the phoneme.

Psychology soon discarded Association Theory as inadequate to explain mental function. Yet its stepchild, apraxia of speech, remains as a viable diagnostic construct in the field of aphasiology. Jakobson (1971) explained such a seemingly paradoxical event when he said:

> Nevertheless, and it often happens in the history of science, even if an outdated theory is abolished, there exist numerous residues (which have) escaped from the control of rational thought. (My translation from the French text.)

The basic flaw in the theoretical and clinical conception of apraxia of speech is its reductionism. Speech is not just movement. Speech is the end result of a complex series of hierarchically related cognitive systems that process linguistic information (Martin, 1974).

Research has supported the argument that, for the brain damaged adult, as for his brain damaged counterpart, articulatory behaviour is not isolated and is affected by a number of factors. Meaning (Martin and Rigrodsky, 1974), grammatical class (Deal and Darley, 1972), part of speech, voice and position (Hardison, Marquardt, and Peterson, 1977), abstraction (Dunlop and Marquardt, 1977), and morphological characteristics (Martin *et al.*, 1975) all have an effect on articulatory performance. This does not mean that apraxia of speech is primarily a linguistic disorder. As I have suggested recently, it may entail a mild form of dysarthria affecting the proprioceptive capabilities of the individual (Martin, 1982).

The most important refutation of the concept lies in the research of its supporters. In what might be called the seminal research for modern investigations of 'apraxia of speech', Johns and Darley (1970) claimed to demonstrate that ten subjects had a motor disorder separate from aphasia and dysarthria. Subsequent studies on these same ten subjects, however, showed that, contrary to the original findings, the subjects did indeed have what might be considered aphasic symptoms, even under the limited operational definitions offered by Johns and Darley (Aten, Johns, and Darley, 1971; Deal and Darley, 1972; Aten *et al.*, 1975). Rather than interpret this as refutation of their original findings, Darley and his colleagues argued it demonstrated that apraxia and aphasia could co-exist.

The problem is in large part one of definition. The need for clear, adequate definitions is a prerequisite in scientific discourse. Theoretical viability as well as diagnostic reliability depend on the adequacy of disorder definition. The lack of a clear definition of apraxia of speech is not a new challenge. Dejerine commented in 1914 that it is easier to define what apraxia is *not*, rather than what it is. Darley, Aronson and Brown (1975) continue the tradition described by Dejerine by defining apraxia of speech primarily with reference to what it is not.

> Apraxia of speech is a distinct motor speech disorder distinguishable from the dysarthrias (speech disorders due to impaired innervation of speech musculature) and aphasia (a language disorder due to an impairment of the brain mechanism for decoding and encoding the symbol system used in spoken and written communication). Apraxia of speech is a disorder of motor speech programming manifested primarily by errors in articulation and secondarily by compensatory alterations of prosody. The speaker shows reduced efficiency in accomplishing the oral postures necessary for production of words. (p. 267)

The addition of speech characteristics to the definition does not clarify the conceptual haziness, since stuttering is also distinct from aphasia and dysarthria and can be described as a disruption of 'motor speech programming' characterized by 'errors in articulation' and 'compensatory alternations of prosody', difficulty assuming 'oral postures' for phoneme production and for the 'sequence of these postures for the production of words'. If a definition that serves as the basis for diagnosis and treatment cannot reliably distinguish between two disorders, that definition is clearly inadequate.

The question of adequate definition is not just a minor academic quibble. One function of diagnostic categories is to organize our observations so that we may more clearly understand the functioning of the braindamaged individual. Unclear and reductionist concepts like apraxia of speech only hinder that search. For example, DeSimoni and Darley (1977) attempted to describe the effect of phoneme duration control of three utterances length conditions in an apraxic patient. The patient studied was diagnosed as having multiple sclerosis with dysarthria but no 'clear' aphasia, even though she did have difficulty expressing ideas. Since we have a disorder that is defined by the lack of both dysarthria and aphasia, it would seem a subject with a definite dysarthria and possible aphasia would not be a suitable source for statements about the nature of the disorder. The researchers solved the problem with tautology, 'Since apraxia for speech is by definition a disorder of motor speech programming, we may assume that the errant speech performance observed in patients with apraxia are attributable to speech programming errors or incapabilities' (p. 257). The individual's other, provable motor disorder was dismissed with 'Dysarthria was considered to be quite secondary'. We find such tautologies and dismissals throughout the literature on apraxia of speech. Again, they reflect not only faulty reasoning but the lack of coherent theory and definition underlying the concept itself.

These objections are not new. Weisenburg and McBride made similar claims when they stated

> ... the disturbances in the executive function mechanisms of speech production ... are not isolated in cases of cerebral lesion with aphasia, but

appear together with extensive changes in language and behavior. No absolute distinction can be made between the simpler and the more complicated disturbances, and it is for this reason as Head rightly contended, that the simpler expressive and receptive speech defects should not be classified as apraxic or agnosic but should be considered as part of the complex aphasic picture. (Weisenburg and McBride, p. 104)

Elicitation of Verbal Behaviour

> Our statements concerning a patient's condition either clinical or anatomical are based on the phenomena observed, i.e., the symptoms. Symptoms do not always come to the fore by themselves. We have to apply definite methods to reveal them . . . there are only a few modifications of behavior we can observe directly and these may not always aid us in recognizing the defect. The patient does not speak or his speech is impaired, but a variety of causes may be operative here. Only if we expose him to definite conditions may we be able to see the real cause . . . Thus the symptoms we find in an individual patient are at least partly determined by our procedure or methods of investigation.
>
> (Kurt Goldstein, 1948, p. 2)

Methods of eliciting verbal behaviour can be divided into three types: retrieval tasks, 'acting upon information' tasks, and free speech. Like all attempts at classification, these divisions are arbitrary since each method includes aspects of the other. For example, acting upon information tasks and free speech must always include retrieval factors.

In the discussion below, illustrative tasks are taken from two standardized tests for aphasia, the Minnesota Test for Differential Diagnosis of Aphasia (MTDDA) (Shuell, 1964) and The Boston Diagnostic Aphasia Examination (BDAE) (Goodglass and Kaplan, 1976). Other tests will be discussed only incidentally for three reasons: Most aphasia tests use the same tasks to elicit behaviour; among all the standardized tests for aphasia the MTDDA and the BDAE are probably the two most complete with reference for elicitation tasks; differences among tests reflect attributes having more to do with psychometrics than the assessment of verbal expression.

One major difference among and within the three categories is the degree to which the examiner has an exact model against which to compare the response. For example, if the aphasic is asked to count, the examiner knows exactly what the response should be but, if she asks, *what do you do with a toothbrush?*, the response can vary acording to both linguistic form and content. The judgement of the response then depends to a large extent on the examiner's expectations, a dependence which may create problems in the overall assessment. One aphasic with a military background answered the question with 'clean the shoes — in between — top and bottom', a response the examiner considered as linguistically deviant and bizarre in content. Actually, old toothbrushes are used in the military to clean and polish the seam between the sole and the top part of the shoe for inspections. While the response was unusual in the sense that it was not what would ordinarily be expected, it was neither bizarre nor incorrect. Indeed, it was helpful in that it gave certain clues to the individual's processing capacities and skills. It seemed bizarre and incorrect because, without a clear-cut unambiguous model for reference, the examiner had to depend on her own experience and expectations, which were not sufficient in this case.

As we shall see, the problem of a referent model within tasks runs through all elicitation procedures.

Retrieval

Retrieval is a basic process in all cognition. Cognitive processing depends on the ability to act on information received which in turn depends on the ability to store and retrieve prior information. Retrieval is used here to characterize those tasks in which there are direct requests for specific information, usually considered to be held in long-term storage.

Automatic speech

Automatic speech is used in almost all aphasia tests as the easiest and most likely to occur of verbal acts. Automatic speech tasks include reciting the alphabet, days of the week, months of the year, nursery rhymes and counting. In informal evaluation clinicians often use singing, prayers, and other highly learned set pieces like the *pledge of allegiance to the flag*. While obscenities and cursing are often automatic, they are usually not used to elicit speech.

Since even the most impaired of patients can, with help, produce the above utterances, their value to assessment is sometimes ignored. Automatic speech can provide valuable diagnostic information about the individual aphasic's ability to initiate speech, to process linguistic elements, especially phonemes, to self monitor or to focus on the task. It can also give the examiner an idea of the degree to which the aphasic responds to facilitation techniques.

Word association tasks, phrase and sentence completion, and similar elicitation tasks can also be considered as forms of automatic speech because of the relative ease with which the examiner can get even the severely impaired aphasic to perform. These tasks allow for a wider degree of acceptable variation in the response. An association to the word 'in', or the completion of phrases and sentences like 'a quart of____', or 'pass the salt and____', may have a high degree of predictive probability but they are not predetermined.

Naming

Naming tasks include visual confrontation naming and responsive naming. In the former, the aphasic names a presented picture or object; in the latter, he responds to characteristics of the object — 'what do you tell time with.' A variation of responsive naming is a form of serial responsive naming in which the task is to name a series of objects centred on a theme. For example, the BDAE asks the aphasic to name body parts and to list as many different animals as possible within a set period of time ('fluency in controlled association'). Naming tasks usually require only single word responses in which the response model is fairly concrete and absolute.

Tasks like answering simple questions (tell me what you do with a hammer?), giving biographical information (what is your name; what kind of work do you do?) defining words (what is a robin?) and so forth, are intrinsically similar to naming in that the basic demand is the retrieval of highly specific linguistically coded information. They are considered different because of the greater complexity involved in both retrieving and coding the information, the greater possibility of acceptable variation in the response and because of the degree to which the examiner can respond to the quality as well as the correctness of the response. 'Hit', 'Bang the nail', 'fix the house', 'work with wood' are correct to certain point. Yet, they are qualitatively different and each has implications for the inferences to be drawn about the individual's retrieval capacities.

Acting Upon Information

As mentioned earlier, one of the difficulties in discussing the assessment of verbal expression is the degree to which verbal expression interacts with other parameters of language behaviour. As will be discussed under modality organization, it is possible to devise a task that elicits behaviour on only one level. This is especially true when we speak of *acting on information tasks*. First, in any exchange between the aphasic and the examiner, there is a demand that the aphasic act on information. Second, in what are generally considered to be comprehensive tasks, verbal expression is always a component of the interaction. There must be a response of some kind no matter the task. Even pattern recognition, as in pointing to pictures or written words named by the examiner, demand the equivalent of saying 'this is the same'. Other so-called comprehension tasks require that the individual express a higher level decision about meaning. (I am including affirmation or negation through head shaking and nodding as a form of verbal expression.) Understanding sentences (should children disobey their parents?); understanding a paragraph, repeating digits and sentences, or handling what the BDAE calls 'complex ideational material', 'Will a board sink in the water', are also expression tasks and difficulty in their performance is related as often to difficulties in verbal expression as to comprehension.

Perhaps the most effective of the *acting on information tasks*, and the one with the clearest relationship to verbal expression, is repetition. Its effectiveness lies in the absolute control the examiner has over the materials to be repeated, thus allowing for control over the model against which to compare the response. Repetition enables the examiner to vary the material in any way deemed appropriate to specific goals. The factors varied may include length, frequency of occurrence, syntactic complexity, articulatory ease, or any other chosen by the examiner. Different factors can be combined 'I stopped at the door and rang his bell' as opposed to 'The phantom soared across the foggy heath'.

Less structured than repetition, yet still within the confines of acting on information, are those tasks like retelling a paragraph that demand paraphrasing. Derived from early research on memory, paraphrasing tasks provide an open ended response model for the examiner based on content.

Free Speech

Free speech, defined here as the speech that occurs in conversational exchange, is the most important and yet the most difficult behaviour to elicit and to valuate.

The most obvious and the most debilitating feature of aphasia lies in the impairment of the ability to participate in free conversational exchange. While the first problem for assessment lies in the characteristic aphasic symptoms themselves, barriers to conversation, apart from aphasia itself, make the natural exchange more difficult. Disability from the recent stroke, the hospital setting with all its factual and emotional connotations, and the test situation provide a context within which the structured task is the more effective means to elicit speech. The structured task, however, is the antithesis of free speech, and can provide only limited information about the individual's capacities for such exchanges. Although the BDAE attempts to lead gradually into conversation through a series of graded steps ranging from automatic speech (How are you?) to describing a picture, open ended conversation can not occur within the confines of standardized test procedures.

There is an additional consideration in the evaluation of free speech. A conversational exchange demands an ongoing interaction dependent on simultaneous as well as preceding stimuli (Muma, 1975; Watzlawick, Beavin and Jackson, 1967). Most of this simultaneous and preceding stimuli, especially that which is linguistic in nature, will come from the other participant in the conversation. Therefore, assessment of the aphasic's conversational performance must include a description and evaluation of the total interaction (Martin, 1981b).

Organizational Criteria

> Not only is it necessary to arrange the tests in sequence, but each set must be placed before the patient in several different ways ... It is also important to graduate the severity of the task before concluding to what extent the patient can read or write.
>
> (Henry Head, 1925, p. 145)

The major functions of organizational criteria are to structure elicitation tasks and to group data for interpretation. For example, a progressive increase of stimulus length for repetition sets predetermined limits on processing demands as it establishes the parameters by which the response will be evaluated. On the other hand, a phonological analysis of all verbal utterances, regardless of how they were elicited, allows for analyses separate from the task itself.

The most common organizational systems used in assessment are: division into modalities, scoring or rating systems, parameters affecting ease or difficulty, and linguistic description.

Modality Organization

> It has been almost universally assumed that the diverse defects of speech which constitute aphasia reveal the elements out of which the use of language is composed. A salt can be broken up chemically into an acid and a base; by analogy it was supposed that the morbid manifestations corresponded to the classification of the clinical phenomena under such categories as 'motor' and 'sensory', 'auditory' and 'visual' or some analogous terminology.
>
> (Henry Head, 1925, p. 143)

Early models of speech and language function were simple and direct. Language had two observable dimensions, passive reception and active expression, and a non-observable, central integrative dimension which handled information received or expressed. Observations were organized accordingly into receptive and expressive modalities, an organization highly compatible with the then recent discoveries of sensory-motor functioning. Even undimensional theorists like Schuell accept the value of modality organization in assessment even though they are derived from and essential to localization theories of aphasia: 'We observe language behavior in the usual modalities, listening, speaking, reading, and writing, because this is what there is to observe about language' (Schuell, Jenkins, Jimenez-Pabón, 1965, p. 169).

For all practical purposes, modality organization in the assessment of verbal expression consists of the examination of speech and writing. The only aphasia test that pays any systematic attention to gesture is the PICA, the most explicit and extreme of the modality organized assessment procedures (Porch, 1967). Unfortunately, in the PICA gesture is equated, to a certain extent, with pantomime, a conception that is limited and limiting. In addition, a rigid adherence to the logic of modality organization and a focus on expressive modalities alone has led to such incongruities as reading tests scored as a gestural activity (Porch, 1967; Martin, 1977).

While almost all standardized tests for aphasia use some form of modality organization, most scholars would agree that the modality model is too simplified to be an adequate construct for language or cognitive functioning. However, while inadequate it is probably the most powerful of the organizational constructs for assessment. Its power lies in its simplicity.

Simplicity is an advantage. Oversimplification is not. The modality construct is an oversimplification of language behaviour. Studies have demonstrated that auditory presentation of material does not necessarily mean auditory processing of the same material. Similarly, visually presented material can engender acoustic coding, especially in short term memory (Lindsay and Norman, 1977). Acceptance of the modality model as a construct of human information processing rather than as an organizational construct for observation has created three interrelated problems: it solidifies the belief that comprehension is separate from expression; it leads to the assumption that it is possible to measure comprehension and expression separately; and it supports the notion of discrete modality impairment. Each belief is incorrect and impedes the advancement of our understanding of aphasia. It is impossible to examine one modality separate from another since, no matter which modality is the focus of attention, another is involved. An auditory or visual comprehension task cannot be given without demanding some expressive act to demonstrate that comprehension. However, if it is accepted that a particular task tests verbal expression and an aphasic makes a mistake on that task, it is only logical to assume that the difficulty lies in verbal expression. Similarly, if a supposedly receptive task is performed poorly, the conclusion usually is that the problem is a receptive one. And if tasks classified according to one modality show more errors than tasks classified as belonging to another modality, it is again only logical to assume that one modality is more impaired than another.

Schuell, though she admitted the possibility of differential impairment according to modality, argued that this different was perhaps only apparent. She wrote, 'Usually in aphasia, the active linguistic processes, speaking and writing, show more impairment than the passive ones, listening and reading. Here *show* may be the important word; it may be that the impairment is only more observable in the active modalities, although this is questionable. However, the same kind of linguistic impairment tends to be apparent in all modalities' (Schuell, Jenkins and Jimenez-Pabón, 1965, p. 104).

Differences according to modality may also stem from the interaction of different stimulus characteristics with different cognitive processes (Martin, 1981c). For example, an auditory stimulus is time constrained, acting upon sensory information storage systems for a limited time (Lindsay and Norma,

1977). Visual presentation of the same material permits longer stimulation of sensory information storage systems, thus allowing other cognitive systems more time to act on the stimulus.

Some problems related to modality organization anticipate the discussion on interpretation of the data. For example, if the aphasic attempts to name a series of pictures instead of pointing to them as asked, the results cannot be interpreted only as a lack of comprehension. The aphasic's verbal utterances demonstrate he has an idea of what is required, although his idea is different from the intention of the examiner. This difference between message intended and message received is not peculiar only to interactions with an aphasic, but is paralleled in normal communication exchanges as well (Muma, 1975; Warzlawick, Beavin and Jackson, 1967). One important implication for assessment of verbal expression, therefore, is that assessment must not be limited to classification of error, that is, one should not just decide whether or not the aphasic understands the specific direction, but rather what is the understanding he has achieved.

Schuell and her colleagues recognized the need to treat observational organization separately from the inferences to be drawn from these observations. They said 'But while we observe behavior [according to modalities], we think in terms of processes that underlie behavior. This is harder because processes cannot be observed but must be inferred' (Schuell, Jenkins, Jimenez-Pabon, 1964, p. 169).

Summary

Modality organization is among the more powerful of organizational constructs in assessment. Its dangers lie in the reification of the construct as a model of information processing rather than as a limited form of organizing and describing observations. Misuse of the modality construct has led to the mistaken impressions that expression is separate from comprehension, that the two can be measured separately, and that discrete modality impairment is possible.

Scoring

The introduction of the standardization test with its reliance on statistical analyses brought about a simultaneous need for means to quantify observations.

Porch (1971) identified four basic scoring methods; description, plus-minus scoring, rating and category scales and multidimensional scoring. It could be argued that the first, description, is not truly a scoring technique in that the data is usually not quantified. However, since all scoring systems are methods of description, Porch's inclusion of description as a means of scoring seems justified, especially since description can be quantified when it is used simultaneously with other organizational means. Accordingly, description will be discussed here as a scoring method.

Description

Description is narrative that permits recording the maximum amount of information about a response. It is best used concomitantly with other means of organization. For example, phonetic transcription allows for exact description and subsequent analysis on a phonological level. The result can be quantified and treated statistically (Martin, Wasserman, Gilden, Gerstman and West, 1975). Similarly, exact description used concomitantly with a semantic or syntactic organization provides a systematic means of recording and analysis on other levels (Crystal, 1982).

Porch (1971) claims that the major disadvantage with description is a lack of standardization and a heavy reliance on the biases and skills of the scorer, objections that can be leveled against any approach. All scoring systems reflect a theoretical perspective and thus are subjective in that they reflect a belief system. In a standardized approach, examiners merely share their subjective perspectives. The belief that a lack of standardization is of necessity a disadvantage arises from an acceptance of the benefits of the psychometric model. Although particularly strong for the researcher's need to compare one individual to another with reference to performance by the group, these benefits are not necessarily paramount in the assessment of performance by the individual. Indeed, if the focus is the individual's performance rather than a comparison to the group, the descriptive method is not only the most complete but probably the most heuristic of all the scoring methods. It is also, at the present time, the best method for describing free speech (*see* above).

Plus–minus scoring

Plus–minus scoring, the decision as to whether a response is correct or not, is the simplest of all the scoring methods. It is most appropriate for those tasks in which there is a clear cut expected response. Visual confrontation naming, repetition, counting, etc. can all be rated fairly unambiguously as correct or incorrect.

One major limitation of plus–minus scoring is that it severely circumscribes observation and, by extension, the whole assessment process. For example, it is difficult if not impossible to put a correct–incorrect label on conversational interchange.

A second major limitation of plus–minus scoring lies in loss of information. The further one goes along a range of response possibility, the more difficult it is to describe a response as correct or incorrect. However, even when it is possible to state clearly that an answer is correct or incorrect, plus-minus scoring can hide important information (Porch, 1971).

The assessment of verbal expression makes sense only if it can tell us something about an individual's ability to process information. Plus–minus scoring limits that endeavour since the fact of error often tells us less than the actual error itself. For example, if an individual says *boy* for *girl*, the nature of the response is as important as its incorrectness.

Goldstein (1948) stressed that plus-minus scoring was deceptive because it could tap into a typical inconsistency of response. Schuell, Jenkins and Jimenez-Pabon (1964) in their defence of the use of plus-minus scoring in the MTDDA, admitted this danger but claimed that by using percentage of error, more than one test, and additional forms of notation, the danger could be averted. Schuell did demonstrate that aphasic performance is consistent, at least with reference to degree of correctness or incorrectness, but this demonstration did not account for either the nature of particular errors or the factors that may have contributed to actual performance.

With major problems like loss of information, lack of a suitable base for drawing inferences, and severe limitations as to what can be observed, the immediate question is why plus-minus scoring is used at all? The answer lies in the demands of the psychometric model. Many standardized tests of aphasia developed after the Second World War relied on factor analysis to examine the nature of aphasic performance. To do so, observations had to be quantified so that data could be entered into the statistical procedures. Even with all its faults, plus-minus scoring is the most efficient and defensible scoring technique for these procedures. This is not meant as a negative comment. The statistical investigations of Schuell (1965), Goodglass and Kaplan (1976), and others have given us a great deal of information about the nature of aphasia. The difficulty lies in the application of this data to the individual. The l;oss of information inherent in a plus-minus system of scoring is not automatically regained for an understanding of the individual aphasic.

Plus-minus scoring, then, while valuable as a research artifact, has limited value in the assessment of verbal expression in the individual aphasic.

Rating and category scales

Rating and category scales are statements of relationships along a continuum of 'goodness' (Porch, 1971). The simplest and most frequently used rating is the mild, moderate, severe classification of impairment. Category scales are ratings applied to specific areas. For example, the MTDDA rates speech on a scale from '0 — No observable impairment' through '3 — Some conversational speech but marked difficulty in expressing long or complex ideas,' to '6 — No functional speech'.

Writing is rated on a similar scale from '0 — No observable impairment' through '3 — Can write short, easy sentences spontaneously and to dictation', to '6 — No functional writing'.

Dysarthria, a motor disorder of expression is also rated from '0 — No observable impairment' through '3 — Intelligible but obviously defective speech', to '6 — Speech usually unintelligible'.

Rating and category scales are valuable in that they give an overall impression of capacities and limitations in the individual aphasic. Such impressions by skilled observers are heuristic and can often serve as an indication of functional changes not picked up by standardized testing, but they are severely limited in that they are usually too vague and imprecise. They also do not give enough information to allow for detailed inferences about the information processing and communicative capabilities of the individual.

Multidimensional scoring

Porch (1971) attempted to deal with problems presented by different scoring methods through the multidimensional scoring of verbal expression. His scoring system was intended to describe the nature of the patient's responses to the tasks and to do so with high reliability and with confidence that small changes in responses were being accurately detected and described.'

Porch's multidimensional scoring is a binary choice system supposedly involving five main dimensions of response: accuracy, responsiveness, completenes, promptness, and efficiency. The scores range from 1 to 15: a score of 15 for an accurate, responsive, complete, prompt, and efficient response, for example, immediately calling a *pen*, a *pen*; a score of 14 if there is distortion; 13 if the response is delayed but correct; 12 if it is incomplete; 11 if it is incomplete and delayed; 10 if there is a self-correction; 9 if the patient gives a correct response after the instructions have been repeated; 8 if he needs additional information to produce an accurate response; 7 if he gives a related response; 6 for an error response; 5 for an intelligible and 4 for an unintelligible reponse; 3 for a minimal reponse; 2 for attending; and 1 for no response.

Porch's claim that the use of this scale specifies the nature as well as the details of the response does not appear to be accurate. For example, a patient, when asked to name a *pen*, might give no response at first, necessitating a repeat of instructions (9); describe the object (5), necessitating additional information or a cue (8); then give, in a distorted manner (14); the related response 'ink' (7); and finally change the response to 'pen', an incomplete response (12). The final score, although the patient has demonstrated behaviours listed in the multidimensional scale from 14 down to 5, is to score 12, and is therefore only one aspect of the response which is reported (Martin, 1977).

Patients sometimes give related responses such as *spoon* or *knife* for the stimulus *fork*, recognize the error but cannot retrieve the correct response, and say 'No! I can't.' The response is scored with a 5, an 'intelligible' response, a classification that also includes perseverative responses and automatic speech. In this particular case, the score would not indicate that the patient had self-corrected, in the sense that he had recognized his own error, or that he had produced a related response (Martin, 1977). Thus, it is not true that, as claimed, '. . . each score entered on the score sheet describes the details of the reponse' (Porch, 1971, p. 790).

Other problems with this test purportedly devoted exclusively to the expressive modalities have been discussed extensively elsewhere (Martin, 1977).

The problem is multidimensional scoring, as in plus–minus scoring and rating and category scales, arises in part from the complexity and variety of human behaviour, even that which is disordered. No system, especially one that attempts to quantify behaviour, can be adequate to this complexity.

Linguistic organization

Goodglass and Blumstein (1973) state 'Beginning with observations on aphasic symptoms made in the middle of the nineteenth century, it was recognized that certain deficits could be defined only in linguistic terms" (p. 5).

While not strictly true, all forms of behaviour can be organized and described according to different parameters, their statement highlights the importance of linguistic organization because of its high reliability, specificity of description, basic validity, and perhaps most importantly, capacity to describe individual verbal behaviour with great detail on several levels with no violation of the interrelatedness of various parts. For example, one can describe the repetition of 'pry the tin lid off' as 'try . . . try . . . take the, you know, the top, the top . . . take it down' on the phonemic, semantic and syntactic levels without the distortion that would result from modality based criteria.

Systematic linguistic investigations are a comparatively recent phenomenon, however, (Lesser, 1978). Accordingly, the most widely used method of assessment, the standardized test for aphasia, makes very little use of linguistic criteria. Except for the BDAE which provides for some linguistic notation, most standardized tests depend on parameters like mode of presentation, length, and frequency of occurrence. Although related, for example, the longer the utterance the more likely it will be syntactically complex, these parameters reflect specific processing capabilities rather than linguistic skills. While additional notations and extra test examination of the data can impose a linguistic organization on observations obtained through standardized tests, linguistic criteria are not basic to their organization.

Linguistic organization usually follows three general hierarchical levels: phonemic, semantic, and syntactic. Some of the more common categories derived from these levels are: literal or phonemic paraphasia (the apparent substitution of one word or phoneme for another); phonetic jargon aphasia (sufficient literal paraphasias whereby speech is rendered unintelligible to the ordinary listener); semantic or verbal paraphasia (the substitution of one meaningful unit for another); semantic jargon (apparently meaningless speech containing numerous verbal paraphasias); anomia; apraxia of speech; and agrammatism, the shortening of speech by omission of many relational elements like prepositions (sometimes called telegraphic speech because of its similarity to messages shortened to save money when sending a telegram). At times, verbal behaviour is described with reference to more complicated forms of linguistic description in terms of transformations from kernel sentences rather than in terms of structural elements alone.

One aspect of linguistic description, suprasegmentals, is not used often in assessment. The major exception is the BDAE which includes melodic line as one of its criteria for diagnosis.

Linguistic categories, like modalities, are merely organizational constructs. When we describe an aphasic as agrammatic or producing phonetic jargon, we are characterizing his production of linguistic information. Linguistic description itself does not say anything about the aphasic's processing skills nor about his communicative abilities. Linguistic organization, like all forms of organization, is simply a system for grouping data for further interpretation.

Performance Parameters

One underlying assumption in the use of performance parameters is that complexity can be equated with relative ease or difficulty. While true for most aphasics, it is not a hard and fast rule. Complexity is the number of operations necessary to complete an act; ease or difficulty, the facility with which an individual can perform these operations. Thus, a complex act may be easy for one individual and more difficult for another. For example, a specific dance step could be very complex but performed with different degrees of ease by various individuals. Therefore, it is important to remember that while complexity can be specified without reference to the individual, difficulty cannot.

The most common performance parameters used to organize assessment procedures are task type, length, frequency of occurrence and probability. With the exception of the PICA, most standardized tests for aphasia start with tasks presumed to be easier and progress to the more difficult.

Type of task

Matching tasks are generally considered to be the easiest of all tasks, and therefore, again with the exception of the PICA, most standardized tests start each section with some form of matching. For example, on the MTDDA, the auditory disturbances section begins with having the aphasic match the examiner's spoken words to a picture; the visual and reading section, matching geometric forms; the speech and language section, matching oral-facial movements of the examiner and repetition; and the visuomotor section, copying.

Following commands, answering questions, paraphrasing, and similar tasks succeed matching. Again, while the relative complexity within and across tasks can be specified, the relative ease or difficulty depends in large part on the specific problems presented by individual aphasics. Thus some aphasics will have more difficulty repeating, while others will experience greater difficulty with answering questions.

Relative ease of difficulty according to task is so much a matter of individual characteristics that it is not the most effective of organizational paradigms, but it should be a guiding principle in the ongoing assessment of the individual, with the examiner noting what types of task appear to give the individual aphasic more difficulty.

Length

For most aphasics, as length increases, difficulty increases, an assumption supported extensively in the literature (Schuell, Jenkins, Jimenez-Pabon, 1965). But length does not operate alone since frequency of occurrence and/or linguistic complexity can interact with length to make an utterance easy or difficult. For example, *cup of coffee* and *ubiquitous* have the same number of syllables, yet the three word phrase would probably be easier for most aphasics. Shorter sentences used for repetition may be linguistically more complex than longer ones (Whitaker and Whitaker, 1972) and thus, perhaps, more difficult.

Frequency of occurrence

Frequency of occurrence apparently affects ease of access to the lexicon. The more frequently a word occurs in the language, the easier it is to retrieve that word.

Again, other factors seem to play a part even in robust findings like the relative ease in processing highly frequent words. Prepositions are among the most frequent of words in the English language, yet many aphasics, especially those characterized as non-fluent aphasics, have difficulty with them. Still, the role played by frequency is so evident and strong that it has become one of the main factors in controlling for relative ease within tasks.

Probability

Probability is here used in the sense of expectation arising from context. One of the more obvious tasks that are highly dependent on probability is the phrase completion task. Only a certain limited number of elements are likely to complete the phrase 'a glass of____ .'

If it were not for context, the processing of linguistic information would be a difficult, almost impossible task. Every word would have to be dealt with as equivalent pieces of data. Through cultural and social experience and the redundancy and regularity of language, however, speaker–listeners of a language are provided a context that enables them to process more easily (Lindsay and Norman, 1977).

Context provides a degree of probability which affects the relative ease of many tasks. Reading, for example, depends in large part on the search for context within the material. When one reads aloud, one searches in advance the material that follows the immediate linguistic unit so as to be able to read the specific unit (Lindsay and Norman, 1977). It may well be that it is this search, with its concomitant increase in processing demand, that makes reading aloud a difficult task for many aphasics.

A major context often ignored in assessment is that which arises from the previous experience of the individual as an aphasic. To use an earlier example, if, when asked to point to a series of pictures named by the examiner, an aphasic immediately begins to try to name them, I can be fairly certain that he has been exposed repeatedly to naming tasks. The placing of the materials in front of him gives a context that elicits a response that is not just symptomatic of a comprehension difficulty.

The Meaning of Assessment

> An account of aphasia . . . must go beyond the description of pathological phenomena and their grouping into clinical types in an attempt to embrace more fully than before, the processes, in order to distinguish pathological and normal happenings from each other or at least to define more clearly the considerations that are necessary for such a dynamic interpretation. It must be an attempt, through an increasingly deeper-penetrating description of phenomenology, to achieve an understanding of the pathological processes and their relationships.
>
> Arnold Pick

Any scientific attempt to examine human behaviour, its disorders, and treatment must answer three questions, what is the nature of normal functioning? what is the nature of the disorder? and finally, what is the nature of therapy? It is within the context of these three questions that inferences must be drawn about the meaning of the elicited behaviour.

The answers will depend primarily on the examiner's chosen level of reference and the theoretical model that underlies the approach to assessment. Different levels of reference will give different although equally valid answers to the essential questions. For example, if the emphasis is on information processing as opposed to communication, normal functioning could be defined as the efficient action and interaction of those cognitive processes which support language behaviour; the disorder as the disruption of efficiency in action and interaction in these processes because of brain damage; and therapy as the attempt to maximize the potential to use these processes. A communication level of reference might define normal functioning as the maintenance, with maximum efficiency, of appropriate receiver sender roles in a conversational exchange; the disorder, as the disruption of this interaction in which one of the participants in the interaction is an aphasic; and therapy, as the improvement in efficiency of role for both participants in their interaction (Martin, 1979, 1981,a,b).

Specification of the level of reference is as essential to an understanding of the behaviour obtained through assessment procedures as it is to the planning and evaluation of the therapeutic process (Martin, 1981,a,b). The chosen level of reference will determine to a certain extent the models used in the assessment of verbal expression. Obviously, if one is assessing communication, one must use a model of communication; if one is assessing cognitive processing, one must use a cognitive model. The underlying theoretical model will in turn determine to a large extent the meaning drawn from the assessment procedure. This explains in large part why skilled examiners observing exactly the same behaviour will come up with entirely different conclusions. Their observations are strained through the sieve of their model. A localizationist model will by necessity lead to conclusions about the site of lesion; an interference model to the effect on information processing; a modality model to the impairment of reception or expression.

Most standardized tests for aphasia are assessments of the aphasic's information processing rather than communication skills. For example, the knowledge that an aphasic can process a three or four word utterance but not a seven word utterance gives us information from which we can perhaps make inferences about his sensory information storage and short term memory capacities. This is not to say that such information has no relevance for communication. Schuell and her colleagues (1964) suggest that one can improve the comprehension of the aphasic in ordinary conversation by speaking short phrases with pauses between them.

All examiners of aphasic phenomena choose a level of reference and have an underlying theoretical model as the context for interpreting their observations. The difficulty lies not so much in whether the model is correct or incorrect; the scientific process with its mandated evaluation of assumptions will take care of that. Rather, a problem occurs when the level of reference and the model are implicit rather than explicit and therefore the assumptions upon which the interpretations are based are not evaluated. When assessment is a matter of technique alone, with no regard for the specification of each of its stages and evaluation of those stages with reference to the obtained data, assessment becomes ritual rather than science.

Acknowledgements

I would like to express my appreciation to my colleagues Harriet Klein and Nelson Moses for their comments and criticisms and especially to Emery S. Hetrick, M.D. for his suggestions and 'ecological' reading of several versions of this chapter.

References

BAY, E. Problems, possibilities, and limitations of localization of psychic symptoms in the brain. *Cortex* (1964), **1**, 92–92.

BENTON, A.L. Problems of test construction in the field of aphasia. *Cortex* (1967), **3**, 32–58.

BIRDWHISTELL, R.L. *Kinesics and Context* (1970). Philadelphia: University of Penna. Press.

BLOCK, N.J. and DWORKIN, G. (eds) *The IQ Controversy: Critical Readings* (1976). New York: Random House.

CRITCHLEY, M. Articulatory defects in aphasia: The problem of Broca's aphemia. In H. Goodglass and S. Blumstein (eds) *Psycho-linguistics and Aphasia* (1973), pp. 51–68. Baltimore: Johns Hopkins University Press.

DARLEY, F.L., ARONSON, A.E. and BROWN, J.E. *Motor Speech Disorders* (1975). W.B. Sanders.

DEAJURIAGUERRA, J. and TISSOT, R. The Apraxias. N P.J. Vinken and G.W. Bruyn (eds) *Handbook of Clinical Neurology: Disorders of Speech, Perception and symbolic behavior.* Volume 4. (1975), p. 48–66. New York: American Elsevier Publishing.

DEJERINE, J. *Semiologie des Affections du System Nerveux* (1914). Paris: Masson.

DESIMONI, F. and DARLEY, F.L. Effect on phoneme duration control of three utterance-length conditions in an apractic patient. *Journal Speech Hearing Disorders* (1977) **42**, 257–264.

GOLDSTEIN, K. *Language and Language Disturbances* (1948). New York: Grune and Stratton.

GOODGLASS, H. and BLUMSTEIN, S. (eds) *Psycholinguistics and Aphasia* (1973). Baltimore: Johns Hopkins University Press.

GOODGLASS, H. and KAPLAN, E. *The Assessment of Aphasia and Related Disorders* (1976). Philadelphia: Lea and Febiger.

HEAD, H. *Aphasia and Kindred Disorders of Speech*. Volume 1 (1926). Cambridge University Press.

JAKOBSON, R. *Child Language, Aphasia and Phonological Universals* (1968). New York: Humantities Press.

JAKOBSON, R. Sur la theorie des affinities phonologique entre les langues. In Roman Jakonson *Selected writings* (1971). The Hague: Mouton.

LESSER, R. *Linguistic Investigations of Aphasia* (1978). New York: Elsevier Inc.

MARIE, P. Aphasics; their clinical examination. Journal de Medicine Interne **9** 219–222 (205) and reproduced in translation in M.F. Cole and M. Coles (eds) *Pierre Marie's Papers on Speech Disorders* (1971), 43–49. New York: Hafner Publishing Co.

MARTIN, A.D. Aphasia testing: a second look at the Porch Index of Communicative Ability. *Journal of Speech and Hearing Disorders* (1977), **42** 547–562.

MARTIN, A.D. An examination of Wepman's thought centred therapy. In R. Chapey (ed.) *Language intervention strategies in adult aphasia* (1981a). Baltimore, Maryland: William and Wilkins.

MARTIN, A.D. Therapy with the jargonaphasic. In J. Brown (ed.) *Jargonaphasia* (1981b). New York: Academic Press.

MARTIN, A.D. The role of theory in therapy: a rationale. *Topics in language Disorders* (1981), **1** 63–72.

MARTIN, A.D. Levels of reference in aphasia therapy. In R. Brookshire (ed.) *Clinical Aphasiology Conference Proceedings* (1979). Minneapolis, Minn.: BRK.
MUMA, J.R. The communication game: Dump and play. *Journal of Speech and Hearing Disorders* (1975), **40**, 296–309.
PICK, A. *Aphasia* (Edited and translated by Jason Brown) (1973). Springfield, Illinois: Charles C. Thomas, Publisher.
SCHEFLEN, A.E. *Communicational Structure: Analysis of a Psycho-therapy Transaction* (1973). Bloomingtin, Indiana: Indiana University Press.
SCHUELL, H. *The Minnesota Test for Differential Diagnosis of Aphasia* (1965). Minneapolis University Press.
WATZLAWICK, P., BEAVIN, J. and JACKSON, D. *Pragmatics of Human Communication* (1967). New York: W.W. Norton.
WEISENBURG, T. and MCBRIDE, K.E. *Aphasia* (1935). Philadelphia, Penna: The Commonwealth Fund.
WEPMAN, J. *Recovery in Aphasia* (1951). Chicago: Ronald Press.
WEPMAN, J. Aphasia therapy: A New Look. *Journal of Speech and Hearing Disorders* (1972), **37**, 203–214.
WEPMAN, J. and JONES, L. *The Language Modalities Test for Aphasia* (1961). Chicago, Illinois: Education Industry Service.
WHITAKER, H.A. and WHITAKER, H. Linguistic theory and speech pathology. *Journal Minnesota Speech and Hearing Association* (1972), **11** 51–56.

17

Assessing Disorders of Gesture

Nancy Helm-Estabrooks

The primary focus of this chapter is the assessment of disorders of gesture associated with acquired brain damage. First, the most common of these disorders will be described. These then will be discussed *vis-à-vis* their relation to other acquired neurobehavioral disorders. Finally, a format for evaluating gestural disorders will be presented.

Definitions of Gestural Disorders

The study of gestural disorders is complicated by at least two factors: (1) the variety of classification terms which have been used by its investigators and (2) the variety of behaviours which are considered to be some form of gesture. A few examples may suffice in making this point. Critchley (1970) distinguishes the use of *pantomime*, in which propositional gestures replace speech, from *gesticulation* in which automatic, emotional gestures accompany speech. Goodglass and Kaplan (1963) class gesture into four types:

1. *Natural gestures*, e.g. holding one's nose when smelling something unpleasant.
2. *Conventional gestures*, e.g. saluting.
3. *Simple pantomimes* comprised of a single, perhaps repetitive movement e.g. playing the piano.
4. *Complex pantomimes* comprised of sequential, different movements, e.g. enacting a jewelry 'hold-up'.

Gainotti and Lemmo (1976) distinguish *symbolic gestures* defined as 'common used conventionalized, communicative movements' (e.g. sign of the cross) from *simple pantomimes* defined as 'direct representations of actions with objects' (e.g. playing the guitar). When discussing gestural disorders in general, these investigators and others use the term 'apraxia'. A description of apraxia is warranted, therefore, in any chapter devoted to gestural disorders.

Geschwind's (1975) definition of apraxia as 'a disorder of learned movements which cannot be accounted for by weakness, sensory loss, incoordination, inattention or comprehension deficit' is commonly cited.

It was Liepmann (1908), however, who first comprehensively defined and delineated apraxia and placed it within a neuroanatonimical framework, although this phenomenon had been described briefly by earlier clinicians such as Jackson (1864). Liepmann described three varieties of apraxia: limb kinetic apraxia, ideational apraxia and ideomotor apraxia.

Limb-kinetic apraxia is 'the loss of kinetic memories for one limb'. Currently doubt exists as to whether this disorder can be distinguished from the motor signs of mild paresis (Hecaen and Albert, 1978).

Ideational apraxia is considered to be a higher level disorder in which individual movements are intact but there is failure to execute complex sequential movements with objects or to misuse an object, e.g. putting the match instead of the cigarette in the mouth. This form of apraxia is considered by many to be a severe form of ideomotor apraxia (Kertesz, 1979).

Ideomotor apraxia is the inability either to imitate, or initiate upon command, movements which may be associated with real or pretended objects. Of the three varieties of apraxia, ideomotor apraxia is the most common, the easiest to investigate, and may be of the greatest importance to aphasia rehabilitation.

The patient with ideomotor apraxia will have difficulty producing upon command or in imitation purposeful learned movements or gestures either with the oral apparatus or with the hand/arm or both. If ideomotor apraxia also impairs the spontaneous or responsive production of symbolic gestures in natural settings, then the patient's communication skills will be compromised. Should this be the case, then careful diagnosis and treatment of the apraxia is warranted. If ideomotor apraxia does not relate to the patient's ability to self-initiate representational movements, then it may be of little more than academic interest to the aphasia therapist. Thus the relationships between aphasia, apraxia, and the natural use of symbolic gestures must be explored more fully. The following review is illustrative of some work directed at resolving these issues.

Apraxia and Aphasia

Investigations of Apraxia and Aphasia

In 1905 Liepmann reported that clinical examination of 89 brain injured patients showed that a high incidence of left hand apraxia occurred in patients with right hemiplegia and aphasia. A much lower incidence of left hand apraxia was found in patients with right hemiplegia without aphasia. Of the 20 cases with left hemisphere lesions and left limb apraxia examined, 14 had aphasia and 6 did not. Liepmann concluded that the left hemisphere is responsible for purposeful movements. More specifically, he associated supracapsular (aphasia producing) lesions of the left hemisphere with apraxia, explaining that such lesions damage commisural fibers from left brain to right brain thus causing abnormal performance with the left hand. Although presence of aphasia was considered to be evidence of a supracapsular lesion site, Liepmann states that lesions between posterior frontal and parietal areas could affect gestural ability independent of the presence or severity of aphasia.

Following Liepmann's study of the relationship between apraxia and aphasia, this subject remained relatively unexplored until 1963 when Goodglass and Kaplan undertook a major investigation of two groups of brain-damaged patients. Group I consisted of twenty predominantly expressive aphasic patients whose scores on subsections of the Boston Diagnostic Aphasia Examination ranged from the moderate to mild levels of impairment. Group II consisted of nineteen, non-aphasic brain-injured control subjects. Three sets of tests were administered to each subject: (1) Gesture-Pantomime Test; (2) Aphasia Examination; (3) Wechsler Adult Intelligence Performance Scale. The gesture pantomime test included verbally presented commands to perform (1) natural expressive gestures, such as covering the ears to show it is noisy; (2) conventional gestures such as the 'okay' sign; and (3) simple pantomiming of an action with an object, such as eating corn off the cob. In addition, one pantomimed expression task was performed while looking at pictures of objects. Patients were also examined for the ability to comprehend complex narrative pantomimes acted out by the examiner. Finally, the patient was asked to imitate natural, conventional and object-pantomimes performed by the examiner. Several of the findings are relevant to the issue of apraxia's relationship to aphasia. First, the gestural performance by aphasic patients was inferior to their brain-injured, intellectual counterparts both in response to commands and in imitation. Second, gestural ability was not related to severity of aphasia when auditory comprehension was controlled. Third, left hemisphere lesioned patients without an associated aphasia were more impaired in gestural performance than right hemisphere lesioned patients. Fourth, gestural performance was directly related to intellectual efficiency (as measured by the performance subsection of the WAIS) in brain injured patients irrespective of aphasia. The authors conclude that although aphasic patients may have an apraxic disorder following a left hemisphere lesion, the findings did not support the concept that apraxia is part of a general, communication disorder.

In the two decades since this landmark study several other investigations have sought to clarify the relationship between apraxia and aphasia by altering both subject and test variables. A few of those studies will be highlighted here. Dee, Benton and Van Allen (1970) for example, studied five groups of right handed, brain damaged patients. Two groups were not aphasic: (1) non-aphasic with right hemisphere lesions; (2) non-aphasic with left hemisphere lesions. Three groups were aphasic: (3) mild; (4) moderate; and (5) severe aphasia according to scores earned on The Token Test (DeRenzi and Vignolo, 1962). Ten skills were tested, first in 32 controls to determine norms and then with the brain damaged groups. Four of the tests measured ideomotor limb apraxia:

1. Production of symbolic actions to verbal command, e.g. 'salute'.
2. Imitation of symbolic actions.
3. Use of actual objects.
4. Manual pantomimed use of unseen objects.

Three tests were used to measure ideomotor oral apraxia:

5. Oral pantomimed use of unseen objects.
6. Production of oral actions to command, e.g. 'whistle'.
7. Imitation of oral actions.

The remaining three tests measured:

8. Imitation of non-symbolic actions.
9. Construction of block designs.
10. Reproduction of drawn designs.

The findings led to the general observation that apraxia is more prevalent among brain-damaged subjects than had been supposed. More specifically, the authors concluded that while ideomotor apraxia and aphasia are associated closely with the left hemisphere and with each other, apraxia cannot be explained in terms of either an aphasic disorder or a motor impairment. They go on to say that the mechanisms which subserve the production of meaningful gestures on command may be closely allied to the mechanisms which subserve language but they are distinguishable from them.

In a gesture study which used the Porch Index of Communicative Ability (Porch, 1971) as the language measure, Pickett (1974) reached a different conclusion from previous investigators. Using the same ten objects employed in the PICA, Pickett carried out 8 experimental tasks with 28 aphasic patients. Six of the tasks examined gesture and pantomime. These included:

1. Producing gestures for the pictured objects.
2. Manipulating the real objects.
3. Matching pictured gestures with the pictured objects.
4. Matching live pantomimes with the gestured objects.
5. Gesturing to command.
6. Imitating gestures.

Two additional tasks were:

7. Naming objects placed in hand
8. Matching object in hand with picture.

Three of these tasks (i.e. tasks 2, 7, 8) closely resemble subtests of the PICA, (i.e. II, III, IV, VIII). Pickett found strong positive correlations between the severity of aphasia and 'gestural ability', and concluded that, because the majority of patients showed improved gesturing with imitation, gestural deficits are part of a total communication problem and do not result from limb apraxia.

Somewhat different conclusions were drawn by Gainotti and Lemmo in 1976, who compared the ability of 53 aphasic, 26 non-aphasic left brain damaged, 49 right brain damaged and 25 normal subjects to recognize and produce symbolic gestures and to discriminate 'verbal sound and meaning'. Interpretation of symbolic gestures was tested by asking subjects to point to the pictured object which related to the pantomime produced by the examiner. Production of symbolic gestures, i.e. the ideomotor apraxia test required subjects to execute symbolic gestures in response to verbal command. If performance was less than satisfactory, a model was presented for imitation. It is unclear how discrimination of 'verbal sound and meaning' was tested, but the task is reported to yield an index of verbal semantic impairment in contrast to the test of symbolic gesture interpretation thought to yield an index of nonverbal semantic disintegration. When performance on all three tests were compared, it was found that:

1. The aphasic group had significantly more difficulty in interpreting symbolic gestures.
2. A significant, positive correlation existed between verbal semantic and non-verbal symbolic scores of aphasic patients.
3. There was no significant correlation between gestural comprehension and gestural production scores of aphasic patients.

In view of the findings, the authors hypothesize that individuals tend to use verbal labels when asked to interpret gestures. If language is impaired at the semantic level, and thus interferes with verbal mediation, then gesture interpretation also may be impaired, that is, a semantic level anomia may influence gestural interpretation scores. Furthermore, the finding that almost two thirds of the aphasic patients could not understand the meaning of simple, symbolic gestures indicated to the investigators that 'a nuclear disintegration' exists in aphasia. Finally, because only a slight relationship was found between interpretation and production of symbolic gestures, Gainotti and Lemmo conclude that gestural production difficulty results from a true apraxic disorder and not from poor comprehension of gestures.

A more recent Italian study examined ideomotor apraxia through response to imitative tasks (DeRenzi, Motti and Nichelli, 1980). A total 280 right-handed patients were asked to imitate sequential and non-sequential, symbolic and non-symbolic gestures produced with either fingers or hands. An example of a sequential, symbolic, finger movement is snapping one's fingers, while an example of a non-sequential, non-symbolic hand movement is holding one's hand, palm down, horizontally, under the chin. In addition to 100 non-brain damaged controls used to establish norms, 80 right hemisphere, 40 non-aphasia left hemisphere and 60 aphasic left hemisphere patients were studied. The aphasic group was further classified as to either Wernicke's, Broca's, global, conduction or anomic aphasia according to a standard aphasia battery and The Token Test. Poor imitative performance was highly associated with aphasia (80% in the apraxic range). When scores were analyzed according to aphasia classification, all global patients, 88% of Wernicke's patients, plus 86% of Broca's patients were apraxic. Of these, all but one global, 56% of the Wernicke's, and 43% of the Broca's patients, were severely impaired. Only one of the five conduction and none of the four anomic patients were impaired. When Token Test scores were correlated with imitation test scores, a significant correlation of 0.56 was found to exist. Comparisons of scores earned on the various categories of movements showed that all were suited to eliciting apraxia. On the basis of these findings, DeRenzi, Motti and Nichelli reached the following conclusions regarding aphasia and apraxia:

1. It is hard to explain impaired ability to imitate movements on the basis of a language disorder, particularly given the similarly poor performance on both symbolic and non-symbolic gestures.
2. Although a significant correlation was found between Token Test scores and imitation scores, it was not high enough to warrant the inference that praxis performance is dependent on language performance. Instead, they state that it is more reasonable to assume that the lesion which produces apraxia often encroaches on cerebral language areas.

In support of these conclusions they cite the clinical observations of patients who have severe apraxia coexisting with mild aphasia.

In two separate papers, Duffy, Duffy and Pearson (1975) and Duffy and Duffy (1981) take a somewhat different approach to investigating the relationship between limb apraxia and aphasia. These investigators distinguish manual apraxia that is 'imitative motor responses' from pantomime, that is, the deliberate use of bodily or manual movements to convey a message in the absence of speech. Their 1981 publication describes three studies, one of which replicates the 1975 study of pantomime recognition, and another examined the relationship between aphasia and the recognition and production of pantomime. The third study examined *four hypotheses* regarding pantomimic deficit: (1) pantomimic deficits are the result of intellectual deterioration; (2) pantomimic deficits are caused by limb apraxia; (3) pantomimic deficits are the result of a central symbolic disorder; and (4) pantomimic deficits are caused by verbal mediation deficits. Duffy and Duffy tested 47 mostly non-fluent aphasic, 27 right brain damaged and 11 control subjects. The pantomime recognition test required subjects to point to 46 pictured objects whose use is pantomimed by the examiner. The pantomime expression test required subjects to produce pantomimes for 23 of the 46 pictured objects. The test of manual apraxia consisted of 80 imitative tasks. The Raven's Progressive Matrices was the test of intelligence. In addition 3 'verbal' tests were used: (1) the entire Porch Index of Communicative Ability; (2) recognition of spoken name of each of the 46 pictured objects used in the pantomime recognition test; (3) naming each of the same 46 pictured items. Based on the findings Duffy and Duffy reach the following *four conclusions*:

1. Pantomimic deficits are not caused by general intellectual deficits in aphasic persons.
2. Limb apraxia may interfere with pantomimic skills but it is not the most potent factor contributing to pantomimic deficits.
3. A central symbolic disorder underlies both verbal and non-verbal (pantomimic) communicative deficits.
4. Pantomimic deficits may be caused by defects in verbal mediation.

Kertesz and Hooper (1982) studied the praxis and language skills of 230 aphasic patients grouped into eight diagnostic categories and 25 controls. The controls consisted of 21 non-brain damaged patients, 72 non-aphasic patients with right hemisphere lesions and 32 non-aphasic patients with left hemisphere lesions. The apraxia test consisted of 20 items in four categories: (1) facial, e.g. put out your tongue; (2) upper limb, e.g. scratch your head; (3) transitive, e.g. use a key; (4) complex, e.g. pretend to play the piano. Subjects were asked to produce movements upon command. If no response or only amorphous, approximate reponses were given, then the examiner modeled the movement for imitation. Real objects were available for eight objects and offered when the patient failed to even imitate an appropriate movement. A four point scoring system was used: a score of 3 indicated a good performance either to command or imitation, 2 indicated that the movement was impaired but recognizable, and a score of 1 was given if the patient performed adequately with a real object. Finally, a score of zero was assigned for no performance, unrecognizable performance or unrelated gesturing, or completely erroneous use of objects. The language exam consisted of the oral subtest (including auditory comprehension) of the Western Aphasia Battery (WAB) and reading and writing tests. In addition, tests of calculation, drawing, block designs and the Raven's Colored Progressive Matrices were given.

Kertesz and Hooper found that apraxia correlated best with comprehension deficit (0.76) and severity of aphasia (0.73). The next highest correlations occurred between the apraxia and the drawing subtest scores. Facial apraxia was significantly correlated with verbal output measures such as fluency and repetition (0.64). Global aphasic patients were the most apractic. The pattern across groups was for transitive and complex movements to be more affected than facial and intransitive upper limb movements. Apraxia was associated with both anterior and posterior aphasia producing lesions. Perhaps surprisingly, non-aphasic patients with left hemisphere damage had slightly better praxis scores than right brain-damaged patients. According to the authors, this suggested that the left hemisphere is not dominant for movements in its entirety, but that apraxia is closely related to those areas of the brain which subserve language. They caution, however, that language impairment and apraxia do not always coincide, but instead there are patients with significant apraxia but no significant language impairment and vice versa.

This review is far from complete. Other studies were published between 1963 and 1986 and because many of the issues concerning apraxia and aphasia remain unresolved, new studies appear yearly.

Summary and Discussion of Apraxia/Aphasia Investigations

Investigators of apraxia generally agree that disorders of learned movement are highly associated with left hemisphere damage. Beyond that, Liepmann (1908), Goodglass and Kaplan (1963), Dee, Benton and Van Allen (1970), DeRenzi, Motti and Nichelli (1980) and Kertesz and Hooper (1982) believe that ideomotor apraxia is closely associated with, but not the result of, aphasia. Gainotti and Lemmo (1976) distinguish gestural production disorders caused by apraxia from gestural recognition disorders caused by a 'nuclear disintegration' associated with aphasia. Finally, Pickett (1974) and Duffy and Duffy (1981) believe that gestural disorders in general are related directly to a central language deficit and are not simply the result of limb apraxia.

At least three factors may account for the differences in opinion regarding the relationship betwen aphasia and apraxia: (1) the aphasia population studies, (2) the aphasia test used, and (3) the apraxia test used. Each of these factors will be discussed.

The Aphasia population

One variable that may account for the different conclusions drawn by the investigators cited above is composition of the aphasia groups. Goodglass and Kaplan (1963) and Duffy and Duffy (1981) examined predominantly expressive or non-fluent aphasic subjects, while DeRenzi, Motti and Nichelli (1980) and Kertesz and Hooper (1982) examined both fluent and non-fluent subjects. Dee, Benton and Van Allen (1980), Pickett (1974) and Gainotti and Lemmo (1976) did not classify their aphasic patients. It is known that specific aphasia syndromes can be correlated with specific neuroanatomical lesion sites (Naeser and Hayward, 1978). It may be that gestural disorders also can be correlated with specific lesion sites so that the population of aphasic patients used in a study of apraxia predetermines, in part, the findings. For example, facial apraxia is more prevalent in non-fluent Broca's aphasic patients with anterior lesions than in those with fluent posterior aphasic syndromes such as Wernicke's aphasia (DeRenzi, Pieczuro and Vignolo, 1966).

The Aphasia test

Another factor which may account for the aphasia/apraxia controversy is the nature of the test used to assess language in these studies. Goodglass and Kaplan (1963) measured aphasia according to Boston Diagnostic Aphasia Exam conversation and narrative speech, object naming and auditory comprehension performance. Performance on the verbal tasks may be influenced by bucco/facial apraxia whereas performance on auditory comprehension tests may be influenced by limb apraxia. Dee, Benton and Van Allen (1970) and DeRenzi, Motti and Nichelli (1980) used the Token Test to measure severity of aphasia. In a discussion which follows the Dee *et al.* report, Geschwind (1970) suggests that the Token Test, which requires patients to manipulate plastic shapes, may itself be a test of praxis. On the basis of this, Geschwind questioned their conclusion that apraxia is significantly correlated with receptive aphasia.

Pickett (1974) and Duffy and Duffy (1981) measured aphasia with the Porch Index of Communicative Ability in which various tasks are carried out with ten common objects. Eight of the sixteen subtests of the PICA are classified as 'gestural'. Of the eight, two subjects (II and III) require 'the patient to demonstrate the function of each test object through pantomime' (Porch, 1971, p. 28). In other words, the aphasia test itself contained pantomimic tasks which may have contributed to the high correlation found between PICA scores and the experimental gestural test. Furthermore, Pickett used the ten PICA objects in his experimental tasks and three of his experimental tasks closely resemble PICA tasks.

Finally, Gainotti and Lemmo used 'a standard test of aphasia' which is not described, so that one cannot determine the extent to which the language test performance may have been influenced by gestural/praxis skills.

The Apraxia test

Not only have investigators of the relationship between apraxia and aphasia utilized different tests of aphasia, they have used a variety of approaches to examination of apraxia. Goodglass and Kaplan tested apraxia by requiring patients to follow commands, imitate gestures, produce gestures to pictured objects and recognize pantomimes. Only symbolic gestures were examined. Responses were scored as adequate (Level I), partially adequate (Level II), inadequate (Level III), and further differentiated into 4 qualitative categories. Dee, Benton and Van Allen used similar tasks employing symbolic gestures but included manipulation of real objects and non-symbolic gestures. Pickett also required patients to manipulate real objects as well as pantomiming but he added a naming and a picture-object matching test. Gestural performance was rated according to a PICA 15 point scoring system. Gainotti and Lemmo limited themselves to recognition and production-upon-command of symbolic gestures which were scored 1 point for correct. DeRenzi, Motti and Nichelli used only imitative tasks but specified gestures as sequential, non-sequential, symbolic and non-symbolic and assigned them scores of 3. 2, 1, 0 points for flawless performance on 1st, 2nd, 3rd, or none of the trials. Kertesz and Hooper (1982) also used a four point scoring system but they tested gestural performance to command, to imitation and with the use of some real objects. They did not penalize the patient for failing to respond, but scored 3 if a good performance was given to either command or imitation. Finally, Duffy and Duffy separated their test of manual apraxia which required patients to imitate 80 upper limb movements from the experimental tasks which tested recognition of pantomimes produced by the experimenter and production of pantomimes for pictured objects. A PICA 16 point multidimensional scoring system was used.

Because these studies yield conflicting results, it may be that the nature of the pantomime tasks called upon differing neuroanatomical regions and pathways. These skills, therefore, may be differentially affected by brain damage. If this is the case, then apraxia should not be regarded as a unitary disorder. Instead, it would appear more profitable to test the ability of patients to produce meaningful gestures in response to imitation, command and pictures with the realization that each task may test different skills along a hierarchy of representational organization. Furthermore, some patients are not particularly apraxic on formal testing, but fail to produce representational gestures in conversation. The opposite may be true of other patients who may be apraxic according to formal tests but produce appropriate gestures in real life situations. DeRenzi, Motti and Nichelli suggest that in these latter patients the motor patterns still exist, but that they are accessible only under highy stimulative conditions. Therefore, when considering gestural disorders, one should note gestures produced in natural settings as well as those produced in response to formal testing.

Spontaneous Gestures and Aphasia

Compared with the study of apraxia relatively little attention has been given to the spontaneous use of gestures by aphasic patients but two such studies were completed in 1979. One investigated the relationship between spontaneous and elicited gesturing and naming performance of 20 aphasic patients, none of who had severe limb apraxia (Helm, 1979), while the other examined spontaneous gestures used by four aphasic patients and four normal controls during structured interviews (Cicone *et al.*, 1979).

The purpose of the first study was to explore a series of questions, two of which are important to us here:

1. Do Broca's, Wernicke's, conduction and anomic patients differentially employ spontaneous gestures during a verbal confrontation naming task?
2. Do these gestures, like aphasic verbal responses, vary in quality?

A videotape format allowed for fine analysis of gestures produced spontaneously while naming 40 items.

Analysis of the videotapes showed that different aphasic groups varied in both the quantity and quality of the spontaneous gestures produced during confrontation naming. While naming, Broca's patients produced at least one gesture in association with the greatest number of pictured items, but these gestures were only of the third highest representational quality of the four groups. The Wernicke's patients rated second to the Broca's group in the frequency of gesturing, but the quality of their gestures exceeded all other groups.

Patients with conduction aphasia produced gestures in association with the fewest number of pictures, but the representational quality of these gestures was very good, second only to the Wernicke's patients. Finally, the anomic patients produced gestures for the third lowest number of pictures and these gestures were the poorest in representational quality. Of particular interest to us here is the fact that the anomic group was the least apraxic according to an independent test of praxis skills. Once again it should be noted that no group was severely apraxic.

Videotapes were used also by Cicone *et al.* (1979). Two Broca's and two Wernicke's patients as well as four non-neurological control subjects were interviewed for 30–45 minuts. Conversational topics were chosen to elicit gestures relating to *time*, e.g. 'How long have you been in the hospital?', *space* e.g. 'How did we get to this floor?' and *self* e.g. 'Do you have any hobbies?' One of the Broca's patients was significantly apraxic. Gestural performance was analyzed according to physical parameters, its temporal relationship to the stream of speech, and its semantic and pragmatic value. It was found that the gestural performance of Broca's and Wernicke's patients closely resembled their verbal performance. The Broca's patients tended to produce simple, unelaborated, highly referential gestures which were generally clear but sparse. Wernicke's patients produced copious gestures, many of which were elaborated, complex and nonreferential. The investigators tentatively concluded that either self-formulated gesturing is dependent directly upon language or that a 'central organizer' underlies both speech and gesture. Damage to this 'central organizer' will affect both speech and gesture equally.

The results of these two studies of spontaneous gesturing in aphasia suggest that different diagnostic groups of aphasic patients have differential capacities for producing self-initiated and self-formulated gestures. While spontaneous gestural behaviours may resemble language behaviours, they may be independent of apraxia and severity of aphasia, when global patients are excluded. It would appear, therefore, that a comprehensive evaluation of gestural skills should include both an apraxia examination and a tool for noting spontaneous use of gestures. Suggested formats for testing both these skills will be presented below.

A Test for Apraxia

The above review showed that praxis may be tested and scored in various ways. The approach described here is that currently in use by the Speech Pathology Service at the Boston Veterans Administration Medical Center. During the years following the deveolopment of our first formal praxis exam, several revisions have taken place. For example, at one time the exam contained a subsection which tested non-representational movements. Because this information did not prove particularly helpful either for prognosing language recovery or for treatment planning, it was eliminated. The present exam, while perhaps not as detailed as others, is relatively easy to administer and score and appears to provide sufficient information regarding apraxia to manage aphasia patients from the rehabilitation perspective.

It includes subtests of facial and limb praxis and pantomime, with limb praxis divided into the subcategories of intransitive movements, transitive movements and finger movements. Items are administered both to command and to imitation and a four point (0–3) scoring system is used (*see* Appendix I).

A Non-vocal Behaviour Rating Scale

The studies by Helm (1979) and Cicone *et al.* (1979) cited above suggest that aphasic patients may have a different capacity for producing spontaneous gestures, than for producing elicited gestures in response to an apraxia test. For this reason a scale for rating spontaneous non-vocal behaviour was developed by Borod, Fitzpatrick, Helm-Estabrooks and Goodglass (1984).

This seven item Nonvocal Communication Scale (NVS) rates behaviours ranging from greetings and pointing to narrative pantomimes which are observed to occur in natural settings. In a feasibility study of the scales, 41 severely aphasic patients were rated by family members, nurses, neurologists, speech/language pathologists and other rehabilitation specialists. The ratings were examined in relationship to a range of cognitive variables. Performance as rated on the NVS appeared not to be dependent on auditory comprehension or general intellectual functioning. Performance, however, was related to limb praxis and constructional ability. The Non-vocal Communication Scale appears in Appendix II.

Gestural Disorders: Summary and Conclusions

Gestural disorders are associated most commonly with left hemisphere brain damage. Because aphasia also is associated with damage to the left hemisphere, the two disorders often co-exist. There are conflicting opinions, however, as to the correlation between the severity of the gestural disorder and the severity of aphasia. As discussed above, part of the conflict may be a result of different approaches to testing gestural disorders and aphasia. Despite the differences of opinion, it probably is safe to conclude that in addition to verbal language problems, aphasic patients also may have difficulty producing gestures and that this difficulty may interfere with or reduce the overall level of communicative effectiveness. It behooves the aphasia therapist, therefore, to examine the patient's capacity for producing a variety of gestures under various circumstances. In this chapter formats for examining praxis, pantomime and spontaneous gesture skills are offered. The aphasia therapist is encouraged to make these or similar tests part of their examination armamentarium along with tests of speech and language functions. In 1975 Geschwind stated 'It is not unreasonable to assume that the more completely we understand some of these (learned movement) disorders, the more likely we will be able to devise rationally designed therapies for many disabilities.' That possibility will be explored in Chapter 19.

Appendix I: Boston Praxis Examination

Pt:............................ Dx:............................ Onset:............................
BDAE Severity Rating............. Examiner............................ Date ....

Facial praxis:	Overall Score:	/30	*Facial apraxia:*
	Command:	/15	Absent (28–30).................
	Imitation:	/15	Mild (20–27).....................
			Moderate (10–19)...........
			Severe (0–9).......................
Limb praxis	*Overall Score:*	*/84*	*Limb apraxia:*
	Intransitive Total:	/24	Absent (80–84).................
	Command:	/12	Mild (65–79.......................
	Imitation:	/12	Moderate (40–64)...........
			Severe (0–39)....................
Hand Used .... Dom. Hand			
	Transitive Total:	/36	
	Command:	/18	
	Imitation:	/18	
	Fingers Total:	/24	
	Command:	/12	
	Imitation:	/12	
Pantomime:	Total Score:	/27	*Pantomimic skills:*
			Good (21–27) ....
			Fair (12–20).......................
			Poor (0–11).......................

General instructions:
1 Test each item first to command. Begin by telling the patient that you are going to ask him/her to do some things without talking. Then say, 'Show me how you . . .'. If the response to command is less than normal (3), then test to imitation while again presenting the verbal command, e.g. 'show me how you cough. Like this (examiner coughs).' If the command score for any item is 3, simply assign 3 to that item for imitation. N.B. Restrain the patient from cueing self with hands, e.g. holding 'a flower' while pretending to sniff.

Scoring System

3 — Normal:	Completely normal performance for the dominant or nondominant hand. There is no notable hesitancy, fumbling or self-correction.
2 — Adequate:	Patient may hesitate or spontaneously self-correct performance, or movement may lack sharpness, although crucial components are present. For example, the patient may 'turn a screwdriver' with the correct holding pattern and movement, but without using empty space to represent the extent of the pretended object.
1 — Partially Adequate:	Some basic components of the gesture are retained but the plane may be incorrect e.g. brushing teeth with finger; or there may the correct holding pattern but no movement; or the patient verbalizes rather than performing silently, e.g. some blowing while saying 'blow, blow'.
0 — Inadequate:	Lacking any of the crucial components of the target, e.g. saying 'cough, cough' without actually coughing; or simply pointing to the head for combing hair; or perseverative reponses.

Limb praxis (intransitive)

Instructions: Use the command 'With your hand, show me how you . . . Do not talk.' If the score is less than 3, repeat the command, but provide a model for imitation. If the score is 3 for any item, simply check 3 for imitation. Note which hand was used.

Task	*To command*				*To imitation*			
	3	*2*	*1*	*0*	*3*	*2*	*1*	*0*
1. Wave 'Goodbye'								
2. Wipe Forehead as if hot								
3. Salute								
4. Stop traffic with hand								

Overall Score: /24 **Command: /12** **Imitation: /12**

HAND USED: . . . . . .

Facial Praxis

Instructions: Test all items first to command. Begin by telling the patient that you are going to ask him/her to do some things without talking. Then say, 'Show me how you . . .'. If the response to command is less than normal (3) then test to imitation while again presenting the verbal command, e.g. 'Show me how you cough. Like this . . . (examiner coughs).' If the command score for any item is 3, simply assign 3 to that item for imitation. N.B. Restrain the patient from cueing self with hands, e.g. holding 'a flower' while sniffing.

Task	*To command*				*To imitation*			
	3	*2*	*1*	*0*	*3*	*2*	*1*	*0*
1. Cough								
2. Blow out a candle								
3. Sip through a straw								
4. Lick crumbs from your lips								
5. Sniff a flower								

Overall Score: /30	Command: /15	Imitation: /15

Finger Praxis

Instructions: The same as limb praxis except the command is 'With your fingers, show me how you . . . Do not talk'. If patient uses the wrong finger, e.g. pointing with the thumb instead of index finger or the wrong number of fingers, assign a score of 1.

Task	*To command*				*To imitation*			
	3	*2*		*0*	*3*	*2*	*1*	*0*
1. Point to the ceiling								
2. Thumb a ride								
3. Make an okay sign								
4. Make a 'V' for victory (peace)								

Overall Score: /24	Command: /12	Imitation: /12
Hand used:		

Limb Praxis (Transitive)

Instructions: Same as for intransitive limb praxis: 'Without talking show me how you would . . .'.

Task	*Command*				*Imitation*			
	3	*2*	*1*	*0*	*3*	*2*	*1*	*0*
1. Brush your teeth with a toothbrush								
2. Comb your hair with a comb								
3. Shave with a razor								
4. Pound a nail with a hammer								
5. Turn a screw with a screwdriver								
6. Stir coffee with a spoon								
Overall score: /36	Command: /18				Imitation: /18			
	Hand used:							

Pantomime

Instructions: Present pictures of the following items and say 'Without talking, show me something about these pictures by pretending they are real. For example, if these scissors (show picture) were real I would pretend to cut like this (demonstrate gesture). Now you try it. (encourage/help patient to produce 'writing' gesture). Okay, now you show me about this one.' (Show picture of hammer). Discourage patient from verbalizing.

Picture	*Score*			
	3	*2*	*1*	*0*
1. Hammer				
2. Large spoon in pot				
3. Screwdriver				
4. Comb				
5. Razor				
6. Toothbrush				
7. Straw in soda bottle				
8. Lighted candle				
9. Flower				
Overall Score: /27	Hand used:			

Appendix II: Non vocal Communication Scale Aphasia Research Center, Boston, VAMC

Patient's name.. SS# ....
Rater's name.. Date ....
Overall NVCS Score .... Onset date................................ BDAE severity rating..........

Directions: For each level of gestural behaviour make a judgement as to whether it occurs on a regular basis, an occasional basis, or never occurs. Circle the appropriate number on each line.

	Never	*Occasional*		*Regular*
1. Gestures to greet or to summon attention Examples:	0	1	2	3
2. Indicates by leading you to something Examples:	0	1	2	3
3. Communicates by pointing Examples:	0	1	2	3
4. Uses pantomime to show states of mind Examples:	0	1	2	3
5. Indicates yes/no correctly Examples:	0	1	2	3
6. Uses pantomime or drawings to show single things/actions Examples:	0	1	2	3
7. Uses connective narrative or drawings to tell stories Examples:	0	1	2	3

References

BOROD, J., FITZPATRICK, P. HELM-ESTABROOKS, N. and GOODGLASS, H. A scale for evaluating non vocal communication in aphasic patients. Paper presented at the *Academy of Aphasia Annual Meeting, Los Angeles, California, October, 1984.*

CICONE, M., WAPNER, W., FOLDI, N., ZURIF, E. and GARDNER, H. The relationship between gesture and language in aphasic communication. *Brain and Language* (1979), **8**, 324–349.

DEE, H.L., BENTON, A.L. and VAN ALLEN, M.W. Apraxia in relation to hemispheric locus of lesion and aphasia, *Transactions of the Neurological Association* (1970), **95** 147–150.

DERENZI, E. and VIGNOLO, L. The token test: a sensitive test to detect receptive disturbances in aphasia, *Brain* (1962), **85**, 665–678.

DERENZI, E., PIECZURO, A. and VIGNOLO, L. Oral apraxia and aphasia. *Cortex* (1966), **2**, 50–73.

DERENZI, E., MOTTI, F. and NICHELLI, P. Imitating gestures: a quantitative approach to ideomotor apraxia. *Archives of Neurology* (1980), **37**, 6–10.

DUFFY, R.J., DUFFY, J.R. and PEARSON, K.L. Pantomime recognition in aphasia, *Journal of Speech and Hearing Research* (1975), 3 18, 115–132.

DUFFY, R.J. and DUFFY, J.R. Three studies of deficits in pantomimic expression and pantomimic recognition in aphasia, *Journal of Speech and Hearing Research* (1981), 70–84.

GAINOTTI, G. and LEMMO, M.A. Comprehension of symbolic gestures in aphasia, *Brain and Language* (1976), **3** 451–460.

GESCHWIND, N. The apraxias: Neurological mechanisms of disorders of learned movements, *American Scientist* (1975), **63, 2**, 188–195.

GOODGLASS, H. and KAPLAN, E. Disturbance of gesture and pantomime in aphasia, *Brain* (1963), **86** 703–720.

GOODGLASS, H. and KAPLAN, E.F. *Boston Diagnostic Aphasia Examination* (1972). Philadelphia: Lea and Febiger.

HECAEN, H. and ALBERT, M.L. *Human Neuropsychology* (1978). New York: John Wiley & Sons.

HELM, N.A. The gestural behavior of aphasic patients during confrontation naming, Doctoral Dissertation, Boston University, 1979.

HELM-ESTABROOKS, N. *Boston Apraxia Exam* United States Copyright, 1986.

JACKSON, H.J. Clinical remarks on cases of defects of expression (by words, writing, signs, etc.) in diseases of the nervous system, *Lancet* (1864), 604–605.

KAPLAN, E.F. and GOODGLASS, H. Aphasia — Related Disorders. In *Acquired Aphasia* M.T. Sarno (ed.) (1981). New York: Academic Press.

KERTESZ, A. *Aphasia and Associated Disorders* (1979). New York: Grune and Stratton.

KERTESZ, A. and HOOPER, P. Praxis and language: the extent and variety of apraxia in aphasia, *Neuropsychologia* (1982), **30, 3**, 275–280.

LIEPMANN, H. *Drei Aufsatze aus dem Apraxiegebeit* (1908). Berlin: Karner.

LIEPMANN, H. Die linke Hemisphere und das Handeln, *Munch. Med. Wschr* (1905), **52**, 2375–2378.

NAESER, M.A. and HAYWARD, R.W. Lesion localization in aphasia with cranial computed tomography and the Boston Diagnostic Aphasia Exam. *Neurology* (1978), **28**, 454–551.

PICK, A. *Studien uber motorische, Apraxie, und ihr nahe stehenden Erscheinurgen* (1905). Leipzig: Deuticke.

PICKETT, L.W. An assessment of gestural and pantomime deficit in aphasic patients, *Acta Symbolica* (1974), **5**, 69–86.

PORCH, B.E. *Porch Index of Communicative Ability* (1971). Palo Alto: Consulting Psychologist Press.

18

The Speech Therapist's assessment of Aphasia

Renata Whurr

Assessment of the aphasic patient may be conducted by neurologists, clinical psychologists, speech pathologists and occasionally by clinical linguists. The approach differs according to the purpose of the assessment. To the neurologist, the purpose of assessment is primarily to determine the nature and symptomatology of the disease, the site of pathology and the response to treatment; to the psychologist it is to discover the nature of the cognitive, memory and perceptual disorders, and to characterize the linguistic disturbances in their broadest aspect; to the linguist, the aim is to provide insights into the language disturbances by constructing linguistic analyses of the patient's oral output in response to stimuli and then to determine the interaction of linguistic levels.

For the speech pathologist the aims of assessment are:

1. To identify aphasia from other possible disorders such as dysarthria, articulatory dyspraxia, dementia, schizophrenia or thought disorders and agnosia (differential diagnosis).
2. To analyse the disorder into subtypes of aphasic disturbance within the four language modalities of listening, speaking, reading and writing.
3. To determine the severity of the disorder.
4. To define fruitful areas for remediation by obtaining a profile of deficient and retained areas of function.
5. To track changes over time.
6. Prognosis

The speech pathologist tries to achieve these aims by using a combination of informal observations together with a standardized aphasia test battery giving objective measures of performance. There are at least 40 published aphasia batteries to choose from. Most are similar in aims, design and construction and are influenced largely by the early tests of Head (1926) which are based on still earlier psychometric batteries.

Formal Aphasia Test Batteries

The characteristics of these batteries can best be examined under a number of headings.

Theory and Classification

The theoretical rationale for any particular test is usually determined by the discipline of the author. Of the published aphasia batteries, eight were developed by neurologists, nine by psychologists, and 11 by speech pathologists. Some recent procedures have been made available by linguists. Theoretical positions basically adopt either the unidimensional or the multidimensional hypothesis of aphasia. For example, Schuell (1965) sees aphasia as a unidimensional disorder, which is not modality specific. In contrast, Wepman and Jones (1961) postulate a heuristic model of language function which implies that there is a modality-bound separation of transmission at every level for both input and output, and a separation of the decoding from the encoding processes. Goodglass and Kaplan (1972) hold that various components of language may be selectively impaired and that this selectivity is a clue to the anatomical organization of language in the brain, localization of the causative lesion, and functional interactions (e.g. inhibitory, regulatory, and selective) of various part of the language system. Despite the fact that the objective of assessment is to investigate language breakdown, none of the standard aphasia examinations is based on linguistic theories.

Surprisingly little of modern linguistics has yet permeated into formal assessments of aphasia. No aphasia assessment battery based on primarily linguistic principles is available (Whitaker and Whitaker, 1972; Lesser, 1978; Crystal, 1981; Whurr, 1982). But linguistic profiling is now providing a relatively new approach to assessment. It is based on a qualitative description and analysis of all language levels in the oral output of the patient and clinician. The aims are to indicate the main differences between normal and abnormal language behaviour, to identify different categories of abnormality, and to provide a view of the systematic nature of disability placed on scales of increasing approximation to linguistic norms. It is necessary to synthesize several different levels of information to achieve these ends. The techniques are explained by Crystal (1981), Coulthard and Montgomery (1981) and Coulthard (1977). The main value of this approach is in providing a principled and rational linguistic basis for hypotheses about remediation and prognosis. Lesser (1978) makes suggestions for linguistically based investigations of aphasia; and there have been many studies investigating one or another level of linguistic operation, usually oral output. Some attempt is being made to incorporate linguistic structure into comprehension tests (e.g. Peuser, 1978; Shewan, 1979; Paradis, 1983), but no battery samples each linguistic level —phonological, prosodic, lexical, syntactic, semantic and pragmatic — on both input and output performance.

The classification system and terminology used in aphasia test batteries are, like their theoretical backgrounds, largely determined by the discipline of the test designers. Systems adopted fall broadly into the following categories.

Localizationist

The emphasis here is on grouping aphasic patients into subtypes on the basis of a constellation of behavioural characteristics which broadly correlate with sites of lesion in the brain. The subtypes usually correspond to Broca's, Wernicke's, conduction, transcortical-sensory and transcortical-motor aphasias — all supposedly produced by circumscribed lesions in the brain. Exponents of the localizationist school in aphasia assessments are Goodglass and Kaplan (1972) and Kertesz (1982).

Neuropsychological

Here the interest is less on localizing the site of lesion and more on identifying the language and non-language characteristics in terms of underlying mechanisms of the language disturbances such as deficits of memory, perception, motor programming, etc. Examples of this approach are seen in Christenson (1974) and Spreen and Benton (1969).

Linguistic

The emphasis here is on determining the linguistic characteristics of the aphasia on all levels of linguistic operation — phonological, prosodic, morphemic, lexical, syntactic, semantic and pragmatic. Testing schemes including this approach can be seen in Crystal (1981) where linguistic analysis is conducted on oral output only. Some batteries include this approach in conjunction with the more conventional dichotomies of expressive and receptive function (*see* Hecaen, 1972; Peuser, 1978; Shewan, 1979; Paradis, 1983).

Functional communication

Here language behaviour is evaluated in a variety of situations and classified in terms of functional ability in each language modality. This approach is seen in Taylor (1969), Holland (1980) and Skinner *et al.* (1984).

Descriptive

In this category aphasic patients are divided into levels of severity — severe, moderate or mild (Eisenson, 1954). This system is also used in conjunction with an overall quantitative rating and then superimposed on the overall qualitative scores (Schuell, 1965; Porch, 1967; Whurr, 1974; Kertesz, 1982).

Organization

The majority of aphasia tests are designed within the receptive/expressive divisions and within the four language-modality framework of listening, speaking, reading and writing. Subtests are usually based on a 'task-orientated' approach. This involves the presentation of stimulus material through the visual, auditory and tactile modalities. Responses can be oral or gestural. Most aphasia batteries contain linguistic components, but few contain prelinguistic components. The linguistic components may include tests of receptive function and of expressive function.

Tests of receptive function

In tests to determine auditory language or comprehension deficits, tasks may include the recognition of gross environmental sound; identifying visually displayed and orally named items, by pointing to objects, colours, shapes, letters, numbers and written words; carrying out simple and complex commands; oral repetition of sounds, words and sentences; orally completing sentences and answering questions. In tests of reading comprehension, most batteries contain tasks involving visual matching (forms, shapes, pictures, colours, objects, numbers, letters, words and sentences); selection via auditory input of visual symbols; reading aloud; comprehension of simple and complex written commands; and answering written questions (in written or oral form).

Tests of expressive function

Tests to assess deficits of oral expression usually include some or all of the following tasks: imitation of oral movements; repetition; reading aloud; completing sentences; confrontation and tactile naming; defining words; formulating sentences by describing objects and picture; giving directions and general discourse, and sometimes singing. In tests of writing, tasks include copying, writing to dictation, writing sequences, names of objects, describing pictures, spelling tasks, crosswords and anagrams.

The prelinguistic components may contain tests for visual disorders, visual perceptual disorders, auditory perceptual function, visual memory, auditory memory, general orientation, cognitive state, praxis, gestures, and calculation ability.

Only a few batteries include items which assess non-language aspects, even though their importance has been stressed (Head, 1926; Benton, 1967). For example, tests of visual, auditory, tactile and olfactory perception, all of which may have some bearing on the aphasic patient's behaviour, are included in the batteries of Monrad Krohn (1921), Halstead and Wepman (1949) and Spreen and Benton (1969). Some batteries include tests of visual, auditory and environmental memory as well as short-term memory (Head, 1926; Butfield, 1952; Goodglass and Kaplan, 1972; and Christienson, 1974). Tests of non-verbal reasoning, such as Raven's Progressive Matrices and Koh's blocks, are included in Butfield (1952), Spreen and Benton (1969) and

Kertesz (1982). Assessment of praxis for non-verbal dyspraxia is included in Monrad Krohn (1921), Head (1926), Brown (1972), Goodglass and Kaplan (1972) and Kertesz (1982).

A few batteries include everyday tasks such as setting a clock, telling the time, handling money, reading maps and playing games such as draughts and cards (Head, 1926). In many respects, these tasks provide insights into the way in which the patient manages his everyday life, despite his language deficits. Head often made his own observations by accompanying his patients from hospital to their homes to detect any abnormalities of behaviour that would escape the notice of an examiner during a formal test. Some tests include the assessment of means of communication other than oral language, such as gesture. Gesture is evaluated specifically by Duffy and Duffy (1978, 1986) and gestural responses are included in the Porch Index of Communicative Abilities (PICA) battery (Porch, 1967). The importance of evaluating gesture as a possible alternative method of communication has been noted by several writers, or if not as an alternative then as an additional method used in conjuction with oral language. Although most aphasia batteries assess all four language skills, a few batteries focus on selected areas of verbal function such as comprehension to detect high level disturbances, as in the tests of De Renzi and Vignolo (1962), Parisi and Pizzamiglia (1970), Shewan (1979), or they concentrate on oral naming (Rochford and Williams, 1964; Oldfield *et al.*, 1965; McKenna and Warrington, 1983).

The total number of subtests within a battery will determine the length of testing time. The range of subtests may be as few as 18 (Porch, 1973), or more than 80 (Spreen and Benton, 1969). Testing time may range from as little as half an hour (Sklar, 1966; Whurr, 1974; Keenan and Brassell, 1975) to a reputed 94 hours for the tests of Weisenburg and McBride (*see* Darley, 1979). Usually the tests last about 1½ hours. The number of items included within subtests ranges from 5 to 32 as in the Minnesota Test for the Differential Diagnosis of Aphasia (MTDDA) and the average number of items in tests is between 6 and 10. The Aphasia Screening Test (AST) controls and limits the number of items to five and the PICA and Aphasia Language Performance Scales (ALPS) limit to ten.

The level of difficulty and complexity of aphasia tests varies from those that assess only high-level auditory comprehension, such as the Token Test (TT) of De Renzi and Vignolo (1962) and the Auditory Comprehension Test (ACTS) of Shewan (1979), to the batteries that include very simple subtests to evaluate the severely impaired patients, such as the AST (Whurr, 1974) and the Examination of Aphasia (EA; Eisenson, 1954). The remaining batteries assess the mid-range of moderately to minimally impaired patients. Not all the tests are graded in difficulty, nor are they necessarily presented in a particular order of difficulty. Some batteries start at a high level of expectation where the patient is asked to produce spontaneous speech as in the Boston Diagnostic Aphasia Examination (BDAE) and the Western Aphasia Battery (WAB) or to respond to a long and complicated auditory command as in the Porch Index of Communicative Ability (PICA) and the Minnesota Test for the Differential Diagnosis of Aphasia (MTDDA).

Quantification

There are four basic methods of scoring: descriptive, plus/minus, rating scales, and multidimensional scoring. The *descriptive* method outlined by Goldstein (1948) involves an examiner recording every response of the patient in as much detail as possible (Head, 1920; Weisenberg and McBride, 1935). The method is still extensively used clinically where standardized tests have not been adopted. *Plus/minus scoring* is the system that divides all responses into categories of correct (plus) and incorrect (minus). The test scores are reported in terms of percentages of plus or minus responses. This method is employed by most aphasia batteries. However, as incorrect responses display a range of distinct qualitative characteristics, *rating scales* were introduced to accommodate these qualitative differences. They rate the severity of the symptom in various modalities as severe, moderate and mild. Porch, critical of the plus/minus system of scoring, developed a *multi-dimensional scoring* system with 16 possible categories of response, based on the original 8-point scale introduced earlier by Wepman and Jones (1961). The objective of multidimensional scoring is to provide a more sensitive measure of how the patients perform on a task rather than on a rigid right/wrong basis.

Charting and Interpretation

Only eight batteries employ specific systems of charting. These vary from plotting performance in comparison with 'average' aphasic patients' performance on a 'z' score profile (Spreen and Benton, 1969) to plotting performance on a + and - scale of average performance (Goodglass and Kaplan, 1972), or plotting performance expressed in percentiles (Porch, 1967) and presenting profiles of retained and deficit areas on histogram displays (Sklar, 1966; Whurr, 1974; Shewan, 1979, 1983). Most test batteries provide simple explanations of results in terms of the severity and type of disorder, levels of impairment, and in some cases prognosis. However, no battery provides instruction in drawing links between the disorders identified and their underlying mechanisms in neuropsychological terms. Discussing the relationship between language breakdown and the structure of the underlying mechanisms remains very much a clinical 'state of the art'. Thus interpretations of test results on the basis of explicit guidance is inadequate — only simple quantitative or descriptive interpretations can be made with any form of consistency. Computerized interpretation is now being introduced. A complete program for interpretation of the PICA will be available in the future, but the value of the method is yet to be established.

Standardization and Factor Analysis

Aphasia tests vary in the extent to which they are standardized. If tests are to be truly standardized, each variable must be specified, but various authors claim that aphasic patients are characteristically too inconsistent in their responses to permit formal scoring standards to be developed and meaningfully applied (Eisenson, 1954; Schuell, 1957; Anastasi, 1982). Moreover, standard scores are meaningless when dealing with heterogeneous aphasic populations. It is unrealistic to expect behavioural homogeneity in the injured brain. But that is not to say that quantification of the data obtained from aphasic populations is not valuable or necessary. As Schuell (1965) said, 'It must be known what a test is measuring, and the validity and internal consistency of a test must be established'. Thus she claimed that standardization and quantification can be defended on scientific grounds.

Of the two main criteria for test standardization, the first is the reliability of the test. This is the extent to which it can be assumed that the test will yield the same results if repeated. The second main criterion is the validity of the test, namely the extent to which the test measures what it purports to measure. Statistical methods of establishing reliability and validity vary, and the suitability of the methods used is the domain of the statistician. Only 10 of the published aphasia test batteries have been subjected to standardization procedures. Six of them have used factor analysis. As yet the methods and techniques of standardization have not been evaluated. The inherent difficulties in the standardization of heterogeneous behavioural variables, and the pressing demand to conform to standardization protocols to give objectivity and credence to the aphasia test batteries, have produced standardization procedures which should not be accepted without some scepticism.

Factor analysis is another method of standardization. The primary aim is to discover common factors to provide the orderly simplification of a number of interrelated measures. It has been applied widely in the behavioural sciences in an attempt to identify factors of 'intelligence' or 'personality' and other multidimensional characteristics of human behaviour. Factor analysis of aphasia test batteries attempts to prove or refute the ideas that aphasia is either a multidimensional or a unidimensional disorder. However, as a method of analysis it is not immune to bias; the results of factor analysis are open to many dangers, such as sampling bias, data manipulation and statistical sophistry. The techniques for extracting the factors generally endeavour to take out as much common variance as possible in the first factor. Subsequent factors are, in turn, intended to account for the maximum amount of remaining common variance until hopefully no common variance remains.

Only seven of the many published aphasia test batteries have been standardized by the factor analysis method: the MTDDA (Schuell, 1957); the Language Modality Test for Aphasia (LMTA; Wepman and Jones, 1961); Approaches to the Study of Aphasia (ASA; Osgood and Miron, 1965); the BDAE (Goodglass and Kaplan, 1972, 1983); the WAB (Kertesz and Poole, 1974); the AST (Whurr, 1974); and the PICA (Porch, 1979). To a large extent, the resulting configurations of these standardization studies are determined by the hypothesis postulated, the structure of the test battery, the subtests selected, the subtest headings, the scoring system, the patient population sampled and the method of analysis applied to the data.

The configurations of the factors in the seven studies provide some support for the hypothesis that aphasia is a multidimensional problem with disturbances of language permeating all factors. In comparing the first factor in each battery, there is evidence of a dominant 'oral language' factor underpinned by a 'symbolic factor'. The first factor in each of the seven studies is shown in *Table 1.*

In the seven studies, factor 2 appears to correlate with three distinct areas: visual, spatial and somatognostic processes; transmission of decoding from encoding and aural to oral modalities and Broca's and global aphasia; graphic modality. Factor 3 appears to divide into: visuospatial and visual-graphic transmission; auditory comprehension; and Wernicke's aphasia; and gestural output. Factor 4 appears to correlate most closely with writing, gross movements of speech musculature and auditory comprehension and transcortical motor aphasia. Only Kertesz and Poole identify more than six factors. This is due to the different statistical techniques applied to the data. They used an attribute and nearest neighbour network analysis, which isolated more distinct categories in their data. All their factors clustered into distinct aphasic syndromes: global, Broca's, Wernicke's, transcortical sensory, and transcortical motor aphasias. Factor analysis of aphasia test batteries is discussed elsewhere by Whurr (1971), Clark *et al.* (1979), Huber *et al.* (1980), Willmes *et al.* (1983) and Goodglass and Kaplan (1983).

Treatment Implications

Defining fruitful areas for treatment is probably the most important objective of aphasia testing to the speech pathologist. Only Butfield (1962) actually states that in her battery, tests are restricted to those thought to be most useful in suggesting cues for re-educational techniques. She considers it essential for the speech therapist to understand the patient's remaining assets and deficits in order to be able to suggest circumvention techniques.

The PICA manual (Porch, 1979) gives guidance on interpretation and analysis which helps to provide a basis for prognosis and treatment. The

Table 1 Factor Analysis of Aphasia Test Batteries

Battery	Factor 1	Factor 2	Factor 3	Factor 4	Factors 5	6	7	8	9	10
Schuell (1957)	Language behaviour	Visual discrimination	Visual-spatial behaviour	Gross movements of speech musculature	Stimulus equivalence	—	—	—	—	—
Wepman and Jones (1961)	Visual to oral transmission	Aural to oral transmission	Visual to graphic transmission	Oral to graphic transmission	Comprehension of symbolic language	Arithmetic	—	—	—	—
Osgood and Miron (1963)	Symbolic versus skill performances	Decoding from encoding	Vocal from manual output	Written from spoken sentence comprehension		—	—	—	—	—
Goodglass and Kaplan (1972)	Broca's aphasia	Spatial quantitative and somatognostic tasks	Wernicke's aphasia	Auditory comprehension	Gerstman's syndrome	—	—	—	—	—
Goodglass and Kaplan (1983)	Visual-spatial	Fluency	Repetition	Auditory comprehension	Writing	✓	✓	✓	✓	✓
Kertesz and Poole (1974)	Global aphasia	Broca's aphasia	Isolation syndrome	Transcortical motor	Transcortical sensory	✓	✓	✓	✓	✓
Whurr (1974)	Verbal output	Visual input matching	Auditory input	Writing — simple output	Writing — complex output	—	—	—	—	—
Whurr (1986)	Verbal output	Comprehension — input	Visual matching — input	— Writing calculation	Writing output	Oral language output				
Porch (1979)	Verbal competency — fluency	Graphic modality	Mainly gestural output	—	—	—	—	—	—	—

highest scores obtained on a given subtest can be interpreted as a potential level of performance on that task. The notion of the ranked communication task continuum is employed as a basis for planning therapy, where treatment is directed at those tasks and skills which are adjacent to the difficult tasks that the patient performs completely successfully. A further feature of the PICA analysis is the aphasia recovery curve. This is computed by taking the patient's overall score, which is converted to an overall percentile (O). The next step is to find the nine highest subtest scores, compute the mean and convert to the nine-high percentile (H) this is repeated for the nine lowest subtest scores which gives the nine-low percentile (L). These three are plotted onto the aphasia recovery curve form. A large high–low gap indicates room for improvement whereas a low high–low gap indicates maximum recovery has been reached.

Although the structured approach to planning treatment on the basis of PICA data is attractive, the remaining batteries do not provide explicit guidance for planning treatment, although the Goodglass and Kaplan rating scale profile of speech characteristics highlights specific features, such as types of grammatical error, semantic word categories and paraphasias, which can be useful in selecting areas for treatment. Most of the authors of aphasia tests have written separately on the subject of treatment (*see* Wepman, 1951; Schuell, 1957; Eisenson, 1973; and Whurr, 1983).

Many clinicians are critical of formal aphasia test batteries. Taylor Sarno (1969) observes that traditional aphasia tests often fail because they can be insensitive to the subtle deficits of the mildly impaired patient and tell very little about the severely impaired. She also notes that patients often respond in unexpected ways, such as by gestural signals and by accurate but inconsistent responses. Many patients find it difficult to perform specific tasks, and yet give evidence in natural language situations of much higher levels of ability. Critchley (1970) and others have referred to the discrepancies noted between performances on formal testing and the use of natural language by aphasics. The formal test situation alone does not reflect all aspects of the patients communication abilities. Most tests have concerned themselves with identifying what the patient said and not to how he communicated. None have attempted to quantify the communication behaviour which a patient actually uses in the course of interaction with others. Taylor Sarno (1969) refers to that dimension as 'functional performance' elicited in formal language tests which often sample artificial behaviours. In her view clinical tests are more a measure of potential rather than actual language use. Lebrun (1983) also feels that the results of standard tests may be misleading; the majority of test tasks in his view are metalinguistic tasks, and 'metalanguage' may be more impaired than 'speech' language in the aphasic patient.

Tests to evaluate a 'functional language' have been designed by Taylor

(1969), Holland (1980) and Skinner *et al.* (1983). Although the Functional Communication Profile (FCP) correlates highly with other standard batteries it is still based on subjective ratings and therefore cannot be considered a reliable measure of behaviour. The Communicative Abilities in Daily Living (CADL) employs role play and other novel features in assessment which are likely to produce unreliable and unrepeatable test performances. However, the investigation of functional communication is an important adjunct to the conventional standard aphasia examination.

Despite these inadequacies in the formal aphasia test battery as a system of evaluating the aphasic patient, it is the system most frequently used by the speech pathologist, and is often the only measure employed (Brookshire, 1978). No one single test can possibly be adequate for the evaluation of all aphasic patients, and therefore it is vital for clinicians to be selective in their choice of battery. However, the decision as to which battery to choose is often based on 'personal choice, rather than on principled and rational selection' (Beele, 1983). There is evidence that clinicians select and continue to use only one battery (usually the battery introduced during their training). For example, Beele (1984) conducted a survey among 162 clinicians in the United Kingdom and found the most widely used batteries in order of preference were the AST followed by the BDAE, and then the short Schuell (Thomson *et al.* 1979). A report in the *American Speech Hearing and Language Association Journal* (December, 1983) listed the order of preference for aphasia test batteries in the USA as: PICA, BDAE and MDDTA. However, most clinicians tend to have a selection of tests available to them. As Müller *et al.* (1981) comment: 'The tests will be chosen to meet their own particular clinical requirements and individual preference.'

Test Selection Criteria

In selecting the most useful aphasia battery or subtests from batteries the clinician needs to be reminded of the main objectives of assessment, namely differential diagnosis, the identification of the type and degree of aphasic disorder, and the determination of potentially fruitful areas for treatment. These objectives can best be met by first screening for the presence of aphasia and then identifying the nature of the disturbances and the level of overall impairment. The selection criteria will be discussed with these objectives in mind.

Screening

Early after the onset of aphasia the patients reponses are known to be inconsistent, thus evaluation at this stage should be essentially of a screening nature. Some clinicians prefer to use their own short informal bedside assessment. A short screening test should be administered when the patient can respond to visually presented materials with interest and consistency. There are several short aphasia batteries suitable for screening purposes; the Halstead and Wepman, adapted by Heimberger and Reitan (1961); short versions of the MTDDA adapted by Schuell (1957, 1966), Thompson and Enderby (1979), and Powell, Bailey and Clarke (1980); the Sklar Aphasia Scale (SAS; Sklar, 1966); the ALPS (Keenan and Brassell, 1975); and the AST (Whurr, 1974); the BEST (West and Sands, 1986); the FAST (Enderby, 1986).

An ideal screening test should be short and practical, yet comprehensive in its coverage. It should sample each language modality. Each subtest should be graded in difficulty with a limited but consistent number of items. It should include some non-language tasks to assess visual and auditory perception, praxis and gesture. The test material should be simple, clear and unambiguous, and consistent throughout the battery, so that patients do not fail tasks because of complicated visual presentation or the introduction of new visual materials. The tasks should be clearly defined, easy to evaluate and easy to score. Ideally, scoring should be on a strict pass/fail basis, so that interpretation of the results is simplified and can finally provide qualitative and quantitative information.

The shortened version of the Halstead and Wepman has been adapted by Heimberger and Reitan (1961). This, according to Lezack (1976), does aid discrimination between patients with left and right hemisphere lesions; for many of the former can copy designs but cannot write, while the latter have no trouble in writing but may not be able to reproduce the designs. Other very short tests which may be suitable for quick formal screening and which assess speaking, listening, reading and writing, but only at one level of difficulty, are the shortened versions of Schuell (1957) — *see* Thompson and Enderby (1979) and Powell, Bailey and Clarke (1980). Most shortened versions of longer tests tend to have an artificial selection of items. The attempt to gather together highly correlated tests leads to the rejection of more difficult subtests and produces a battery which can only assess moderate levels of impairment, missing the severe and mild levels of impairment, and so is not suitable for screening levels of impairment. The SAS (Sklar, 1966), which consists of four subtests representing the four language areas, is a longer test and useful for screening patients. Each subtest contains 25 items. According to Halpern (1979) the SAS compares favourably with other tests used in aphasia evaluation, although it has limitations in not reporting types of error quantitatively, and in failing to assess dysarthria and apraxia of speech. The ALPS (Keenan and Brassell, 1975) consists of 40 items with 10 items in each subtest. Items within subtests are heterogeneous, and in general order of increasing difficulty within subtests. Responses are scored as 'correct', 'prompted' or 'incorrect'. Ritter (1979) found the ALPS a good screening instrument but noted that it failed to provide helpful information for planning therapy.

The AST (Whurr, 1974) is a battery that is short but comprehensive. It samples all four language modalities, but includes some non-language tasks to assess visual and auditory perception and praxis. There are 20 tests of receptive function and 30 tests of expressive function. There are five items in every subtest, each scored on a simple pass/fail system. Tasks are clearly defined and responses easy to evaluate. The test is graded in difficulty, within each modality sampled, and screens all levels of impairment. It is useful therefore to define the area and level of deficit as well as the retained areas. A profile is obtained of retained and lost abilities within eight language components: visual perception, reading comprehension, reading aloud, auditory comprehension, speech production, oral language, writing and calculation. The AST provides a defect scale which indicates severity along four dimensions on overall total scores, and also separately on perceptive and expressive functions. The scale defines very severe, severe, moderate and mild defects. The materials used are large, clear and unambiguous, and are consistent throughout the whole battery. The AST has been discussed by Skinner (1971) and Beele (1984) who found that it failed to take into account automatic verbal responses and gestural skills in social situations. However, it was thought to be useful as a screening instrument, and for the assessment of the severely impaired patient, as it contained graded tasks starting at a very simple level.

Assessing the Severely Impaired Patient

As Brookshire (1978) observed, the speech pathologist may find when examining the severely impaired patient that most test items of the standardized aphasia examination are too difficult, so that most subtests are failed completely and none are performed without error. The examiner thus knows what the patient cannot do, but not what he can do. The standardized examination administered to the severely impaired patient should be the same as that administered to the mildly impaired patient. The tasks should sample performance in a number of stimulus modalities at lower levels of complexity.

A battery to assess the severely impaired patient must conform to certain criteria. Severely impaired patients may have visual field or perceptual defects which will prevent them from responding to visually presented materials. As most formal aphasia testing involves the presentation of visual materials, those materials should be large, clear and unambiguous. Moreover, the visual modality is the first that should be assessed to determine whether the patient is capable of responding to test materials at all. The next important step is to avoid oral spoken test instructions as the patient may be unable to respond to auditory stimuli, and so may fail tests because he has not understood the instruction. The best way to cicumvent this problem is to use gestural demonstration, as far as possible. As the severely impaired may be unable to produce speech, the emphasis during the initial stages of testing should be on non-language gestural outputs, i.e. pointing, matching and selection. The total number of responses should be limited to avoid fatigue.

In summary, the severely impaired patient should be assessed in a strict order of inputs and outputs to determine whether any functions exist, even to a slight degree, in any language modality. The order should be:

1. Visual matching + gesture response
2. Auditory comprehension + gesture response.
3. Speech production + oral response.
4. Oral language + oral response.
5. Writing + written response.

Aphasia test batteries that are useful in the evaluation of severely impaired patients are the Neurosensory Center Comprehensive Examination for Aphasia (NCCEA; Spreen and Benton, 1969), the EA (Eisenson, 1946), and the AST (Whurr, 1974). The NCCEA was evaluated by Greenburg (1979) who thought it useful for the severely impaired brain-injured adult if administered by a skilled and experienced examiner. The EA (Eisenson, 1946) is particularly useful for the evaluation of agnosias. However, it requires too many responses to make it practical, as the severely impaired patient fatigues quickly. The AST fulfills many of the criteria and was specifically designed for the assessment of the severely impaired patient. The MTDDA commences with assessment of the auditory modality, the PICA commences with too high a level of auditory instruction, the BDAE and WAB start with the emphasis on spontaneous speech. Visual material in most batteries is too small and basically unsuitable for this group of patients.

Assessing the Moderately Impaired Patient

The moderately impaired patient will have some functional understanding and use of language in all four modalities. The objective of aphasia testing for this group is specifically to identify treatment areas and to highlight language disturbances in depth. The most widely used batteries for the evaluation of the moderately impaired aphasic patient are the MTDDA, the BDAE and the PICA. All three have been evaluated by Brookshire (1978), Darley (1979) and Müller *et al.* (1981).

The *MTDDA* contains a larger number of test items than any other battery and will probably give a more complete inventory of the patient's language abilities. Zubrick and Smith (1979) recommend it as a thoroughly researched and refined tool. Müller *et al.* (1981) comment on its simple administration of scoring as well as its comprehensiveness and predictive power. The diagnostic categories have prognostic significance in that each category carried a prediction regarding the amount and nature of recovery of speech and language abilities, although its value for prognosis and prediction in acute aphasia needs further study. Zubrick and Smith (1979) and Müller *et al.* (1981) describe the main shortcomings of the MTDDA as no assessment of gesture, pantomime or articulatory dyspraxia; no measures of non-language sensory and motor function or other non-language deficits; and no test of right hemisphere function, so that it is therefore of limited use with mild and severe aphasic patients. It is too comprehensive and many of its 47 subtests are thought to be redundant and to duplicate information; there are unequal numbers of items in each section; it uses a plus/minus scoring system based on an error score and as there is no statistical treatment of raw scores, examiners have to convert error scores into correct scores before planning treatment; and there are no illustrated graphs, the test stimulus material being somewhat dull.

The *BDAE* is comprehensive, distinguishes between patterns of performance, and contains unique scales for measuring qualitative aspects of speech output. It contains a systematic and extensive sampling of input and output modality combinations at several levels of complexity. In addition, it provides a large sampling of performance on non-language tasks in the section on 'supplementary non-language tests'. Its main value is to clinicians who wish to speculate about the localization of lesions, and Duffy (1978) commends it for defining and standardizing types of aphasia based on presumed anatomical substrates. Its weaknesses lie in its limited use with the severely impaired patient, and its failure to include assessment of gesture, pantomime or articulatory dyspraxia. It is lengthy to administer and much of the test is thought to be redundant from the diagnostic standpoint as the rating scale on oral speech serves to classify the type of aphasia. There is a lack of prognosis and of treatment planning. There is limited information about test–retest and interjudge reliability. There are doubts about the accuracy of the inferences drawn concerning the site of the lesion. Finally, the stimulus material is small and cramped.

The *PICA* has been regarded as a highly standardized psychometrically designed aphasia test battery (McNeil, 1979). The emphasis is placed on processing rather than on linguistic deficits. Its major uses have been for planning therapy and predicting recovery. It appears to provide the most sensitive measure of patient performance. It has evoked much negative and positive comment. Its weaknesses have been observed as a lack of theoretical depth and poor basic test construction. For instance, factor analysis produced unclear factors. It fails to assess comprehension and only provides a narrow range of subtests for assessment of the auditory modality. As there is not evaluation of spontaneous speech and no measure of functional communication, it is of limited use with the severely impaired patient. It requires over 40 hours training time and because of its quantifiable nature it is open to misuse and misinterpretation.

Whichever battery of tests is used on the moderately impaired patient, the information based on those batteries needs to be supplemented with additional data. Neuropsychological tests of memory, perception, learning and cognitive function, which help to define further the underlying mechanisms or strategies adopted by the patient, are important in the planning of remediation. Linguistic description is another important source of information to complete the profile of language breakdown.

Assessing the Mildly Impaired Patient

The mildly impaired aphasic may well succeed on most subtests in most aphasia batteries. Most items are not sufficiently complex to tap the upper limits of the high level patient's capabilities, so that the patient may show only minimal defects and yet still have language impairments which affect his social and vocational life. No one battery is specifically designed for the evaluation of the mildly impaired patient. Only the TT (De Renzi and Vignolo, 1962) is designed to assess high-level comprehension disturbances and gives no information on reading, speaking or writing. Clinicians intent on evaluating subtle impairments in auditory and reading comprehension, oral and written language of high-level patients need to select subtests within formal batteries, or look to neuropsychological and psychometric batteries. High-level assessment of auditory and reading comprehension needs to take into account aspects such as memory and cognitive processing as well as linguistic complexity. Lesser (1978) observes that research into these areas is underway. Cognitive neuropsychological research is now dealing with all the major aspects of language processing (Coltheart *et al.*, 1986).

There are several subtests in various aphasia batteries that are useful for assessing high level auditory comprehension disturbances. For instance, the MTDDA contains tests for identifying items named serially, understanding sentences, following directions and understanding paragraphs. The WAB contains tests of sequential auditory commands. The BDAE has subtests involving complex ideational material. The QUALT (Queensland University Aphasia Language Test) (Tyrer and Eadie, 1978) includes tasks selecting from five spoken words. The QUALT also includes more difficult tasks where patients have to select spoken sentences (descriptions) to fit best visually presented pictures. The Auditory Comprehension of Sentences (Shewan, 1979) usefully assesses various syntactic components at sentence level. Lesser (1978) describes linguistic investigations to assess high-level disturbances in all language modalities. Assessment of high-level auditory disturbances should tap phonological, prosodic, lexical syntactic and semantic levels. Complex reading comprehension is assessed in the MTDDA, BDAE, WAB and QUALT. Reading rate, spelling and comprehension can be assessed by the Nelson National Adult Reading Test, the Gates and McGintie Test and the Jastak Tests. However, Coltheart (1980,

1981, 1985, 1986) describe the most thorough investigation of acquired reading disturbances, as does Ellis (1984), Patterson (1982), Funnell (1983), Coltheart (1980, 1985, 1986).

The MTDDA includes tests for defining words, retelling paragraphs, completing sentences, answering questions, and describing pictures. The BDAE assesses speech on a rating scale of speech characteristics which include fluency, naming, reading aloud and repetition; further analysis involves melodic line, phrase length, articulatory agility and paraphasia. The WAB rates spontaneous speech on the basis of the information content, fluency, grammatical competence and paraphasias on a 0–10 scale. Prins, Snow and Wagenaar (1978) produced a spontaneous speech analysis based on 30 rateable variables. The main problem in evaluating oral language is the method by which it is elicited. Whichever method is used, it needs to be made clear whether it is discourse, picture description, answering questions and so forth. Ideally oral output should be tape-recorded and analysed on all linguistic levels (Crystal, 1981; Whurr, 1982). Writing can be assessed at various levels; graphemic, morphemic, phonotactic. Some research conducted in this area is discussed by Lesser (1978), Hatfield (1976) and Whurr (1986). The mildly impaired patient needs to be evaluated in neuropsychological terms to determine his memory, learning, conceptual and cognitive levels. Only a combination of all of the above information can provide a basis for planning treatment.

Summary and Conclusions

The criteria for a technically adequate test to evaluate language disturbances after brain damage has been discussed by Marie (1902), Head (1920), Weisenburg and McBride (1935), Schuell (1965), Weigl (1966), Benton (1967), Green (1970) and Brookshire (1978). A clinically useful aphasia test battery should:

1. Be comprehensive in range.
2. Measure patients' responses to stimuli in all four language modalities.
3. Include a selection of non-language tasks.
4. Clearly define tasks and grade them in difficulty from simple to complex.
5. Provide an even distribution of simple, moderate and complex level subtests to evaluate severely, moderately and minimally impaired patients.
6. Contain a sufficient number of items within each subtest.
7. Contain clear materials which should be unambiguous and free of bias (e.g. IQ, social class, nationality, education).

8. Be consistent and uniform in scoring.
9. Be easy to administer.
10. Be easy to evaluate in terms of responses.
11. Be simple to interpret, chart and profile.
12. Contain profile analysis and charting systems for visual display.
13. Be sufficient in yielding qualitative and quantitative information.
14. Provide clear guidelines for treatment and prognosis.

The extent to which these criteria are fulfilled is discussed in part by Darley (1972), Lezack (1976), Brookshire (1978) and Müller *et al.* (1981). No one aphasia battery can fulfil all the listed criteria. Aphasic patients need different types of assessment at different points in time between the onset of their aphasia and the later stages. Ideally there should be at least four batteries available to the clinician — the first to screen for aphasia, and three others to assess in depth the three levels of impairment, severe, moderate and mild. The 'family' of batteries should have a cross-disciplined theoretical basis with a balanced influence of neurological, cognitive neuropsychological and linguistic elements. All four batteries should be consistent in design, construction, organization and scoring and controlled for level of difficulty. Progress could be tracked by uniform methods of assessment. This would facilitate the planning of treatment and help to provide realistic prognostic pointers. However, at present clinicians need to select from a wide range of those batteries or parts of batteries which best fulfil clinical requirements.

Table 2 represents the author's suggested selection of the main formal aphasia examinations over a 6-month period post-onset. Time post-onset from 1 week to 24 weeks is represented on the horizontal axis. The three levels of impairment are represented on the vertical axis. Tests are selected to fit best the needs of the patient from the first week post-onset at a severe, moderate or mild level of impairment. During this stage the patient will need an informal word assessment. At about the second week, the patient requires some form of objective screening system to identify the type and degree of disorder. Treatment at this stage will be based on the screening information. The high-level patient will need additional in-depth testing and the moderate patient may need assessment of functional communication. The severe patient may need assessment of gesture or pantomime. The assessment may take place at 2 months and then again at 6 months after the initial assessment. Reassessment may be conducted on the same battery or on a selection of subtests from other batteries. The purpose of reassessment is to track progress, evaluate the effectiveness of treatment and to modify treatment according to the patient's changing needs.

The formal aphasia examination is necessary as a method of producing

Level of severity	*Time post-onset*							
	Months 0			*1*		*2*	*3 4 5*	*6*
	Weeks 0	*1*	*2*	*4*	*6*	*8*	*10 12 14 16 18 20 22*	*24*
Mild		AST ALPS SAS	WAB	QUALT BDAE WAB	TT ACTS QUALT	AAT		TT AAT QUALT BDAE WAB
Medium	Informal ward assessment	Screening tests AST	EA SAS ALPS AST	MTDDA	PICA	FCP CADL AST		PICA MTDDA AAT WAB AST
Severe	Informal ward assessment	Screening tests AST	AST ALPS SAS EA			AST		AST

AAT = Aachen Aphasia Test
ACTS = Auditory Comprehension Test of Syntax
ALPS = Aphasia Language Performance Scales
AST = Aphasia Screening Test
BDAE = Boston Diagnostic Aphasia Examination
CADL = Communicative Abilities in Daily Living
EA = Examination of Aphasia
FCP = Functional Communication Profile
MTDDA = Minnesota Test for the Differential Diagnosis of Aphasia
PICA = Porch Index of Communicative Abilities
QUALT = Queensland Aphasia Language Test
SAS = Sklar Aphasia Scale
TT = Token Test
WAB = Western Aphasia Battery

objective and measurable information about the aphasic patient's lost and retained abilities. As a measuring instrument, the formal battery is insensitive to subtle changes and is useful only for specific purposes, namely the identification of language disturbances from a background of other types of disorder and identification of the degree of impairment within each language modality. More detailed accounts of language behaviour, and non-language behaviour, require descriptive analysis at all linguistic levels — phonological, prosodic, morphological, lexical, syntactic, semantic and pragmatic. The relative inadequacy of the modality framework task-orientated approach of aphasia examination has been noted, but it is the only method that produces objective qualitative information for the specific purposes described. The dilemma is how to decide how much objectivity has to be sacrificed in order to provide more in-depth qualitative accounts of aphasic behaviour. A 'trade-off' is undesirable. The only way both to achieve objectivity and to obtain descriptive information is to use two complementary systems, one adopting a conventional input/output test framework with quantifiable and repeatable performances, providing albeit a narrow, restricted but measurable view, and the other using an analytic procedure which describes the patient's language in linguistic, neuropsychological and pragmatic terms. In due course aphasia testing will be based on an integrated amalgamation of all the disciplines involved. 'There needs to be a correlation of clusters of linguistic, psychological and neurological symptoms' (Whurr, 1982). The achievement of this will depend on the progress of inter-disciplinary research in the field of disability after brain damage.

Aphasia Test Batteries and Examinations 1898–1987

BASTIAN, H.C. (1898) Diagnosis in speech defects. In *A treatise on Aphasia and Other Speech Defects*. London: H.K. Lewis.

MARIE, P. (1902) Marie's paper test. *Rev. Neurol.*, **16**, 611–974.

HEAD, H. (1920) *Methods of Examination in Aphasia and Kindred Disorders of Speech*. Vols. 1 and 2. London: Cambridge University Press.

MONRAD KROHN, G.H. (1921) Examination for Aphasia in *The Clinical Examination of the Nervous System*. London: H.K. Lewis.

THOMASON, H.C. and RIDDOCH, G. (1925) *Diseases of the Nervous System*. 4th Ed. Cassell & Co.

WEISENBURG, T. and MCBRIDE, K.E. (1935) *Aphasia. A Clinical and Psychological Study*. New York: Commonwealth Fund.

EISENSON, J. (1946) (Rev. 1954) *Examining for Aphasia*. New York: The Psychological Corporation.

HALSTEAD, W.C. and WEPMAN, J.M. (1949). The Halstead and Wepman Aphasia screening test. *J. Speech Hearing. Dis.* **14**, 9–15.

HALSTEAD, W.C., WEPMAN, J., REITAN, R.M. and HEIMBURGER, R.F. (1949) *Halstead Aphasia Test Form, M.* University of Chicago Industrial Relations Centre.

BUTFIELD, E. (1952 — Revised 1964) The Assessment of the Aphasic Patient *Speech* Oct. 1952.

SCHUELL, H. (1957) A Short Examination For Aphasia. *Neurology*, 7, 625–634.

HEIMBERGER, R.F. and REITAN, R.M. (1961) *Testing for Aphasia and Related Disorders*. Indiana University Medical Centre.

WEPMAN, J. and JONES, L. (1961) *The Language Modalities Test for Aphasia (L.M.T.A.)* Chicago Education Industry Services.

DERENZI, E. and VIGNOLO, L.A. (1962) *The Token Test — a sensitive test to detect receptive disturbances in aphasics. Brain 85*: 556–678.

FAWCUS, R. and FAWCUS, M. (1963) *Adult Aphasia Assessment*. Self publication.

SCHUELL, H. (1965 — revised 1940) *The Minnesota Test for the Differential Diagnosis of Aphasia*. University of Minnesota Press.

DUCARNE, DE RIBAUCOURT, B. (1965 and 1972). *Test pour l'examen de l'Aphasie* Centre de Psychologie Appliquée, 48 Ave. Victor Hugo, Paris.

SKLAR, M. (1966) *Sklar Aphasia Scales*. Western Psychological Services.

PORCH, B. (1967). *The Porch Index of Communicative Ability*. Palo Alto Consulting Psychologists Press.

SARNO, M.T. (1969). *Functional Communication Profile*. Institute of Rehabilitation Medicine, New York University Medical Centre.

SPREEN, O and BENTON, A.L. (1969). *Neurosensory Centre Comprehensive Examination of Aphasia*. British Columbia Neuropsychology Laboratory, University of Victoria, B.C.

PARISI, D. and PIZZAMIGLIO, L. (1970). *Syntactic Comprehension in Aphasia. Cortex 6, 2* 204-216.

GOODGLASS, H. and KAPLAN, E. (1972) (1983) 2nd Ed. *The Assessment of Aphasia and Related Disturbances. Boston Diagnostic Aphasia Examination* (B.D.A.E.) Philadelphia Lea and Febiger.

WHURR, R. (1974) *Aphasia Screening Test*. Whurr Publishers Ltd., 2 Alwyne Road, London N1 2HH, England.

CHRISTIENSON, A.L. (1974) *Luria's Neuropsychological Investigation*. Copenhagen: Munksgaard.

KEENAN, J.S. and BRASSEL, E.G. (1975) *Aphasia Language Performance Scales*. Murfeesboro Pinnacle Press.

MCNEIL, M.R. and PRESCOTT, T.E. (1978) *Revised Token Test*. Baltimore: University Park Press.

TYRER, J. and EADIE, M.J. (1978) *The Queensland University Aphasia and Language Test*. Hawthorn, Victoria: The Australian Council for Education Research.

DERENZI, E. and FERRARI, C. (1978) *The Reporters' Test — a Sensitive Test to Detect Expressive Disturbances in Aphasics. Cortex*, **14** 279–93.

THOMPSON, J. and ENDERBY, P. (1979) *Is All Your Schuell Really Necessary? British Journal of Disorders of Communication*, **14**, 195–201.

SHEWAN, C.M. (1979) *Auditory Comprehension Test for Sentences*. Chicago Biolinguistics.

PEUSER, G. (ed.) (1979) Allgemeiner Deutscher Sprachtest Steinert (1975) in G. Peuser (ed.) *Studien zur Sprachtherapie*. Patholinguistica 4, München: Fink.

POWELL, G., BAILEY, S. and CLARKE, E. (1980) *A very short version of the Minnesota Aphasia Test. Brit. J. Soc. Clin. Psych.*, **19**, 289–94.

HOLLAND, A. (1980) *Communication Abilities in Daily Living* (CADL). Baltimore: University Park Press.

KERTESZ, A. (1982) *Western Aphasia Battery*. New York: Grune & Stratton.
PARADIS, M. (1983) *Multilingual Aphasia Battery*. Paper presented at the American Speech Hearing and Language Association Miniseminar: Cincinnati.
SKINNER, C., WIRZ, S. and THOMPSON, I. (1984) *The Edinburgh Functional Communication Profile*. Bicester: Winslow Press
POECK, K. and WILLMES, K. (1984) *The Aachen Aphasia Test* — A New Multilingual Aphasia Test Battery. Aachen: International Neuropsychological Society Workshop.
HELM, N. (1984) *Screening the Severe Aphasic Patient.* San Francisco. Paper presented at the American Speech Hearing and Language Association.
WEST, J. and SANDS, E. (1986) *Bedside Examination Screening Test*. Rockville: Aspen Publishers Inc.
ENDERBY, P. (1987) *Frenchay Aphasia Screening Test*. Windsor: NFER Test Publications.

References

American Speech Hearing and Language Association Journal, December 1983.
ANASTASI, A. *Psychological Testing* 5th edn. (1982) New York: Macmillan.
BEELE, K.A., DAVIES, E. and MULLER, D. Therapists' Views on the Clinical Usefulness of Four Aphasia Tests. *British Journal of Disorders of Communication* (1984), **19**, 169–178.
BENTON, A.L. Problems of Test Construction in the field of aphasia. *Cortex* (1967), **3**, p. 32.
BIBER, C. *Same/Related and Unrelated Condition Test*. Unpublished observations.
BISHOP, D. *The Reception of Grammar* (T.R.O.G.), (1984). Department of Psychology, University of Manchester.
BROOKSHIRE, R. *An Introduction to Aphasia* (1978). Minneapolis: BRK Publishers.
BROWN, J.W. *Aphasia, Apraxia and Agnosia — Clinical and Theoretical Aspects* (1972). Illinois Charles C. Thomas.
BUTFIELD, E. *The Assessment of Aphasia*. Self-Publication.
BYNG, S. *Sentence Processing Deficits in Aphasia: Investigations and Rehabilitation* (1986). Unpublished PhD Thesis. University of London.
CHIAT, S., JONES, E.V. Processing Language Breakdown. In M. Ball (ed.) *Theoretical Linguistics and Disordered Speech and Language* (in press). London: Croom Helm.
CHRISTIENSON, A.L. *Luria's Neuropsychological Investigation* (1974). Copenhagen: Munksgaard.
CLARK, C.I., CROCKETT, D. and KLONOFF, H. Factor Analysis of the PICA — Porch Index of Communicative Ability. *Brain and Language* (1979), **7**, 1–7.
COLTHEART, M. Cognitive Neuropsychology and the Study of Reading. In M.I. Posner and O.S.M. Marin (eds) *Attention and Performance XI* (1985). Hillsdale, New Jersey: Lawrence Erlbaum Associates.
COLTHEART, M., SARTONI, G. and JOB, R. (eds) *The Cognitive Neuropsychology of Language* (1986). Hillsdale, New Jersey: Lawrence Erlbaum Associates.

COLTHEART, M., MASTERSON, J., BYNG, S., PRIOR, M. and RIDDOCK, M.J. Surface Dyslexia. *Quarterly Journal of Experimental Psychology* (1983), **35A**, 469–95.

COLTHEART, M., PATTERSON, K. and MARSHALL, J. (eds.) *Deep Dyslexia* (1980). London: Routledge, Kegan Paul.

COULTHARD, M. An introduction to Discourse Analysis. In C.N. Candler (ed.) *Applied Linguistics and Language Study* (1977). Harlow: Longman.

COULTHARD, M. and MONTGOMERY M. (eds) *Studies in Discourse Analysis* (1981). London: Routledge and Kegan Paul.

CRITCHLEY, M. *Aphasiology and Other Aspects of Language* (1970). London: Edward Arnold.

CRYSTAL, D. Clinical Linguistics in Disorders of Human Communication, G.E. Arnold, F. Winkel and B.D. Wyke (eds). New York: Springer-Vorlag.

DARLEY, F. The Efficacy of Language Rehabilitation in Aphasia. *JSHD*, **XXXVII**, 13–21.

DARLEY, F. *Evaluation of Appraisal Techniques in Speech and Language Pathology* (1979). Reading, Mass.: Addison-Wesley Publishing Co.

DERENZI, E. and VIGNOLO, L.A. The Token Test: A sensitive test to detect receptive disturbances in Aphasia. *Brain* (1962), **85**, 665–78.

DUFFY, J.R., WATT, J. and DUFFY, R.J. Deficit of Non-verbal Communication in Aphasic Patients: A Test of Some Current Causal Theories. In *Clinical Aphasiology Conference Proceedings* (1978). Minneapolis: BRK Publishing.

EISENSON, J. *Examining For Aphasia* (1954). New York Psychological Corporation.

EISENSON, J. (Rev. 54) *Examining for Aphasia* (1946). New York Psychological Corporation.

EISENSON, J. *Adult Aphasia Assessment and Treatment* (1973). New Jersey: Prentice Hall.

ELLIS, A.W. *Reading, Writing and Dyslexia* (1984). London: Lawrence Erlbaum Associates. Hillside, New Jersey.

ENDERBY, P. *Frenchay Aphasia Screening Test* (1986). Windsor, England: NFER-Nelson Test Publications.

FUNNEL, E. Physiological Processes in Reading: New Evidence from Acquired Dyslexia. *British Journal of Psychology* (1983), **74.2**, 159–180.

GATES, and MCGINTIE, *Reading Test* (1965). Houghton Mifflin Co.

GOODGLASS, H. and KAPLAN, E. *The Assessment of Aphasia and Related Disorders* (1972). Philadelphia: Lea and Febiger.

GOODGLASS, H. and KAPLAN, E. *The Assessment of Aphasia Related Disorders* (1983) 2nd edn. Philadelphia: Lea and Febiger.

GREEN, E. On the Contribution of Studies in Aphasia to Psycholinguists. *Cortex*, **6** 216–235.

GREENBURG, R.F. In F. Darley (ed.) *Evaluation of Appraisal Techniques in Speech and Language Pathology* (1979). Reading, Mass.: Addison-Wesley Publishing Company.

HALPERN, H. In F. Darley (ed.) *Evaluation of Appraisal Techniques in Speech and Language Pathology* (1979). Reading, Mass.: Addison-Wesley Publishing Company.

HALSTEAD, W.C. and WEPMAN, J.M. The Halstead and Wepman Aphasia Screening Test: *Journal of Speech and Hearing Disorders* Vol. 14. (1949). pp. 9-15.

HATFIELD, M. Aspects of Acquired Dysgraphia and Implications for Reeducation. In C. Code and D.J. Muller (eds) *Aphasic Therapy* (1982). London: Arnold.

HEAD, H. *Methods of Examination for Aphasia and Kindred Disorders of Speech* Vols. 1 and 2. (1926). London: Cambridge University Press.

HECAEN, H. Studies of Language Pathology. In T.A. Sebeok (ed.) *Current Trends in Linguistics 81*, (1972). The Hague: Mouton.

HEIMBERGER, R.F. and REITAN, R.M. *Testing for Aphasia and Related Disorders* (1961). Indiana University Medical Centre.

HOLLAND, A. *Communication Abilities in Daily Living* (CADL), (1980). University Park Press.

HOWARD, D. and PATTERSON, K. *Pyramids and Palm Trees Test*. Unpublished observations.

HUBER, W., WENIGER, D., POECK, K. and WILLMES, K. Der Aachener Aphasic Test: Aufbau und Uberprufung der Konstruktion. *Der Nervenarzt* (1980), **51**, 475-482.

HUBER, W., POECK, K. and WILLMES, K. The Aachen Aphasia Test. In F. Clifford Rose (ed.) *Advances in Neurology. Progress in Aphasiology* (1984). New York: Raven Press.

JONES, E.V. Word Order Processing in Aphasia: Effect of Verb Semantics. In F. Clifford Rose (ed.) *Advances in Neurology. Progress in Aphasiology* (1984). New York: Raven Press.

JASTAK, S.F. and JASTAK, S.R. (eds) *Wide Range Achievement Tests* . Wilmington: D.E. Guidance Associates (1965).

KEENAN, J.S. and BRASSELL, E.G. *Aphasia Language Performance Scales* (1975). Pinnacle Press.

KERTESZ, A. and POOLE, The Aphasia Quotient: The Taxonomic Approach to Measurement of Aphasic Disability. *Canadian Journal of Neurological Sciences* (1974), **1**, 7-16.

KERTESZ, A. and PHIPPS, J. Numerical Taxonomy of Aphasia. *Brain and Language* (1977), **4**, 1-10.

LEBRUN, Y. Aphasia Testing: Some Neurolinguistic Concerns (1983). Unpublished observations.

LECOURS, A.R., LHERMIITTE, F. and BRYANS, B. (eds.) The Assessment of Aphasia. In *Aphasiology* (1983). Balliere Tindall.

LESSER, R. *Linguistic Investigations of Aphasia* (1978). London: Edward Arnold.

LESSER, R. and REICH, S. Language Disorders. In A. Burke (ed.) *The Pathology of Cognition* (1986). London:Methuen.

LEZACK, M. *Neuropsychological Assessment* (1976). New York: Oxford University Press.

MARIE, P. *Revue Neurologique* (1902), **16**, 611-974.

MCKENNA, P, and WARRINGTON, E. *Graded Naming Test* (1982), Windsor: NFER-Nelson Test Publishers.

MCNEIL, M.R. Porch Index of Communicative Ability. In F.L. Darley (ed.) *Evaluation of Appraisal Techniques in Speech and Language Pathology* (1979). Reading, Mass.: Addison-Wesley.

MONRAD KROHN, G.H. Examination for Aphasia. In *The Clinical Examination of the Nervous System* (1921). London: Lewis.

MÜLLER, D., MUNRO, S. and CODE, C. *Language Assessment for Remediation* (1981). London: Croom Helm.

NELSON, H. *National Adult Reading Test* (1982). Windsor: NFER-Nelson Test Publishers.

OLDFIELD, R.C. and WINGFIELD, A. *A Series of Pictures for Use in Object Naming* (1965). M.R.C. Psychology. Reserved Unit Special Report No. PLU/65/19.

OSGOOD, C. and MIRON, M. *Approaches to the Study of Aphasia* (1963). University of Illinois Press.

PARADIS, M. and LECOURS, A.R.Aphasia in Bilinguals and Polyglots. In A.R. Lecours, F. Lhermitte and B. Bryans (eds) *Aphasiology* (1983). London: Balliere Tindall.

PARISI, D. and PIZZAMIGLIO, L. Syntactic Comprehension in Aphasia, *Cortex* (1970), 204–15.

PATTERSON, K.E. Neuropsychological Approaches to the Study of Reading. *British Journal of Psychology* (1982), **72**, 151–174.

PENN, C. *Syntactic and Pragmatic Aspects of Aphasic Language* (1983). Unpublished PhD Thesis. University of Witwatesrand.

PEUSER, P. *Aphasia — Patholinguistics 3* (1978). Munich: Wilhelm Fink Verlag.

PORCH, B. *The Porch Index of Communicative Ability* (1967). Palo Alto: Consulting Psychologists Press.

POWELL, G., BAILEY, S. and CLARKE, E. A very short version of the Minnesota Test for the Differential Diagnosis of Aphasia. *British Journal of the Society of Clinical Psychologists* (1980), **19**, 189–194.

PRINS, R., SNOW, C and WAGENAAR, E. Recovery from Aphasia: Spontaneous Speech Versus Language Comprehension. *Brain and Language* (1978), **6,** 192-211.

RITTER, G.E. In F.L. Darley (ed.) *Evaluation of Appraisal Techniques in Speech and Language Pathology* (1979). Reading: Addison-Wesley Publishing Company.

ROCHFORD, G. and WILLIAMS, M. The Measurement of Language Disorders. *Speech Pathology and Therapy* (1964), **7**, 3–21.

SCHUELL, H. A Short Examination for Aphasia. *Neurology* (1957), **7**, 625–634.

SCHUELL, H. *The Minnesota Test for the Differential Diagnosis of Aphasia* (1965). Minneapolis: University of Minnesota Press.

SCHUELL, H. *Aphasia Theory and Therapy* (1974). Selected Lectures — Papers of Hildred Schuell. Baltimore: University Park Press.

SHEWAN, C.M. *Auditory Comprehension Test for Sentences* (1979), Chicago: Biolinguistics.

SKINNER, C. Personal Communication (1971).

SKINNER, C., WIRZ, S.L. and THOMPSON, I. *Edinburgh Functional Communication Profile* (1984). Winslow Press.

SKLAR, M. *Sklar Aphasia Scales* (1966). Western Psychological Services.

SPREEN, O. and BENTON, A.L. *Neurosensory Centre Comprehensive Examination for Aphasia* (1969). University of Victoria, B.C.

TAYLOR, M. *Functional Communication Profile* (1969). Institute of Rehabilitation Medicine, New York: University Medical Centre.

THOMPSON, J. and ENDERBY, P. Is all your Schuell really necessary? *British Journal of Disorders of Communication* (1979), **14**, 95–201.

TYRER, J.H. and EADIE, M.J. *University of Queensland Aphasia Language Test*. The Australia Council for Educational Research Ltd, Queensland University, Hawthorn, Victoria, 3122 Australia.

WEIGL, E. On the Construction of Standard Psychological Test in Cases of Brain Damage. *Journal of Neurological Sciences* (1966), **3**, 123 (5).

WEISENBURG, T.H. and MCBRIDE, K.E. *Aphasia, A Clinical and Psychological Study* (1935). New York: Commonwealth Fund.

WEPMAN, J.M. *Recovery from Aphasia* (1951). New York: Ronald Press Co.

WEPMAN, J.M. and JONES, L.V. *Language Modalities Test for Aphasia* (1961). Chicago: Education Industry Service.

WEST, J. and SANDS, E. *Bedside Examination Screening Test* (1986). Rockville: Aspen Publishers Inc.

WHITTAKER, H.A. and WHITTAKER, J.L. Linguistic Theory and Speech Pathology. *Journal of the Minnesota Speech and Hearing Association* (1972), **11**, 51–65.

WHURR, R. *An Aphasia Screening Test* (1974). Whurr Publishers Ltd. 2 Alwyne Road, London N1 2HH, England.

WHURR, R. Towards a linguistic typology of aphasic impairment. In D. Crystal (ed.) *Linguistic Controversies* (1982). London: Edward Arnold.

WILLMES, K., POECK, D., WENIGER, D. and HUBER, W. Facet Theory Applied to the Construction and Validation of the Aachen Aphasia Test. *Brain and Language* (1983), **18**, 259–276.

ZUBRICK, A. and SMITH, A. In F. Darley (ed.) *Evaluation of Appraisal Techniques in Speech and Language Pathology* (1979). Reading, Mass.: Addison-Wesley Publishing Company.

V

Treatment

19

Non-vocal Approaches to Aphasia Rehabilitation

Nancy Helm-Estabrooks and Patricia A. Emery

Introduction

Aphasia is an acquired language disorder that manifests itself most apparently through the primary language modalities of speech production and comprehension. Traditionally, aphasia therapy has focused on remediation of these primary language skills but, as Schuler and Baldwin (1981) pointed out, there is a growing awareness that language is not just a vocal–auditory phenomenon, that speech behaviour does not necessarily imply language skills, and that language can be expressed through modalities other than speech. Although Schuler and Baldwin were referring specifically to the remediation of childhood autism, their observations has significance for aphasia rehabilitation.

Speech typically is the preferred mode of communication and the end goal of our therapeutic efforts in aphasia. Non vocal approaches may be used transitionally as the patient regains functional speech skills, or augmentatively to enhance restricted natural communication skills on a more permanent basis. The purpose of this chapter is to discuss these non-vocal approaches to rehabilitating aphasic individuals.

Assessment of Candidacy for Non-vocal Communication Systems

Decisions as to candidacy for a non vocal system and the selection of the appropriate system are based on a careful differential diagnosis of the patient's disorder(s). This differential diagnosis should identify retained skills and positive performance features as well as defective skills and negative performance features. It is not limited to language but will include neurological and cognitive test results as well.

Practic functioning is of crucial importance to the choice of a non-vocal system. Apraxia is a disorder of purposeful, learned movements that cannot be accounted for by weakness, paralysis or incoordination. Apraxia has obvious implications even for the use of the simplest communication aids. In its severest form, limb apraxia may affect 'pointing', that is, indicating with the index finger. Milder forms of apraxia may interfere with the acquisition or execution of a manual gesture system. In addition, virtually every test of an individual's cognitive and language skills depends on a reliable output pathway. It is possible that severe oral and gestural/limb apraxia will compromise the reliable use of any voluntary motor output channel in aphasic individuals. In these cases, it may be difficult to assess the patient's cognitive and language deficits including auditory comprehension. The clinician must creatively explore reliable reponse modes. For example, some patients who cannot articulate, write or point to 'yes' or 'no' may be able to indicate these concepts reliably by grasping the arm of a wheelchair where the words 'yes' and 'no' accompanied by frowning and smiling faces have been taped.

Any potential candidate for a non-vocal system must have the capacity for symbolic representation. The most basic level of symbolic skill may be assessed by asking the patient to perform a match-to-sample task. This can be evaluated informally or formally by such tests as subtest VIII of the Porch Index of Communicative Ability (PICA), (Porch, 1967). In this subtest, simple line drawings of ten objects are matched with their real object counterparts. As in all testing, it is important for the clinician to determine that the patient has understood what is expected of him and that any failure to perform accurately is not due to confusion.

Even when a patient can perform match-to-sample tasks, suggesting at least a basic appreciation of symbolic representation, other variables such as general memory and intelligence may interfere with the successful learning and/or implementation of a new form of communication. Wechsler (1958) defines intelligence as the global capacity of the individual to act purposefully, to think rationally, and to deal with his environment. Evaluation of intelligence in a severely aphasic individual is always difficult. One must rely on tests that do not require production or understanding of verbal messages. The Raven's Progressive Matrices (1960), involving the selection and matching of designs, is one way of measuring non-verbal reasoning. The clinician must be aware, however, of any visuo-spatial or visual scanning problems that could interfere with the patient's performance on this test. A poor performance on the Raven's, whatever the reason, may be predictive of poor treatment response.

Once the clinician has established that the aphasic patient has retained capacity for symbolic representation, a non-vocal communication system can be considered. Non vocal systems can be grouped into two broad categories: (1) manual sign systems; and (2) visual symbol systems and communication aids. Both of these categories will be discussed below in terms of their theoretical basis and clinical application.

Manual Sign Systems

Theoretical Basis for Manual Sign Systems

Many researchers have studied the gestural abilities of aphasic patients. Interest in this topic dates to 1870 when Finkelnburg theorized that aphasia was not only a disorder of speech, but a central symbolic disorder that effects non-verbal behaviour as well. Support for Finkelnburg's theory is found in the work of such investigators as Pickett, 1974; Duffy *et al.*, 1975; Duffy and Duffy, 1981; and Cicone *et al.*, 1979. In contrast, other studies support the view that aphasia and apraxia are overlapping but independent phenomena (e.g. Goodglass and Kaplan, 1963; Kimura and Archibald, 1974; Geschwind, 1975; Varney, 1978; Seron *et al.*, 1979; Daniloff *et al.*, 1982). The view of aphasia/apraxia will influence the decision as to non vocal treatments. Proponents of the central symbolic disorder theory of aphasia question the efficacy of non-vocal treatment approaches (e.g. Duffy *et al.* 1975; Cicone *et al.*, 1979). In contrast, such investigators as Daniloff *et al.*, who found better gestural skills than speech skills in their aphasic patients, recommend manual communication therapy. This important controversy is discussed in more detail elsewhere in this volume and should be reviewed by clinicians considering non vocal intervention.

In manual communication systems, words and ideas are replaced by gestures. The term 'sign language' frequently is used to refer to all manual systems including American Sign Language, American Indian Sign, Paget-Gorman Sign and Signing Exact English. Not all of these, however, contain the elements of grammar which, strictly speaking, qualify them as a language. For example, American Indian Sign (Amer–Ind) is not a language, but a signal system or 'gestural code' (Skelly, 1979) consisting mostly of concrete signs that look like the concepts they represent. In this respect, Amer–Ind differs from systems such as American Sign Language (ASL) which utilises arbitrary signs having little or no relationship to their referents.

The degree to which a manual sign system can be considered a language is a critical issue for aphasia rehabilitation. Because aphasia is a disorder of language, it is logical to expect that the more closely a manual system resembles a spoken and written language, the greater challenge it will present to the aphasic individual. This important point is underscored by the repeated finding that deaf users of sign language become aphasic in sign following left hemisphere brain damage (*see* for example, Sarno *et al.*, 1969;

Underwood and Paulson, 1981). Furthermore, these deaf persons may display sign language behaviours that resemble those seen in classic aphasia syndromes such as Broca's or Wernicke's aphasia (Poizner *et al.*, 1984).

Despite the fact that sign language skills may become compromised in deaf persons with left hemisphere brain damage, a manual gesture approach to rehabilitation of hearing aphasics is not without theoretical rationale. Gestures, for example, can be produced independently of vocal communication and may be easier to process than the temporally faster and shorter auditory signals. Furthermore, the hand movements required for manual systems are less motorically refined than the articulatory movements required for speech. Finally, the hand and arm, unlike the oral apparatus, can be manipulated by the therapist and visually monitored by the patient.

Clinical Application of Manual Sign Systems

The notion of replacing defective speech output with manual gestures has long held appeal for aphasia rehabilitation specialists. Goldstein and Cameron (1952) devised a "Hand Talking Chart" consisting of 20 iconic and arbitrary signs. Chen (1968) combined a manual alphabet with gestures, (e.g. the letter 'W' with a gesture toward the mouth for 'water'), in what she called the Talking Hand approach. Chen's method was challenged by Eagelson *et al.* (1968) who found the approach difficult to teach and inadequate for the communication needs of their patients, and developed an alternative programme that combined deaf sign language and American Indian signs. According to Eagelson, Vaughn and Knudson (1976), their programme, which consisted of 12 'self care' signs, was used by 31 "expressive dysphasic" patients until verbal communication improved.

The fullest application of a system based on American Indian sign is seen in the work of Skelly and her colleagues (Skelly *et al.*, 1972, 1973; Skelly *et al.*, 1974; Skelly, 1979). Although originally applied to non-aphasic disorders, e.g. glossectomy, it was adapted for oral/verbal apraxia and later for severe aphasia. Skelly (1979) stated that experience with this latter group has shown that performance was best when training was limited to the gestural modality in the early stages of therapy. Even when the patient has acquired some signs and has improved in auditory comprehension test scores, she suggested sequential and not simultaneous presentation of gestural and verbal stimuli.

Rao *et al.* (1977) used a version of Amer–Ind with ten severely aphasic patients who failed to achieve the expected gains from traditional therapy. Approximately 150 signs were introduced in a group therapy setting. Verbalization was neither encouraged nor discouraged, but appropriate, intelligible verbal responses were positively reinforced. After 4–20 months ($\bar{x}$ = 9.5) of training, 7 of the 10 patients showed improvement on a standardized aphasia test.

A combination of Amer–Ind and American Sign Language (ASL) was used by Kirshner and Webb (1981) to treat a patient with muteness and impaired auditory comprehension after bitemporal infarctions. The patient had intact visual matching-to-sample skills and her reading comprehension exceeded her auditory skills. In a 7 month period she learned 127 signs which she produced in one or two sign 'utterances'.

Hoodin and Thompson (1983) compared the effects of three randomly administered treatment procedures on two non-fluent subjects: (1) Amer–Ind gesture training alone; (2) Amer–Ind with verbalization; and (3) verbalization alone. Three groups of nouns were randomly assigned to the three treatment procedures. It was found that a combination of gesture plus verbalization was the best facilitator of verbal labeling although there was variability across the two subjects. Generalization to untrained items was negligible.

Relative to the attention given Amer–Ind there are few reports of the exclusive use of American Sign Language (ASL) with aphasic patients. Bonvillian and Friedman (1978) described the response of a single patient to a rehabilitation programme based on ASL. Because the patient suffered a head injury rather than a stroke the generalization of the findings to aphasic stroke patients is tenuous.

The relative ease of acquiring and using Amer–Ind versus ASL was examined by Guilford *et al.* (1982). Eight aphasic adults learned and used the two systems with equal ease. Production of gestures in either system was significantly related, however, to auditory comprehension as measured by the Boston Diagnostic Aphasia Exam (Goodglass and Kaplan, 1972) a finding explained, in part, by the verbal in-put nature of the training programme.

The confounding problem of auditory comprehension deficits is circumvented in a method called Visual Action Therapy (Helm-Estabrooks, Fitzpatrick and Barresi, 1982). No verbalization is used in this hierarchically structured programme that trains global aphasic patients to produce representational gestures for hidden visual stimuli. Helm-Estabrooks *et al.* described the effects of VAT on eight patients who had failed to respond to traditional language treatment approaches. All eight subjects exhibited significant improvement on pantomime and auditory comprehension subtests of the Porch Index of Communicative Ability (PICA) (Porch, 1967) upon completion of the programme. This improvement was independent of time post onset of aphasia.

Subsequent investigation showed that some global aphasic patients were unable to complete the VAT programme. In 1983 Biber *et al.* analyzed the neuropsychological test results as well as BDAE scores of 20 patients who participated in VAT. The test scores, that best predicted whether a patient would complete VAT, were those involving memory for designs and visuospatial/construction ability. Performance on the following tests correlated with VAT completion at the 0.001 level of significance: (1) Wechsler Memory Scale, Delayed Recognition for Designs; (2) WAIS Object Assembly; (3) Boston Diagnostic Aphasia Exam 'Parietal Lobe Battery' Stick Designs from Memory; and (4) Drawing to Command and Copy. Of the thirteen BDAE and PICA subtests analyzed, only the BDAE Symbol/Word Discrimination subtest correlated significantly with VAT completion. This subtest requires patients to match letters and words that are written in lower and upper case print and script. These findings suggest once again that factors extrinsic to language or aphasia may be important in teaching aphasic patients to produce even highly representational gestures such as those used in VAT.

Although our purpose here is to describe specific gesture training approaches for aphasia patients, the work of Schlanger, Schlanger and their colleagues using pantomimic role playing with aphasic patients bears mention; they (Tannenbaum and Schlanger, 1968; Schlanger and Schlanger, 1970; Schlanger, 1976; Schlanger and Frieman, 1979) have found role-playing to be useful in reducing frustration, anxiety, and inhibition, and in improving self-confidence and insight. Furthermore, pantomime approaches may lead to increased verbalization in some patients.

Based on her observation of aphasic patients in natural settings, Holland (1977) has pointed out that they 'probably communicate better than they can talk'. Certainly, the best measure of any gestural treatment is the extent to which the newly acquired signs are used to communicate in natural settings. Without evidence of functional generalization, there is no assurance that the patient has not merely seen the therapeutic task as 'a set of patterns to be memorized or a game to be played at stated times during the day' (Gardner *et al.*, 1976). It is difficult, however, to measure functional use of skills acquired in treatment. This is best accomplished through observation of the patient within various environmental settings with a variety of other persons. The Functional Communication Profile (Sarno, 1969) contains a measure of gestural skills. The Boston Non Vocal Communication Scale (Borod *et al.*, 1984) is specifically designed as a rating of non vocal strategies in natural settings.

Holland's Communicative Abilities in Daily Living (CADL, 1980), which involves acting out naturally occurring situations, is a more formal approach to assessing the use of gestures than the FCP or BNRS. In the CADL, credit is given when a patient communicates a correct idea through any means. For example, in response to the question 'How many children do you have?' the patient may receive full credit for saying, writing or gesturing the correct number. Aten *et al.* (1982) found that the CADL was sensitive to changes in chronic aphasic patients receiving functional communication therapy, whereas the PICA was not. This suggests that the CADL may be used as a dependent measure of functional generalization of manual sign systems.

Visual Symbol Systems and Communication Aids

Theoretical Basis

Visual symbol systems may consist of photographs or iconic line drawings, arbitrary signs that stand for concepts, or orthographic, written language. For example, a cigarette can be represented by an iconic line drawing, whereas a concept such as 'not allowed' can be represented by the arbitrary symbol of a circle containing a diagonal line. When the two symbols are combined, the message becomes 'no smoking'. This same message, of course, can be orthographically conveyed in any written language. The success of visual symbol systems with other non-speaking populations prompted investigations of their use with aphasic adults., For theoretical and practical reasons, these have been explored largely with globally aphasic patients.

Two landmark studies used symbol systems in an effort to determine whether patients who do not produce or appear to understand natural language retain the symbolic and the computational skills necessary for language (Glass *et al.* 1973; Gardner *et al.*, 1976). In each of these theoretically motivated studies, the subjects were severely aphasic but well-oriented and motivated. Pre-testing showed that the patients could sort words from non-words (Glass *et al.*) or match objects with representational line drawings (Gardner *et al.*). Glass *et al.* used arbitrary symbols, cut from coloured paper, for objects such as 'juice' and concepts such as 'not the same'. When arranged from left to right, these symbols formed 'sentences'. Level I of the nine step training hierarchy involved selection of the correct symbol (same or different) to describe the relationship between two items, e.g. spoon:cup. The highest level involved the observation of an activity performed by the clinician followed by the selection and arrangement of symbols that accurately described that activity, e.g. 'Andrea drink water'.

Gardner *et al.* used index cards upon which simple representational or arbitrary symbols were drawn. This system, called VIC for Visual Communication, contained proper nouns, common nouns, verbs, prepositions, markers, interjections, adjectives and locations plus activities, such as 'go home'. Cards were arranged from left to right in a task hierarchy that included: (1) understanding and responding to commands; (2) answering questions; (3) describing events; (4) expressing feelings; (5) expressing immediate needs; (6) expressing desires.

Both the Premack *et al.* and the Gardner *et al.* studies showed that globally aphasic patients can learn to select and arrange non-orthographic symbols in a way that suggest that language is not lost in this syndrome. The authors concluded that globally aphasic patients may retain a rich conceptual system and at least some of the cognitive operations necessary for natural language. While these landmark studies did not explore the therapeutic use of symbol systems, Gardner and his colleagues found that some patients showed notable improvement in BDAE auditory comprehension scores following VIC despite the fact that no verbalization was used during the training programme. The concept that natural language may be deblocked in aphasia through the use of another symbol system is an intriguing concept that has some support (*see* for example, Johannsen-Horbach *et al.*, 1985).

The concept of using electronic devices and computers as both therapy tools and communication aids dates to the early 1960s when teaching machines such as the Grolier Min–Max 11 were combined with Programmed Instruction methods. In 1965, Taylor and Sands used programmed, mechanical instruction with twenty-five severely impaired aphasic adults. Twenty-one of these patients completed the program with varying degrees of success. The investigators concluded that Programmed Instruction was a potentially effective means for teaching language to aphasic adults and that computers held great promise for patients with verbal impairment secondary to brain damage.

Edwards and Rosenberg (1965) reported positive results with 'automated training' with five aphasic patients. Their subjects were required to visually discriminate nonverbal stimuli on a screen by pushing a button. All five were able to effectively complete the program. The authors noted that this type of structured, nonverbal program was a preliminary step to future training programmes using verbal materials.

Clinical Application of Visual Symbol Systems

Few studies have explored the use of symbol systems with aphasic patients as a means of functional communication. The system that has received the most attention is Blissymbolics, originally developed as an international communication system (Bliss, 1965). The 100 basic symbols contain iconic pictures representing concrete objects such as 'house' and arbitrary symbols representing concepts such as 'plural'. Signs may be combined to yield additional vocabulary as when the iconic picture for 'house' is combined with the arbitrary symbol for 'plural' to indicate 'city'. In the 1970s, three preliminary studies of the use of BLISS with aphasic patients were reported (Hughes, 1976; Kirby, 1978; Saya, 1978).

Trunzo (1981) chose to use Blissymbols rather than manual sign or other pictographic systems. She stated that, with gestural systems, whoever communicates with the aphasic patient must have prior knowledge of the symbols, whereas with BLISS the written words are presented beneath each symbols. BLISS seemed preferable to other pictographic approaches because Blissymbols can represent whole concepts and not just single units of meaning. Trunzo implemented a 20 hour training programme with four adult aphasics with severe oral/verbal apraxia. She found that: (1) Although all subjects learned Blissymbols, they showed varying degrees of proficiency, (2) The patients capacity for acquiring Blissymbols appeared related to their receptive language skills, (3) Speech intelligibility improved by pointing to Blisssymbols.

Lane and Samples (1981) used a combination of Blissymbols and their written and spoken representation in treating four patients with severe verbal apraxia as well as aphasia. Patients were seen in hourly group sessions held once a week over 8 months. Approximately ten symbols were introduced or reviewed in each session. The tasks required the patients to draw the symbols, write their corresponding word, and attempt to say the names. The therapist then said the words and the patients pointed to the corresponding symbols/written words. No patient appeared to have used BLISS for functional communication. Two subjects could not retain Blissymbols from session to session, but the two remaining patients reportedly benefitted from BLISS in so far as their use seemed to facilitate writing.

Johannsen-Horbach *et al.* (1985) used BLISS with four globally aphasic patients who had previously received at least six months of traditional treatment. Individual sessions were conducted twice a week for at least two months. The goals were for patients to acquire a basic lexicon of Blissymbols, to produce and understand simple BLISS sentences, and to use BLISS to communicate in the home environment. The written equivalents were displayed beneath each symbol and their verbal realization was neither reinforced nor restricted. The patients' performances were assessed after twelve sessions. Although all four patients reportedly acquired a symbol lexicon, one patient with extensive left hemisphere brain damage, including the thalamus, was discontinued because of extreme perseveration. In the other three, perseveration was milder with the symbols than with natural language. Two patients were able to use BLISS to communicate with relatives and one of these produced some phrases. BLISS facilitated verbal output in two patients, one of whom regained some functional speech. One of the four patients used BLISS for daily communication.

Like Lane and Samples, Johannsen-Horbach *et al.* combined BLISS with natural language, so it is difficult to differentiate the effects of the Blissymbols from the effects of the written and spoken stimuli. It would appear that no study has explored BLISS in the same manner that Gardner *et al.* (1976) explored VIC, that is, without verbal or written language. Nevertheless, the available evidence suggests that even globally aphasic patients can acquire at least a rudimentary visual symbol system, that may to some degree substitute for, or deblock, natural language.

Drawing is another potential means of non-vocal communication, although it is a relatively unexplored area. One notable exception is the 1974 study by Hatfield and Zangwill, who investigated the ability of a non-fluent aphasic patient to produce drawings to convey the following: (1) short stories narrated to him; (2) events acted out by the clinician; and (3) events in the patient's own life. The results of this study as well as informal work with other aphasic patients were encouraging. Hatfield and Zangwill concluded that the patients' drawings indicated the relative integrity of ideational processes in patients with predominantly expressive language disorders.

Pillon *et al.* (1980) used drawing to rehabilitate a globally aphasic patient who had been an artist and caricaturist. Over a three year period, the patient reportedly progressed through a wide range of drawing tasks from simple, e.g. drawing objects to copy, to complex, e.g. drawing sequences of pictures depicting events in his life. The authors concluded that the use of drawing, which taps right hemisphere functioning, is a viable method of nonvocal communication for certain aphasic patients and merits further investigation.

Clinical Application of Communication Aids

Communication aids can range from a few pictures of items of personal relevance to the patient, (e.g. 'toilet') to a computer. Whatever the aid, selection of an appropriate device will depend upon the patient's symbolic, visuo-spatial, cognitive and motor skills as well as practical considerations of communication needs. An ambulatory patient who travels around the community may require a highly portable system for functional use, whereas a bedridden patient with good language and cognitive skills may use a computer. Ultimately, however, the patient's willingness or motivation to use an aid should be assessed, particularly before an expensive device is purchased.

In her 1947 chapter on aphasia rehabilitation, Backus suggested that clinicians provide severely aphasic persons with a set of visual cues such as a picture of a car, family snapshot, or written words, so they can make themselves understood more easily. Such simple, customized communication boards/notebooks may be particularly useful in the early stages of recovery (*see*, for example, Beukelman, Yorkston and Dowden, 1985). Occasionally, a patient is motivated to develop a nonvocal aid for himself. The small notebooks full of personal information that some patients carry in their pocket are a form of communication aid.

There appear to be no formal studies of the effectiveness of simple aids, perhaps because the benefits seem obvious. It may be the case, however, that aids commonly remain in the drawer or patient's pocket or that they are used only when someone other than the patient initiates the activity. As suggested above, the degree to which a device is put to use becomes a particularly relevant issue when considering the more costly, electronic aids that are commercially available (Vanderheiden, 1978). In 1981, Shane stated that it is unclear as to whether augmentative systems, which have proven helpful to patients with motor speech disorders, will provide aphasic patients with a more useful communication system. Beukelman and Yorkston's patient with severe verbal apraxia progressed from the use of a picture board to the electronic Handivoice 130 with synthesized speech, but he was unable to use this device to formulate grammatically complete sentences. Often, he preferred to select single words rather than the available phrases and would use these words to introduce topics that he then communicated through his own speech and gestures.

One study compared the responses of thirteen aphasic patients to five non-aphasic, speech-impaired controls with an electronic aid called SPLINK (Helm-Estabrooks and Walsh, 1982). Earlier Perry, Gawel and Rose (1981) showed SPLINK to be an effective mode of communication for patients with motor neuron disease. This instrument consists of a large word board (16″ × 26″) and microprocessor that can be linked by infra-ray to any television set. The board contains 950 commonly used words and phrases, the alphabet, and numerals. The patient communicates by pressing an 11/16″ × 5/16″ space for target stimuli which then appear on the television screen. A pre-established, ten-step training protocol was followed to the highest level of each patient's ability. It was found that no aphasic patient achieved a more effective level of communication with SPLINK than with his own spoken, written and/or gestural systems. In contrast, all five of the controls were able to progress to step ten (using the SPLINK for conversation) despite the presence of severe neurological disease in three cases. These results suggest that electronic communication tools may not significantly aid the communication of patients whose disorder is primarily one of language rather than one of speech production. However an instrument such as SPLINK might be used for practicing language skills.

Of the available communication hardware, computers, in particular, are being used for language rehabilitation (Katz, 1984). Mills (1982) described a computer program for improving auditory comprehension skills, while Seron *et al.* (1980) developed a program for treatment of aphasic writing disorders. Loverso *et al.* (1985) adapted their syntax training approach for computer use.

Colby *et al.* (1981) programmed a portable microprocessor to 'find' words for an anomic patient. Called ISP (Intelligent Speech Prosthesis), the program used the following search strategy: (1) Topic Areas, e.g. *food*, (2) First letter of the word, e.g. *S*, (3) Last letter e.g. *K*, (4) A middle letter, e.g. *A*, (5) A related or GOESWITH word, e.g. *MEAT* = the target word *STEAK*. The GOESWITH words are individualized for each user. Among the special features of this system is a 'respeller' program that converts phonetically spelled words such as 'enuf' to their conventional spelling.

Colby *et al.* described the response of one patient with thalamic anomia to ISP. The patient had good reading comprehension but mild to moderate verbal apraxia and sentence level agraphia. Further, he had difficulty monitoring his own output which interfered with his successful use of ISP, for example, he would choose the appropriate word but continue his search. The major problem presented by ISP was its small memory which limited the number of words in the lexicon. The investigators pointed out, however, that microprocessors, with the ability to store thousands of words and their associations, were rapidly becoming available. For a catalogue of currently available computer soft-ware the reader is referred to the International Software–Hardware Registry at the Trace Center, University of Wisconsin in Madison.

After reviewing the available literature, however, Prescott and Loverso (1985) concluded that little efficacy data is currently available regarding computerized aphasia treatment programs. They encourage clinicians to collect or await more efficacy data before wholeheartedly endorsing computerized aphasia rehabilitation.

Summary

Nonvocal communication systems may facilitate communication skills in some aphasic patients. These systems can be broadly grouped into two categories: (1) Manual Sign Systems; and (2) Visual Symbol Systems/ Communication Aids. Nonvocal systems may be used transitionally until the patient regains functional speech, or permanently in cases where verbal output remains severely compromised.

The choice of a nonvocal system for any aphasic adult at any stage in the recovery process is based on careful assessment of the patient's motor, linguistic, and cognitive skills. Among these are: (1) limb praxis and movement; (2) auditory and reading comprehension; (3) visual scanning, matching and discrimination; (4) memory; (5) problem solving; and (6) orientation and motivation.

As in all aphasia rehabilitation, the true measure of nonvocal systems is the extent to which the patient uses newly acquired skills to communicate successfully within natural settings. Therefore, a dependent measure of functional generalization must be used to determine treatment success.

References

ATEN, J.L., CALIGIURI, M. and HOLLAND, A. The efficacy of functional communication therapy for chronic aphasia patients. *Journal of Speech and Hearing Disorders* (1982), **47**, 93–96.

BACKUS, O. The rehabilitation of persons with aphasia. *The Pathology of Speech* (1947). New York: Harper and Brothers.

BEUKELMAN, D., YORKSTON, K. and DOWDEN, P. *Communication augmentation: a casebook of clinical management* (1985). San Diego, CA: College Hill Press, Inc.

BIBER, C., HELM-ESTABROOKS, N. and FITZPATRICK, P. Predicting response to an aphasia treatment program with neuropsychological test results. Paper presented to the Academy of Aphasia (1983). Minneapolis, MN.

BLISS, C.K. *Semantography: Blissymbolics* (1965). Sydney, Australia: Symantography Publications.

BONVILLIAN, J.D. and FRIEDMAN, R.J. Language development in another mode: The acquisition of signs by a brain-damaged adult. *Sign Language Studies* (1978), **19**, 111–120.

BOROD, J., FITZPATRICK, P., HELM-EASTBROOKS, N. and GOODGLASS, H. A scale for evaluating non-vocal communication in aphasia patients (1984). Paper presented at the Academy of Aphasia, San Diego, CA.

CHEN, L. 'Talking Hand' for aphasic stroke patients. *Geriatrics* (1968), **23**, 145–148.

CICONE, M., WAPNER, W., FOLDI, N. ZURIF, E. and GARDNER, H. The relation between gesture and language in aphasic communication. *Brain and Language* (1979), **8**, 324–349.

COLBY, K.M., CHRISTINAZ, D., PARKINSON, R., GRAHM, S. and KARPF, C. A word-finding computer program with a dynamic lexical-semantic memory for patients with anomia using an intelligent speech prosthesis. *Brain and Language* (1981), **14**, 272–281.

DANILOFF, J., NOLL, J.D., FRISTOE, M. and LLOYD, L. Gesture recognition in patients with aphasia. *Journal of Speech and Hearing Disorders* (1982), **47**, 43–49.

DUFFY, R.J., DUFFY, J.R. and PEARSON, K. Pantomime recognition in aphasics. *Journal of Speech and Hearing Research* (1975), **18**, 115–132.

DUFFY, R.J. and DUFFY, J.R. Three studies of deficits in pantomime expression and pantomimic recognition in aphasia. *Journal of Speech and Hearing Research* (1981), **24**, 70–84.

DUFFY, R.J. and DUFFY, J.R. *New England Pantomime Tests* (1984). Tigard, Oregon: C.C. Publications, Inc.

EAGELSON, H., HENSON, D., BRADLEY, H. and TANNER, J. The use of mimicry in self care hand signs by aphasic patients. *American Archives of Rehabilitation Therapy* (1968), **16**, 2:39-44.

EAGELSON, H., VAUGHN, G. and KNUDSON, A. Hand Signals for Dysphasia. *Archives of Physical Medicine and Rehabilitation* (1970), **51**, 111–113.

FINKELNBURG, D.C. Niederrheinische Gesellschaft, Sitzung vom 21. Marz 1870 in Bonn. Berlin. *Klinische Wochenschrift* (1870), **7**, 449–450; 460–462.

GARDNER, H., ZURIF, E., BERRY, T. and BAKER, E. Visual communication in aphasia. *Neuropsychologia* (1976), **14**, 275–292.

GESCHWIND, N. The apraxias: neural mechanisms of learned movements. *American Scientist* (1975), **63**, 188–195.

GLASS, A., GAZZANIGA, M.S. and PREMACK, D. Artificial language training in aphasia. *Neuropsychologia* (1973), **14**, 275–292.

GOLDSTEIN, H. and CAMERON, H. New method of communication for the aphasic patient. *Journal of Arizona Medical Association* (1952), **9**, 17–21.

GOODGLASS, H. and KAPLAN, E. Disturbance of gesture and pantomime in aphasia. *Brain* (1963), **86**, 703–720.

GOODGLASS, H. and KAPLAN, E. *Boston Diagnostic Aphasia Examination* (1972). Philadelphia: Lea and Febiger.

GUILFORD, A., SCHEUERLE, J. and SHIREK, P. Manual communication skills in aphasia. *Archives of Physical and Medical Rehabilitation* (1982), **63**, 601–604.

HATFIELD, F.M. and ZANGWILL, D.L. Ideation in aphasia: the picture-story method. *Neuropsychologia* (1974), **12**, 389–393.

HELM-ESTABROOKS, N., FITZPATRICK, P. and BARRESI, B. Visual action therapy for global aphasia. *Journal of Speech and Hearing Disorders* (1982), **44**, 385–389.

HELM-ESTABROOKS, N. and WALSH, M. The response of aphasic patients to an electronic communication aid. Paper presented to *The American Speech-Language-Hearing Association Convention*, Toronto Canada (1982).

HELM-ESTABROOKS,, N. Treatment of subcortical aphasias. In W. Perkins (ed.) *Current Therapy of Communication Disorders* (1984), pp. 97–103. New York: Thieme-Stratton.

HOLLAND, A.L. Some practical considerations in aphasia rehabilitation. In M. Sullivan and M.S. Kommers (eds) *Rationale for Adult Aphasia Therapy* (1977), pp. 167–180. Lincoln, N.E.: University of Nebraska Medical Center.

HOLLAND, A.L. *Communication Abilities in Daily Living* (1980). Baltimore, M.D.: University Park Press.

HOODIN, R.B. and THOMPSON, C.K. Facilitation of verbal labeling in adult aphasia by gestural, verbal, or verbal plus gestural training (Abstract). In R.H. Brookshire (ed.) *Clinical Aphasiology Conference Proceedings* (1983), p. 62. Minneapolis, MN.: BRK Publishers.

HUGHES, E. Symbols for adults. *Blissymbolics Communication Newsletter*, 2 (1976).

JOHANNSEN-HORBACH, H., CEGLA, B., MAGER, U., SCHEMPP, B. and WALLESCH, C.W. Treatment of chronic global aphasia with a nonverbal communication system. *Brain and Language* (1985), **24**, 74–82.

KATZ, R. and TONG NAGY, V. A computerized treatment system for chronic aphasic patients. In R.H. Brookshire (ed.) *Clinical Aphasiology Conference Proceedings* (1982), pp. 153–160. Minneapolis, MN.: BRK Publishers.

KATZ, R. Using microcomputers in the diagnosis and treatment of chronic aphasic adults. *Seminars in Speech and Language* (1984), **5**, 1.

KIMURA, D. and ARCHIBALD, Y. Motor functions of the left hemisphere. *Brain* (1974), **97**, 337–350.

KIRBY, J. Blissymbolics and an aphasic patient. *Alberta Speech and Hearing Association Journal* (1978), **3**, 4.

KIRSHNER, H.S. and WEBB, W.G. Selective involvement of the auditory-verbal modality in an acquired communication disorder: benefit from sign language therapy. *Brain and Language* (1981), **13**, 161–170.

LANE, V.W. and SAMPLES, J.M. Facilitating communication skills in adult apraxic: application of Blissymbolics in a group setting. *Journal of Communication Disorders* (1981), **14**, 157–167.

LOVERSO, F., PRESCOTT, T., SELINGER, M., WHEELER, K and SMITH, R. The application of microcomputers for the treatment of aphasic adults. In R.H. Brookshire (ed.) *Clinical Aphasiology Conference Proceedings* (1985), pp. 189–195. Minneapolis, MN: BRK Publishers.

MILLS, R. Microcomputerized auditory comprehension training. In R.H. Brookshire (ed.) *Clinical Aphasiology Conference Proceedings* (1982), pp. 147–152. Minneapolis, MN: BRK Publishers.

PERRY, A.R., GAWEL, M. and ROSE, F.C. Communication aids in patients with motor neurone disease. *British Medical Journal* (1981), **282, 23**, 690–692.

PICKETT, L. An assessment of gestural pantomime deficit in aphasic patients. *Acta Symbolica* (1974), **5**, 69–86.

PILLON, B., SIGNORET, J.L., VAN EECKHOUT, P. and LHERMITTE, F. Le dessin chez un aphasique. *Revue Neurologie* (1980), **136, 10**, 699–710.

PORCH, B.E. *Porch Index of Communication Ability* (1967). Palo Alto, CA: Consulting Psychologists Press.

POIZNER, H., BELLUGI, U. and IRAQUI, V. Apraxia and aphasia for a visual-gestural language. *American Journal of Physiology* (Regulatory Integrative Comp. Physiol. 15) (1984), **246**, R868–883.

PRESCOTT, T. and LOVERSO, F. Computerized aphasia rehabilitation: state of the art. Paper presented to the American Speech-Language-Hearing Association Convention, Washington, D.C. (1985).

RAO, P.R., BASILI, A.G. HORNER, J. and KOLLER, J. Amer-Ind with aphasics. (Fort Howard V.A. project). In M. Skelly *Amer-Ind Gestural Code* (1977). New York, NY: Elsevier.

RAVEN, J.C. *Guide to the Standard Progressive Matrices* (1960). London, England: H.K. Lewis.

ROSENBERG, B. and EDWARDS, A.E. An automated multiple response alternative training program for use with aphasics. *Journal of Speech and Hearing Research* (1965), **8**, 415–419.

SARNO, M.T. *The Functional Communication Profile: manual of directions* (1969). New York, NY: New York University Medical Center — The Institute of Rehabilitation Medicine.

SARNO, J., SWISHER, L. and SARNO, M.T. Aphasia in a congenitally deaf man. *Cortex* (1969), **5**, 390–414.

SAYA, M.J. Bliss and the adult aphasic. *Alberta Speech and Hearing Association Journal* (1978), **3**, 8.

SCHLANGER, P. and SCHLANGER, B. Adapting role-playing activities with aphasic patients. *Journal of Speech and Hearing Disorders* (1970), **35**, 229–235.

SCHLANGER, P. Training an adult aphasic to pantomime. Paper presented to the American Speech-Language-Hearing Association Convention, Las Vegas, NV (1976).

SCHLANGER, P. and FREIMAN, R. Pantomime therapy with aphasics. *Aphasia, Apraxia and Agnosia* (1979), **1**, 34–39.

SCHULER, A.L. and BALDWIN, M. Nonspeech communication and childhood autism. *Language Speech and Hearing Services in Schools* (1981), **12, 4**, 246–257.

SERON, X., VAN DERKAA, M.A., REMITZ, A. and VAN DER LINDEN, M. Pantomime interpretation in aphasia. *Neuropsychologia* (1979), **17**, 661–668.

SHANE, H. Working with the nonspeaking person. *Asha* (1981), **23(8)**, 461–464.

SKELLY, M., SCHINSKY, L., DONALDSON, R. and SMITH, R. *Handbook of Amerind Sign* (1973). St. Louis, MO: V.A. Workshop.

SKELLY, M., SCHINSKY, L., SMITH, R. and FUST, R. American Indian Sign (Amerind) as a facilitator of verbalization for the oral verbal apraxic. *Journal of Speech and Hearing Disorders* (1974), **39**, 445–456.

SKELLY, N., SCHINSKY, L., SMITH, R., DONALDSON, R. and GRIFFIN, J. American Indian Sign: a gestural communication system for the speechless. *Archives of Physical and Medical Rehabilitation* (1975), **56**, 156–160.

SKELLY, M. *Amer–Ind Gestural Code Based on Universal American Indian Hand Talk* (1979). New York, NY: Elsevier.

TAYLOR, M. and SANDS, E. Application of programmed instruction techniques to the language rehabilitation of severely impaired aphasic patients. Paper presented to the *American Speech–Language–Hearing Association Convention* (1965). Chicago, IL.

TRUNZO, M. Assessment of Blissymbolics in adult apraxic-aphasics. Poster session presented at the American Speech–Language–Hearing Convention, Los Angeles, CA (1981).

UNDERWOOD, J. and PAULSON,; C. Aphasia and congenital deafness: a case study. *Brain and Language* (1981), **12**, 285–291.

VANDERHEIDEN, G. *Nonvocal Communication Resource Book* (1978). Baltimore, MD: University Park Press.

VARNEY, N. Linguistic correlates of pantomime recognition in aphasic patients. *Journal of Neurology, Neurosurgery, and Psychiatry* (1978), **41**, 564–568.

WECHSLER, D. *The Measurement and Appraisal of Adult Intelligence* (4th ed) (1958). Baltimore, MD: Williams and Wilkins.

20

The Management of the Aphasic Patient

David J. Mulhall

Introduction

This chapter is mainly concerned with the impact of aphasia on personal relationships. Since marriage is its focus, the discussion appropriately includes 'something old, something new, something borrowed and something blue'. The first of these refers to rehabilitation, an activity pursued on a multidisciplinary basis after the acute phase of illness is over and the patient's clinical state has stabilized, a process which prepares patients to leave hospital and return to the community.

All things are relative and, certainly, this applies to the new material, which concerns a counselling technique helpful in working families and the spouse in particular. Although the focus of health and social care is on the patient, too little attention has been paid to the needs of the spouse, whose burden of day-to-day care is often onerous and can be stressful. The spouse can facilitate adaptation to changed circumstances or can erode progress made in retreat; there is a clear need to nurture the former and discourage the latter.

'Borrowed' is the work of Dr David Griffiths who made available certain unpublished work on rehabilitation; Mrs Madge Wicks was kind enough to allow the text of certain of her public addresses to be used.

With regard to 'blue', or, more accurately, 'blues' the management of aphasic patients is difficult for professional staff and close relatives, in particular, the initial shock of the illness and confrontation with the possibility of death. Later, there is the inevitable frustration of aphasia, the anguish many relatives experience and the feelings of failure which erode self-confidence.

Aphasia infrequently presents in the absence of other disabilities so that this chapter is widely based, with practical suggestions regarding management, discussion of methodological issues in relation to counselling, and case studies in order to exemplify certain points.

Management in Hospital — Rehabilitation

When in the mid- and late 1940s, the National Health Service was being planned and introduced in the United Kingdom, there was the belief that disease could successfully be combated. What was not clearly foreseen was that, as infantile mortality dropped, allowing increasing numbers of people to survive until their full biological potential, the frontiers of health care would shift from acute life-threatening diseases of the young to chronic and disabling conditions of the mature and elderly. Many of the major health care problems have multiple causes and damaging effects which erode individual autonomy and continue to require management long after active treatment has been abandoned. In these circumstances, it is the quality of existence rather than life itself which is endangered, so that questions of management, the first stage of which is rehabilitation, deserves active consideration that in most sorts of enduring disability, and not only to aphasia, which infrequently presents in the absence of other disabilities.

We shall first define rehabilitation, then consider a model which categorizes disabilities and to conclude the discussion with consideration of five major principles, the emphasis of which will be on how theory can be translated into practice.

Goldberg (1974) provided a clear statement of the aims of rehabilitation when he defined it as 'the process of restoring a handicapped person, if not to the level of function and the same social position which he had achieved before the onset of illness, then at least to a situation in which he can make best use of his residual capacities within as normal as possible a social context'. An advantage of this definition is that it includes the biological, social and psychological components of a patient's functioning, giving a whole-person approach to rehabilitation.

With respect to the model of disability, Wing (1977) gave a three-tiered categorization:

1. 'Intrinsic' or primary disabilities i.e. the signs and symptoms arising directly from an accident or illness, and refer to problems of mobility, co-ordination, sensory function, cognition and language. Losses in any of these areas may have profound repercussions for self-help skills, communication and social functioning.
2. 'Adverse secondary reactions' are not part of the illness but represent maladaptive reactions and include loss of self-esteem, negative self-evaluation, low motivation, anxiety, depression etc. Such difficulties compound the problems generated directly by illness and reduce still further the quality of a patient's existence.
3. 'Extrinsic disadvantages' or 'premorbid disabilities' include both lifelong and more immediate factors. The former include limited intellectual

ability and educational and social disadvantage, the impact of which may be reflected in limited social and practical skills. The more immediate factors include lack of support from the family and, in some cases, the effects of prolonged institutionalization.

Again, this categorization refers to the biological, social and psychological levels of functioning which interact with each other in the presentation of multiple handicaps which characterize so many aphasic patients. It makes clear the far-reaching nature of disabilities and encourages those in the field to take a broad view.

In rehabilitation, the following considerations are worthy of close attention: (1) assessment, (2) goal setting and monitoring, (3) environment, (4) long-term follow-up and (5) the organization and management of services.

Assessment

Rehabilitation should be planned, organized and provided on the basis of a detailed knowledge of individual needs, so that a comprehensive assessment is required. This is by no means synonymous with a diagnosis, global statements such as IQs, or overall scores of other tests, which are usually too general to provide information upon which direct action can be taken. The need is for a detailed record of functional performance in the areas listed above under 'intrinsic' disabilities viz., mobility, sensory function, personal care, communication, cognition and social and occupational functioning. Whilst thse requirements seem obvious, the relevant research has not been done so that assessment tend not to be based on a rational basis (Townsend, 1974). Whenever possible, functional information should be based on recent observable behaviour, free from jargon and not unduly concerned with aetiology.

Goal Setting and Monitoring

Having determined specific needs, both long- and short-term goals should be specified, action orientated and recorded in an accessible form. Change should be monitored to determine if the patient has improved, remained the same or deteriorated. Every effort should be made to prevent stagnation, so that it may be necessary to modify goals and strategies of intervention. Precise prognosis is difficult because of wide individual differences both between and within patients. The rate of change may vary and, even if gains are short-lived, the patient's motivation and staff morale are more likely to be maintained if there is a continuing sense of purpose and direction derived from regular review.

Environmental Considerations
The environment of a disabled person must be planned, organized and arranged so as to encourage those functions which the patient is either unable or unwilling to perform but as much emphasis should be placed on capabilities as on disabilities. Suitable levels of stimulation and activity must be available as their absence often leads to deterioration, hence the involvement of the family, if there is one, or alternatively, to the milieu of the ward or hostel.

Long-term Follow-up
After the acute phase and the patient having regained self-confidence, reacquired lost skills and learned new skills, the patient should be ready to transfer from the hospital to the community. If there is insufficient, or inappropriate, community care the gains made may be lost and, even when conditions are good, success in rehabilitation is often related to long-term maintenance, so that there must be good liaison between the hospital and social and community based health services and all necessary arrangements should be made in anticipation of discharge. Once in the community, contact with the rehabilitation service via one of its members should be retained and although it is difficult to predict how long follow-up should continue, access should be available when the need arises.

Services
A considerable amount of skilled organization and management is required, the aims of management being to ensure that existing provisions are adequate and that the separate components e.g., nursing, physiotherapy, occupational therapy, speech therapy, are co-ordinated. It is particularly important that the patient does not experience time gaps or sudden jumps between stages. No one profession has a monopoly on skills, insight or wisdom; each makes a unique contribution but all are united in sharing the common aspiration of helping the patient. Progress in rehabilitation may be slow and, as this can be detrimental to morale, active consideration should be given by the co-ordinator of the multidisciplinary team, usually the Consultant, to staff support.

Rehabilitation focuses on the patient and the effects of illness but once the patient leaves hospital the specific needs of the family must be considered in greater detail.

Management and the Family

Many patients experience considerable distress because of their disabilities, as do those most closely associated with them. In many cases little help is given to close relatives, sometimes ascribed to lack of resources but often because of uncertainty about how to proceed. There are various general points which are relevant to the management of difficult situations. First, however, comments from the wife of an aphasic patient will be quoted in order to illustrate some of the difficulties which confront those who find themselves having to provide day-to-day care for disabled relatives. The following statement is from Mrs Madge Wicks who has been an ardent campaigner on behalf of aphasic patients. Now in her mid-seventies Mrs Wicks has cared for her husband for nearly 7 years. He has 'a complete paralysis of the right side', is 'speechless and incontinent'. She wrote:

> '... I think that, except for the very rare occasions, all companionship between us is lost; we just endure. He endures my nagging, criticism and irritability caused, let me say in self-defence, not entirely by him but by the fairly constant nagging pain of arthritis, but it seems sometimes the last straw that in addition I have to endure his oddities — I love him much but I don't like him a bit. I think it is almost impossible, unless you are a very exceptional person, which I certainly am not, to fully adjust to the personality change, or rather personality exaggeration. One just feels lost, you marry one man for all the reasons one does and, after 50 years, you find yourself married to a totally different person but still in love with the man he was. You have a great compassion and your loyalties are as strong as ever but, how can you have true companionship when you cannot exchange thoughts and read the same books and discuss them, the odd snide remark, the arguments and discussion, the humour; all are gone with the lost speech — his humour is mostly now of the custard pie variety; how sad I think, that the old dryness and subtlety are gone. We are together, thank God, but no longer true companions; often I think life has become a long shouting match ...'

Much depends on how suddenly the accident or illness occurs, as on the stage in life at which it happens. Strokes and head injuries by their nature are sudden and usually without warning so that the initial reaction is one of shock, throwing people off balance so that they become preoccupied with trivia. An example of this was a woman, whose husband had had a stroke, demanding to see the hospital Consultant. She left the ward staff in no doubt that she was not to be diverted from her purpose and that her mission was one of pressing importance. When she saw the Consultant it transpired that her main concern was about the sitting-room curtains which she had recently ordered. Was she to cancel the order or proceed with the plan to improve the decor? Such incidents as this are relatively common and, almost certainly, reflect the way in which vulnerable people divert themselves from issues that are too big to confront by preoccupation with incidentals.

When confronted by serious and damaging illnesses, relatives, and patients if sufficiently alert, are often concerned about the possibility of death. Anxiety born of uncertainty has to be endured because outcome cannot always be determined in the early stages. When there can be little doubt that the responsibility for providing or withholding this information remains with medical staff, a matter not to be delegated to others nor, indeed, neglected. The majority of terminally ill patients prefer to be told the truth about their condition (Kubler-Ross, 1969). There may be difficulties with those who have a loss of comprehension, but many people approaching death have a certain awareness of the fact, so that direct confrontation may be gratuitous. It may be more helpful to respond to the patient, for example, if the patient asks 'Am I dying?' it may be appropriate to answer 'Is that something on your mind?', which gives the patient an opportunity to talk about fears and crystallize feelings and thoughts. At any one time, the matter may not be pursued and may re-emerge later. The principle of handling this delicate topic is to take it as far as the patient wishes and to recognize that feelings of vulnerability may be presented in different forms and under different guises. What appear to be questions are sometimes no more than the vocalization of thoughts, perhaps to see what they sound like. If so, the patient will not be aided by a direct answer but will derive more benefit by being encouraged to explore the underlying ideas at whatever depth is acceptable and tolerable.

Closely allied to this is informing the spouse and other family members. Sometimes only the spouse or parent etc., is informed and is asked not to reveal the truth to the patient, which places the family under the double burdens of preparing for bereavement and hiding this reality from their sick relative. In caring for children with terminal illness (Burton, 1971), parents aspire to give their child, in the remaining months, the life which he or she will not now have and, in so doing, inadvertently create unnecessary pressures. The breaking of bad news is difficult for both givers and recipients, and specific circumstances will dictate how this delicate matter should be handled in order to be as sympathetic as possible.

When death itself is not threatened, close relatives are the recipients of good wishes etc., from others who are greatly concerned. Sometimes those who send good wishes do so as much for their own benefit, by way of seeking expiation and comfort, as for the benefit of the other person. When weighed down with doubt and realistic worry it can be burdensome to have to respond to well-wishers, so that it is better to wait until approached by the anxious person and then to respond sympathetically rather than to volunteer regrets, a strategy to be discussed more fully later.

As time passes the implications of the disabilities will gradually be assimilated, and this will be aided by involving the spouse in discussions regarding treatment, rehabilitation and eventual discharge from hospital or, if the patient is at home, about to return to as normal as possible a way of living. Speech therapists can offer invaluable help by acting as role models in demonstrating how to communicate with aphasic patients, demonstrating this to colleagues in other professions who are less knowledgeable about aphasia. It is often easier to imitate a good example than to learn from instructions, no matter how clearly presented.

At this stage the spouse has three needs: first, to learn more about the nature and likely outcome of the illness; secondly, to be given clear instructions about what to do and what not to do and, thirdly, help in crystallizing thoughts and feelings regarding how to proceed. Much has been written about the difficulty of communication between medical practitioners and patients or, in this case, relatives (Ley and Spellman, 1967; Ley, 1977). Social classs differences in the use of language, inability to retain information in stressful situations, failure to understand specialized terminology, possession of preconceived notions etc., are among the difficulties which militate against adequate communication. It is particularly important to ensure that whatever information is conveyed has been correctly understood, and it may be necessary to repeat the same message on several occasions. Another important principle is that the various members of a multidisciplinary team, whether working in hospital or the community, must be consistent. If an anxious relative or patient receives contradictory messages, confidence will be undermined, and it is the responsibility of the co-ordinator of the clinical team to ensure that consistency is maintained.

While the young are quick to adapt to changed circumstances, this is not the case for those of more mature years, who need time to assimilate new ideas and skills and may have little insight into this fact. It is particularly important to convey information clearly, for example, by giving them every opportunity to supplement information gain by watching the speaker's face. Because older people are slower to learn new skills, they need more practice; whenever possible, tasks should be broken down into a series of simple steps and presented in a graded sequence so that the acquisition of one step follows naturally from previous steps. The learning must be accurate because older people find it difficult to unlearn mistakes.

Before the patient's discharge from hospital, it is helpful to give relatives some insight into their new commitments by allowing the patient to spend ocasional days at home and then a weekend, an experience that often reveals unanticipated problems which can be dealt with before final discharge. Relatives should be informed on the timing and pattern of follow-up procedures and should be informed who to contact should difficulties arise; in particular, assurances should be given that the General Practitioner and Social Services will continue to offer help and support.

Only experience and time can fully acquaint a family with the reality of coping with a disabled relative, for example, coming to terms with frustration born of inactivity, the embarrassment and discomfort of incontinence, the restrictions imposed by immobilty and the resentment engendered by diminished autonomy. Sleep patterns may be disturbed, there may be a loss of short-term memory, with difficulty holding attention for more than a few minutes; in general, there may be a sense of helplessness. Although many of these disabilities are common, not all aphasic patients are so severely afflicted but coping may be particularly difficult when those concerned have been married for as much as three or four decades, since patterns of behaviour become so well-established that change is difficult. When circumstances force change, older people can only draw upon actions already in their behavioural repertoires, for example, the wife of a disabled man may become over-protective and even tend to infantilize him, because her previous experience of managing dependency may have been only with her children. Difficulties within a marriage tend to become magnified at times of crisis, particularly if they have been long-standing and resolved. Under these circumstances, disability can become a pretext for rejection, particularly if the spouse has a low tolerance for frustration. Over-protection or rejection compound the problems and put the disabled person's morale and quality of life at even greater risk. Marriages and family life is dynamic, people reacting to each other so that there is a constant interchange. One particularly sad example of this arose in the marriage of an aphasic man whose wife claimed to be the dominant partner. The children had left home and she had developed her own career. She therefore greeted the prospect of caring for a disabled spouse with disquiet — it would, after all, keep her from her job. At the time of his discharge from hospital he was very limited in what he could manage and his obvious dependency must have encouraged his wife to invest greater interest in his care than she had expected. Gradually, the man emerged further from his illness and therefore required less supervision. It was found that he had improved to a point at which day care could not, in the light of limited resources, be justified; yet his state was such that he could not be left alone at home without supervision. Possibly because of his evident improvement his wife became progressively less tolerant of caring for him. Both of them were subject to frustration. He because he was nearly, but not quite, independent and she, because of her lack of freedom to return to work. She asked for help in coping with this difficult situation but seemed not to find it and, eventually, took an overdose of drugs, fortunately without causing herself serious damage.

The partners of aphasic patients would not regard themselves as having a marital problem yet most of them have a feeling that they are, in some sense, failing without being able to identify the source of their disquiet. It is in this context that the need for counselling arises.

Counselling

Counselling can be defined in several ways but, in the present context, fundamental distinction is from treatment, although the two types of activity overlap. Therapy requires that the patient or client adapts to the therapist's way of working and frame of reference, for example, those who receive psychotherapy based, no matter how tenuously, on the principles of dynamic psychology, will find that interpretations are made of their unconscious processes and that references are made to defences etc., the aim being to promote personal growth and to increase insight. Although it is difficult to define these terms, or to determine when the aims have been attained, there could be little success if the client is unprepared to be guided by the therapist's perspective and way of working.

Another, but distinctly different, approach to psychological therapy is the application of behavioural techniques which also require that patients accommodate to certain principles and assumptions, in particular, emphasis is placed by the therapists on observable behaviour and on the contingencies of reinforcement which influence it. Although these two types of intervention are conceptually distinct, it is generally possible to determine which treatment patients have received by listening to how they conceptualize their difficulties, which suggests that recipients of treatment assimilate the language and way of thinking of their therapists.

In contrast to therapy, counselling attempts to work within the patient's frame of reference. Assumptions and aspirations, expressed by the patient are the focus of interest, but there are important differences of approach, the two most important being the phenomenological and the problem-solving approaches. The former emphasizes personal growth, self-realization and self-actualization; it derives from existential philosophy and phenomenological psychology and is concerned with alienation and man's search for meaning. The uniqueness of each individual's perception of reality is emphasized, and the focus is on the present rather than the past or future, it being assumed that a person's drive is towards growth and integration. The theories from which such an approach is derived is referred to as 'client-centred' and Rogers is generally regarded as the founder of this non-directive style of counselling, of which the most significant therapeutic element is the equality of the counselling relationship. The client is believed to have the capacity and motivation to solve his or her own problems and these will emerge from the safety of a relationship with the counsellor. Rogers (1942) argued that counselling is a 'definitely structured permissive relationship which allows the client to gain an understanding of himself to a degree which enables him to take positive steps in the light of his new orientation'. Great emphasis was placed by Rogers on the personal qualities and attitudes of the counsellor. Genuineness, unconditioned positive regard and accurate sympathetic understanding were identified as being the key attributes.

In contrast, the problem-solving approach to counselling derives from a change of focus which occurred in the United States in the nineteen-sixties and resulted from increasing interest in behavioural psychology. The counsellor was seen as a behaviour changer concerned with the 'facilitation of human effectiveness, or more succinctly, the degree of control which an individual is able to exert over his environment' (Blocher, 1966). The name Krumboltz is most often associated with this shift of emphasis, since he described the counselling process as 'whatever ethical activities a counsellor undertakes in an effort to help the client engage in those types of behaviour which will lead to a resolution of the client's problems' (Krumboltz, 1965). A year later, he wrote 'As a result of consulting a counsellor a person with problems ought to be better able to find solutions. In addition, he ought to be able to solve future problems independently and effectively. In short, the counsellor is interested in helping to promote a more adaptive problem-solving kind of behaviour' (Krumboltz, 1966).

More comprehensive and general theories of counselling have been developed (Carkhuff, 1972, 1973; Carkhuff and Berenson, 1976; Egan, 1980), the main premise being that an effective helping strategy with individuals is to perceive helping as teaching clients basic life skills in order that they can solve their own problems. Another is that the counselling relationship is a necessary, but not sufficient, condition for helping. The counsellor aids the client through the cyclical processes of exploration, understanding, action and evaluation. The relationship is necessary in order that the counsellor may be able to work from within the patient's frame of reference and that the patient should trust the counsellor sufficiently to enter into a working alliance.

Common to these various perspectives is the importance of the relationship between patients and counsellors and, in contrast to medical models of intervention, patients are expected to take responsibility for themselves. These two fundamental principles appear to be incompatible but this is not the case. Many of those seeking help find themselves going round in circles; fail to put pieces of the jigsaw puzzle together to form an integrated picture, and the counsellor's task is to facilitate this acting as a neutral sounding-board. Most personal interaction is characterized by mutual influence but not so in counselling as patients should gradually find their own solutions in what is reflected back by the counsellor.

Those concerned with behaviour change often argue that counselling is too subjective, as goals are not specified and outcome is not easily evaluated but, if intervention focuses on a frame of reference and the expectation that he or she will formulate and execute personal strategies, two of the three criteria for claiming that a counselling approach is being used have been fulfilled.

The particular technique presented here is compatible with this way of working, being focused on the relationship between patient and spouse, or any other person with whom the patient is closely associated on a day-to-day basis on a personal level. Patients themselves will often not be involved in counselling because, by definition, they would probably be unable to express themselves with the kind of precision required. Despite this, equal weight is given to both patient and spouse albeit that only the spouse's descriptions and views are available. This is unimportant because the technique, known as the Personal Relations Index or PRI for short (Mulhall, 1977, 1978), is always confined to the individual perspectives of the two people being considered. In marital or family counselling this is an asset because, where husbands and wives are in contention, it is most beneficial not only to confront each with a clear view of themselves but also to confront both with the views of the other. In the management of those with aphasia there is a particular need, emphasized earlier, to consider how best to help the spouse, on the grounds that the patient will already have been the main focus of treatment and rehabilitation with the spouse often having received little or no attention.

Before presenting details of the PRI, which is a highly structured technique, certain background considerations need to be reviewed, the first of which is a precise statement of what the technique is designed to achieve. One of the many concerns confronting the wife of an aphasic patient is an awareness that her influence may, in some sense, be compounding the problems, even though her intention is usually to facilitate adjustment; this feeling is often ill-defined which may in itself contribute to greater worry and frustration. The PRI is addressed to this, seeking to clarify the wife's view of the relationship and to feed back a clear picture of the relevant processes.

Often informants have come to believe that the situation is beyond them and that they have lost control. Rather than making a positive contribution to adjustment they feel that they can only react. The picture produced by the PRI presents an easily understood, dispassionate description of what tends to happen, without in any sense casting aspersions or challenging the integrity of either partner; it clarifies the nature of mutual influences and reveals that control has not been lost; and also suggests to the informant what action could usefully be taken.

The second consideration is why a structured technique is necessary to achieve this end. Whilst a skillful and experienced practitioner would reach the same point, it is a costly process in terms of the number of manhours required. Resources are so limited that it is often not possible to offer the intensity of service required as an acceptable minimum. It is also often difficult to produce convincing evidence of outcome. For these two reasons it is necessary to employ expeditious means so that more people can be offered a service which can be evaluated. In addition the PRI offers structure to both professional and patient, the former knowing precisely what type of information to collect and then how to use it, and the latter being sympathetically helped to introduce coherence into a mixture of hitherto disordered impressions.

The last consideration concerns the methods used. Social interaction can be conceived of as a dynamic system, the elements of which are the interactions between the two people under investigation. The purpose is to study how the system operates, and this involves detailed discussion with them in order to establish what these elements are, which is conceptually distinct from analyzing responses to a standard set of questions.

An important part of the PRI is that patients, having provided the bricks, are given the wherewithal to construct their own buildings, a process of synthesis as opposed to analysis, which is the usual purpose of psychological tests.

It will be helpful to consider the ways in which the PRI is and is not compatible with a *systems approach*. In general, the term system is used to describe complex (i.e., multivariate) dynamic processes some of which are natural while others are man-made. Disciplines concerned with the study of natural systems include meteorology, ecology and biochemistry, whilst man-made systems include tele-communications, computer technology, automatic navigational devices etc. In each of these areas there are numerous interacting variables with constantly changing values but in many systems the notion of homeostasis is fundamental. This implies feedback loops which trigger action should the value of certain variables change so as to disturb the equilibrium. An example of this is found in colonies of animals living in an environment of finite size; assuming that there is a plentiful supply of food, reproduction continues until a critical population density is reached whereupon decreased fertility and cannibalism of the young are among the means by which further expansion of population is prevented. A comparable example in a man-made system is the thermostat used to regulate temperature: When the temperature is below the setting of the thermostat heat is produced but, once it reaches the setting, the heat source is shut off until such time as the temperature again drops below the critical value.

The study of systems is relatively new but presents great methodological challenges. Progress in science has been heavily dependent on developments in mathematics, which have enabled scientists to ask new questions, a reciprcal relationship between mathematicians and scientists which is as important in the study of systems as it was in relatively simpler processes. Whilst there are relatively few mathematical tools available for studying systems the advent of computers has offered many new possibilities. For the first time man has available a dynamic system which is not too complex to understand and with which other processes can be studied. Growing recognition of the need to study systems has led to the development of systems theory and, from this, the systems approach. Boulding (1956) argued that 'General Systems Theory is the name which has come into use to describe a level of theoretical model building which lies somewhere between the highly specialised endeavours of pure mathematics and the specific themes of the specialised disciplines.'

The PRI is concerned with interpersonal systems and as a technique builds models; to this extent it is compatible with a systems approach but there are other features which are not compatible. Let us consider an imaginary system which is difficult to control manually; a systems engineer is asked to study the system and to produce an automated means of control, and his tasks will be to study inputs, intervening processes and outputs, measuring the relevant variables and, in particular, their upper and lower limits. In developing the control box the engineer may need to install sensory devices to determine relevant values, the information collected will become input to the control box and the functioning of the system will be modulated by outputs from the box. Operations of the box itself may involve electronic circuitry or a computer but, in either case, a precise specification of the relevant processes will be required.

In the case of the PRI it is generally not possible to distinguish between inputs and outputs, for example, in a dyadic (i.e., two person) relationship one of the two people may be kind. At times this will be something to which the other person will react but, at other times, it may be a reaction to that other person. Kindness is therefore both a stimulus and a response, its specific status being dictated by the immediate context in which it arises. The same lack of clarity applies to any state included in the model and reflects the fact that a particular relationship is a small, although not necessarily unimportant, part of a person's total system. In recognition of this the representations constructed by the PRI do not exclude the influence of other variables, even though no explicit reference to them is made.

Another factor in contrasting the PRI with the systems approach involves measurement of the variables. In physical systems this is achieved with greater or lesser difficulty but in social and psychological systems, there are often great difficulties, particularly if the variables relate to personal experiences with no obvious external referents. Various scaling techniques are available but, in the present context, the advantages of employing these have to be weighed against the capacity of those under investigation to cope with what would inevitably be long, and probably complex, questionnaires. The strategy employed in the PRI is to ascertain the relative likelihood of occurrence of each of a limited set of possibilities.

An important feature of the PRI is that it is idiographic. Most psychological tests are nomothetic or dependent for their interpretation upon normative data, for example, the measurement of intelligence usually involves determining the testee's standing in relation to the rest of the population. An idiographic technique does not depend on norms but produces results which can be understood in their own right and without reference to other people. At a clinical level, this type of single case approach is helpful because the purpose is to focus on the specific needs of the individual but, at a research level, it may be important to make general statements about patient groups. Whilst this possibility is not excluded by the PRI, it involves certain strategies which will not be further discussed here.

The technique of PRI can now be presented more concretely by reference to clinical case studies, the purpose of which is to illustrate difficulties and problems which arise and to demonstrate how counselling can be used to ameliorate them.

The first case is of a woman, Margaret, in her mid-sixties whose husband had a stroke leaving him aphasic and with a hemiplegia. The couple had been married for thirty-four years and he had recently retired from a senior position in commerce. She was first seen four months after her husband's illness and, although she was acquainted with the implications of his disabilities, this was the first time she had been given the opportunity to talk freely about her difficulties although she had been closely associated with hospital staff who had tried to advise her and to allay her anxieties. She was asked to describe typical feelings, attitudes and behaviour which characterized both her husband and herself in their daily lives. Initially, she was asked about the difficulties her husband had experienced following his stroke, how she responded to each of these and then how he reacted to her, and how they responded to each other. It was often necessary to feed back what she had said so that she could corroborate, refute or elaborate upon her own statements. Examples of behaviour and the particular situations in which it occurred were encouraged. In effect, she was helped to negotiate with herself in order to clarify her own thinking.

Discussions of this kind are informal and in no sense intended to pressurize the informant. In these cases, care is taken not to suggest what should be said except to ensure that the set of psychological states used to describe the two people should include both positive and negative attributes. In general, there is no difficulty in collecting information on the negative side but there is often considerable difficulty getting people to comment positively about themselves or indeed their partners.

The purpose of the discussion is to obtain seven descriptions of each of the two people; a total of fourteen states. No departure from this number is acceptable which, in itself, imposes a helpful discipline on both staff and clients. The reason for choosing this number is technical, as will become apparent later, but it does require that redundancies and duplications are excluded. This often leads to the difficulty of too few states being suggested whereupon the scope of the discussion should be widened to cover a broader range of areas. Throughout, the person conducting the discussion is aware of the client's vulnerability so that, at the end, the informant is satisfied that the picture constructed is a full and accurate reflection of the relationship.

Individual differences between clients are apparent, since some are lucid and insightful, whilst others are constrained and inarticulate. Differences in educational experience, social level, word power etc., play a part in this but the model underlying the system is sufficiently flexible to accommodate wide variation.

Margaret's descriptions were as follows:

Wife (Self-description)	*Husband (as described by wife)*
A. I feel worried.	*1. He is frustrated by his symptoms.*
B. I become tense.	*2. He suffers from headaches.*
C. I am happy.	*3. He has difficulty with his vision.*
D. I encourage him to help himself.	*4. He is considerate.*
E. I am sympathetic to his problems.	*5. He finds little things irritating.*
F. I am loving.	*6. He is patient.*
G. I feel depressed within myself.	*7. He is cheerful.*

The tone of these states suggest that her view is that there is much mutual respect and devotion, they appear to have even temperaments but to have been blighted by his disabilities. She was in a state of distress about her perceived inability to cope and yet she was unable to identify the source of this, and the list of states did not immediately suggest what her difficulty was or where it arose.

The next stage is to construct a unique questionnaire, exclusively comprised of the information derived from Margaret. Such a questionnaire must give equal weight to the husband and wife and to the various states ascribed to each of them; it must collect a maximum of information with the minimum number of questions; it must be simple to answer and its format must reduce bias to low levels. These criteria are achieved by employing a highly systematic but flexible model which is implemented by computer. The data are the various states and the role of the computer is to schedule the contents of questions, then rapidly and accurately to print them out. Examples of the questions, of which there are 98, are shown in *Table 1*.

In some questions, wife responds to husband and, in others, he responds to her. The various states are sometimes used as actions and sometimes as reactions, for example, in the second question his action is to be happy whilst, in the first question, it is presented as a reaction to her. Margaret's task in answering the questionnaire, which was sent to her through the post together with instructions, was to decide for each question which was most likely of the three reactions and which the least likely. She was asked to indicate this by circling the M adjacent to the most likely reaction and the L

Table 1

WHEN YOUR HUSBAND SUFFERS FROM HEADACHES DO YOU	A)	FEEL HAPPY	M	L
	B)	BECOME TENSE	M	L
	C)	ENCOURAGE HIM TO HELP HIMSELF	M	L
WHEN YOU ARE HAPPY DOES YOUR HUSBAND	A)	REACT WITH PATIENCE	M	L
	B)	FIND LITTLE THINGS IRRITATING	M	L
	C)	SEEM CHEERFUL	M	L
WHEN YOUR HUSBAND IS CONSIDERATE DO YOU	A)	EXPRESS SYMPATHY ABOUT HIS SYMPTOMS	M	L
	B)	ENCOURAGE HIM TO HELP HIMSELF	M	L
	C)	SHOW THAT YOU ARE LOVING	M	L

adjacent to the least likely one. Typically, it takes between twenty and thirty minutes to complete the questionnaire. The instructions make it clear that, whereas the same ideas are used many time in different combinations, no question is repeated. They also point out that answers are a matter of opinion and cannot be correct or incorrect.

When the completed questionnaire is returned, responses are encoded and processed by the computer to produce results of the type shown in *Table 2*.

In explaining the interpretation of these results it will be helpful to outline the model underlying the PRI. Within each question the respondent is placing, in order of likelihood of occurrence, three reactions to a given action. At best, this information is partial because it is necessary to know, for each action, the relative likelihood of occurrence of all seven possible reactions. To achieve this it is necessary to present the same action several times but, each time, with a different set of reactions. It is then necessary to combine the various responses to produce an overall ordering of reactions ranging for each action, for example, row 1 (horizontal) of the upper matrix corresponds to 'Frustrated by his symptoms' and the values in the adjacent columns (labelled A to G) indicate the relative likelihood of the responses. The letters refer to Margaret's states (A corresponds to 'worried', B to 'tense' etc.) and the numbers to his state (1 corresponds to his being 'frustrated by his symptoms', 2 to his 'suffering from headaches' and so on, to 7 which corresponds to his being 'cheerful'). Returning to Margaret's reactions to her husband's frustration, the larger the value, the more likely the reaction. The most likely reaction(s) in each row have been circled so that, in row 1 it occurs in column D and this corresponds to wife 'encouraging him to help himself'. Without realizing it, Margaret has produced a complete and separate ordering of her reactions to each of his states (upper matrix) and a complete and separate ordering of his reactions to each of her states (lower matrix).

The penultimate stage in the synthesis of a structure representing the relationship involves linking each state with its most likely outcome(s), for example, the most likely outcome in row 6 occurs in column C i.e., 6→C and the most likely reaction to C (lower matrix) occurs in column 7 i.e., 6→C→7 etc. This process is continued until each of the various states is incorporated into the final dynamic structure which is shown in symbolic form (i.e., as letters and number) in *Figure 1*.

The final stage involves presenting the structure in a form which can easily be understood by the patient. The numbers and letters are simply replaced by the names or titles of the people and the states to which they correspond; this is also performed by computer but the preceding stage of constructing the graph has not been programmed because the potential variety of connection exceeds 1.6 million even when there is only one most likely outcome per state and, as can be seen from the circled items in rows 2, 3 and 5

Table 2

husband's actions		wife's reactions A	B	C	D	E	F	G
1	Frustrated by his symptoms	2	1	0	(6)	5	4	3
2	Suffering from headaches	4	2	0	1	(5)	4	(5)
3	Having difficulty with his vision	2	1	0	(5)	(5)	3	(5)
4	Considerate	1	0	5	3	4	(6)	2
5	Finding little things irritating	3	1	0	(5)	(5)	(5)	2
6	Patient	1	0	(6)	4	3	5	2
7	Cheerful	0	2	4	(6)	3	5	1

wife's actions		husband's reactions 1	2	3	4	5	6	7
A	Worried	4	1	2	5	3	(6)	0
B	Tense	4	2	2	(6)	2	5	0
C	Happy	3	1	2	5	1	3	(6)
D	Encourage him to help himself	(6)	0	4	2	4	4	1
E	Sympathetic to his problems	(6)	1	3	4	1	5	1
F	Loving	3	0	2	5	1	4	(6)
G	Feeling depressed within herself	4	2	1	(6)	3	5	0

of the upper matrix in *Figure 1*, this does not apply. The model is capable of representing an almost infinite variety of structures and this has defied logical analysis sufficient to develop the relevant computer programs albeit that each structure can rapidly be constructed manually. Margaret's graph is shown in *Figure 2*.

By following various pathways around the graph, an impression of the dynamics of the relationship can easily be obtained, for example, despite his handicaps, Margaret's husband is still able to offer emotional support; when she is depressed or tense he is considerate and when she is worried he is patient. Likewise, Margaret is trying to offer her husband comfort, for example, when he finds little things irritating, she is sympathetic to his problems and loving, and she encourages him to help himself, as when he is

Figure 1

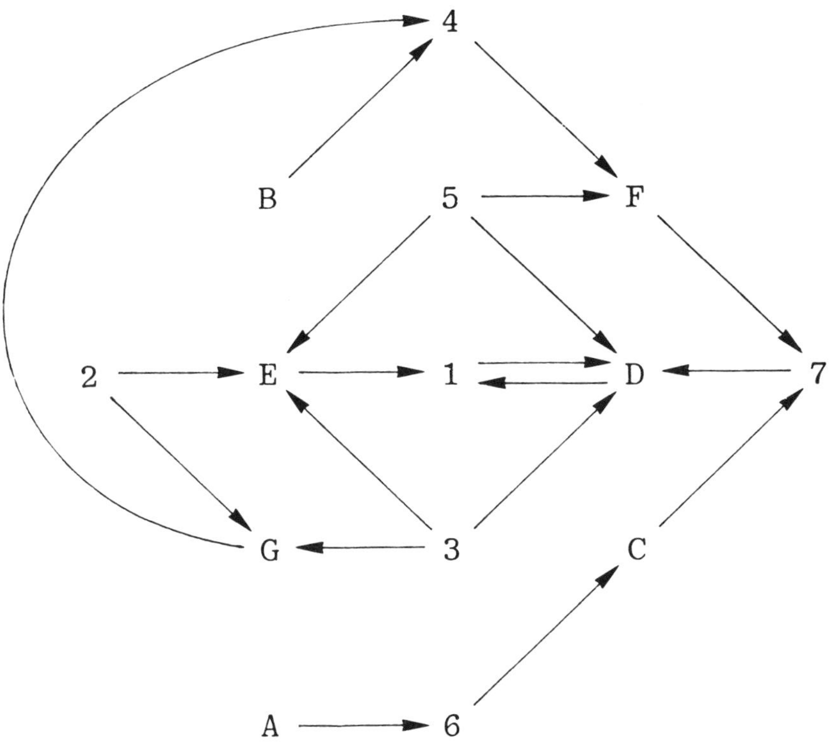

frustrated by his symptoms. Despite her best intentions, sympathy and encouragement have the unintended effect of heightening and maintaining his frustrations; his condition is, of course, intrinsically frustrating but, in as much as the graph accurately reflects Margaret's view, the results of her efforts are contrary to her intentions. When she saw the graph, this was put into perspective and identified the source of her nagging doubts but, more than this, she was able to suggest that it would be more productive if encouragement was contingent upon his attempts to use his remaining capability. She recognized that hitherto her sympathies had tended to reinforce his negative attributes but now she resolved to use reinforcement positively.

The second case study, also involving the use of the PRI, concerns a man in his late twenties who, less than a year after getting married, had a sudden onset of vertigo and tinnitus and a grand mal fit. He developed a severe communication problem and was said to have undergone a marked change in character. Investigations revealed that he had a cerebral tumour, of uncertain pathology, in the left lobe. He received a course of radiotherapy to the brain which involved ten treatments over a period of nineteen days. Psychological investigation after these treatments suggested that the patient was of average intellectual ability; there was a gross loss of short-term memory and the communication difficulty was confirmed. Prior to his illness the patient worked as a technician and his wife was a Junior School teacher.

Younger patients with malignant tumours generally have a poor prognosis. During the acute phase of this patient's illness, survival seemed unlikely but his response to radiotherapy was positive and he showed improvement. His wife had been very anxious about the outcome of his illness, and she attended a group run by Social Workers for the families of newly disabled patients but, so defensive were her reactions, she was discouraged from further attendances. It was apparent, seeing the woman with her husband, that her forthright manner was not confined to the group; she tended to infantatize him and to direct his every action. This continued after he was discharged from hospital and, apart from the social problems arising from lack of income and running the home alone, she had difficulty coping with his frustration, memory loss and lack of communication. She was reluctant to accept help or talk about the situation but was eventually persuaded that she might find it easier to manage if she could see matters more clearly. She described herself and her husband as follows:

Wife	*Husband*
I am afraid to leave him alone.	He's forgetful.
I get frustrated with him.	He lacks self-confidence.
I tend to mother him.	He fails to understand.
I'm worried that I can't cope.	He's dependent on me.
I feel comfortable with him.	He becomes stubborn.
I find it difficult to be sympathetic.	He shows outward affection.
There are times when I'm happy.	In general he's satisfied with life.

A questionnaire was produced and she had no apparent difficulty in answering it. The graph constructed from the results is shown in *Figure 3*.

There are here two separate and unconnected sub-graphs, the lower of which is uninformative and reflects the inappropriateness of exerting pressure on subjects to contrive positive statements. The upper graph reveals that all pathways eventually converge on a series of three small loops focused

Figure 2

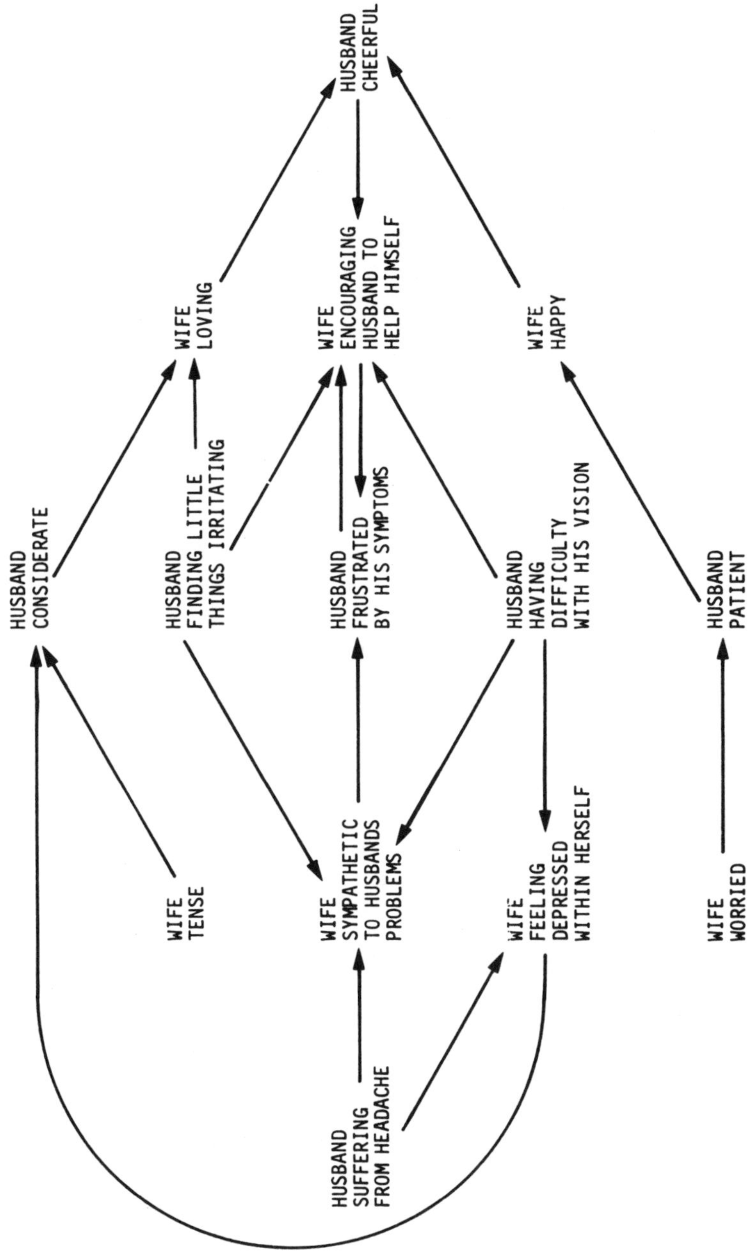
HUSBAND CHEERFUL
WIFE LOVING
WIFE ENCOURAGING HUSBAND TO HELP HIMSELF
WIFE HAPPY
HUSBAND CONSIDERATE
HUSBAND FINDING LITTLE THINGS IRRITATING
HUSBAND FRUSTRATED BY HIS SYMPTOMS
HUSBAND HAVING DIFFICULTY WITH HIS VISION
HUSBAND PATIENT
WIFE TENSE
WIFE SYMPATHETIC TO HUSBANDS PROBLEMS
WIFE FEELING DEPRESSED WITHIN HERSELF
WIFE WORRIED
HUSBAND SUFFERING FROM HEADACHE

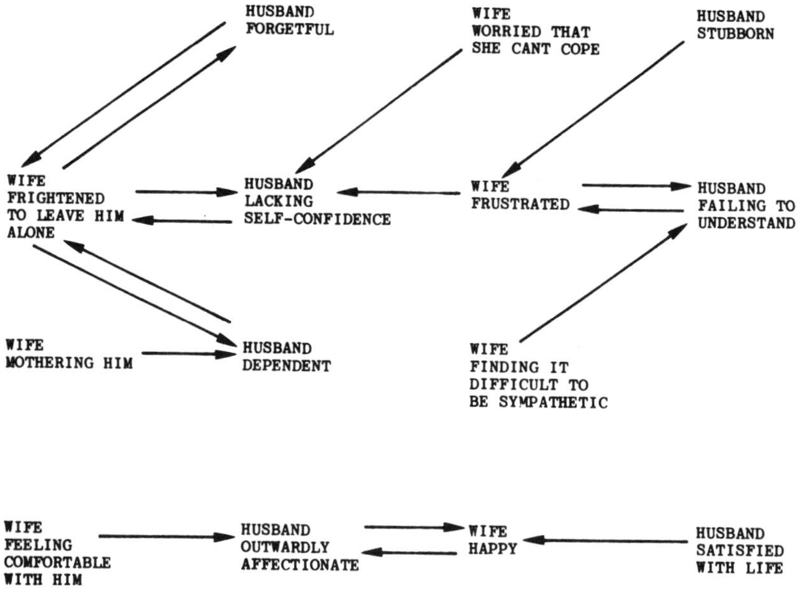

Figure 3

on her fear of leaving him alone, which means she appears inadvertently to reinforce his dependency, memory loss and lack of self-confidence and, in so doing, erodes his already diminished autonomy. On seeing these results, which she initially claimed not to understand, she volunteered that her influence was unhelpful and that he should be encouraged to use his remaining capacities lest he lose them. She suggested that 'he could be more active in clearing up the flat and with the washing up and we could go shopping together'. She seemd to think that he would enjoy preparing a few simple meals and would, in general, benefit from taking a more active role.

During discussion it emerged that she had been reared by rather rigid parents with whom she had lived until she was married. Her father had done most things for her and, possibly because of parental autocracy and limited social skill, she held herself in low self-esteem. So significant was this that she had probably come to believe that her only chance of sustaining an enduring relationship was with someone even less self-confident than herself who would rapidly become dependent on her. Thus she had probably misperceived her own needs which represented a premorbid disability with grave repercussions for both herself and her husband and may have been the origin of her evident ambivalence.

The next clinical example refers to a 57-year-old aphasic stroke patient

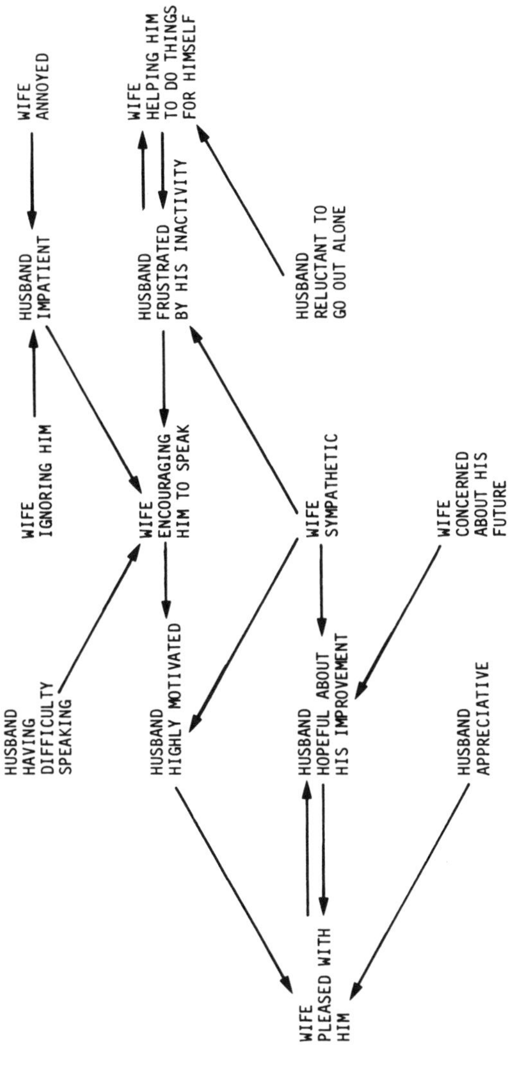

Figure 4

who, in partnership with his wife, ran a highly successful business. She was in her early 50s and had many talents; she recognized that her husband needed encouragement and, in an apparently abusive manner, left him in no doubt that this would only be forthcoming if he was seen to be helping himself — a tactic employed with considerable skill was to appear annoyed, even though she did not feel it. Her husband's functional capacity and speech had shown slow but progressive improvement and they were both determined to further this trend. In reality, the damage caused by the stroke was probably not very great but her decisive and positive approach to management seemed to potentiate the process of recovery. *Figure 4* shows the graph from her PRI responses.

Ignoring or being annoyed with him made him impatient, which she encouraged him to express verbally, and this seemed to have motivated him. In contrast, sympathy and helping him to do things for himself may not always have been beneficial, again suggesting that, as in *Figure 1*, kindness can at times have the unfortunate and unintentional effects of confronting patients with their disabilities.

The final example is from a 69-year-old man who was found to be dementing, his behaviour was disturbed and he had little speech. The graph for this patient is shown in *Figure 5*.

This example has been chosen so as to illustrate the great difficulties families sometimes have in caring for demented relatives. It can be seen that the patient is truculent and self-willed most of the time, so that his wife can do little than react to him and she seems to feel that, even this, is usually ineffective.

In view of this, and evidence from the general practitioner, hospital specialist and the social service, consideration had to be given to offering the patient full-time nursing care in hospital, a suggestion greeted with mixed reactions by his wife. She was relieved but felt herself to be a failure and recognized with sorrow that his departure was probably the end of the most important chapter in their mutual lives. Part of her ambivalence emerged from a question about how nurses could cope with him when she could not. It was put to her that she had been called upon to manage him and the home for 24 hours a day whereas nurses had the dual advantages of working finite shifts and being able to have a personal life after work. Reference was also made to the importance of maintaining regular contact by visiting him. Again, it was necessary to recognize her vulnerability in conducting these delicate negotiations and to give her every opportunity of expressing herself.

In drawing together the threads of the foregoing discussion it is clear that there are wide individual differences in biology, psychological make-up and social experience, but the unifying strand has been the disadvantage inflicted by aphasia. Those who have been presented live, like everyone else, in a world which is as much social and symbolic as it is physical. Yet for them the essence of social contact and the stimulation it provides has at best been obliterated and at worst destroyed. Some had lost hope, others had retained it; some managed with much skill, others with little; most had limited insight and all, in varying degrees, felt vulnerable. The specific difficulties they had were inadvertent reinforcement of negative behaviour, erosion of already

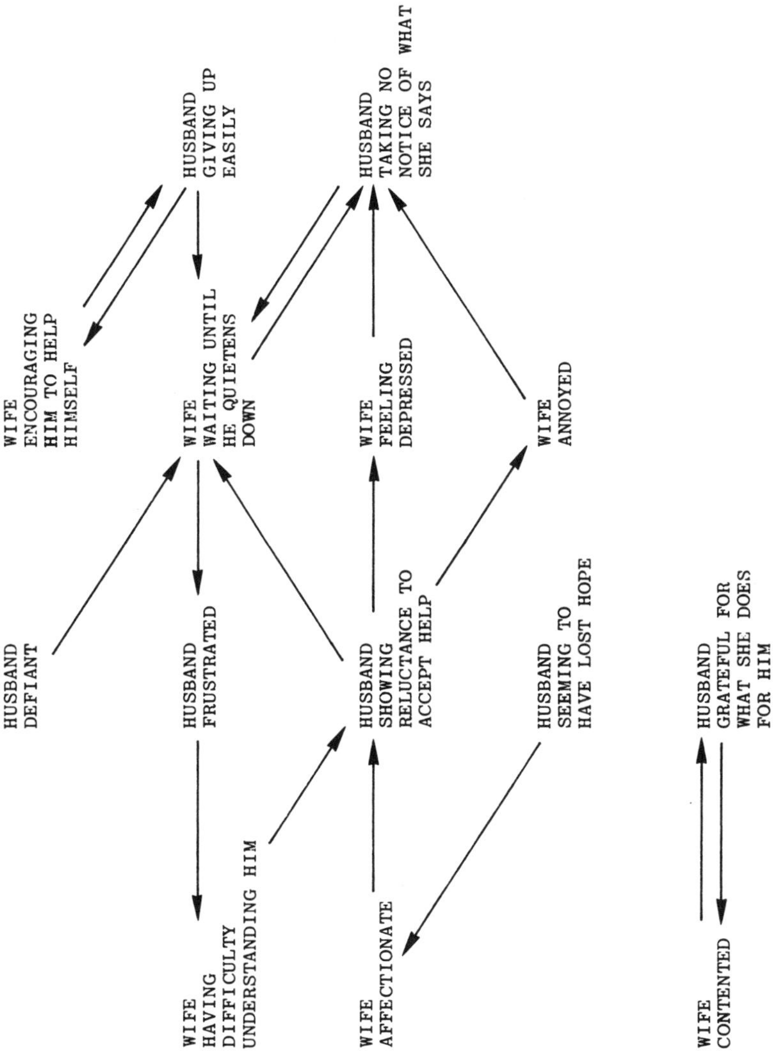
HUSBAND DEFIANT
WIFE ENCOURAGING HIM TO HELP HIMSELF
HUSBAND GIVING UP EASILY
WIFE WAITING UNTIL HE QUIETENS DOWN
HUSBAND FRUSTRATED
WIFE HAVING DIFFICULTY UNDERSTANDING HIM
HUSBAND SHOWING RELUCTANCE TO ACCEPT HELP
WIFE FEELING DEPRESSED
HUSBAND TAKING NO NOTICE OF WHAT SHE SAYS
WIFE AFFECTIONATE
WIFE ANNOYED
HUSBAND SEEMING TO HAVE LOST HOPE
HUSBAND GRATEFUL FOR WHAT SHE DOES FOR HIM
WIFE CONTENTED

Figure 5

diminished autonomy and difficulty in recognizing that continued management had become untenable.

What remains uncertain is the extent to which they had made previous attempts to obtain help. Certainly, they had been informed about the nature of their spouses' illnesses and attempts had been made to allay their anxieties. The opportunity of attending clubs for patients and families had been open to each of them but, somehow, their specific needs seem to have remained obscure.

The two major issues emerging from this are the importance of sensitizing those working in the Health and Social Services to what is probably a large and important area of unmet need and, secondly, what strategies should be adopted in meeting it. Many relatives and probably patients require advice but the difficulty seems to be that, even when given, compliance is limited. The likely reasons for this include lack of understanding, poor memory, especially if the timing is wrong, and preconceived ideas which are often unhelpful or inaccurate. Under these circumstances, the case for working within the clients' frame of reference is particularly strong. By helping them to examine and elaborate their own ideas and to develop their own strategies, the chances of success are likely to be increased. In the cases presented, any solutions which emerged came directly from the subjects, suggesting that advice-giving should be a process of drawing out information rather than imparting it. Perhaps the most important rider to add it that, whereas it may be comforting to discuss difficulties at an affective or feeling level, the need is to know what action to take for the rest of today and tomorrow or, put another way, to be useful, strategies must be translated into behaviour.

Conclusions

The intention of this chapter has been to raise issues which relate directly to clinical practice and, in particular, to emphasize the notions of continuing care and management. Such an emphasis diverges from an approach to health care preoccupied with treatment and cure of acute illnesses and, in so doing, it departs from the so-called medical model. The difficulty arises that, in an era of scientific medicine which is only now emerging from the search for specific aetiologies, there has sometimes been a certain reluctance to pay attention to the social and psychological dimensions of illness. Fortunately for the recipients of health care this too is beginning to change but still the imprint of the medical model is clearly visible in the training and subsequent practice of many non-medical health care professions, as exemplified by over-concern with diagnosis and far too little concern with observable function and consideration of how independence can be enhanced. The best evidence of this is the lack of agreed measures of function which in itself limits the scope for adequate studies of outcome. Possibly because of this, there is often a lack of precision in stating what goals should be achieved by a particular patient at any particular stage in his or her management. Kushlick (1973) drew a helpful distinction between 'a performance' and a 'fuzzy'. He recommended the use of the 'Hey Dad' test for deciding into which of these two categories a desired treatment goal fell. For example, 'Hey Dad, let me show you how I can . . .

1. Increase this client's potential.
2. Change his attitudes.
3. Provide a supportive environment.'

are fuzzies because Dad will not be able to observe whether or not I have done what I told him I would do. In contrast 'Hey Dad let me show you how I can . . .

1. Record the number of single word utterances this patient produces spontaneously when his wife visits him this afternoon.
2. Get her to walk ten metres before lunch.
3. Encourage him to use more eye contact when conversing with others.'

are examples of performances because Dad will be able to observe the outcome.

Most people use fuzzies most of the time, which probably contributes to the lack of agreement between the members of multidisciplinary teams about the patients for whom they are providing care. Not uncommonly this degenerates into territorial disputes about who should be doing what, especially when co-ordination of the team is deficient, as unhappily is sometimes the case. An alternative is, wherever possible, specify goals as performances by stating them with precision. This calls for close observation of behaviour and can lead to much greater clarity of purpose which, whilst necessitating a slower pace, lends itself to co-operative working and greater job satisfaction for the team members.

There is, of course, scope for debate about where particular therapeutic activities are to be located on the fuzzy-performance continuum. Counselling for example is an activity which has probably been largely towards the fuzzy end but, as has been demonstrated, there is reason to believe that it can, with advancing technology, be nudged progressively towards the other end. The same applies to many other relevant activities in the continuing care of aphasic patients provided that active attempts are made to break each task down into separate but linked stages.

Finally, two points must be re-emphasised. First, that skills in approaching speechless patients are rare and most significantly found amongst speech therapists. For them these skills are often stock in trade and it may sometimes be the case that sight of this is lost so that they forget to act as models for others. It will be unfortunate if those who, by dint of long and repeated practice have acquired specialized skills, fail to use them to the advantage of all concerned. Secondly, and in some ways related to this, is the difficulty relatives, who unlike staff have the burden of 24-hour a day care, have in knowing how to proceed. Often, they are shown what to do but, as it is frequently found that patients' functional levels fall off when they return home, it must be that the training members of the family are given is deficient. Whilst there has been growing recognition of the social and interpersonal implications of aphasia, there is still far too little invested in establishing how best to train family members. Perhaps they too will benefit from being taught specific tasks broken down into small, but linked, stages. At each stage they should observe and then practice until proficient before moving on to the next one.

This kind of training will often be necessary but may not be sufficient, hence the need for helping relatives to develop their own strategies by the process of counselling. Such an approach has ubiquitous application and is certainly not restricted to particular types of two-person relationships nor, indeed, to health care problems. Most relatives welcome an opportunity to discuss the problems before them and will in fact make approaches to the member of the team with whom they believe they have a certain rapport. The need is to recognize these approaches when they are made and to respond to them with sensitivity. One of the advantages of the PRI is that the initial discussion can be conducted spontaneously in the course of conversation, which is likely to generate a more helpful outcome than deliberately bombarding the client with allusions to a formal technologically based assessment procedure. Such an introduction would probably be alarming and may reflect the apprehensions of a team member who is diffident about how to use the technique. The need is to be at ease in order to put the client at ease, again a case for skill acquisition.

References

BLOCHER, D. *Development Counselling* (1966). New York: Ronald Press.

BOULDING, K. *General Systems Theory — the Skeleton of Science. Management Science* Vol. 2 (1956).

BURTON, L. Cancer children. *New Society* (1971), 17th June.

CARKHUFF, R.R. *The Art of Helping* (1972). Amberst, Mass.: Human Resource Development Press.

CARKHUFF, R.R. *The Art of Problem Solving* (1973). Amberst, Mass.: Human Resource Development Press.

CARKHUFF, R.R. and BERENSON, B.G. *Teaching as Treatment* (1976). Amberst, Mass.: Human Resource Development Press.

EGAN, G. *The Skilled Helped: A Model for Systematic Helping* (1980). Monteray, Brooks Cole Publishing Co.

GOLDBERG, D. Principles of rehabilitation. *Comprehensive Psychiatry* (1974), **15**, 237–248.

KRUMBOLTZ, J.D. Behavioural Counselling: Rationale and Research. *Personnel and Guidance Journal* No. 44. (1965).

KRUMBOLTZ, J.D. *Revolution in Counselling* (1966). Boston: Houghton Mifflin.

KUBLER-ROSS, E. *On Death and Dying* (1969). London: Tavistock.

KUSHLICK, A. Some ways of setting, monitoring and attaining objectives for services for disabled people. *British Journal of Subnormality* (1975), **XXI**, 84–102.

LEY, P. and SPELMAN, M.S. *Communicating with the Patient* (1967). London: Staples Press.

LEY, P. Communicating with the patient. In J.C. Coleman (ed.) *Introductory Psychology* Chapter 12 (1977). London: Routledge & Kegan Paul.

MULHALL, D.J. The Representation of Personal Relationships: an Automated System. *International Journal of Man–Machine Studies* (1977), **9**, 315–335.

MULHALL, D.J. Dysphasic Stroke Patients and the Influence of their Relatives. *British Journal of Disorders of Communication* Vol. 13 (1978), **2**, 127–134.

ROGERS, C.R. *Counselling and Psychotherapy* (1942). Boston: Houghton Mifflin.

TOWNSEND, P. The Disabled in Society. In D.M. Boswell and J.M. Wingrove (eds) *The Handicapped Person in Society* Chapter 3 (1974). London: Tavistock.

WING, J.K. In Wirt *et al.* (eds) *Life History Research in Psychopathology* Vol. 4 (1975). University of Minnesota Press.

21

Assessment of Treatment in Aphasia

Renata Whurr

Treatment, therapy and rehabilitation are ill-defined areas. Treatment may mean anything from social contact with patients to the execution of specific therapeutic techniques, such as Melodic Intonation Therapy. As yet, there is no theory of language pathology disability and so no coherent theory for therapy (Crystal, 1981). However, in the absence of such a theory, the treatment and rehabilitation of aphasic patients are performed by speech therapists, volunteers, family and friends. Whether these activities change the patient's abilities, attitudes or way of life, is open to question. Moreover, it is not clear whether these activities are best handled by the highly trained speech therapist or a well-motivated volunteer or nurse. As the nature of the treatment is infrequently specified, so the idea of what it may be has led to a variety of misconceptions. Thus, Edwards (1973) stated the following:

> 'A good deal of emotional heat is generated about the treatment of dysphasia, most of which concerns whether or not it is of any use rather than the relative merits of various devices. Neurologists on the whole take an agnostic view, speech therapists naturally have some degree of belief in their powers in this particular field, whilst most other disciplines tend to take a calm, uncritical view. The therapist points to the difference beytween the patient a week after the installed stroke and 3 months or so later, claiming the livelier mind and a few additional words, better strung and more clearly pronounced as her due. As with many of her medical colleagues in the whole disease she tends to accept any improvement as testimony to her skill, its absence as not her fault and rejects the natural history of events. Her critics see comparable results without treatment. They claim that it is the fortuitous preservation of some of the anatomophysiological necessity and its stimulation by the environment and the repetitive practice that comes from it, that produces the difference. At the best, they say, speech therapy is an occupation for the patient; at the worst an expensive indulgence for the relatives and a source of irritation to the patient. Certainly a number of patients whose thinking and emotion are relatively

> preserved are angered by the indignity of being pressed to say their pitiful few words in a way to please their teacher. The speech therapist is as useful and useless and as near or as far from the damage she is trying to overcome as her physiotherapeutic sister treating hemiplegia. To her the recovering lower motor neurone dysarthria or dysphonia is on a par with the similarly recovering peripheral nerve paralysis or the fracture; the stammer much like the dyspraxia of a hand; the muscles of dysphasia as far removed from the lesion as the paresis is from the ischaemic brain. However, most patients are more naturally inclined to exercise their damaged speech than the weight of paralysed limbs so that assistance is more valuable to recovery of movement than of speech. If this is understood and acknowledged and no false claims made the speech therapist can be useful to the management of a difficult total situation that includes relatives as well as the patient and his profession.'

Edwards' views are outdated and there is evidence that there are many specific treatment techniques which can be and are selectively applied to specific problems:

1. Treatment of naming disorders: Wiegel-Crump 1973, Seron 1973, Brookshire 1975, Linebaugh, 1977, Rosenbek 1977, Thompson 1981, Howard 1984, 1985, 1986, Morton 1985.
2. Treatment of Comprehension Disorders: West 1973, Holland 1974, Kusher 1978, Whurr 1983, Marshall 1984, Byng 1986, Marshall 1986, Shewan 1986.
3. Treatment of Verbal Production: Beyn 1966, Berman 1967, Shewan 1975, Sparks 1974, 1976, Naesser 1975, Helm-Eastbrooks 1980, 1981, 1984a, 1984b, 1986, Weniger 1980, Albyn-Davies 1981, Whurr 1983, Prescott 1983, Kearns 1984, Shewan 1986, Jones 1986.
4. Treatment of Gestural Communication: Holland 1972, 1984, Sparks 1974, Skelly 1974, Rao 1978, 1986, Helm-Estabrooks 1982, Kearns 1982, Shewan 1986.
5. Treatment of Reading Disorders: Shewan 1986, Webb 1986.
6. Treatment of Writing Disorders: Leischner 1957, Schwartz 1973, Hatfield 1976, 1982, 1983, Shewan 1986, Whurr 1986.
7. Treatment of Functional Communication: Aten 1982, 1986, Holland 1982, Shewan 1986, Albyn-Davies 1986.
8. Generalization of Treatment: Stokes and Bauer 1977, McMullen, 1986.

Treatment, rehabilitation and management are all part of a process that needs co-ordination over time. Usually the speech pathologist acts as the co-ordinator and director of the process, in conjunction with others. The effectiveness of those many-faceted aspects of treatment and rehabilitation is a contentious issue, and serious doubts are often expressed about the value of speech therapy itself (Hopkins, 1975, 1984). The main problem raised by the evaluation of the recovery of function after aphasia is connected with the fact that as yet there is no comprehensive, reliable, quantifiable or reproducible method for measuring aphasic disability. Attempting to measure changes in language performances solely on the basis of the traditional aphasia battery or functional communication questionnaire is inadequate and insensitive. Another problem for the validation of treatment in aphasia is that treatment is rarely defined. Few of the studies conducted on treatment specify what is meant by treatment, how it is conducted or how the patient responds.

There have been nearly forty documented studies of treatment in aphasia. The outcome has not produced unequivocal or entirely convincing results either to support or reject the hypothesis that treatment is effective or otherwise. Most of the studies have been comparative:

1. Treated patients versus untreated controls (Vignolo, 1964; Smith, 1972; Hagen, 1973; Basso *et al.*, 1975, 1979; Kertesz and McCabe, 1977; Whurr, 1983; Shewan, 1983; Lincoln *et al.*, 1984).
2. Treatment by speech therapists *v.* treatment by volunteers (Griffiths, 1974, 1975; Lesser *et al.*, 1978; Meikle *et al.*, 1979; Griffiths *et al.*, 1980; David *et al.*, 1982).
3. Treatment by speech therapists *v.* treatment by nurses (Shewan, 1983.
4. Language orientated therapy *v.*, cognition based therapy (Shewan and Kertesz, 1983).
5. Programmed instruction *v.* language therapy (Sarno *et al.*, 1970).
6. Intensive treatment *v.* less intensive treatment (Smith, 1972).
7. Individual *v.* group treatment (Wertz *et al.*, 1978).
8. Treatment in hospital *v.* at home (Wertz *et al.*, 1979).

None of these studies provides statistically convincing differences. From these studies, it appears that patients seem to change over time regardless of whether they are treated by speech therapists or volunteers, treated intensively or once a week, treated on their defective or on their retained areas of function, treated by cognitive therapy or language therapy or programmed instruction or even left untreated. Most studies are group studies, and the numbers in the group ranges from 20 to 100. A possible conclusion is that comparing large numbers of patients produces unwieldy statistical data which disguise more than they reveal. To counteract this, researchers have examined single cases with the patient acting as his own control (Davies, 1978; Chapey, 1981; Coltheart, 1983; Howard 1985; Byng, 1986). Certainly, a detailed study of one patient across many parameters using descriptive techniques as described by Crystal *et al.* (1982) would provide more qualitative information. The evidence sought by researchers is that aphasic patients improve overtly and measurably when treated. The stress on objective measurement has made researchers resort to the only tools available for objective quantification of performance — namely the formal aphasia batteries.

Subjective Ratings of Aphasia Treatment Research Studies

Most studies have used one or more of the formal aphasia assessment batteries as measures of patients 'before' and 'after' performances, but all have inherent weaknesses and none is an entirely reliable indicator of performance. Alternative subjective and impressionistic ratings by family doctors, volunteers or even speech therapists have been used in several research projects. Griffiths (1974, 1975, 1980) investigated the benefits derived by patients from volunteers who 'with common sense, ability to observe and a desire to help' aimed at 'bringing stimulation and return of hope and confidence' in a club situation supplemented with weekly home visits. Overall improvement was assessed by the family doctor. Specific modalities such as comprehension, reading and writing were assessed by speech therapists, volunteers and supervisors. Aspects such as memory, money, numbers, shapes, calendar, time and colour, concentration, alertness, use of hands and general confidence (for which there was no professional assessment) were gauged by the volunteers. Griffiths concluded that the scheme contributed to confidence, general happiness and general attitude with improvement in morale. She thought that it stimulated and broadened life for each patient. Results were based on good neighbour approach, no official judgement, encouragement of independence and continuous stimulation. This produced a good basis for professional help which Griffiths never claimed it replaced. She also makes clear that it was not a controlled study. None the less, speech therapists also confirmed improvement in speech of 70% of patients. It seems that non-language parameters such as motivation and confidence are more observable entities in the evaluation of progress even though the system of analysis is subjective.

There are other research studies on treatment of aphasia which involve subjective ratings. For example, in the Butfield and Zangwill (1946) study senior staff members judged speech, reading, writing and calculation performance of severe aphasics on a three point scale. Specific treatment techniques were described and the results of re-assessment were expressed on an overall rating of both expressive and receptive function. Severely impaired patients made the smallest gain during the initial recovery period. Wepman (1951) adopted the Progressive Achievement Tests which provided more objective scores in reading, writing, spelling and arithmetic in terms of school grades. Comparisons of results among different studies are complicated because improvement was sometimes referred to both normal standards and pre-training defect (Wepman, 1951; Taylor, 1964) and sometimes to pre-training defect alone (Butfield and Zangwill, 1946). Other studies (e.g. Leischner, 1960) have rated improvement along a scale but the initial degree of impairment is sometimes not reported. The early studies of Weisenburg and McBride (1964) often adopted an expressive–receptive–

global–amnesic type of clinical classification to define types of aphasia but the definition was seldom precise.

Vignolo (1964) stressed the need for objective evaluation to assess the degree of impairment and hence improvement. Additionally, he stated that spontaneous evolution of aphasia must be studied to see if it exists and whether it shows any quantitative or qualitative trends. Vignolo examined the records of 69 adult aphasics who were tested at least twice by a standard aphasia examination used in his clinic; this preliminary study investigated only three language performances — oral description, oral naming and comprehension of oral commands — which were rated on a 0–3 scale. There were 42 treated aphasics and 27 non-treated controls. The control group was composed of those patients who were unable to attend for therapy or who defaulted from attending. Patients had one treatment session each week for at least 20 sessions and the methods of treatment were specified.

The results show that in general the groups did not differ although there was a trend towards more and quicker improvement in the treated group. Vignolo, questioning this result, comments that effects of rehabilitation are 'too subtle to be assessed through our method of examination'. The study gave no hint of any differential influence of treatment in one type of aphasia rather than another. However, disturbances of oral expression and comprehension seemed more likely to improve spontaneously, particularly the latter. Severe expressive disturbances were more likely to impede restitution of overall verbal communication than receptive disturbances. Improvement of oral expression was not influenced by the initial level of auditory comprehension. Articulatory dyspraxia had a significant retarding effect on the recovery of expression. Treatment seemed to have a specific effect provided that it continued for more than 6 months.

Basso *et al.* (1975) carried out an extended study in an attempt to verify the 1964 findings: 185 aphasics, 91 treated and 94 untreated controls, were submitted to the same assessment scheme. The Goodman statistical analysis established that language rehabilitation had a positive effect on the improvement of oral expression, whilst the duration of aphasia at the time of the first examination had a negative effect on improvement. These results differed from those of 1964 because of the different method of analysis rather than the different methods of assessment.

Basso *et al.* (1979) further studied the influence of language rehabilitation on specific language skills (speaking, understanding, reading and writing) in 281 patients — 162 treated and 119 controls — who were reassessed 6 months after the initial assessment. The aphasia was assessed by the standard language examination used since 1962 by Basso and Vignolo (unpublished observations). The type of aphasia was rated on the Goodglass and Kaplan (1972) fluency/non-fluency dimension. The statistical analyses comprised four separate analyses of oral expression, auditory comprehension, reading and writing. The complex contingency tables resulting from these subdivisions were analysed by means of a log-linear model to estimate the significance of the effect of each variable. The results indicated a relative improvement of the four modalities with a consistent trend across aphasic syndromes and across both treated and untreated controls. Comprehension improved more than expression, and oral language improved more than written. The rank order of the four language modalities appeared the same in the two groups. This suggests that rehabilitation accelerates the course of restitution without altering its pattern. Basso *et al.* found that the simple tests used 'measured the symptoms of consequence to the patient in his personal working life' and the scores reflected functional communication ability. Standard administration in a laboratory setting makes tasks somewhat more difficult than similar tasks encountered in real life.

Wertz *et al.* (1986) in a comparison of clinic, home and deferred language treatment for aphasia found that aphasic patients who met stringent selection criteria were assigned randomly to three groups: clinic treatment by a speech pathologist for 12 weeks, followed by 12 weeks of no treatment; home treatment by a trained volunteer for 12 weeks, followed by 12 weeks of no treatment; or deferred treatment for 12 weeks followed by treatment for 12 weeks by a speech pathologist.

The results after 12 weeks showed that the treated patients did significantly better on their language measures than the deferred treatment patients. However, at 24 weeks after entry — and after the deferred treatments had received treatment — there were no significant differences among groups. The authors conclude that clinic treatment for 12 weeks does not compromise ultimate improvement. They argue that the change in the deferred group at 12 weeks supports the belief in spontaneous recovery, and delaying treatment still resulted in an 11% overall improvement, and therefore appears to have no irrevocable influence on improvement. Yet none of the group differences was significant ($p > 0.05$). This observation contrasts with the general belief that language therapy should be initiated early, probably before 2 months post-onset. However, advocates of early intervention support their suggestion with data from treatment trials at least 3 months longer than this study. Moreover, their groups were of mixed types of aphasia who have different recovery curves; Broca's aphasia may take initially longer to show improvement. There were 12 cases of Broca's aphasia, two of mixed type and six of Wernicke's aphasia.

Formal Aphasia Test Batteries in Aphasia Treatment Research Studies

In the 40 research studies investigating aspects of treatment, the batteries most frequently used to measure the type and degree of aphasia are the

Functional Communication Profile, the Porch Index of Communicative Abilities, the Minnesota Test for the Differential Diagnosis of Aphasia, the Boston Diagnostic Aphasia Examination, the Western Aphasia Battery, and the Aphasia Screening Test (see Table). The remaining studies have used adaptations of these or have constructed their own batteries. All these batteries have inherent weaknesses when used specifically for research purposes. The strength and weaknesses of the aphasia battery are discussed below.

The Functional Communication Profile

The Functional Communication Profile (FCP) is a clinical tool which attempts to measure spontaneous language ability based on an estimate of the patient's pre-morbid language level. It comprises 45 communication behaviours considered to be common language functions of everyday life. Ratings are made on a 9-point scale in five areas; speaking, reading, understanding, movement, and a miscellaneous category which includes writing and calculation. These ratings are based on informal interactions with the patient in conversation. So the evaluation is subjective. The examiner's observations are plotted on a questionnaire. An overall score reflects the sum of the weighted part scores and can be used as a single measure of a patient's communicative effectiveness — 100% represents the estimated pre-morbid communication efficiency. Comparisons between the FCP and the MTDDA (Sands *et al.*, 1969) showed a high degree of statistical agreement between the two. The results are not surprising since correlations were being made across similar language activities in both tests.

In a study evaluating the responses of aphasic adults to a structured language test and the FCP, Greenberg (1966) found high inter-examiner reliability. However, the author's caution that the test has been devised for use by 'experienced clinicians having access to hundreds of aphasic patients in any given year'. They stress that the test may have little validity when used by inexperienced personnel having only intermittent contact with aphasics or access to a limited case load. Sands and co-workers recognized that one major obstacle to the systematic study of recovery of language has been the lack of measures sensitive to small changes in performance. Unfortunately, the FCP with its subjective rating system is not a reliable or sensitive clinical tool to measure subtle changes.

The FCP has been used in several research studies. Sands, Sarno and Shankweiler (1969) investigated the long-term assessment of language function in aphasia after stroke. 30 stroke patients, median age 56 years, who had received at least 7 months speech therapy were followed up over 4–12 months after the termination of therapy. 13 months after the termination of treatment, patients demonstrated a modest but significant gain of 15% on the FCP. Sarno, Silverman and Sands (1970) compared the effects of two methods of treatment, programmed instruction and non-programmed instruction, and of no treatment on 31 patients with severe expressive-receptive aphasia due to a stroke. They were assessed 3 months after onset and randomly assigned to the three groups. All patients were re-assessed after 80 hours treatment. Gains were small and similar in all groups, including the untreated controls. The authors concluded that patients with severe aphasia do not benefit from speech therapy.

In another study, Sarno and Levita (1971) investigated 28 untreated stroke patients on admission, at 3 months and at 6 months after onset. They found that the period of most significant spontaneous recovery was completed by 3 months. Sarno (1969), critical of using only one measure to detect changes in language performance, decided to use the FCP and the NCCEA in the evaluation of language after stroke. Sarno and Levita (1971) examined recovery in treated aphasic patients during the first year after stroke. They divided 43 patients into three categories — fluent, non-fluent and global. Three measures were used — the FCP, the Token Test and the NCCEA. The results showed that individual types of aphasic patient recovered at different rates. Sarno noticed the discrepancy between the striking changes on task-orientated performance and functional ratings. Some changes in chronic aphasics can be accounted for by extra-linguistic compensatory mechanisms and not by specific language processing changes aone. These results provided much greater specific detail than the earlier results, presumably because of the additional testing parameters of TOA, FCP and category ratings.

The 1969 study, where Sands stated that severe aphasic patients assessed on the FCP do not benefit from speech therapy, needs to be viewed with caution. The FCP is particularly inappropriate for the assessment of severely impaired patients, since subtle remaining abilities cannot be captured purely on the basis of a subjective questionnaire.

Other studies using the FCP as the only measure of language performance also should be viewed with caution. For example, David *et al.* (1982) compared the effects of treatment by two different groups, qualified speech therapists and untrained volunteers. The results were unequivocal. Patients in both groups made small gains which were not significantly different from one another. The FCP was an unfortunate choice of testing instrument to measure the effects of treatment. Obviously, it was selected because of its simplicity and high degree of inter-score reliability with the MTDDA. 43 speech therapists in 14 different centres were involved in the trial of David and her co-workers. All were trained in the use of the test on the basis of five video-recordings and most also examined one or two patients. It is worth noting that Taylor Sarno stresses the importance of training time before using the FCP. The reliability of 43 different speech therapists assessing patients on the FCP after only limited experience must be questioned, and this is a further weakness added to what is a subjective system of assessment.

The FCP correlates well with other formal aphasia batteries especially the MTDDA (Greenberg, 1966; David, 1979). However, all aphasia batteries are bound to correlate highly with one another. All batteries consist of more or less the same subtest tasks and so the comparison is between constituents of language which contain sufficient homogeneity to provide high correlation. All patients entered into the research studies where the FCP is used appear to progress over time regardless of whether they are severely impaired, treated by two different methods, treated late after onset, tracked over 6 months of treatment, or treated by volunteers or speech therapists. These data call into question the suitability of the FCP as a research tool when used without any other battery. The most it can be expected to reveal is the direction of fairly gross changes in performance. It cannot reveal subtle changes and so it is not adequate as a research tool.

The Porch Index of Communicative Ability

The PICA was designed to assess the aphasic patient's entire ability to communicate not just his ability to use speech and language (Porch, 1967). The test is constructed on the basis of sampling all aspects of communicative behaviour, including that of gestural response. The system of scoring is multi-dimensional, rather than the dichotomous plus/minus system used by most batteries. The score considers five dimensions: accuracy, responsiveness, completeness, promptness and efficiency. Its main weakness as a research tool is its complicated multi-dimensional scoring system which requires 40 hours of training time. The system itself is cumbersome since it operates on a 16-point scale. The scale indicates qualitative differences in performance on a quantitative basis. It is not a system that can be easily understood by other professionals, unless they have undergone training. Although multi-dimensional scoring is a useful method for observing subtle behavioural changes it is unsuitable for research purposes.

Two research studies have involved the PICA. Meikle *et al.* (1979) compared treatment by volunteers and speech therapists, and Lincoln (1984) compared treated patients with untreated controls. Neither study found any significant difference. In the former, 31 patients were assessed on the PICA and on a simple unpublished test which assessed comprehension, verbal expression, writing and spelling. Serial assessments of each patient were made at 6 weekly intervals using the PICA. Analyses were made of the change in PICA scores from initial to final assessment and of the percentage change from the initial value. The time between initial and final assessments and the initial PICA scores were used as covariants. A two-factor analysis of variance (patients × PICA overall percentiles) with repeated measures on the PICA overall percentiles confirmed that there was no significant difference between the two forms of treatment and established that appreciable improvement between initial and final assessment occurred in both groups of patients.

Lincoln *et al.* (1984) performed a randomized control trial to determine whether speech therapy produces a better language outcome than natural recovery alone. Patients were assessed on the PICA 4 weeks after a stroke. During the next 2 weeks they were allocated to the treatment or the no-treatment group. All patients were seen at 6-weekly intervals by assessors. Patients were assessed on the PICA and FCP at the pre- (10 weeks after stroke), mid- (22 weeks) and post- (34 weeks) treatment assessment, and with a shortened version of the PICA at 16 and 28 weeks. The groups were compared at each assessment using tests for independent data and no significant differences were found on any measure. The study claims to indicate that speech therapy did not improve language abilities beyond what was achieved by spontaneous recovery. The authors state that speech therapists need to place more emphasis on the assessment of the type of communication problem.

Martin (1977) raises a number of questions concerning the PICA. He points out that sometimes the multidimensional scoring fails to capture details of a patient's response. Support for this criticism has come from factor analysis which showed that not all the factors loaded 'clearly' (Clark *et al.*, 1979). The test in its standard form does not directly assess comprehension, nor does it provide an evaluation of spontaneous speech. Once again, the failure of the two studies to find significant differences questions the validity of the measuring instruments and the methods of assessment.

The Minnesota Test for the Differential Diagnosis of Aphasia

The MTDDA is based on the hypothesis that aphasia is a unidimensional disorder which in its 'pure' form entails a reduction of available vocabulary and an impaired auditory verbal retention span evident in all language modalities without specific perceptual or apraxic disturbances. The underlying *aphasic* element permeates seven diagnostic and prognostic categories identified by factor analysis of 155 aphasic subjects and scaled on a severity basis of total, severe, simple, mild and global. It does not distinguish between types of aphasia. Scoring is on a plus/minus basis expressed in numbers of errors — i.e. an error score. There are unequal numbers of items within each subtest, ranging from 5 to 32 items. Numerical conversion is required to translate the error scores and also to obtain mean performance scores for each group of subjects. Because of its unidimensional hypothesis it provides a consistent assessment of language function within each language modality. However, the method of scoring produces a clumsy method of measuring change. Despite these disadvantages, the two research studies using the MTDDA to investigate the performances of treated and untreated patients demonstrated that the MTDDA was sensitive to differences in performance between the groups.

Smith (1972) compared the progress of treated chronic aphasic patients with untreated controls, and Hagen (1973) also compared treated patients with untreated controls. The extensive study of Smith and co-workers investigated diagnosis, intelligence and the effects of language rehabilitation on 126 left hemisphere stroke patients whose mean age was 46.7 years. They were examined up to 21 weeks after the stroke on a large battery of tests of language and non-language function. All were assessed on a selection of 21 subtests from the MTDDA which sampled each language modality. In addition they were extensively assessed on standardized measures of non-language function which involved a complete neuropsychological battery, tests of motor function, tests of visual and auditory short-term memory, visual retention tests, simultaneous (face–hand) stimulation of sensory function, tests of tactile stimulation, the coloured progressive matrices and the Wechsler Adult Intelligence Scale. Sixty-seven patients received treatment from final year speech pathology students under the supervision of their clinical tutors for an average of 395 hours over 15.8 weeks. Fifteen control patients who were assessed but not treated were included in the trial. The controls were not entirely matched since they had a higher mean age, they were more severely impaired, and they had evidence of bilateral cerebral dysfunction with lower mean scores on the non-language tests. All patients were reassessed at the end of the trial and the authors state that the results 'clearly indicate that language rehabilitation results in measurable gains in language function beyond what can be expected to occur as a result of spontaneous recovery'. Treated patients made highly significant gains in language function over the controls. Moreover, they noted that all four language components, digit span, oral and written substitution showed a consistent pattern of greater gains after 40 weeks than after 5 weeks. They concluded that intensive residential language therapy results in significant improvement in chronic aphasia.

Hagen (1973) investigated the effects of treatment versus no treatment in a group of 20 males with communication disorders after stroke. The results showed that both groups improved spontaneously during the first 3 months but the treatment group continued to progress beyond the point of spontaneous recovery to attain functional communication ability. Patients for the project were carefully assessed to conform to strict criteria for entrance to the trial, including assessment on the MTDDA, so that they were matched for type and degree of language impairment. The first 10 patients referred who conformed to the criteria constituted the treatment group and the next 10 acted as untreated controls. During the first 3 months all patients received physical rehabilitation only. For the next 12 months all were assigned to long-term care wards. Those receiving communication therapy received 4 hours of individual, 8 hours of group, and 6 hours of independent therapy per week. The subjects were reassessed at 3, 6 and 12 months.

Inspection of the data indicates a significant increase in auditory retention, visual comprehension, and visual motor abilities of both groups. Comparison of the treated and untreated patients on each of the language subtests showed an improvement across time for the treatment group in comparison with the control group on reading comprehension, language formulation, speech production, spelling and arithmetic. Hagen observed that only those communication processes that have bilateral cerebral representation appear to recover spontaneously to functional level. Left hemisphere processes continue to improve spontaneously up to 9 months after the onset but not subsequently. Speech production and reading comprehension improve only up to 6 months after onset. He concluded that treatment is a process of 'channelling' spontaneous recovery and compensating for deficits, a conclusion corroborated by both Basso (1975) and Whurr (1983).

The Boston Diagnostic Aphasia Examination

The aim of the BDAE is to aid in the localization of cerebral damage (Goodglass and Kaplan, 1972, 1984). The view that specific aphasic syndromes can be attributed to damage in specific locations and to specific mechanisms is implicit to the approach of Goodglass and Kaplan. Most research studies which have used the Boston classification and brain scans confirm that in general sites of lesion can be correlated with type of aphasia. Scoring on the BDAE is plus/minus with points deducted for delay of response or partially corrected responses. A qualitative assessment of articulatory difficulties, paraphasic errors and jargon is made on a present or absent system. The scores are expressed through a combination of Aphasia Severity Rating, Rating and Speech Characteristics and a 'Z' score profile of subscores. Many patients may fall into one or two of the six major diagnostic categories but the system of classifying the remaining four categories remains elusive and unrealistic.

Lesser *et al.* (1978) examined the contribution that rehabilitation made to aphasic patients language abilities and their social confidence when treated by volunteers in a club situation. 16 patients with a duration of aphasia of at least 11 months were assessed on the BDAE, the FCP, tape recorded conversations and a social situation questionnaire. The patients met on one day a week in a club situation where they were reassessed after 22 weeks. There was no significant evidence of improvement on the tests of the BDAE that used objective scoring. The results of this trial suggested that language disorder did not improve measurably in these patients, although their sociability and motivation to communicate did improve.

Western Aphasia Battery

Kertesz and Poole (1974) modified the BDAE to suit their basically clinical and neurological approach to taxonomic groupings of aphasics. The modified battery — the WAB (Kertesz, 1982) — was designed to evaluate the main clinical aspects of language function: content, fluency, auditory comprehension, repetition, naming, reading, writing and calculating. The scoring system provides overall measures of severity, the aphasia quotient which was the oral portion of language assessment and the cortical quotient which includes the non-verbal scores. The subscores allow a practical classification of the aphasia according to a taxonomic table (Kertesz, 1979) which includes seven cortical sites rated on fluency, comprehension, repetition and naming.

Kertesz and McCabe (1977) using the WAB investigated recovery patterns and prognosis in 93 aphasic patients. Recovery rates were higher in post-traumatic than in stroke cases. The greatest recovery was seen in Broca's aphasia, followed by the conduction group. Anomic aphasia appeared to be a common end-stage of recovery. Long-term follow-up showed that global aphasics have a poor prognosis, while Broca's and Wernicke's have intermediate ones. Complete recovery occurred frequently among anomic, conduction, and transcortical aphasics and in more than half of the traumatic cases. Initial severity and outcome correlated significantly. Younger patients recovered better. Although some patients recovered well while having therapy, there were no significant differences between the treated and untreated groups.

Shewan (1983) compared the effects of three different types of treatment on language recovery and investigated whether they were more effective than no treatment (Shewan and Kertesz, 1985). 100 aphasic patients were examined on the WAB, the Auditory Comprehension Test for Sentences (Shewan, 1979) and on Raven's Coloured Progressive Matrices 2–4 weeks after stroke and 3, 6 and 12 months after the first tests. The three treatment groups involved Language Orientated Therapy, Stimulation Facilitation Therapy, and 'treatment' from untrained nurses. There were untreated controls. All treated patients had three 1-hour sessions weekly for 1 year in a clinical setting. The patients receiving all three forms of treatment did better than untreated controls when evaluated on the Language Quotient which is a composite index of oral and written subtests. However, when oral skills were examined using the Aphasic Quotient as the outcome measure, none of the results reached significance, highlighting the importance of including both oral and written language performance in measuring language recovery. The patients receiving treatment by non-professionals approached statistical significance. As a measure of performance the WAB produced evidence of significant differences between treated patients and untreated controls when both oral and written language subtests were combined. However, it did not demonstrate significant differences between types of treatment.

The Aphasia Screening Test

The AST is a simple, sensitive and comprehensive test which assesses language disturbances in all four language modalities on a task orientated approach. The tasks are graded in difficulty from simple to complex within each modality. There are only five items in each subtest. The scoring is on a strict pass/fail system with a possible score of 5 on each subtest. There are 20 receptive and 30 expressive tests giving a maximum possible overall combined score of 250, and individual overall scores for receptive and expressive functions can be derived. A deficit scale of severe, moderate and mild is obtained by calculating the overall combined score and the individual receptive and expressive scores.

The AST has been used in a study comparing the effects of directing treatment at 'deficit areas' as opposed to the 'retained areas' (Whurr, 1983); 31 aphasic patients were assessed 1–4 months after having a stroke. They were divided into two groups on the basis of their geographical location. Another 15 patients who did not have speech therapy available to them at the time were also assessed to act as an untreated control group, in order to compare changes in function over time. Patients in each group were divided into three levels of impairment — severe, moderate and mild. These three levels were compared and contrasted on overall combined scores, on receptive function scores and on expressive function scores. The data were then divided into eight modalities so that more detailed investigation could be conducted of the modality recovery curves at all levels of impairment in all three groups of patients.

The data supported the view that treatment should be directed at deficit areas. Improvement in overall function may be effected by a reconstruction approach — that is building up the lost links, stage by stage, until a functional level is reached. However, the results were not clear cut. More detailed investigation of separate language skills and their recovery curves at the three levels of impairment showed that severely impaired patients seemed to respond to both methods of treatment but more to that directed at deficit areas.

Moderately impaired patients made a significantly greater improvement across all language modalities with this method and indeed with the alternative method they regressed on oral language and calculation. The minimally impaired patients seemed to gain with both methods and there was no significant difference between the two. Receptive and expressive functions seem to have different recovery curves.

Summary and Conclusions

Many of the 40 aphasia research studies into treatment efficacy have had weaknesses in test design. The measuring instruments have had inconsistencies within the planning of test items, a lack of gradation of tasks, and dubious systems of scoring. These are some of the elements in the aphasia test batteries used that need to be considered. These flaws in aphasia test batteries may be further compounded by statistical manipulation and factor analysis. The aphasia test battery, the functional communication profile and detailed linguistic analysis can provide only limited qualitative information. Likewise results from the use of such batteries and methods must be viewed in the context of these limitations. Such results may be both equivocal and unreliable, yet subjective ratings, let alone single case studies, are likely to produce even less reliable conclusions. However, aphasia treatment research to date has produced the following tentative suggestions.

Treatment Versus No Treatment

The most controversial issue in the study of treatment of aphasia is whether it produces any objective improvement. One obvious method to investigate whether aphasic patients respond to treatment is to compare treated patients with untreated controls. Only 10 studies have done so. The small number is due to the ethical problems of denying patients treatment facilities for research purposes. The 10 studies have involved overall the comparison of about 751 treated patients with 428 untreated controls. No conclusion can be drawn from any of the studies because of weaknesses in the research design particularly concerning the nature of treatment and patient selection. The type, duration, intensity, focus and rationale of treatment received is often not specified completely (Culton, 1969; Smith, 1972; Lincoln, 1984).

Basso (1975, 1979, 1982, 1987), Vignolo (1964), Hagen (1973), Rusk (1970), Whurr (1983) and Marks (1957) attempt to specify either the type of treatment, its duration or its focus. However, not one of their studies can be considered seriously because the treatment and control groups in all but Hagen's are in some way unmatched, or the assessment is based on some subjective rating system. Hagen admits that, because of the small number of subjects in his study, his findings of measurable gains in the treatment group compared with controls cannot be generalized to all patients with a communicative disorder following a stroke.

Despite these inherent weaknesses the studies of Hagen (1973), Basso (1979), Vignolo (1964), Whurr (1983) and Wertz (1985) do reflect a trend that treatment may help to speed up a normal recovery process. The treated patients reached a higher level of functional performance more quickly than the controls. Only Hagen (1973), Lincoln (1984) and Wertz (1986) enter control patients matched by type and degree of language impairment along with at least 12 other selection criteria, and Lincoln's and Wertz controls were not only matched but also randomly selected.

Basso *et al.* (1979) and Vignolo (1964) had 230 controls selected on the basis of default, i.e. they were patients who could not manage to attend for treatment or who opted out of treatment. Smith (1977) and Whurr (1983) had control patients matched on the basis of level of impairment but not matched for age or time since the stroke occurred. Marks *et al.* (1957), Rusk *et al.* (1968) and Culton (1969) did not match patients by aetiology or type of aphasia which was in itself assessed on a subjective rating in their studies.

Aetiology

Prognosis and recovery differ according to aetiology (Kertesz, 1977). Complete recovery from aphasia after stroke is unusual (Vignolo and Basso, 1979; Whurr, 1983) but it is more common with other aetiologies such as trauma (Kertesz, 1977; Frazier and Ingram, 1920; Butfield *et al.*, 1952).

Evolution of Type of Aphasia and Response to Treatment

Kertesz and McCabe (1977) found that the extent of recovery was good in anomic, conduction, transcortical motor and sensory aphasics. Broca's and Wernicke's aphasia made a moderate recovery. Global aphasia made little recovery. Shewan (1983) found that the extent of the improvement varied according to the type of aphasia — Broca's 85%, global 79%, Wernicke's 72%, anomic 40% and conduction 37.5%. Improvement in oral and written language was better in conduction aphasia than Broca's.

Overall Improvement over Time

Most aphasics appear to improve with time regardless of whether the improvement is due to spontaneous recovery or treatment (Griffiths, 1974, 1975, 1980; Lesser, 1978; Meikle *et al.* 1979;m David *et al.* 1982; Shewan, 1983), and treatment may simply accelerate this natural process of improvement (Hagen, 1973; Basso, 1979; Whurr, 1983).

Differential Recovery of Expressive and Receptive Functions

There is agreement that receptive and expressive function recover at different rates (Lebrun, 1976; Basso, 1982; Whurr, 1983) but not about which recovers most. Butfield and Zangwill (1946) and Godfrey (1959) found that expressive function recovered more. Others have found that receptive function improves more than expressive (Vignolo, 1964; Leischner, 1972, 1976; Kenin and Swisher, 1972; Schneider, 1975; Lebrun, 1976; Hanson and Cicciarelli, 1978; Lomas and Kertesz, 1978; Prins, 1978; Basso, 1979; Whurr, 1983; Shewan, 1983). In these studies, expressive function appeared to improve with treatment and regressed without it. Receptive function appeared to improve with time but recovery was hastened by treatment (Basso, 1979; Whurr, 1983). Henri and Cantor (1975) found that receptive function improved before expressive function. The study of Whurr (1983) indicated that receptive function was improved by treatment in mild and moderately aphasic patients but not in severe aphasics. Expressive function improved at all levels of impairment. Kertesz postulated that as expressive function is heterogeneous its recovery cannot be studied as if it were a single factor. Measuring overall scores, as in the Aphasia Quotient, does not allow conclusions to be drawn about changes in the various components of language.

Specific Modality Recovery of Language Skills

According to Kenin and Swisher (1972) language skills recovered at different rates and evolved as follows — copying, auditory and reading comprehension, speech, oral and written naming. According to Henri and Cantor (1975) the order was listening, reading, speaking and writing. Whurr (1983) studied the recovery curves of eight language components on three levels of impairment — severe, moderate and mild — in three groups of patients: those treated on their retained areas of function, those treated on their defective areas of function, and untreated controls. The modality changes after 6 months showed differential orders of improvement in each group. Treatment directed at the deficit areas produced most improvement in reading, auditory comprehension, speech production and oral language.

Hagen (1973) described modality specific spontaneous recovery in patients receiving treatment who acquired functional abilities in reading, comprehension, language formulation, speech production, spelling and arithmetic but auditory and visually mediated abilities recovered to functional levels without treatment. These results indicated that treatment in aphasia needs to be conducted with some specificity. Each language component, at each level of impairment, seems to respond differentially to the method of treatment and whether it is directed at the lost or intact function areas. As aphasic patients do not form a homogeneous group it is clear that each individual patient requires a carefully designed treatment programme based on detailed assessment of their initial profile of lost and retained areas in all language modalities.

Conclusions

Several issues in aphasia therapy research remain unresolved even after 40 studies. First there is the problem of objective measurement. Darley (1972) laid down the now classic protocol for conducting research into the treatment of aphasia. He stated that: 'reliable quantitative data must be gathered with rigorous objectivity. However, in addition, one must add that the tools used to gather the data must be powerful and subtle enough to detect subtle changes in language performance'. The prerequisite for a research tool to evaluate subtle changes in language performance is that it must provide quantitative, qualitative and pragmatic information. Quantitative information should be obtained on a task-orientated approach which assessed all language modalities and which includes pre-linguistic tasks.

The tasks should be ordered in graded difficulty. Scoring should be on a pass/fail correct score system. There should be uniformity and equal numbers of items in each subtest, as well as equal numbers of subtests in each language modality to simplify scoring. The overall quantitative score should indicate the level of overall severity of impairment. Qualitative evaluation should be based on these data and should provide a multidimensional profile of lost and retained abilities, as well as an analysis of all linguistic levels, plus a neuropsychological account of the disorders underlying language disturbances. Pragmatic analysis should involve observation of the patient in non-test situations. A composite profile of all three areas should be produced to provide a comprehensive exploration of all parameters of the natural course of recovery.

The research design should take account of the many variables that must be considered in aphasia treatment research, including aetiology, site and size of lesion, age, sex, education, intelligence, handedness, laterality, time after onset and all those variables concerned with treatment. It is not possible to include and control for every variable and so the research projects must specify which variables are included, which are excluded and why. Group research presumes that the members of the group possess a set of important characteristics in common, such as a deficit of the same processing mechanism. This assumption of homogeneity is a priori impossible in aphasia because of the multiple variables involved. Group study research usually involves grouping patients on the basis of classification criteria that are not detailed enough to ensure that patients are homogeneous in terms of the components of processing that are impaired. Patient grouping is normally accomplished on the basis of classic syndromes or by site of lesion. Patients in groups based on classic syndromes could have impairment of different psychological mechanisms and thus 'violate the requirements of homogeneity in group research' (Caramazza, 1984).

Research studies have involved a range of several hundreds of patients to comparisons of less than ten. The arguments against large-scale studies have been clearly stated by Coltheart (1983) and others. The alternative, to obviate the problems posed by large-scale studies, is the single case study. The single case study is based on single subject experimental design where it is possible to explore one variable at a time, and to create a wide variety of paradigms to answer many very specific questions. There are obvious advantages.

According to Caramazza (1984) single case studies involve replications and extensions which implicitly assume a typology or classification of aphasia. That is, replications and extensions are intended to generalize to particular types of aphasia. The generalization is not to a particular pattern of symptoms but to a patient type defined in terms of a disruption to some processing component.

The pendulum has swung in favour of the single case study method because large-scale group research has been expensive, time consuming and disappointing. However, the single case study approach, although providing explicit detailed description of a patient's performance, does not allow extrapolation of the results to other patients. The individual patient acting as his own control may produce valuable insights but the problem of such an approach is that it may produce another source of well documented, anecdotal descriptions rather like the classic case studies of the early twentieth century neurologists. A practical compromise has been offered by Caramazza (1984) who proposes a combination of 'the group/case study' approach where groups of patients are studied extensively and individual differences are pursued.

Another major problem in evaluating recovery after treatment is that treatment is rarely defined or specified. Few of the group studies say clearly what is meant by treatment, how it is conducted and how the patient responds, even though therapists are constantly urged to have specific long- and short-term goals with treatment plans for each session and clearly documented reports of patients' responses. Ideally, treatment should start with a careful plan based on the interpretation of the patient's performance on a formal test battery. The test results should be analysed. A profile of retained and disrupted areas of function should be computed by noting all the high scores (retained areas) and all the low scores (deficit areas). They should be divided further into retained and deficit language modality groups, linguistic levels — phonological, prosodic, syntactic and semantic — and subtest orders of difficulty. Treatment must be specified on the basis of the following:

1. The objective or goals of treatment.
2. The technique used and its rationale.
3. Individual or group treatment.
4. The frequency of treatment.
5. The length of each treatment session.
6. The duration of treatment.
7. The number of therapists and their qualifications.
8. The extent of involvement of other hospital personnel, family and friends.

As none of the 40 documented accounts of research into aphasia therapy has been based on studies which have fulfilled the basic minimum criteria it would seem premature at this point to conclude that treatment does not produce measurable or functional improvements in performance. What is clear is that further research must be conducted. It must confirm to the requirements of rigorous scientific protocols which means at least (1) objective and detailed measurements of the disorders presented, (2) specification of the variables measured including the reasons for the inclusion of those variables and the exclusion of others, (3) specification of the patients entering the trial, and (4) complete specification of the treatments provided.

Many patients have gone through research studies over the last 40 years — over 3000 treated patients and 350 untreated controls — the position appears that neither the single case study, the large group study, non-randomized control trials have provided completely satisfying answers to our questions. This does not mean we have to reject all the data made available to us, on the contrary, what is proposed by Fitzgibbon (1986) and Nye (1986), is that we combine and co-ordinate this vast amount of available information and conduct a meta-analysis, which is a system of analysis of analysis, a quantitative method for research synthesis and an efficient way to summarize large literature. Meta-analysis is helpful in highlighting gaps in the literature, provides insights into new directions for research, and for finding mediating or interactional relationships or trends too subtle to see, or that cannot be hypothesized and tested in individual studies. Meta-analysis may well enable us to summarize the 'state of knowledge' of the field of treatment of aphasic patients and this is planned for the future. Until then we are urged by Caramazza (1984) to conduct the 'small group case study approach' in which a small group of patients is studied extensively and individual differences pursued.

Aphasia therapy is on trial and for the sake of those patients suffering from a condition which by definition prevents them from putting their own case, those in charge of their welfare should be urged to research more carefully and precisely into the nature of the condition and into the factors that may ameliorate it. We are looking towards specificity of measurement matched by specificity of treatment. Until these two areas can be included satisfactorily into our research, we are not in a position to say treatment is not effective, any more than we can say with full confidence that it is effective. Aphasia therapy research must proceed.

> 'Perhaps until we understand more about dysphasia, we would do better to concentrate on small well-defined groups, comparing one mode of treatment with another, gradually building in this way a hard core of firm facts' (Lancet, 1977).

Treatment Studies of Aphasia Therapy 1946–1986

Study	*Assessment used*	*Specifies treatment*	*No of patients*	*Untreated controls*
Butfield and Zangwill, 1946	Subjective rating	✓	70	
Eisenson, 1949	Subjective rating	—	68	
Wepman, 1951	Subjective rating	—	203	
Marks, Taylor and Rusk, 1957	FCP	—	38	
Godfrey and Douglas, 1959	Exam ratings	Occupational Therapists		
Leischner, 1960		?	105	
Schuell and Jenkins, 1964	MTDDA	—	155	
Vignolo, 1964	Observation	✓	42	27
Rusk and Taylor, 1968	FCP	—	31	
Kreindler and Frandis, 1968	Observation	—	?	
Culton, 1969	Observation Ravens	—	10	11
Sands, Sarno, Shankweiler 1969	FCP	✓	30	
Sarno, Silverman and Sands, 1970	FCP	✓	31	8
Sarno and Levita, 1971	FCP and NCCEA	✓	—	28
Hagen, 1973	MTDDA	✓	10	10
Eaton-Griffith, 1974	Subjective rating	Volunteers	31	
Basso, Faglioni and Vignolo, 1974	Observation	✓	41	94
Eaton-Griffith *et al.*, 1975	Subjective rating	Volunteers	552	
Leischner, 1976	Observation	✓	430	
Rose *et al.*, 1976	Observation	—	50	
Broida, 1977	Observation	—	14	
Kertesz and McCabe, 1977	WAB	—	93	14
Lesser *et al.*, 1978	BDAE	Volunteers	16	
Levita, 1978	FCP	—	?	
Wertz, 1978	PICA +	✓	?	
Sarno and Levita, 1979	FCP Token NCCEA	—	43	
Basso, Capitani and Vignolo, 1979	Observation	✓	281	14
Meikle *et al.*, 1979	PICA	Volunteers	31	

Treatment Studies of Aphasia Therapy 1946–1986 (continued)

Wertz *et al.*, 1979	PICA +	✔	?	
Eaton-Griffith *et al.*, 1980	Observation	Volunteers	397	
David *et al.* 1982	FCP	Volunteers	96	
Aten *et al.*, 1982	PICA CADL	✔	7	
Shewan, 1983	WAB ACTS Ravens	Nurses	77	23
Whurr, 1983	AST	✔	31	15
Lincoln *et al.*, 1984	AST BDAE PICA	—	97	74
Shewan and Kertesz, 1984	WAB ACTS Ravens	Nurses	77	23
Wertz *et al.*, 1986	PICA FCP BOAE CADL Token	Relatives	64	29

Treatment Studies of Aphasia Therapy 1946–1986

Measurements and assessments used:		
Subjective ratings	=	4
Observation	=	12
Exam ratings	=	1
Objective tests:		
FCP	=	10
PICA	=	5
MTDDA	=	3
BDAE	=	3
RPM	=	3
NCCEA	=	2
TT	=	2
AST	=	2
WAB	=	2
ACTS	=	1
CADL	=	1

Key

FCP = Functional Communication Profile.
PICA = Porch Index of Communicative Abilities.
MTDDA = Minnesota Test for the Differential Diagnosis of Aphasia.
BDAE = Boston Diagnostic Aphasia Examination.
RPM = Ravens Progressive Matrices.
NCCEA = Neurosensory Centre Comprehensive Examination of Aphasia.
TT = Token Test.
AST = Aphasia Screening Test.
WAB = Western Aphasia Battery.
ACTS = Auditory Comprehension Test of Syntax.
CADL = Communicative Abilities in Daily Living.

References

ALBYN DAVIS, G. *A Survey of Adult Aphasia* (1983). New Jersey: Prentice Hall.

ALBYN DAVIS, G. and WILCOX, J.W. *Adult Aphasia Rehabilitation — Applied Pragmatics* (1985). NFER — Nelson.

ALBYN DAVIS, G. and WILCOX, M.J. Incorporating parameters of natural conversation in aphasia treatment. In R. Chapey (ed.) *Language Intervention Strategies in Adult Aphasia* (1981). Baltimore: Williams and Wilkins.

ATEN, J., CALIGUIRI, M and HOLLAND, A. The efficacy of functional communication therapy for chronic aphasic patients. *Journal of Speech and Hearing Disorders* (1982), **47**, 93–96.

BASSO, A. and VIGNOLO, L. Unpublished data (1962).

BASSO, A., FAGLIONI, P. and VIGNOLO, L. Etude controlée de la réducation du language dans l'aphasie. Comparison entre aphasiques traité et non traités. *Revue Neurologique (Paris)* (1975), **131**, 607–614.

BASSO, A., CAPITANI, E. and VIGNOLO, L. Influence of rehabilitation on language skills in aphasic patients. A controlled study. *Archives of Neurology* (1979), **36**, 190–196.

BASSO, A., CAPITANI, E. and ZANOBIA, M. Pattern of recovery of oral and written expression and comprehension in aphasic patients. *Behavioural Brain Research* (1982), **6**, 115–128.

BASSO, A. Approaches to Neuropsychological Rehabilitation Language Disorders. In M. Meir, A. Benton and L. Diller (eds) *Neuropsychological Rehabilitation* (1987). Edinburgh: Churchill Livingstone.

BERMAN, M. and PEALLE, L.M. Self generated cues: A method of aiding aphasic and apractic patients. *Journal of Speech and Hearing Disorders* (1967), **32**, 372–376.

BEYN, E.S. and SHOKHOR-TROTSKAYA, M.K. The preventive method of speech rehabilitation in aphasia. *Cortex*, (1966), **2**, 96–109.

BROIDA, H. Language Therapy Effects in Long Term Aphasia. *Archives of Physical and Medical Rehabilitation* (1977), **58**, 248–253.

BROOKSHIRE, R.H. Effects of Prompting on Spontaneous Naming of Pictures by Aphasic Subjects. *Human Communications* (1975), **3 (2)**, 63–71.

BUTFIELD, E. and ZANGWILL, O. Re: Education in Aphasia: A review of 70 cases. *Journal of Neurology, Neurosurgery and Psychiatry* (1946), **9**, 75–79.

BYNG, S. *Sentence Processing Deficits in Aphasia: Investigations and Remechation*. Unpublished PhD Thesis (1986). University of London.

BYNG, S. and COLTHEART, M. Aphasia therapy research: methodological requirements and illustrative results. In E. Hjelmquist and L.B. Nilsson (eds) *Communication and Handicap. Aspects of Psychological Compensation and Technical Aids* (1986). Amsterdam: North Holland.

CARRAMAZZA, A. The Logic of Neuropsychological Research and the Problem of Patient Classification in Aphasia. *Brain and Language* (1984), **21.1**, 9–20.

CHAPEY, R. What do we need to know? Future issues. In R. Chapey (ed.) *Language Intervention Strategies* (1981). Baltimore: Williams and Wilkins.

CLARK, C.I., CROCKETT, D. and KLONOFF, H. Factor Analysis of the Porch Index Communicative Ability. *Brain and Language* (1979), **7**, 1–7.

CLIFFORD ROSE, F., BOBY, V. and CAPILDEO, R. A Retrospective Study of Speech

Disorders following Stroke with particular reference to the value of Speech Therapy. In Y. Lebrun and R., Hoops (eds) *Recovery in Aphasics — Neurolinguistics*, Vol. 4 (1976), pp. 189–197. Amsterdam: Svets and Zeitlinger.

COLTHEART, M. Aphasia therapy research — a single case study approach. In C. Code and D.J. Muller (eds) Aphasia Therapy, *Studies in Language Disability and Remediation 6* (1983). London: Edward Arnold.

CRYSTAL, D. *Clinical Linguistics* (1981).Vien: Springer-Verlag.

CRYSTAL, D. *Profiling Linguistic Disability* (1982). London: Edward Arnold.

CULTON, G.L. Spontaneous Recovery from Aphasia. *Journal of Speech and Hearing Research* (1969), **12**, 825–832.

DABUL, B. and HANSON, W.R. The Amount of Language Improvement in Adult Aphasics related to early and late treatment. Paper presented at *the Annual Convention of American Speech* (1975). Hearing Association. Washington, D.C.

DARLEY, F. The Efficacy of Language Rehabilitation in Aphasia. *Journal of Speech and Hearing Disorders* (1972), **37**, 3–21.

DARLEY, F. *Aphasia* (1982). Philadelphia: W.B. Saunders Co.

DAVID, R., ENDERBY, P. and BAINTON, D. Treatment of Acquired Aphasia: Speech Therapists and Volunteers Compared. *Journal of Neurology, Neurosurgery and Psychiatry* (1982), **45**, 957–961.

DAVID, R. *A Final Report*: Personal Communication (1979).

DEAL, S.L. and DEAL, L.A. Efficacy of Aphasia Rehabilitation: preliminary results. In R.H. Brookshire (ed.) *Clinical Aphasiology Conference Proceedings* (1978). Minneapolis, Minn.: BRK (Prognosis in aphasia *Lancet* (1977), **ii**, 24.)

EDWARDS, C.E. *Neurology of Ear, Nose and Throat* (1973), p. 265–266. London: Butterworth.

EISENSON, J. Prognostic factors related to language rehabilitation in aphasic patients. *Journal of Speech and Hearing Disorders* (1949), **14**, 262–264.

EISENSON, J. *Adult Aphasia* Ed. 2 (1984). Englewood Cliffs, N.S.: Prentice-Hall.

FITZGIBBON, C. In defence of randomized controlled trials, with suggestions about the possible use of meta analysis. *British Journal of Disorders of Communication* (1986), **1**, 117–124.

FRANKLIN, S. A Cognitive Neuropsychological Approach. In *Approaches to the Treatment of Aphasia* (1986). London Hospital Medical College.

FRAZIER, C.H. and INGHAM, D. A Review of the Effects of Gunshot Wounds of the Head. *Archives of Neurology and Psychiatry* (1920), **3**, 17–40.

GODFREY, C. and DOUGLAS, E. The Recovery Process in Aphasia. *Canadian Medical Journal* (1959), **80**, 618–624.

GOODGLASS, H. and KAPLAN, E. *The Assessment of Aphasia and Related Disorders* 2nd edn. (1984), Philadelphia: Lea and Febiger.

GREENBURG, F.R. *Functional Communication Ability and Responses to a Structured Language Test in Dysphasic Patients* (1966). American Congress of Physical and Medical Rehabilitation, San Francisco.

GRIFFITHS, V.E. Stroke and the Family. *British Medical Journal* (1974), **iv**, 122.

GRIFFITHS, V.E. Volunteer scheme for dysphasia and allied problems in stroke patients. *British Medical Journal* (1975), **iii**, 633–635.

GRIFFITHS, V.E. and MILLER, C.L. Volunteer stroke scheme for dysphasic patients with stroke. *British Medical Journal* (1980), **281**, 1605–1607.

HAGEN, C. Communicative abilities in haemiplegia. Effect of speech therapy. *Archives of Physical and Medical Rehabilitation* (1973), **54**, 454–463.

HANSON, W.R. and CICCIRELLI, A.W. The time, amount and pattern of language improvement in adult aphasics. *British Journal of Disorders of Communication* (1978), **13**, 59–63.

HATFIELD, F. Re-training in writing in severe aphasia. In Y. Lebrun and R. Hoops (eds) *Recovery in Aphasics* (1976). Amsterdam: Swets and Zeitlinger.

HATFIELD, F. Aspects of acquired dysgraphia and implications for re-education. In C. Code and D. Muller (eds) *Aphasia Therapy* (1983). London: Edward Arnold.

HELM, N.A. and BARRESI, B. Voluntary control of involuntary utterances: a treatment approach for severe aphasia. In R.H. Brookshire (ed.) *Clinical Aphasiology Proceedings* (1980). Minneapolis: BRK.

HELM-ESTABROOKS, N., FITZPATRICK, P.M. and BARRESI, B. Response of an agrammatic patients to a syntax stimulation programme for aphasia. *Journal of Speech and Hearing Disorders* (1981), **46**, 422–427.

HELM-ESTABROOKS, N., FITZPATRICK, P. and BARRESI, B. Visual action therapy for global aphasia. *Journal of Speech and Hearing Disorders* (1982), **44**, 385–389.

HELM-ESTABROOKS, N. Treatment of Subcortical Aphasia. In M. Perkins (ed.) *Current Therapy of Communication Disorders* (1984). New York: Thieme-Stratton.

HELM-ESTABROOKS, N. Severe Aphasia. In A. Holland (ed.) *Language Disorders in Adults* (1984). San Diego: College Hill Press.

HELM-ESTABROOKS, N. and RAMSBERGER, G. Treatment of Agrammatisation in Long Term Broca's Aphasia. *British Journal of Disorders of Communication* (1986), **21.1**, 39–45.

HENRI, B.P. and CANTOR, G.J. A longitudinal investigation of patterns of language recovery in eight recent aphasics. Paper presented at *The ASHA Convention, Detroit* (1975).

HOLLAND, A.L. Case studies in aphasia rehabilitation using programmed instructions. *Journal of Speech and Hearing Disorders* (1972), **37**, 3–21.

HOLLAND, A.L. and SONDORMAN, J.C. Effects of a programme based on the Token Test for teaching comprehension skills to Aphasics. *Journal of Speech and Hearing Research* (1974), **17**, 589–598.

HOLLAND, A.L. *Language Disorders in Adults Recent Advances* (1984). San Diego: College Hill Press.

HOPKINS, A. The need for speech therapy for dysphasia following stroke. *Health Trends* Vol. 7 (1975), 58–60.

HOPKINS, A. Practical help. *Lancet* June 23 (1984), pp. 1393–1396.

HOWARD, D.and HATFIELD, F.M. *Aphasia Therapy: Historical and Contemporary Issues* (in press). London: Laurence Erlbaum Associates.

HOWARD, D. and PATTERSON, K. Methodological issues in neuropsychological therapy. In X. Seron and G. Deloche (eds) *Neuropsychological Rehabilitation* (in press). London: Laurence Erlbaum Associates.

HOWARD, D., PATTERSON, K., FRANKLIN, S., ORCHARD LISLE, V., and MORTON, J. Treatment of Word Retrieval Deficits in Aphasia: A Comparison of Two Therapy Methods. *Brain*, (1985), **108**, 817–829.

JONES, E.V. Building the foundation for sentence production in a non-fluent aphasic. *British Journal of Disorders of Communication* Vol. 21 (1986), **1**, 63–81.

KEARNS, K.P., SIMMONS, N.N. and SISTERHEN, C. Gestural sign (Amer-Ind) as a facilitator of verbalization in patients with aphasia. In R.H. Brookshire (ed.) *Clinical Aphasiology Conference Proceedings* (1982), pp. 183–190. Minneapolis: BRK Publishers.

KEARNS, K.P. and SALMON, S.J. An experimental analysis of auxiliary and copula verb generalization in aphasia. *Journal of Speech and Hearing Disorders* (1984), **49**, 152–163.

KENIN, M., SWISHER, L.P. A study of pattern of recovery in aphasia. *Cortex*, 1972), **8**, 56–68.

KERTESZ, A. and MCCABE, P. Recovery patterns and prognosis in aphasia. *Brain* (1972), **100**, 1–18.

KERTESZ, A. and POOLE, E. The aphasia quotient: the taxonomic approach to measurement of aphasic disability. *Canadian Journal of Neurological Sciences* (1974), **1**, 7–16.

KERTESZ, A. *Western Aphasia Battery* (1982). New York: Grune and Stratton.

KERTESZ, A. *Aphasia and Associated Disorders*, Taxonomy and Recovery (1979). New York: Grune and Stratton.

KREINDLER, A. and FRADIS, A. *Performance inAphasia — A Neurodynamic, Diagnostic and Psychological Study* (1968). Gauthier: Villars, Paris.

KUSHNER, D. and WINNITZ, H. Extended Comprehension Practice Applied to an Aphasic Patient. *Journal of Speech and Hearing Disorders* (1977), **42**, 296–305.

LEBRUN, Y. and HOOPS, R. *Intelligence and Aphasia* (1974). Amsterdam: Swets and Zeitlinger.

LEBRUN, Y. Recovery in Polyglot Aphasics. In Y. Lebrun and R. Hoops (eds) *Recovery in Aphasics* (1976). B.V. Amsterdam: Swets and Zeitlinger.

LECOURS, A.R., HERMITTE, F. and BRYANS, B. (eds) Aphasia Therapy. In *Aphasiology* (1983). Balliere: Tindall.

LEISCHNER, A. *Die Storangen der Schnftsprache* (1957). Stuttgart: Thieme.

LEISCHNER, A. Zur Symptomatologie und Therapie der Aphasier. Der *Nervenarzt* (1960), **31**, 60–67.

LEISCHNER, A. Aptitude of aphasics for language treatment. In Y. Lebrun and R. Hoops (eds) *Recovery in Aphasics* (1976). Amsterdam: Swets and Zeitlinger.

LENDRUM, W. and LINCOLN, N. Spontaneous Recovery of Language in Patients with Aphasia between 4 and 34 weeks after Stroke. *Journal of Neurology, Neurosurgery and Psychiatry* (1985), **48**, 743–748.

LESSER, R. and WATT, M. Untrained Community Help in the Rehabilitation of Stroke Sufferers with Language Disorders. *British Medical Journal* (1978), **ii**, 1045–1048.

LESSER, R. Application of psycholinguistic research to rehabilitation in Aphasia. Paper presented at *The Second International Aphasia Rehabilitation Congress* (1986). Goteborg: Sweden.

LEVITA, E. Effects of Speech Therapy in Aphasic Responses to the Functional Communication Profile. *Motor Skills* (1978), 47–151.

LINCOLN, N.B., MCQUIRE, E., MULLEY, G.P., LENDREM, W., JONES, A.C. and MITCHELL, J. RA The effectiveness of speech therapy for aphasic stroke patients: a randomised controlled trial. *Lancet*, **i**, 1197–1200.

LINEBAUGH, C.W. and LEHNER, L.H. Cueing Hierarchies and Word Retrieval: A

Therapy Programme. In R.H. Brookshire (ed.) *Clinical Aphasiology Conference Proceedings* (1977), pp. 19–29. Minneapolis: BRK Publishers.

LOMAS, J. and KERTESZ, A. Patterns of Spontaneous Recovery in Aphasic Groups: A Study of Adult Stroke Patients, *Brain and Language* (1978), **5**, 388–401.

MARKS, M., TAYLOR, M. and RUSK, H. Rehabilitation of the Aphasic Patient. A Survey of 3 years' experience in a Rehabilitation Setting. *Neurology* (1957), **7**, 837–843.

MARSHALL, R.C., TOMPKINS, C.A. and PHILLIPS, D.S. Improvement in Treated Aphasia Examination of Selected Prognostic Factors. *Folio Phoniatrica* (1982, **34**, 305–315.

MARSHALL, R.C. and NEUBERGER, S.I. Extended Comprehensive Training Reconsidered. In R.H. Brookshire (ed.) *Critical Aphasiology Conference Proceedings* (1984), pp. 181–187. Minneapolis: BRK Publishers.

MARSHALL, R.C. Treatment of Auditory Comprehension Deficits. In R. Chapey (ed.) *Language Intervention Strategies* 2nd edn (1986). Baltimore: Williams and Wilkins.

MARTIN, A.D. Aphasia Testing. A second look at the PICA. *Journal of Speech and Hearing Disorders* (1977), **42**, 547–562.

MCGUIRK, E. Efficacy of Speech Therapy and Dysphasic CVA Patients. Paper presented *The International Association of Logopaedics and Phoniatrics Conference, Edinburgh* (1983).

MCMULLEN, M. Evidence of Generalisation in Aphasia Treatment. Paper presented at *The British Aphasiology Conference* Preston (1986).

MEIKLE,, M. WECHSLER, E., TUPPER, A., BENENSON, M., BUTLER, J., MULHALL, D and STERN, G. Comparative Trial of Volunteer and Professional Treatments of Dysphasia after Stroke. *British Medical Journal* (1979), **ii**, 87–89.

MORTON, J. A Treatment of Word Retrieval Deficits in Aphasia. *Brain* (1985), **108**, 817–829.

NAESER, M.A. A Structured Approach Teaching Aphasics Basic Sentence Types. *British Journal of Communication Disorders* (1975), **24**, 127–133.

NEWCOMBE, F., MARSHALL, J., CARRIVICK, P. and HIORNS, R. Recovery Curves in Acquired Dyslexia. *Journal of Neurological Sciences* (1975), **24**, 1127–133.

NYE, C. Quantifying Language Recovery in Adult Aphasics. Paper presented at *The ASHA Convention* Detroit (1986).

PACKMAN, A. and INGHAM, R.J. Contingency management in the Treatment of Adult Aphasia. A Review. *Australian Journal of Human Communication Disorders* (1977), **5**, 110–117.

PENN, C. Compensation and Language Recovery in the Chronic Aphasic Patient. Paper presented at *The 2nd International Aphasia Rehabilitation Congress* (1986). Goteborg, Sweden.

POECK, K. Paper presented at *The Academy of Aphasia* Nashville (1986).

PORCH, E. *Porch Index of Communicative Ability* (1967). Palo Alto, Calif: Consulting Psychologists Press.

PRESCOTT, T.E., SELINGER, M. and LOVERSO, F.L. An analysis of Learning, Generalization and Maintenance of Verbs by an Aphasic Patient. In R.H. Brookshire (ed.) *Clinical Aphasiology Conference Proceedings* (1983), pp. 178–182. Minneapolis: BRK Publishers.

PRINS, S., SNOW, C.E. and WAGENAAR, E. Recovery from Aphasia: Spontaneous Speech versus Language Comprehension. *Brain and Language* **6** 192–211.

RAO, P. and HORNER, J. Gesture as a deblocking modality in a severe aphasic patient. In *Clinical Aphasiology Proceedings* (1978), pp. 180–187. Minneapolis: BRK Publishers.

DE RIBACOURT-DUCARNE, *Reducation Semiologique de l'aphasie* (1987). Paris: Masson.

ROSENBEK, J.C., GREEN, E.F., FLYNN, M., WERTZ, R.T. and COLLINS, M. Anomia: A Clinical Experiment. In R.H. Brookshire (ed.) *Clinical Aphasiology Conference Proceedings 1977* (1977), pp. 103–111. Minneapolis: BRK Publishers.

RUSK, H.A. and TAYLOR, M.S. *Speech Therapy and Language Recovery in Severe Aphasia. A Final Report* (1970).

SALVATORE, A. and THOMPSON, C. Intervention for Global Aphasia. In R. Chapey (ed.) *Language Intervention Strategies in Adult Aphasia* 2nd edn (1986). Baltimore: Williams and Wilkins.

SANDS, E., SARNO, M.T. and SHANKWEILER, D. Long Term Assessment of Language Function in Aphasia due to Stroke. *Archives of Physical Medicine and Rehabilitation* (1969), 202–106.

SARNO, M., SILVERMAN, M. and SANDS, E. Speech Therapy and Language Recovery in Severe Aphasia. *Journal of Speech and Hearing Disorders* (1970), 607–623.

SARNO, M. and LEVITA, E. Evaluation of Language Improvement after Completed Stroke. *Archives of Physical Medicine and Rehabilitation* (1971), **52**, 73–78.

SARNO, M.T. *Functional Communication Profile* (1969). Institute of Rehabilitation Medicine, New York University Medical Centre, 400 East 34th Street, New York.

SARNO, M.T., SILVERMAN, and SANOS, E. Speech Therapy and Language Recovery in Severe Aphasics. *Journal of Speech and Hearing Disorders* (1970), **13**, 607–623.

SARNO, M.T. and LEVITA, E. Recovery in Treated Aphasia during first year post Stroke. *Stroke* (1971), **10 (6)**, 663–670.

SCHUELL, H.M. *Differential Diagnosis of Aphasia with the Minnesota Test* (1965). Minn: University of Minnesota Press.

SCHWARTZ, L., NEMEROFF, S. and REISS, M. An investigation of writing therapy for the adult aphasic: the word level. Presented at *The ASHA Convention* Detroit (1973).

SERON, X., DELOCHE, G., BASTARD, V., CHASSIN, G. and HERMAND, N. Word-finding difficulties and learning transfer in aphasic patients. *Cortex* (1979), **15**, 149–155.

SHEWAN, C.M. Facilitating sentence formulation: a case study. *Journal of Communication Disorders* (1976), **9**, 191–197.

SHEWAN, C.M. Recovery from Aphasia: Effects of Different Language Treatment Types. Presented at *The ASHA Convention* November, Concincinnati (1983).

SHEWAN, C.M. and KERTESZ, A. Effects of Speech and Language treatment on recovery from Aphasia. *Brain and Language* (1984), **23**, 272–299.

SHEWAN, C.M. and BANDUR, D.L. *Treatment of Aphasia. A Language Orientated Approach* (1986). London: Taylor and Francis.

SKELLY, M., SCHINSKY, L., SMITH, R.W. and FUST, R.S. American Indian Sign (Amerind) as a Facilitator of Verbalisation for the Oral Verbal Aprxic. *Journal of Speech and Hearing Disorders* (1974), **39**, 445–456.

SMITH, A. *Diagnosis, Intelligence and Rehabilitation of Chronic Aphasics* (1972). Ann Arbor, University of Michigan, Department of Physical Medicine, Rehab.

SPARKS, R.H., HELM, N. and ALBERT, M. Aphasia rehabilitation resulting from melodic intonation therapy. *Cortex* (1974), **10**, 303–316.

SPARKS, R.H. and HOLLAND, A.L. Melodic intonation therapy for aphasia. *Journal of Speech and Hearing Disorders* (1976), **41**, 287–297.

STOKES, T.F. and BAUER, D.M. An implicit technology of generalization. *Journal of Applied Behaviour and Analysis* (1977), **10**, 349–367.

TAYLOR, M. Language Therapy. In H.G. Barr (ed.) *The Aphasic Adult: Evaluation and Rehabilitation* (1964). Charlotsville, Va.: Wayside Press.

THOMPSON, C.K. and KEARNS, K.P. An experimental analysis of acquisition, generalization and maintenance of naming behaviour in a patient with anomia. In A.H. Brookshire (ed.) *Clinical Aphasiology Conference Proceedings 1981* (1981) pp. 35–42. Minneapolis: BRK Publishers.

VIGNOLO, L.A. Evaluation of Aphasia and Language Rehabilitation: A Retrospective Exploratory Study. *Cortex* (1964), 344–367.

WEBB, G.W. and RUSSEL, J.L. Therapy for Retraining Reading. In R. Chapey *Language Rehabilitation Strategies in Adult Aphasia* 2nd edn (1986). Baltimore: Williams and Wilkins.

WEISENBURG, T. and MCBRIDE, K. *Aphasia, a Clinical and Psychological Study* (1964). New York: Hafner.

WENIGER, D., HUBER, W., STACHOWIAK, F.J. and POECK, K. Treatment of Aphasia on a Linguistic Basis, pp 149–157. In M. Taylor-Sarno and O. Hook (eds) *Aphasia. Assessment and Treatment* (1980). Stockholm: Almqvist and Wiksell International.

WEPMAN, J.M. *Recovery from Aphasia* (1951). New York: Ronald Press.

WERTZ, R.T., COLLINS, M., WEISS, D., BROOKSHIRE, R.H., FRIDEN, T., KURTZKE, J.F. and PIERCE, J. Veterans Administration Co-operative Study on Aphasia. Paper presented at *The American Association for Advancement of Science* (1978). Washington D.C., February 1978.

WERTZ, R.T. *et al.* Veterans Administration Co-operative Study — Comparison of Hospital and Home Treatment Programmes for Aphasic Patients (1979).

WERTZ, R.T., DAVID, G.W., ALTER, J. *et al.* Comparison of Clinic, Home and Deferred Language Treatment for Aphasia. A Veterans Co-operative Study. *Archives of Neurology* (1985), **43**, 653–658.

WEST, J.A. Auditory Comprehension in Aphasic Adults: Improvement through Training. *Archives of Physical Medicine and Rehabilitation* (1973), **54** 78–86.

WIEGEL-CRUMP, C., and KOENIGSKNECHT, R.A. Tapping the Lexical Store of the Adult Aphasic Analysis of the Improvement made in Word Retrieval Skills. *Cortex* (1973), **9**, 410–418.

WHURR, R. *An Aphasia Screening Test* (1974). Whurr Publishers, 2 Alwyne Road, London N1, England.

WHURR, R. Deficits or Retained Areas — Which to treat in Aphasia? Paper presented to *The ASHA Convention*, November (1983), Cincinnati.

WHURR, R. *Contrasting Patterns of Recovery in Acquired Dysgraphia*. Paper presented to the Aphasia Committee. IALP. (1986).Brussels, Belgium.

WHURR, R. An Evaluation of Research Studies Conducted into the Treatment of Aphasia. Paper presented at *The Second International Aphasia Rehabilitation Congress* (1986). Goteburg, Sweden.

Name Index

Page numbers in italics indicate figures or tables. Those followed by 'n' refer to notes.

Subject Index

Page numbers in italics represent figures or tables. Those followed by 'n' refer to notes.